THE HANDBOOK OF FOOT AND ANKLE SURGERY

THE HANDBOOK OF FOOT AND ANKLE SURGERY

An Intellectual Approach to Complex Problems

Editor

John S Gould MD

Professor of Surgery
Division of Orthopedic Surgery
Section Head, Foot and Ankle Surgery
University of Alabama at Birmingham (UAB)
Birmingham, Alabama, USA

Managing Editor

Mason N Florence MD

Foot and Ankle Fellow
Division of Orthopedic Surgery
Section of Foot and Ankle
University of Alabama at Birmingham
Birmingham, Alabama, USA

Foreword

Judith F Baumhauer MD MPH

JAYPEE BROTHERS MEDICAL PUBLISHERS (P) LTD

New Delhi • London • Philadelphia • Panama

Jaypee Brothers Medical Publishers (P) Ltd

Headquarters

Jaypee Brothers Medical Publishers (P) Ltd
4838/24, Ansari Road, Daryaganj
New Delhi 110 002, India
Phone: +91-11-43574357
Fax: +91-11-43574314
Email: jaypee@jaypeebrothers.com

Overseas Offices

J.P. Medical Ltd
83, Victoria Street, London
SW1H 0HW (UK)
Phone: +44-2031708910
USA
Email: info@jpmedpub.com

Jaypee-Highlights Medical Publishers Inc.
City of Knowledge, Bld. 237, Clayton
Panama City, Panama
Phone: +507-301-0496
Fax: +02-03-0086180
Email: cservice@jphmedical.com

Jaypee Brothers Medical Publishers Ltd
The Bourse
111 South Independence Mall East
Suite 835, Philadelphia, Pennsylvania,
Fax: +507-301-0499 19106, USA
Phone: + 267-519-9789
Email: joe.rusko@jaypeebrothers.com

Jaypee Brothers
Medical Publishers (P) Ltd
17/1-B Babar Road, Block-B
Shaymali, Mohammadpur
Dhaka-1207, Bangladesh
Mobile: +08801912003485
Email: jaypeedhaka@gmail.com

Jaypee Brothers
Medical Publishers (P) Ltd
Shorakhute, Kathmandu
Nepal
Phone: +00977-9841528578
Email: jaypee.nepal@gmail.com

Website: www.jaypeebrothers.com
Website: www.jaypeedigital.com

Inquiries for bulk sales may be solicited at: jaypee@jaypeebrothers.com

The Handbook of Foot and Ankle Surgery: An Intellectual Approach to Complex Problems

First Edition: **2013**

ISBN 978-93-5090-501-2

Printed at: Ajanta Offset & Packagigns Ltd., New Delhi

Dedicated to

The two Pioneers in Academic Medicine and Foot and Ankle—J Leonard Goldner MD *and Nathaniel Gould* MD, *my father. Their devotion to learning, teaching, compassionate care of patients and meticulous surgical technique has been an enormous positive influence on my career.*

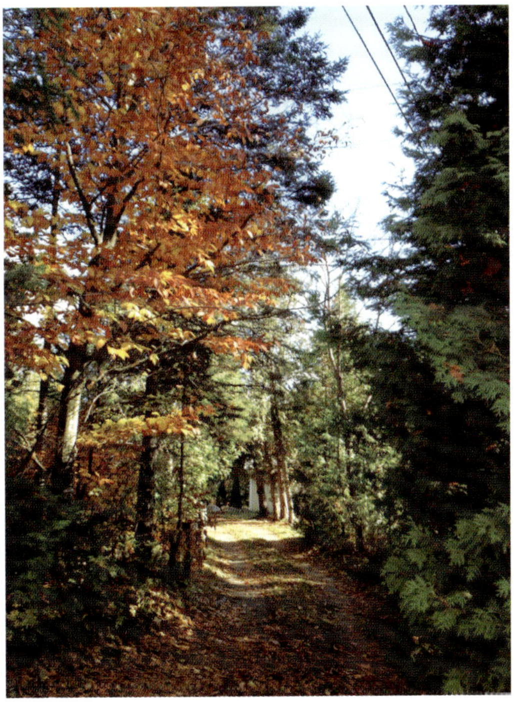

"The Road Less Traveled"
Autumn: Joe's Pond. West Danville
Vermont, USA

Contributors

Sonya Ahmed MD
Assistant Professor
Department of Orthopedic Surgery
University of Texas Medical School of Houston
Houston, Texas, USA

Judith F Baumhauer MD MPH
Professor
Orthopedic Surgery
Department of Orthopedic Surgery
University of Rochester
Rochester, New York, USA

Bruce Cohen MD
Assistant Program Director
Department of Surgery
Director, Foot and Ankle Fellowship
OrthoCarolina Foot and Ankle Institute
Charlotte, North Carolina, USA

Michael Conklin MD
Assistant Professor
Orthopedic Surgery
Division of Orthopedic Surgery
Department of Surgery
University of Alabama at Birmingham
Birmingham, Alabama, USA

Robert M Crabtree BS MS
Administrative Director of Orthopedics
Department of Surgery/Division of Orthopedic Surgery
University of Alabama at Birmingham
Birmingham, Alabama, USA

Catherine Cunningham
Medical Student
UMDNJ-New Jersey Medical School
Newark, New Jersey, USA

Beatriz Garcia-Cardona MD
Foot and Ankle Fellow
Division of Orthopedic Surgery
Section of Foot and Ankle
University of Alabama at Birmingham
Birmingham, Alabama, USA

John S Gould MD
Professor of Surgery
Division of Orthopedic Surgery
Section Head, Foot and Ankle Surgery
University of Alabama at Birmingham
Birmingham, Alabama, USA

Joseph G Khoury MD
Chief of Orthopedic Surgery
Children's of Alabama
Residency Program Director and Assistant Professor of Orthopedic Surgery
University of Alabama at Birmingham
Birmingham, Alabama, USA

John S Kirchner MD
Assistant Professor
Division of Orthopedic Surgery
Section of Foot and Ankle
University of Alabama at Birmingham
Birmingham, Alabama, USA

Sheldon S Lin MD
Associate Professor
UMDNJ-New Jersey
Department of Orthopedic Surgery
Newark, New Jersey, USA

Jason Lowe MD
Assistant Professor
Division of Orthopedic Surgery
Section of Traumatology
Department of Surgery
University of Alabama at Birmingham
Birmingham, Alabama, USA

Katherine C Ma MD
Department of Orthopedic Surgery
University of Rochester
Rochester, New York, USA

William McGarvey MD
Associate Professor of Orthopedic Surgery
Director, Foot and Ankle Surgery
University of Texas Health Science Center
Houston, Texas, USA

Siddhant K Mehta MD
Resident, Department of Orthopedic Surgery and Rehabilitation
University of Mississippi Medical Center
Jackson, Mississippi, USA

Shana N Miskovsky MD
Assistant Professor
Orthopedic Surgery
Case Western Reserve University School of Medicine
Head, Division of Orthopedic Foot and Ankle University Hospitals of Cleveland
Cleveland, Ohio, USA

William Min MD MS MBA
Assistant Professor
Orthopedic Surgery
Division of Orthopedic Surgery
Section of Traumatology
Department of Surgery
University of Alabama at Birmingham
Birmingham, Alabama, USA

Christopher Orr PA-C MMS
University Hospitals Case Medical Center
Department of Orthopedics
Cleveland, Ohio, USA

Cristian Ortiz MD
Professor
Universidad del Desarrollo
Foot and Ankle Unit
Orthopedics and
Traumatology Department
Clinica Alemana
Santiago, Chile

Stephen F Pehler MD
Orthopedic Resident
Department of Surgery
Division of Orthopedic Surgery
University of Alabama
at Birmingham
Birmingham, Alabama, USA

James J Sferra MD
Center Director, Foot and
Ankle Surgery
Department of
Orthopedic Surgery
Orthopedic and
Rheumatologic Institute
Cleveland Clinic
Cleveland, Ohio, USA

Judith W Smith MD MBA
Ferrell-Duncan Clinic
Department of
Orthopedic Surgery
Springfield
Missouri, USA

Emilio Wagner MD
Assistant Professor
Universidad del Desarrollo
Foot and Ankle Unit
Orthopedics and Traumatology
Department
Clinica Alemana
Santiago, Chile

Pablo Wagner MD
Foot and Ankle Fellow
Universidad del Desarrollo
Foot and Ankle Unit Orthopedics
and Traumatology Department
Clinica Alemana
Santiago, Chile

Foreword

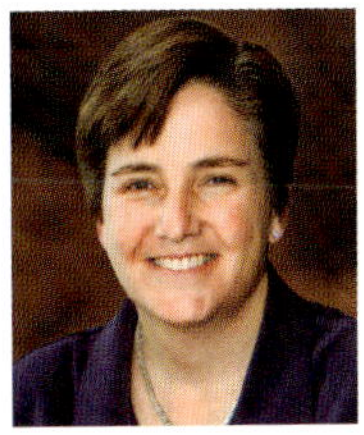

John S Gould is an icon in Orthopedic Surgery. He really has "done it all".

Gould was destined to write this book. He is not simply a teacher and educator, nor is he just a clinician and researcher; he has years of experience as a Department Chairman, a manager, an academician and a leader. Gould has also been in private practice in a small group, as well as a large high profile sports medicine practice providing care for professional athletes. He has drawn from his life's experiences to write a book that covers clinical foot and ankle topics in a logical, common sense fashion while also imparting practical knowledge like operating room instrumentation, the use of surgical assists, and follow-up care and outcomes.

Gould is not afraid to go where no surgical textbook has gone before. Topics like Training Residents and Fellows, How to Discharge a Patient from your Practice?, and Ethical Issues with Referring Physicians are just a few of the dicey topics he addresses in *The Handbook of Foot and Ankle Surgery*.

A graduate of Exeter and Harvard, former Editor-in-Chief of Microsurgery and the American Journal of Orthopedics, Gould is a gifted writer. He has demonstrated these skills in multiple ways: firstly, he successfully authored three prior books, and has over 200 additional editorials and peer-reviewed publications to his credit. Secondly, he is an expert clinician trained in Hand Surgery, Plastics and Microvascular techniques, and Foot and Ankle. As the son of Nathaniel Gould, a founder of the American Foot and Ankle Society, foot and ankle care practically runs in his veins. He has successfully trained hundreds of residents and fellows in Orthopedic Foot and Ankle Surgery.

As a well-recognized leader, Gould has been president of 10 national and regional societies, including the American Orthopedic Foot and Ankle Society (AOFAS), Mid-America Orthopedic Association and the Clinical Orthopedic Society. His acumen at organizing and communicating with groups and his success at getting these groups to work together is a topic addressed in his book. He has been a visiting professor in 99 institutions in the US and abroad, and has given over 400 scientific and clinical presentations.

The Handbook of Foot and Ankle Surgery is a culmination of Gould's nearly 41 years of clinical research and leadership experience in a diverse variety of domains. It will help medical students, residents, fellows and clinicians answer tough questions with clarity. This is a "must have" handbook to read and share.

Judith F Baumhauer MD MPH
Professor of Orthopedic Surgery
Department of Orthopedic Surgery
University of Rochester
Rochester, New York, USA

Preface

The Handbook of Foot and Ankle Surgery contains a logical approach and school of thought in Orthopedic Foot and Ankle which was developed through the training influences and experience of the senior author and editor's 41 years in academic and private medicine. During 37 of these years, the author worked directly with Orthopedic Residents and Fellows, primarily at the University of Alabama at Birmingham, USA and the Medical College of Wisconsin, in Milwaukee, USA. The approaches to diagnosis and management of these complicated problems were developed working with patients, carrying out clinical and basic research, ongoing awareness of the world literature, collaboration and discussion with colleagues in the Orthopedic Foot Club and the American Orthopedic Foot and Ankle Society, and travel to five continents as a Visiting Professor and Lecturer.

Contributors to this book are all colleagues at the University of Alabama at Birmingham, USA or former Foot and Ankle Fellows at UAB or MCW, who are engaged in teaching their own residents and fellows at this time.

This handbook is unique, in that it also contains a large section on the actual practice of medicine in this field, a discussion of office management, a career as an academic surgeon, and the senior author's philosophy concerning patient management, and interactions with colleagues, residents and fellows gleaned from his editorials during his tenure as Editor-in-Chief of The American Journal of Orthopedics.

The text is not comprehensive historically or even currently, on all approaches to foot and ankle orthopedic problems. It presents an approach and techniques used by the authors as their preferred methodology for these various issues. Many of the techniques are unique to these practices, while others are essentially the "gold standard" and used throughout the United States and abroad. If there is a common thread to these techniques, it is that after extensive experience with most of the acceptable alternatives, the proposed approach is logical, is based on good clinical research, and has worked effectively over a sufficient follow-up period, in our opinion, to be the best option in the year, 2012–13. With all these years of experience and acknowledging the rapidity of advancing orthopedic knowledge and technology, the author readily admits that we will continue to progress to techniques providing improved function and durability. Nothing is forever. Hopefully, the authors have not been, and will not be, resistant to change in a positive direction, and applaud every effort and accomplishment bettering our care of patients. Our foremost philosophy must be to improve their lot, to advance our capabilities, and to teach this knowledge to those who follow.

John S Gould MD

Acknowledgments

I am very grateful to the multiple Fellows and Residents whom I have worked with over the years at the University of Alabama at Birmingham, the Medical College of Wisconsin, and the University of South Alabama who have constantly stimulated and prodded me to increase my knowledge and hone my skills so that I could be the best teacher possible for them.

I would like to express great appreciation for the contributions of my colleagues and former Fellows, and particularly to Mason N Florence MD, my Managing Editor, for his countless hours of work with editing and providing extensive reference research throughout the manuscript.

I am also indebted to our dedicated Development Editor, Ms Payal Bharti, and her team at M/s Jaypee Brothers Medical Publishers (P) Ltd, New Delhi, India, for their conscientious efforts to produce a high quality publication in a timely manner for worldwide distribution.

Finally, it is imperative that I thank my wife, Sheryl Hartford Gould—my best friend and confidant, who has endured and encouraged me for almost 50 years.

Contents

Section 1: General Considerations

Section 2: Forefoot Problems

Section 3: Midfoot Problems

Section 4: Hindfoot Problems

Section 5: Ankle Problems

Section 8: The Rheumatoid Foot

Section 9: The Diabetic Foot

Section 10: Special Fracture Problems of the Foot and Ankle

SECTION 1

General Considerations

Chapters Outline

1 General Workup of the Foot and Ankle Patient

John S Gould

HISTORY TAKING

At this point in time, there is enormous pressure on clinicians to see patients as rapidly as possible and find time-saving measures which will expedite the patient visit. Consequently, patients are asked to complete a history form on their own prior to the actual encounter with the physician; and, in the clinic setting, for a student, nurse, or other attending physician extenders to take the history and, with the electronic medical record, to check appropriate boxes in a template for patient history. While a substantial portion of the history can be done in this expeditious manner, the "history of the present illness" remains an essential responsibility of the "attending physician".

While a patient's litany of prior physician visits, diagnoses and treatments provides some helpful information, it is more useful to determine the "chief complaint" as is traditional, and to ask about details of the onset of symptoms and to ask the patient to characterize the details precisely. When and how did the problems arise, as well as you can remember: acute onset vs insidious beginning? If there was pain involved, describe the type of pain and where it was located. What were you doing at the time when the problem occurred? With that information, you can then ask, what happened next, including the medical visits, treatments and the response to the attempted management. Now you want to know how the problem affects the patient at the present. Does it occur at night? Do you have pain with the first step in the morning or does it come on gradually through the day? Is it aggravated with increased activity, etc.? As you take the history, you attempt to characterize the complaints as mechanical, infectious, oncologic, neurogenic, vasogenic, etc. More questions are asked as the data is revealed. Even if a diagnosis is not obvious, you can determine the type or types of problem and ask more searching questions. There are patients with arthritic problems, for example, which include nerve irritation as well, even if the primary issue is arthritic. There are also patients who began with one diagnosis and it has now evolved into another, such that the picture is more complex and sometimes confusing. *Never start the physical examination until you have listened to the patient and asked the searching questions which will take you to the diagnosis.*

PHYSICAL EXAMINATION

The physical examination includes all the systems of the foot and ankle; namely skin, bones, joints, ligaments, vessels and nerves; and observation of the patient weight bearing, non-weight bearing, and walking, from various perspectives. It also requires a precise knowledge of surface anatomy.

With the patient standing, an observation of gait including the entire extremity and special attention to the foot from heel strike, foot flat, to toe-off. Observation of the arch and the heel position from the front, back and medial perspectives is important. In certain situations, single leg stance and the ability to rise onto the toes during single leg stance (without leaning forward and leaning on the hands), while observing the movement of the heel during this maneuver may be essential. Joint ranges of motion, including abnormal motion or evidence of instability should be noted. Manual motor strength is noted. Of particular interest, palpation of specific joints and ligament locations is very critical, especially to determine if symptoms and signs correlate. When neurogenic symptoms are present, palpation of the peripheral nerves and likely locations of entrapment or injury is critical (This point is further emphasized in the chapter on peripheral nerve entrapments). The evaluation of sensory and motor deficits are made and one should also note rugal patterns on the toes, and feel for autonomic changes such as dryness or smoothness, indicating nerve dysfunction. To determine nerve injury and regeneration, Tinel's signs or proximal and distal Tinel's and the distance between them should be noted. The vascular status includes not only the palpation of pulses, but also the capillary refill, color and turgor should be noted. *The correlation of physical findings and history are very essential. When they do not correlate, one needs to review the history again, think more broadly about central nervous system and more systemic conditions, as well as the possibility that the complaints may be factitious.*

ORDERING AND INTERPRETATION OF APPROPRIATE LABORATORY AND IMAGING EXAMINATIONS

Regarding the ordering and interpretation of laboratory and imaging studies, it is notorious in orthopedic circles, in general, to have patients referred with spurious diagnoses based on the reading and diagnosis from an imaging study, which was done in the absence of a good history and physical examination. It is also easy to be pressured by a patient, a patient's agent, insurance or governmental guidelines for a diagnosis to order ancillary tests. In fact, a part of "defensive medicine" created by litigious situations forces us to obtain as much objective data as possible to support or deny our diagnosis. This is understandable, but not an excuse for ordering inappropriate testing for the mere purpose of "checking a box", or to avoid the far more critical good history or physical examination. The studies which can confirm and localize better a suspected diagnosis or rule out a critical alternative diagnosis are appropriate. Electrodiagnostic studies are essential, for example, to confirm or deny radiculopathy or generalized neuropathy, but may not confirm or deny an entrapment syndrome, which is not advanced, or in which the sensitivity of the testing method is not high enough. X-rays are standard fare when studying the foot and ankle, but high quality digital resolution and appropriate views to make a proper determination of the suspected clinical diagnosis is essential. While a standard series of films may be satisfactory for the hospital radiologist, the foot and ankle specialist often requires additional and more specific information. The standard views are the anterior-posterior (AP), lateral and oblique for the foot; and the AP, and lateral of the ankle. Most surgeons want the AP and lateral films in both areas to be weight bearing, but in postoperative patients, this is usually not applicable early on. When assessing the toes and metatarsophalangeal joints, the X-ray beam should be centered on the area of interest. Various oblique views are helpful for certain suspected fractures. Heel alignment requires a tangential view of the os calcis. The subtalar joint is best viewed with Broden's views (the X-ray beam is directed cephalad 30°, 45° and 60° with the foot internally rotated at the ankle) so that one can fully see the posterior facet. To image the alignment of the heel relative to the tibia, a tangential view of the heel, which includes the tibia proximally, provides the needed information. Such imaging requirements will be discussed in the appropriate sections of the text.

The same concept is true with magnetic resonance imaging (MRI) and computed tomography (CT) scans. A diagnostic center without good musculoskeletal radiology supervision and high quality scans are not only misleading but also dangerous. As an orthopedist, one must be able to recognize the pathology and to read and not over-read the images. It is always essential to remember that signal changes on MRIs may have numerous interpretations and the diagnosis must correlate with the clinical picture. Diagnostic ultrasound has also become a useful and far less expensive tool than MRI to aid the diagnosis in a more precise way for superficial lesions. In the face of possible infections, it is always helpful to have systemic indicators such as the elevated sedimentation rate, C-reactive protein and an elevated white cell count. Imaging studies such as labeled white cell scans can be useful, and positron emission tomography (PET) scans which can localize collections of white cells can, when available, aid in surgical planning.

2 Making the Diagnosis and the Discussion of Management with the Patient

John S Gould

COLLATION OF DATA AND INDUCTIVE REASONING

As stated previously, the patient history determines whether the diagnosis is based upon a mechanical, neurogenic, vascular, infectious, oncologic, or even functional etiology. The physical examination often confirms this impression, but also helps to localize the site of the lesion. Some diagnoses may be purely clinical and are based only on this information, but in many instances, objective testing will document or assist in sorting out the differential diagnosis. As one collates the data, it is essential that all the components are all compatible with the diagnosis. A laboratory result or imaging study, which is not in keeping with the clinical findings, should be looked upon with suspicion. For example, when an over-reading of an X-ray or a bone scan by a radiologist is not compatible with either the history or physical examination, one needs to remember that these studies may not be specific and are frequently misinterpreted. Asking the right questions, listening to the patient, knowing your surface anatomy, and understanding the significance and limitations of the special studies will, with the collation of this data, lead to an accurate diagnosis. This is known as inductive reasoning.

DISCUSSION WITH THE PATIENT AND RECOMMENDED MANAGEMENT

The history of prior care, exactly how it was administered and the patient's description of compliance, helps determine the plan of management. It may be clear that the conservative management was inadequate, either due to inappropriate prescription or simply poor patient understanding or compliance. This might lead one to again prescribe a conservative approach which should be more likely to succeed if the patient will comply.

On the other hand, if the patient has been trying conservative measures for the past six months or a year, which are not necessarily those which you would prescribe, but are considered appropriate by many, it may be ridiculous to start with a nonoperative approach just out of principle. This is particularly true when it is obvious that the patient is convinced that nothing short of surgery is a consideration and will not comply with your conservative recommendations. A significant part of the art of medicine is to determine the patient's expectations from his or her visit to you. This is not to imply that you should recommend surgery when the patient suggests or demands it. There is simply a point in time when the patient is ready for the joint fusion, arthroplasty, or even amputation, and you, as the surgeon, should recognize that.

In addition, there are times when the definitive procedure may be indicated, but the patient is not emotionally ready, and your responsibility is to "plant the seed" for a later procedure, but to defer for the moment, staying with a nonoperative approach. Finally, there are times when nonoperative treatment or an inadequate procedure would be injurious to the patient, and it is your obligation to convince the patient to proceed with the definitive procedure, accepting no lesser option. An example for this may be in the case of osteomyelitis where an aggressive surgical approach may be essential to preserve life or limb and to acquiesce to a conservative approach, even when the patient wants it, is to practice subpar medicine.

WAYS TO PRESENT YOUR APPROACH TO CARE IN A TIERED MANNER, EXPLAINING ALTERNATIVES, BUT CLEARLY STATING YOUR OPINION AND THE DATA WHICH SUPPORTS THE PREFERRED OPTION FOR THE INDIVIDUAL PATIENT

The author's approach is to initially explain the diagnosis and to answer any questions concerning the etiology, pathodynamics and natural history of the condition. This discussion is tailored to the patient's apparent level of understanding and/or interest in knowing the information. Surprisingly enough, the individual's profession, socioeconomic class, or intelligence does not necessarily have a direct correlation to his or her interest in these matters. The author has had advanced education professionals simply want to know what to do about the problem and care less about the details. Based on his assessment of the problem and the patient's past treatment, the author then makes his recommendation for management. The author will describe other options to treat the problem, but does not provide a comprehensive list. For example, if he has diagnosed pure acute plantar fasciitis, he recommends his regimen of tissue specific stretching, oral anti-inflammatories and some form of an orthotic device. The author knows fully well that there are also taping schemes, other orthoses, injections, night splinting, extracorporeal shock wave therapy and more. He may simply note that there are other techniques, but that this has been successful for more than two thirds of his patients within a six week span of treatment. The patient is given a follow-up appointment at that interval.

More commonly, the author sees patients with chronic disorders that have not responded to regimens prescribed elsewhere. These patients often indicate that they have either been referred for surgical intervention or have come to this state of readiness on their own. The author recognizes that his regimen may not always be more successful than any other, and that patient compliance is likely to be suboptimal, and thus moves rapidly to a surgical discussion.

There are patients in this group that by dint of their age or by their sad history clearly need to make the next operation their last. Parenthetically, there are operations that offer potentially an outcome closer to normal function and those that provide satisfactory function but nothing close to normal. Those procedures providing a more normal functional result sometimes are less durable or may have a higher likelihood of failure, whereas another procedure provides less function but is definitive and may be more durable, relieve pain more reliably, and be the last operation needed. For instance, with the same presenting pathology in the ankle, we may do a simple arthroscopic cleanout in one patient, a total ankle in another and an arthrodesis in a third.

At times, it is essential for the patient to enter into the decision-making process, given the options and the odds for success. At other times, as stated earlier, this is inappropriate. Some time ago, the author was referred a diabetic lady with neuropathy and osteomyelitis of the distal and proximal phalanges of the great toe from a plantar ulcer. She was being treated with minor debridement and oral antibiotics based on surface cultures. The condition was progressive; she was systemically ill; the toe was swollen and red; and the X-ray demonstrated total destruction of the phalanges with sparing of the metatarsal. She did not want an amputation. The only option the author recommended was an amputation, hopefully a disarticulation at the MTP joint. The author was sensitive to her objections and attempted to be as understanding and kind as possible. She was explained that her function would be minimally disturbed based on the author's experience with toe to hand transfers as a microsurgeon. The author also discussed the typical acceptability of her potential appearance based on his prior experience, recognizing that any patient with a missing portion of the anatomy is very conscious of this loss, mourns it, and is certain that it is obvious to others.

The point to be understood is that the author believes it is inappropriate to agree to a less definitive procedure and allow the disease to progress with reasonably certain more dire consequences. When these untoward events do occur, the patient is more likely to blame you than to admit that your initial advice was to do otherwise. She was provided the only reasonable recommendation, with the alternative to seek advice elsewhere. She did acquiesce and had the disarticulation which healed promptly. Despite an ideal medical outcome and very good appearance in the author's opinion, she is content, albeit not overjoyed with the appearance. She respects the author and has had a safe and proper outcome.

SUMMARY

To summarize, advice to patients must be based on wide experience, a thorough knowledge of the field, the literature and known outcomes of the therapy proposed. It must be tailored to the individual patient and his or her needs. As a thoroughly educated physician and surgeon you do not have limited knowledge or skills. You have the personal capability to provide any therapy, surgical or medical, and thus are not biased by limitations in your education, training, practice, or intelligence. Consequently, your approach will be ethical and appropriate.

For many problems of the foot and ankle there is an algorithm for treatment that begins with the simplest and least invasive approach and escalates in complexity through the realm of conservative measures in terms of more complex bracing, physical therapy and medications. Beyond this are surgical procedures, again with progressive interventions. The ladder of progression depends on the patient's prior treatment, stage of the disease and response to your measures once he or she is under your care. One may begin at various levels of treatment based on these considerations; and medications, therapy, orthoses and surgery may be combined in various ways. The important consideration is that the measures taken are progressive, if necessary, and are not a random group of therapies which are all at the same level as in an empiric "try this" and "try that" approach. This issue will be covered further in the chapter on "Follow up Clinic".

3

Dealing with Referring Physicians

John S Gould

COMMUNICATING WITH THE REFERRING PHYSICIAN

With most versions of the electronic medical record, there is a space for the "referring physician" and a note is generated from the record to the individual, stating the diagnosis and intended management. When this is a standard fare, it is satisfactory to use, especially for referrals from primary care physicians. In contrast to this, most of the author's referrals are from orthopedic surgeons and a few are from Foot and Ankle specialists. When the author has determined that the referral follows an effort at diagnosis or failed management, he feels an obligation to send a personal letter or to call the physician. He believes this is appropriate when his findings or treatment plan may be of benefit to the referring physician's future management of patients or may be helpful in his ongoing provision of care for the patient or family.

DEALING WITH CONTRARY ADVICE

As an academic specialist, it is very likely that the author will determine a diagnosis and/or develop a plan of treatment which may be contrary to that of prior doctors. It is also possible that a diagnosis for which the patient has been treated in the past or on an ongoing basis may not be one with which he agrees. How does one present that to the patient in a way that he is convinced that you are correct and you do not denigrate the prior physician? This requires an artful approach as a result of which neither physician is sullied and the patient is happy and content with both the prior and current management. In some instances, this can be done easily. If the prior doctor is a primary care provider, you can indicate that your expertise as a specialist accounts for your approach and that the initial efforts would not be inappropriate. When the referral is from a general orthopedist, the same argument can be made. As an academic as opposed to a private practitioner, one can explain that the problem is complex or has evolved and that in your position at the end of the referral chain, you are far more likely to encounter the esoteric or confusing problems. The same argument can be made when the patient has been treated by a non MD practitioner such as a physical therapist, pedorthist, or nurse practitioner. Here it is only fair to say that an individual made an attempt to help and was astute enough to refer the patient when the treatment rendered was not effective. With other alternative medicine providers, The author does his best to approach these issues in the same manner. *You will never improve your reputation, continue to receive referrals, or improve patient care overall, by taking the negative approach that "you are brilliant, while everyone else is stupid". A positive approach to your actual or potential referral base will help everyone, including* your *patients.*

ETHICAL ISSUES

When a former resident or fellow of the author refers a patient or the author sees such a patient who has obtained an appointment through another route, he always sends a comprehensive note and calls the doctor to explain his diagnosis and treatment plan. If this is contrary to the other doctor's approach, the author lets him figure it out by himself.

When a patient disagrees with the author concerning a recommended plan of action, he never becomes indignant. The author will attempt to understand alternative point of view, and, if it is reasonable, but he disagrees, he will attempt to explain his rationale. If the patient's argument is illogical, he suggests the patient take it up with his referring physician. The author neither gets into arguments with patients, nor "does it the patient's way", as that has never been an effective approach.

4

When to Refer a Patient?

John S Gould

CIRCUMSTANCES WHEN PATIENT REFERRAL TO ANOTHER PHYSICIAN IS INDICATED OR APPROPRIATE[1]

Just how specialized are you? Can or should you treat every patient? Should you feel humiliated when a patient asks for a second opinion? To whom do you refer? J Leonard Goldner defined various categories of orthopedic specialization: the designated generalist (an orthopedist who covers most of the field but excludes certain areas, such as the hand or complex spine cases); the subspecialist (a generalist with a special interest—sports, foot and ankle, etc.); and the superspecialist (who restricts his practice to only one or two areas—as hand, foot and ankle, sports, etc.).In the private sector, most orthopedists fall into one of the first two categories and, in foot and ankle, most truly superspecialists are in the academic sphere.

From the author's perspective, it is obvious that one refers a problem which is outside one's specialty. The author strongly defers to a rheumatologist, endocrinologist or diabetologist. He also refers dermatologic problems of the foot, including warts and other skin lesions, to dermatologists. He confers with vascular surgeons concerning the large vessels and plastic surgeons, when appropriate. Many local tissue rearrangements and microsurgical procedures are within the author's personal expertise or that of a colleague in orthopedics, but this may not be the case for many foot and ankle specialists. Peripheral nerve surgery is also within the author's realm, but for many in the field, these cases should be referred to a plastic surgeon with such expertise or occasionally to a neurosurgeon with peripheral nerve experience. A musculoskeletal radiologist can be of significant help in interpretation of MRIs, ultrasound studies and even for an opinion on a plain X-ray.

It is fairly clear that you should refer a patient who is in need of a surgical procedure with which you are not fully familiar. If this is a problem which you may encounter frequently, it is reasonable to enlist the help of an associate to assist until you become proficient, or to obtain a mini fellowship, visit experts and scrub on multiple cases, and acquire all the technical assistance possible on your first solo procedure. A weekend course is not sufficient, but is a good start. There are excellent technical courses available now through the American Academy of Orthopaedic Surgeons, the Orthopaedic Learning Center and various industry sponsored courses. *If, on the other hand, the procedure is one that you would not expect to encounter often, it is prudent to refer the case and not have any regrets!*

A more ambiguous territory are those cases in which you do not know the diagnosis or the patient fails to respond to a treatment which you feel is appropriate. Failure of a patient to respond is due to either the wrong diagnosis, inappropriate treatment, or a lack of patient compliance. Unless the underlying problem can be identified and rectified, this is an indication for referral.

When a patient's relationship to you is too close: a relative, an associate, or a close friend, you may prefer referral. Rendering such care, however, may be appropriate, if, for example, the need for care is urgent or you are clearly the most qualified of those readily available.

Referral is always appropriate if the problem is complicated, many options exist and you would like another opinion before initiating treatment. Perhaps the patient holds the same opinion. Are second opinions always valid? Certainly not! Some patients, insurance companies, and health maintenance organizations (HMOs) and possibly governmental insurers feel that it is appropriate to always question any doctor's opinion. When the issue is controversial, then the author agrees.

The key is to find a superspecialist whose interest focuses on the specific diagnosis at hand. For the patient to bounce around among general orthopedists, subspecialists, podiatrists and family practitioners is not to make forward progress. The author advises patients to choose their consultants wisely and often provides a list of those who should be knowledgeable, regardless of whether they will agree with the author or not.

When you send a patient to a consultant you should make it absolutely clear in your letter, and call, that you are sending the patient for "an opinion only", "for an opinion with an option to treat"; if you would be happy to receive the patient back for treatment, or if you would be happy to provide aftercare if this would be beneficial for the patient. This leaves no ambiguity regarding your intent and keeps the consultant and you happy. The author always provides any and all information he has for a consultant. If the patient chooses to seek care from the consultant, you should agree and confer your blessing.

To seek advice or assistance in the care of a patient is a wise step; good for both you and the patient when the consultant can potentially help. Patients admire and often praise the physician who knows when to refer!

REFERENCE

1. Gould JS. "When to refer" in My First Love: The Art, the Practice, and the Ethics of Medicine. Birmingham: Seacoast Publishing, Inc; 2004.p.38.

5 When and How to Discharge a Patient from Your Practice?

Robert M Crabtree, John S Gould

DISCHARGE OF THE PROBLEMATIC PATIENT

There are circumstances when you may need to terminate your care of a patient. This chapter has been written with University-based risk management legal advice; the authors provide the usual steps taken for this matter.

There are patients in one's practice, periodically, who become problematic. When and how you can disassociate them from your practice is a ticklish issue, and the management of this has to be done for appropriate reasons, and without alienating your colleagues, abandoning your patient, and inciting a law suit. Neither a complication nor a bad result is an appropriate cause to discharge a patient, although a referral may be a legitimate option after discussion with the patient and a potential consultant. The more likely "problem patient" is one who has not responded to conservative measures, but refuses referral and insists on further appointments with you after being told that you have no further reasonable options. Another is the chronic pain patient with whom you have exhausted legitimate remedies. Finally, there is the patient with a healed surgical procedure who is dissatisfied for one reason or another and simply does not want discharge or referral.

The advice of a risk management professional with experience in the surgeon's state laws relative to "abandonment" should be consulted to avoid legal problems. A letter to the patient from the administrator of the practice should be composed, stating that "you have no further options for management of the patient and that further appointments will not be provided by your practice." There should be no further discussion about the details of the patient's problem or any other reasons for discharge of the patient. A list of every other orthopedic surgeon in the region should be provided along a statement of the practice's willingness to forward copies of all the medical records, X-rays or other studies pertinent to the patient's care from the doctor's office to a future caregiver. The simple statement that you can and will no longer provide care, and the openness indicated to provide any information garnered, should be sufficient to not create ill will or legal action. Nonetheless, it is essential to have your risk management person sign off on the action. In these situations, it is critical to "swallow your pride", be nonaccusatory and proceed with the action. Continuing to see the patient, and to grow increasingly antagonistic, is likely to provoke an unsatisfactory outcome to the relationship.

6

The Operating Room

John S Gould

INTRODUCTION

The precise roles and background experience of persons assigned to assist a surgeon in the operating room have become increasingly ill defined and confused by modern technology. Requirements for the documentation on an electronic data base by a registered nurse have made her other roles seems of secondary importance. Nonetheless, the author will define the roles expected of these people, by many and certainly traditional surgeons.

OPERATING ROOM PERSONNEL

The Circulating Nurse

The circulating nurse traditionally sets up a case by assuring that all the required instruments and special materials such as *implants* and *osteobiologics*, synthetic grafts and the like are actually in the operating room (OR) or, at least, are in the hospital and readily available when needed. There are numerous steps and persons involved who assist initially in this process, but it is ultimately the responsibility of the "circulator" to make sure that "the stage is properly set". In addition, this individual is the proper one to tie the backs of gowns of the operating surgeons, make sure the lights are turned on and grossly properly positioned, that the electrocautery is on, properly set, and that the foot pedal is attached and placed adjacent to the designated foot of the designated operator of the device (surgeon or first assistant). She (or he) properly applies the tourniquet cuff, and sets the machine to the requested time and pressure. She also positions the patient, adding bolsters to maintain the position, and adds protective devices to elbows, neck of the fibula, and other bony prominence areas and vulnerable nerves. She may also be called upon to assist an anesthetist or anesthesiologist, or insert a urinary catheter, on occasion. During the procedure, she may be called upon to provide unanticipated materials from outside the operating room. *Most importantly, however, her primary role during a procedure is to be the "supervising general" of the operating room, making certain that there are no breaks in sterile technique by anyone in the room, or any unsafe activities or distractions by anyone in the room, including any visitors or technical personnel. This role cannot be overemphasized and cannot be employed if the circulator is out of the room (With all this responsibility, it is not surprising that requiring this nurse to do data entry during a case, is unacceptable to many surgeons).* At the end of the procedure, this nurse must assist the team in preparing the patient for transportation to the recovery area and provide the "hand off" information to the nurses in this area. Finally, she starts over again with the next case, with as rapid a turnover as possible. In an outpatient operating facility, this nurse may also be involved in room cleaning and proper care of used instruments.

The Scrub Nurse

The Scrub nurse traditionally was a registered nurse who not only knew all the instruments and in what order they were to be handed to the surgeon, but also knew each procedure so well that she could anticipate the next step and have the proper instrument ready before being asked for it. In addition, this nurse knew how to handle emergency situations with the proper instruments for the management of a lacerated vessel or essentially other such unanticipated events which can occur during the surgical procedure at hand. Scrub technicians have frequently supplanted the knowledgeable registered nurse (RN), but they should also be capable of the same skills. The ability to do the back table assembly of complex instruments and implants; management of ill-functioning power tools; and the ability to help the surgeon when a better choice of instrument may be of value at a difficult moment of the procedure makes this individual a valuable member of the surgical team.

The Radiology Technologist

The radiology technologist provides the fluoroscopic assistance which has, at this point in time, become an essential asset for foot and ankle, and other orthopedic specialists. This person must be quick, knowledgeable and efficient along with everyone else in the team. The video monitors must be available for the surgeon to see without turning around. The technologist must be able to position his camera in perfect planes perpendicular to the object being studied and position the device and obtain the resolution ideal for the surgeon's interpretation. He needs to know all the views expected of him by both the surgeon and subsequently by the radiologist who will review the images. Finally, he must understand and maintain sterility, and minimize radiation to the patient and surgical team. The use of surgeon-operated small imaging machines plays a role in some procedures and may decrease radiation when used properly. However, less than proper positioning of the camera and its use for larger anatomical areas proximal to the digits and metatarsals may lead to erroneous interpretations. Again, the author would emphasize the role of the technologist in assuring that everyone in the operating room use proper radiation shielding for critical anatomy.

Technical Assistants

Technical assistants are increasingly used by surgeons during complex procedures using new devices and implants. While their help to the scrub nurse, circulating nurse, and the surgeon is unquestioned, they must be cognizant of sterile technique including sterile areas and pathways in the OR, and the circulating nurse must be ever vigilant while they are in the "theater". Essentially, they must understand their role and focus strictly on their purpose at hand. Socializing and discussions of matters outside of the case at hand is generally unacceptable. Using LASER pointers and maintaining their discussions with the nurse and surgeon in a nondistracting manner is essential.

Nurse Anesthetists

Nurse anesthetists are typically the primary persons at the head of the table, utilizing the anesthesiologists during induction and emergence; and for problems which may occur during the maintenance of anesthesia. They can also advise on positioning issues which can adversely affect the patient's anesthesia, particularly related to chest expansion; and can advise the surgeon on any issue related to patient welfare, including the lapse of tourniquet time.

Surgical Assistants

Surgical assistants may be orthopedic residents or fellows, physician assistants, registered nurse first assistants and surgical technicians. Two assistants, perhaps including a medical student, can increase efficiency in some cases. It is the surgeon's responsibility to position the assistants in such a way to provide maximal help and to not hinder the free passage of instruments between the surgeon and the scrub nurse.

FOOT AND ANKLE TRAYS AND "PULL TICKETS"

For all intents and purposes, each surgeon should have multiple trays made up with standard basic equipment for every case. Multiple sets are needed to avoid having to clean and sterilize a set between cases. The foot tray is essentially a "hand tray" which is usually well known in most ORs today. This tray contains the standard retractors—double narrow and double wide skin hooks; small narrow and wide right angle retractors; small Hohmann's; Senn retractors; Army-Navy's; and various sized self-retaining blunt devices (Weitlaner's and the like). A selection of periosteum elevators: Key, Cushing, and Freer's are needed. Various forceps, including delicate Adson's, smooth Adson's and multitooth Adson's (Brown-Adson's) are needed including longer handled delicate tipped forceps (Gerald's) for vessel and nerve work. The author prefers curved tenotomy scissors for dissection and straight tenotomy for cutting sutures. Each set should have heavier scissors as well for coarser suture and heavy tissue such as curved and straight Mayo's. The author's trays all have small Hoke osteotomes and a small and large mallet; and a

K-wire cutter. They also have Jurgen's pinballs for standard 1.6 mm or 0.062" K-wires. For the standard incision; he uses a #15 blade scalpel; and for deeper dissection, a Beaver blade, typically the #64 (one sided with one safe blunt side). The author uses larger needle holders for large (00, 0) and larger suture and small Webster needle holders for 4-0 and 5-0 suturing, on the subcutaneous and skin. He has a special nerve tray and a special vessel tray with microinstruments and clamps which he requests for specific cases. Young surgeons should go over trays initially and periodically to add instruments which they often request and have to be added to a case and to delete instruments which are used infrequently.

"Pull tickets" or cards should be completed by every surgeon detailing the typical instrument needs for a particular type of case above and beyond the standard tray. Some ORs have "standard lists", but these are frequently inadequate for the foot and ankle surgeon. With specialty specific circulating and scrub nurses, these cards should be updated frequently for efficient surgery. In addition to the standard tray and the specific "case card or pull ticket", when each case is scheduled, all implants and insertion equipment; and osteobiologics, whether kept in stock in the hospital, or items which are brought in on a contingency basis need to be specified. More and more hospitals have oversight committees which approve certain implants and osteobiologics to be used based on actual research as to efficacy, surgeon preference, and cost or a combination of these factors, so that it is important for the surgeon to be aware of hospital practice prior to the onset of a surgical procedure.

SETTING UP AND PATIENT POSITIONING[1]

Without a doubt, this is one of the most critical issues which make some cases go well and others to be a struggle. It is also something that residents seem to learn more slowly than other aspects of surgery; perhaps, because many practicing surgeons ignore these issues as well. The author prefers to sit during most foot and ankle procedures and position the patient so that he can work in this position and rest his forearms on the table for balance, steadiness and precision. The foot does not go to the end of the table for foot and ankle surgery and if the patient is tall, the extension is added to the head. A rolled blanket may be added under the hip to roll the foot to a neutral position with the toes pointed straight up; rolled over further and a roll placed under the knee to work on the outside of the foot or ankle; or simply to use no bolster to allow the hip to externally rotate to promote access to the medial foot. The author uses a bean bag to maintain the person in a lateral position for access to the lateral foot, ankle, or calcaneus; especially for osteotomies of the heel and ease of passing pins through the heel with fluoroscopic guidance. This is far easier than holding the foot up in the air for this purpose. When we wish to go anterior or medial, we complete the lateral procedure, even closure, and release the bean bag, rolling the patient back to the neutral or even externally rotated position. Posterior heel approaches and even plantar foot procedures are usually done in the prone position. The plantar approach to a Morton's neuroma is typically done with the patient placed in Trendelenburg position, and a sterile drape placed over the end of the table. Arthroscopic procedures have a special setup which will be discussed in the particular section.

Finally, positioning of the lights is done with one placed proximal to the field and the other placed distal, so that the beams pass between the surgeon and his assistants' heads and are not blocked as either moves in and out. Procedures begin after the surgeon is assured that he is operating on the proper patient and proper sided limb; that the lights are properly positioned; that the electrocautery is attached and ready for use and the foot pedal in position; that the suction is on the field; that he is comfortable and that the anesthetist is aware that he is to start. Skin markings are drawn, the tourniquet is inflated, and then the procedure is initiated. It goes without further emphasis that the surgeon is certain that he has the proper equipment for the procedure and that all implants are present.

REFERENCE

1. Gould JS. "The Master's Touch" in My First Love: The Art, the Practice, and the Ethics of Medicine. Birmingham: Seacoast Publishing; 2004.p.63.

7

The Follow-up Clinic

John S Gould

THE LEARNING LABORATORY[1]

The benefits gained by seeing patients in a follow-up clinic are immense. The author considers it a "learning laboratory." For residents only rotating on a service for a month or two, they only have a brief glimpse of an individual patient's progress; but the combination of vignettes provides a complete picture of the anticipated outcome of a specific surgical procedure at each stage of the course. This allows the trainee as well as the surgeon to relate the usual course anticipated from one's own experience when discussing a procedure with a new patient. It also allows the surgeon, the trainee and the clinic nurse to know honestly when seeing or answering a patient call whether the situation recounted by the patient is really to be expected at this point in time or whether it is abnormal. There are no textbooks which can really provide this kind of information and why only a surgeon who personally follows his own patients can truly be relied upon to provide proper information to patients before and after procedures.

POSTOPERATIVE EARLY CARE

In the postsurgical follow-up clinic, the author likes to review, at intervals, how each element of the original symptoms and signs are faring. Patients may still be complaining that they are not "normal" yet, but as the author goes over their original complaints, many have resolved. From this, the author not only learns the sequence of improvements to reiterate to others, but can point out the improvements and reassure patients that they are getting better. This precise information is valuable clinical research and informs you more about the effectiveness of your surgical maneuvers. This provides ongoing learning and eventually translates into "experience".

CONTINUED CONSERVATIVE CARE

Ongoing care must be purposeful. For surgical patients, you are following a patient, typically, until he or she is healed and can resume normal activity. This may include a period of rehabilitation as well as primary healing. If a deformity may have a tendency to recur, either due to growth, as in a cerebral palsy child, or to potential biomechanical imbalance, as in bunions, longer term follow-up must be considered until growth is complete or until after a historic data interval deformities usually do not recur—such as a year, or two years. When a patient has a joint implant, long-term follow-up of many years is indicated to deal with wear or deterioration of the device, especially when these signs are subtle and may not produce clinical symptoms early in the process.

Conservative treatment care continues until a patient reaches a plateau of recovery. This plateau may constitute either "recovery" to a normal state or to a condition deemed satisfactory to the patient, or the patient has failed to respond to this mode of care. When the situation is the latter, a decision needs to be made on the next course of action. The reason for failure has to be determined, as discussed below, and the options discussed with the patient.

THE PATIENT WHO IS NOT RESPONDING TO CONSERVATIVE CARE[2]

Reasons for Failure to Respond

When a patient fails to respond to a prescribed treatment, there are three possible reasons: (1) an inaccurate diagnosis or one which has evolved; (2) an inappropriate treatment plan or; (3) to the patient's failure, for one reason or another, to follow your plan. All of these possibilities carry equal weight.

All plantar heel pain, for example, is not "plantar fasciitis" and when it is the correct diagnosis, it may evolve into a neurogenic condition, "traction neuritis", which will be explained in the relevant chapter. If the treatment has not evolved with the diagnosis, the original care will fail. When inadequate treatment is the culprit, it may be due to the wrong medication or an inadequate dosage, an improperly prescribed or fabricated appliance; or an inadequate duration of treatment. Finally, the patient may not be complying due to a misunderstanding, ignorance, or even purposeful self-neglect. Many of these issues can be detected during follow-up visits, including a review of the actual appliance or review of the details of the treatment plan with the patient. A brace or orthotic device should be inspected by the physician soon after the patient receives it. Patient compliance also requires careful questioning: it is not adequate to simply ask if the patient is following the prescribed regimen.

On each follow-up visit, the author does not review all components described above; however, when the plateau has been reached and the time for typical resolution of symptoms has occurred and the patient has not responded, each detail noted above is considered.

Review of the diagnosis returns to the history, physical examination and ancillary studies. Were they accurate and were they interpreted properly? If you are certain that you have the right diagnosis, the correct treatment plan and patient compliance, but the patient has failed to respond, you now have several options which should be discussed with the patient. If there has been a failure in any of the three components, you again need to confer with the patient concerning your next steps.

If the diagnosis is incorrect, a new treatment plan is devised. If the diagnosis is not clear, either further ancillary testing may be indicated, or this may be an indication for referral. If the diagnosis is correct, and the treatment has not been effective, although the patient is compliant, an escalation of conservative care may be indicated. On the other hand, a surgical procedure may be indicated. A discussion with the patient should include details of the escalated treatment plan (such as a potentially more effective brace) and the likelihood of success with it. Realistic surgical options and expectations should also be considered. For some patients, medical issues and other factors may pre-empt surgical options and the more advanced conservative care is a required option.

WHEN TO DISCHARGE THE PATIENT?

The patient who is recalcitrant to your efforts by being noncompliant requires a decision whether to make further efforts with him. Options here include referral to another physician or simply discharge from your care.

Patients should be discharged from conservative care when they have reached the plateau level and are either well, well enough to be satisfied, or if you have nothing further to offer. This may mean referral to someone with, perhaps, more expertise, to another approach to care, such as a pain clinic, or to wherever or whomever the patient chooses. This is not always a failure of care. Some patients will be grateful for your efforts and willing to "live with their problem".

REFERENCES

1. Gould JS. "The Learning Laboratory" in My First Love: The Art, the Practice, and the Ethics of Medicine. Birmingham: Seacoast Publishing; 2004.p.65.
2. Gould JS. "Failure" in My First Love: The Art, the Practice, and the Ethics of Medicine. Birmingham: Seacoast Publishing; 2004.p.29.

8

Managing Complications

John S Gould

ETHICAL APPROACHES TO DEALING WITH COMPLICATIONS[1]

"Complications" occur in all medical care, including surgery. By legal definition, complications are not malpractice. There are numerous etiologies which can include an inaccurate diagnosis, improper indications, an inadequate surgical procedure, an incorrectly performed surgical procedure, errors occurring during surgery, patient factors including physiology, general health, exogenous agents, and compliance, and numerous undetermined etiologies. *It is important to appreciate that even when a diagnosis and the chosen surgical procedure are current and the operation has been done correctly, complications may occur which are neither the fault of the surgeon nor the patient.* Only when the "standard of care" for a given community is breached, should there be a determination of malpractice.

WHEN TO INTERVENE AND WHEN TO CONTINUE A NONOPERATIVE APPROACH?

While all parties involved in the patient's care, including the physician and his staff, and the patient are unhappy with the result, the physician's obligation is not to assign blame, but to take an objective approach to the resolution of the problem and to encourage the patient. One must not ignore a complication, but to put it into a proper perspective. If it is minor and easily resolved, that should be emphasized. If it is serious and potentially limb or life threatening, it should be approached promptly and vigorously. When a nonoperative approach is appropriate, it is used, but when it would be radical to withhold a surgical intervention, the author will recommend that initially. Several contrasting examples should be illustrative. Superficial skin infections including a stitch abscess, despite culturing some form of *Staphylococcus*, should respond well to simple conservative treatment. In contrast, a small wound slough in an anteromedial incision for a total ankle replacement requires vigorous surgical debridement as part of successful treatment. Simple dressing changes may lead to a much more serious condition. When you know that a "conservative" approach will, in all likelihood, not have a successful outcome, it is not appropriate to initiate it. *The point to emphasize is to be knowledgeable, forthright and vigorous in management.*

When conservative treatment is making measurable progress, it should be continued. This might be applicable to wound infection or slough care, to a nonunion of an osteotomy or joint fusion, or to the resolution of pain. If progress is not being made, a more vigorous approach should be entertained. A surgical intervention, which has a reasonable likelihood of success, should be considered, or a referral warranted, if an interval is reached at which the patient should rightfully have responded, and does not. To continue empirical treatments in the face of no improvement is inappropriate.

REFERENCE

1. Gould JS. "Blaming the Other Guy", "Blaming the Patient" in My First Love: The Art, the Practice, and the Ethics of Medicine. Birmingham: Seacoast Publishing; 2004. pp.42, 4.

9 Working with Residents and Fellows

John S Gould

RECOMMENDATIONS FOR WORKING WITH TRAINEES

When working with "trainees", it is always important to remember one's obligations to the patient, primarily, and secondarily to the education of the "students" and finally, to the institution in which one is working. The welfare of the patient is always to be considered, yet the benefits accruing to the patient by having a team helping the surgeon, observing the surgeon and challenging him cannot be underestimated. The teaching surgeon or "pro" has to always be at his best. He leads by example and by integrity. The student helps by gathering data which is reviewed constructively and an algorithm for treatment is established. The leader, or surgeon, has to plan the approach using established techniques proved by well-documented evidence. If he cannot explain the rationale for the approach and the subsequent surgery, if that is warranted, he will be challenged. In the operating room, having additional knowledgeable support makes procedures easier and outcomes more predictable.

Didactic teaching by the attending surgeon, both related to the clinic and the operating room, as well as background reading by the student is essential. After that, close apprentice teaching is the standard course of study. The author expects junior residents to understand disease processes and how to work up a patient problem. From there, they should be able to develop a plan of care. The senior resident should know the conservative and surgical options in more detail and, by the end of a rotation, know how to do most of the standard procedures. A fellow needs to know the fine points of management, and a more detailed capability in the operating sphere of care. Generally, the author believes that within two months, all levels of trainee should be very competent in the clinic. Each level of trainee is given graduated responsibility in the operating room.

GRADUATED RESPONSIBILITY

Each trainee must be familiar with the patient and his problem before the surgical procedure and know, at least theoretically, how the procedure is done. Preoperative planning for the specific patient is done in a conference shortly before the actual procedure: in a recent prior clinic or even the day prior to surgery. Positioning of the patient on the operating table, draping and the sequence of steps should be understood. Surgeons have to do procedures to become competent and this is allowed in a graduated fashion under strict supervision. With increased training and after demonstrated competence, the resident surgeon is given more leeway and more responsibility. From the surgical incision to the closure and the postoperative dressing, each step requires demonstration and supervision, even repetitively, until a level of capability is reached. The ability to carry out a procedure and to do it in an expert manner takes more than time and repetition. It requires mental attention and acuity. When one struggles with a step of any procedure, that problem should be reviewed to determine whether it is a matter of technique, dexterity, or instrumentation. A younger surgeon may be as good as or better than an older surgeon because he has thought through the problems with the details and found solutions.

EVALUATION OF THE TRAINEE

Each resident and fellow requires a written evaluation following a rotation and a semiannual conference with his advisor and annually with his program director. The author thinks it is essential to discuss all areas of the resident's endeavor as is done today in American programs following the guidelines of the Residency Review Committee of the Accreditation Council of Graduate Medical Education. Such a process does not exist for fellows, and here it behooves the Fellowship Director to meet at least semiannually with each fellow to advise on his achievements and areas requiring improvement. Further study, more time in a Skills Laboratory, or better concentration on detail may all be recommendations. This may also help the attendings know which fellows may need more exposure to certain procedures.

WHEN TO RECOMMEND FIRING OF A TRAINEE?

Orthopedic residents have five years of training, while foot and ankle fellows have training only for one year, after their residency. Residents have multiple rotations on the various subspecialties and may excel in one or another, or many. The fellow only has one rotation and needs to excel in that one alone. There are clear-cut situations which require dismissal: unethical behavior and dishonesty. Inappropriate intervention in the operating room or not following the specific directions of an attending surgeon may be others. The difficult question is when to sever the fellowship arrangement due to lack of competence or failure to learn. This can be an extremely difficult situation and harkens back to the criteria one uses in selecting the fellow in the first place. Unless the fellow has had his orthopedic training in your program, you cannot be certain of his level of competence. When one goes back to the application and reviews the Letters of Recommendation, one can usually find clues and innuendos which were ignored or not appreciated at the time of application or interview. This is where most of the mistakes are made and the wrong person selected. Let us assume that all indications in the fellow's background indicate that he was competently trained and received good recommendations for your fellowship, but he is not performing up to your standards. The author thinks it is important to determine if the problem is internal; that is, with your program or with the fellow's response to it, or whether there was something else in his history which you may have missed. At this point, it is essential to speak with someone you feel is trustworthy in the individual's original training program, and, in detail, with your faculty. Finally, you must interview the individual and attempt to understand the discrepancies between your expectations and his performance. In the author's experience, they have been discovered to have an unknown physical illness, marital strife on several occasions, a learning disability situation, an undisclosed faculty conflict situation, and a severe lack of confidence in the operating room when not working under close supervision. Some of these situations are correctable; others have led to career changes. In any case, an abrupt severance of the contract was not done and help for the individual provided. It would appear to be rare that an individual who can successfully navigate an orthopedic residency would not be competent to do the same with a fellowship.

10 Administration and Organization of the Subspecialty Office

Judith W Smith

PATIENT CENTERED CARE AND THE TEAM APPROACH

The subspecialty office has a unique opportunity to consolidate many services into one visit in a unified, efficient fashion. This is a concept that greatly enhances the patient experience, and at the same time really motivates "the team", the office personnel, because they realize the significance of their contribution in bringing the patient quality care and excellent service. The most important concept for the personnel to grasp is that the office has a patient centered approach to care. The patient is in the middle of the circle, and personnel are there to circle around them and take care of their needs.

This is not only a philosophy of care. If there is an opportunity to have input into the physical layout of the office, the physical space can be designed from blueprints to completion with this concept in mind. Patient flow is the key concept, so the space should be designed to avoid choke points where patients experience delays. It is not a good experience if the surgeon sees the patient in a timely fashion, but then there is a 45 minute delay to obtain an X-ray. The physical layout can contribute greatly to this ability to maintain flow, and architects/designers should keep in mind ways to expand areas where flow is constricted. For example, an office in the blueprint stages might mark in a lead lined waiting area adjacent to an X-ray suite in case a second X-ray room is needed as the office expands. If the waiting area is always jammed with patients needing an X-ray, it might be prudent at that point to put in more X-ray capacity. This is far more efficient than constructing a second X-ray room after the fact while the office is physically in operation.

PERSONNEL

Cooperation and cross training is essential in the subspecialty office. Employees must be willing to multitask, and to take on jobs normally handled by other personnel. The patient essentially cycles through the office entering from the lobby area, moving through the examining area, X-ray and physical therapy or durable medical equipment (DME) sites before exiting back to the lobby. As they journey through this loop each patient will interact with varying sets or subsets of these employees. It is the sum of these experiences that makes the final impression. A patient may not interact for a long period of time with a physician, but perceives that he had an excellent and productive experience because of the time spent with a dedicated physical therapist, for example.

Front Office: Entering

The first person the patient will encounter, who will set the tone for the entire visit, is the receptionist. The receptionist needs to be personable and pleasant while obtaining appropriate paperwork and demographic information. In some offices the receptionist will collect co-pays or money due from prior visits. In many offices the patient will fill out demographic and medical information regarding the purpose of the visit. This information can be filled out in advance if the office has forms available online or is able to include forms with an initial mailing. As more offices move to an Electronic Medical Record, there is the possibility of a patient entering his medical information directly into the chart, which is more efficient than having office personnel enter it once he is in an examining room. This can be done by installing computer kiosks in the lobby. Finally, patient portals are being developed that are Health Insurance Portability and Accountability Act (HIPAA) compliant. These portals allow patients to ask questions electronically directly to the doctor or nurse, and to receive their laboratory results or other communications. If a patient has computer access and signs up for such a program, they could fill out the past medical history and other pertinent information online in advance of an appointment.

Middle Office

The patient will then move to the middle portion of the visit where he or she will encounter the nurse (medical assistant) and the physician, as well as some of the following personnel: certified pedorthist, physical therapist, X-ray technician and cast technician. The "hand off" is very important in maintaining flow. The physician might leave the room and order an X-ray and an orthosis. The X-ray technician and certified pedorthist need to know that they have orders to see that patient. In the author's office, these services are offered in a middle hallway, and the providers are notified of the order through a system of colored flags on the doors. If a patient has an X-ray and then needs to go to the pedorthist following the X-ray, he does not come back into the physician examining area, but will go next door in the middle hallway to the next step in his plan of care.

At this point in the office visit, communication about the plan of care to the patient is very important. In a complex case, the physical therapist can join the physician in the examining room to discuss the management of the problem, or the physician can review the outside films with the X-ray technician to discuss what additional views are needed. When these conversations take place in front of the patient, there is often greater compliance with going to physical therapy or obtaining the orthoses because the patient heard the conversation outlining the customized plan of care for their problem.

Front Office: Exiting

On leaving the office, there are different paths that the patient may take. If the patient needs to speak to a surgery scheduler, the physician would ideally fill out a surgery booking sheet (electronic or paper) which would include the International classification of diseases (ICD-9) codes and Current procedural terminology (CPT) codes for the planned procedures. Prior to booking, the patient should speak to a financial adviser, who can advise the patient about estimated costs based on their insurance plan. Most patients want to understand what surgery will cost them and are very grateful to receive this estimate in order to prepare financially. Many patients are confused about the differences between elective and nonelective surgery and are concerned that their insurance plan will deny coverage. Once they understand that elective surgery is covered by their insurance company, they want to go forward with the procedure. The office should have a formula for what percentage of estimated money owed needs to be collected prior to performing elective surgery and this task is usually performed by the financial advisor. In most offices, nonelective (emergency or time-sensitive cases) will go forward with surgery scheduling even if the individual does not have an ability to pay in advance. Those patients should still be advised regarding their financial obligations. This would include cases like fractures that may not need to go to the operating room that day, but need to be fixed in a timely fashion.

The surgery scheduler will then explain the entire process around the surgery, including obtaining the preoperative history and physical examination, the preadmit appointment with the hospital, and medical clearance if needed, directions for the day of surgery, and dates for the initial postoperative appointment.

Patients who are not scheduling surgery generally need a follow-up appointment, and will exit along the same hall stopping by the appointment secretary's desk. That individual can perform a variety of different tasks, depending on how the office is structured. For example, the appointment secretary may have time to handle forms such as Family and Medical Leave Act (FMLA), short-term disability, work status, etc. She may be answering phones, or scheduling tests that were ordered.

The financial advisor, surgery scheduler and appointment secretary play an important role: they set the tone as a patient leaves the office with a final impression of his experience. In addition, the timely follow-up of these individuals after the patient leaves is critical, as the patient may not be able to collect a check until FMLA is completed, or their life is on hold while they wait to get a call regarding the date of surgery.

Back Office

The back office consists primarily of the billing and collections personnel. In some offices these functions will be outsourced. The author feels that it is prudent to maintain significant oversight in this area regardless of whether the function is maintained in-house or outside the office. Metrics comparing the performance of this office function to a national or regional standard, such as, Medical Group Management Association (MGMA) is important. This is an area where it may be prudent to obtain consultant overview on a periodic basis, or invest in continuing education for the staff so that they maintain competence in the ever changing world of health care reimbursement. Compliance with government regulations is a key issue, with the potential for significant financial penalties for coding errors, even if unintentional. A Revenue Cycle Scorecard or similar auditing tool is helpful in evaluating performance over time. A contract with an outside agency is often based on performance using these types of metrics.

The office may or may not have a dedicated office manager depending upon the size of the operation. The office manager should be a jack of all trades, able to substitute for any other employee should they be sick, on vacation, or just behind and creating a slowdown in the office flow on a given day. The concept of the working manager is critical—someone who is active and visible in the work environment, and is willing to put in the same hours or more as staff. Performance metrics are often an important motivator. In most cases, even managers need to be managed.

The Problem Employee

Finally, the employer should never feel that an employee is indispensable. Key employees are extremely valuable, but the practice should never be held hostage by anyone who feels the operation will fail without them. Conversely, the employer should never extend the employment of personnel who are not performing. Although managing personnel is difficult, and finding new employees is time consuming, marginal employees should not be kept on. Although at times that seems to be the easiest thing to do, it is even more time consuming to counsel and manage those employees. This is an area where the 80/20 rule applies: the lower performing twenty percent of the staff will occupy eighty percent of management's time!

COMPUTERIZING YOUR PRACTICE

Computerizing your practice allows you to:

- Collect and analyze demographic data, including patterns of referring physicians
- Maintain a digitalized medical record
- Potentially interact with the hospital if the system can be integrated
- Submit claims and monitor collections electronically
- Participate in government programs with incentives for "meaningful use".

DURABLE MEDICAL EQUIPMENT

There are pros and cons to managing durable medical equipment (DMEs) in the office setting. On one hand the physician can order anything she wants using multiple different vendors. On the other hand inventory management is not a core expertise of most medical offices. Maintaining inventory can tie up needed cash and space. Billing and collections for these items can be missed, and it is often unclear whether the patient will be responsible for the payment, or whether this is an item that will be reimbursed by the insurance company. Finally, inventory counts are necessary on occasion to maintain accuracy and usually there will be some amount of inventory that is "lost".

If DMEs are outsourced, the office can charge fair market value for the rent of the office space to the DME company. This provides independent service, but still gives the patient that centralized care with "one stop shopping". They are given a prescription for an item, but do not have to drive across town to get the item. This also frees up office personnel, as the patient moves on in the flow of the office to the independent DME provider.

OFFICE FLOW

Medical offices are "People movers". Like an airline, a medical office needs to courteously but efficiently move people through the visit while still giving them good service and the sense that they have had a good experience. Also like the airline, when the system gets bogged down and there are long wait times, people become frustrated and dissatisfied.

In order to maximize flow, each team member needs to know where each patient is in the visit. Some type of communication system, like flags or lights outside the doors will indicate what is needed next in that patient's room, be it X-ray, physical therapy, a cast tech, or the doctor. Usually, the nurse has the "big picture" and can direct traffic effectively. Being flexible and proactive is key. If X-ray is backed up, physical therapy can proceed first. Avoid linear thinking.

If there is a constriction in the patient flow, add additional resources to help. If the receptionist is overwhelmed, the patient scheduler can double up with reception. Everyone should be able to multitask, to cover when it is busy, or when someone is sick or on vacation. If rooms are being blocked by patients waiting to talk to the surgery scheduler, those patients can wait in the lobby or talk to the scheduler by phone, so others can get into the examining rooms. Again, the nurse is the key person to keep the flow moving. She should not get distracted by unnecessary phone calls or side issues, during clinic. The manager should be monitoring the flow and helping at constriction points.

Delays need to be actively managed to retain patient satisfaction. If the office is running behind, communication to the patient about what to expect is key. This will often diffuse the situation and give the patient the more control of the situation. They can decide to wait, come back after lunch, or reschedule. A television in the waiting room, wireless internet access, or an offer to get a patient a cup of coffee can be very helpful in minimizing the patient's frustration.

11

Clinical and Basic Research

Catherine Cunningham, Siddhant K Mehta, Sheldon S Lin

INTRODUCTION

With ongoing innovations in biotechnology, orthopedic surgery is a rapidly evolving field. Given the continual demand to improve current treatment options and quicken recovery from musculoskeletal problems, research plays an integral role in advancement of the field of orthopedic surgery. Basic science and clinical research projects allow for improvement in the understanding of various musculoskeletal diseases and permit the exploration of novel methods to accelerate bone and soft tissue healing. Research is also a key component for a successful academic career in orthopedic surgery. However, it is often challenging for young investigators to pursue research endeavors, even after an interest has been developed. The need to obtain funding becomes apparent when taking into account the resources necessary to conduct basic science and clinical research (e.g. laboratory space, supplies, support staff, imaging, etc.). Furthermore, given the time commitment required to oversee research activity, an appropriate balance between clinical duties and academic responsibilities must exist. This chapter aims to describe the role of the orthopedic clinician scientist and presents considerations that should be made when choosing to pursue an academic career in orthopedic surgery.

THE ORTHOPEDIC CLINICIAN-SCIENTIST: A DYING BREED?

The academic orthopedic clinician-scientist has been characterized as an orthopedic surgeon-scientist, by the virtue of being active in research and having the ability to apply scientific discoveries made from bench-top to bedside in an effort to improve patient care. With the unique capacity to translate basic science, clinical, or biomechanical research into practical applications of orthopedic medicine, orthopedic clinician-scientists can significantly impact the field of orthopedic surgery.

Since as early as 1979, multiple articles[1-13] have lamented the gradual decline and dearth of the clinician-scientist. For the orthopedic field in particular, another observation has been a harbinger of future shortages. While numerous studies[14-18] have shown that MD-PhD trainees have achieved significant academic success (defined as progression in rank with published papers and attainment of extramural funding), few individuals from this cohort have chosen a surgical career in general, and out of these even fewer choose orthopedic surgery.[6] This fact provides the orthopedic community with an impetus to explore multiple key questions. Is the concept of academic orthopedic clinician-scientist dying? Are there certain characteristics that are prognostic of success? Lastly, and perhaps most importantly, what are the barriers that exist for an orthopedic clinician-scientist's success and can these barriers be overcome?

RECRUITING FUTURE RESEARCHERS

Using his proposed criteria, Brand et al. estimated that approximately 560 active orthopedic clinician-scientists existed in 2002-2003, of which only 25% reported spending more than 50 days per year on research activities.[12] Therefore, the number of active clinician-scientists is very small (less than 5%) when compared to the total number of orthopedic surgeons in the United States. One recent article attempted to address this issue and analyzed a cohort of 868 students from 13 MD-PhD training programs.[19] Their survey demonstrated a relatively strong interest in the orthopedic field (regarding both patient care and research) among MD-PhD students nationally. The authors suggested the solution to bolstering the number of orthopedic clinician-scientists lay in the active recruitment of more MD-PhD students to orthopedic surgery. Based on the data, they extrapolated that even modest recruitment could lead to over 100 new orthopedic clinician-scientists every eight years, potentially doubling of the number of orthopedic clinician-scientists over the next fifty years. Atesok et al. suggested not only actively recruiting, but incorporating research and clinician-scientist career pathways into current orthopedic residencies.[20] Although tapping into this already small pool is critical, other issues that need to be addressed include the identification of factors that influence an individual's intent to perform research as well as the real and potential barriers to a successful career as a clinician-scientist.

EARLY RESEARCH TRAINING

It is clearly impossible to conduct research without first attaining appropriate knowledge of research methods and developing the ability to test logical, well-developed, and clinically relevant hypotheses. Experience in research can be attained during formal or informal, pre- or postdoctoral training as well as throughout residency and fellowship.

Summer research programs afford medical students the opportunity to become involved with research at their medical schools. They are usually 1–2 months in duration, and allow students to design short, but meaningful projects and learn the "basics" of the research process. Involvement in such programs provides the students early exposure into research, which may be influential in future career decisions.

Predoctoral research fellowships are also useful in training young clinician-scientists. These programs are usually one year in duration, and require full commitment of the student in scholastic and research activity prior to graduation from medical school. Opportunities presented by predoctoral research fellowships are vast. With involvement in clinical and/or basic science research, the student acquires an in-depth understanding of research techniques and is able to develop research interests early in his/her career. Additionally, there is an opportunity to develop a mentoring relationship that will facilitate career development and residency/fellowship placement.

Postdoctoral fellowships are also a valuable means of research training. Several orthopedic surgery residency programs offer a research track, in which trainees dedicate 1–2 years (in addition to traditional 5-year clinical training) to conduct basic science and/or clinical research. Research training is initiated before or in between 1st year and 2nd year of the clinical training, where the resident has minimal clinical responsibility. The overall goals of these programs are to introduce residents to various clinical and laboratory research methods and to provide experience in grant writing, manuscript preparation, and dissemination of research results at conferences. Hence, these programs are designed for scholars who demonstrate a commitment to research and education, and desire to become orthopedic clinician-scientists. However, Segal et al.[21] showed that although the number of publications during and after completing residency were greater in residents with advanced research training, no difference was observed between residents with a research year and those without, with respect to the number of residents entering private or academic practice. Similarly, Bernstein et al.[22] described the experience of the University of Pennsylvania's research program during residency between 1978 and 1993 and reported that 59% took faculty positions in an academic setting. These studies show that advanced research programs during residency may not necessarily ensure the number of residents that choose the orthopedic clinician-scientist path.

FOSTERING THE YOUNG CLINICIAN-SCIENTIST

The importance of clinician-scientists in the field of orthopedic surgery was reconfirmed with a survey of both the residents and chairs of 16 orthopedic departments.[23] Both groups agreed that research was important to the clinical practice of orthopedics and should be conducted by orthopedic surgeons. Unfortunately, following on the heels of this was the observation that few practice what they preach, or in other words few orthopedic residents had intentions of entering into an academic research career. Analysis of the resident pool showed that potential interest in pursuing research could reach as high as 70% (if including both interested residents and those unsure of their interest), but only 25% would like to perform basic science research. This begs the question, what is the major deterrent?

As reported by a number of papers,[3,7,11,18,24,25] the barriers facing a junior clinician-scientist are vast and result in a vicious cycle. Faced with insufficient funding, clinician-scientists are not well-compensated for their time and hence increase patient contact to make up the difference. Doing so interferes even more with research activity, prevents professional recognition and makes research funding more difficult to obtain. Increased documentation requirements, decreased reimbursements and excessive malpractice insurance costs worsen an already tenuous situation. Clinical practice becomes too demanding, financial responsibilities mount and they are forced to choose: pure clinician, or pure scientist? Due to competition with PhDs, too often the scientific aspect is neglected, causing the already small number of clinician-scientists to dwindle.

However, Ahn et al. also found that prior research experience, lower debt and primary authorship of a manuscript were all associated with a higher degree of interest in performing research. This knowledge was then utilized to determine various incentives for becoming an academic orthopedic clinician-scientist. When surveyed, residents identified protected research time and ample funding as the incentives they favored most during residency, with salary support and debt forgiveness as those they favored after residency. Department chairs, on the other hand, reported the incentive they were most willing to support was protected time both during and after residency. The authors concluded "the optimal set of incentives may indeed be found by combining the results from both groups into a hybrid concept: a combination of protected time, increased access to funding, salary support and debt relief." This echoes an earlier survey of all clinician-scientists by Donath et al. (Fig. 1),[26] which recorded similar sentiments.

THE PRESSURE OF CLINICAL PRODUCTIVITY

As stated above, the potential of an orthopedic surgeon to generate a greater amount of annual revenue compared to that of their nonsurgical colleagues creates a significant difference in salary between the full-time orthopedic clinician and the orthopedic clinician-scientist (Fig. 2).[27] Often described as the "golden handcuff," annual salaries of the more clinically-oriented orthopedic surgeons put many a department chair in quite the predicament. If an orthopedic clinician-scientist spends 50% of the given work week in the laboratory not seeing patients, not generating relative value units (RVU's) and therefore not obtaining monetary reimbursement, should their salary be equal to the full time equivalent (FTE) of a practicing orthopedic surgeon? Sadly, if it is equal, collegial resentment of protected research time and "not carrying a fair share" of the clinical workload is often encountered.[8]

Hurwitz, in 1999, has stated that unless there is financial equity between the two cohorts of an orthopedic department, a financial disincentive occurs.[5] He did acknowledge that less call with equal pay could lead to ill-will, but felt that practice-oriented clinicians must understand the need for financial sacrifices in order to advance the field of orthopedics, improve our educational materials, and ultimately benefit patient care. These concepts may be considered noble, however a recent survey provided the actual reality. Less than 50% of residents and 25% of clinicians feel the sacrifice should come from department funds, and even less so from their individual pocket.[23] One potential solution may be to compromise: if a clinician-scientist spends 50% of given FTE in the laboratory, then their salary may be a combination of 50% FTE of orthopedic surgery and 50% FTE of orthopedic research. Obviously, this controversial dilemma will continue to play out during the currently changing financial and social pressures of a new healthcare system.

IMPORTANCE OF A RESEARCH PROGRAM AND MODEL FOR FUTURE DEVELOPMENT

One of the key understated concepts in becoming a successful clinician-scientist is the need to identify a focused area of research. This clinical question, whether far-reaching and affecting millions of people such as diabetes mellitus (DM), or only a chosen few (i.e. Lou Gerhig's disease), must provide a challenge and spark ongoing interest for the researcher. For example, the authors' personal research program focuses on the well known issue of impaired bone healing (double that of normal fracture healing) in patients with DM[28] and the high complication rate (more than 30%) observed with attempted foot-ankle fusion in the DM population.[29-33] With over 21 million Americans with DM in 2011, the authors feel that a disease that affects so many patients and loved-ones provides the motivation to study and understand this clinical quandary.

Balance Between Research/Clinical Work/Family/Administrative Tasks

"You need a primary focus. To wake on Monday and be a doctor and then on Tuesday to be a researcher is a lot more difficult than to self-identify a primary activity." (#5)

"The clinical demands are always here and now and you're forever putting off the research until tomorrow…." (#7)

"My contract stipulates 50/50 distribution between clinic and research.... It is not difficult to manage the balance—you find things difficult if you don't like them." (#8)

"Research gets squeezed between administrative work, clinic, and teaching, and it's hard to say no if you're a junior faculty so you end up agreeing to do a wide variety of different things, and it's really hard to figure out how to balance all these things and properly advance yourself and find satisfaction in what you're doing. There is no one to help figure out exactly how to properly allocate my time—no authority figure to say I shouldn't be spending more than this amount of time in that or that in this, etc…" (#12)

Difficulties in Obtaining Grants/Proposing Research as a Clinician-Scientist

"The biggest challenge to being a clinician-scientist is not the clinic part, it's the research part—because you have to compete against PhDs who do nothing else." (#2)

"There is a difference grant committees have in terms of expectations from clinician-scientists and researchers. Primary researchers are more likely to propose developing a brand new system whereas clinician-scientists are more likely to want use the existing system to answer the following problem." (#5)

Economic Disincentives to Pursuing This Pathway

"One of the reasons I was able to stick with research was because I was either too stupid or too uncaring about how much money I made." (#2)

"If you're interested in becoming a clinician-scientist, you can't be a person for whom financial reward is your first priority." (#2)

Exposures to Research

"It's very important to get med students/residents exposed to research, because you will catch the 10%-15% of med students that have the right attributes for research." (#2)

"You need to have passion. I think you have to inoculate that passion during the first 1-2 years of med school. I would arrange for these students to go to the best-mentored labs/environment and get them the best exposures possible to give them the bug and then you hope that those who get the bug keep it—because throughout med school you don't have time to do anything—and then want to do research later on. Because you can't be told to do research, it will never work." (#11)

Fragile Early Career Environment

"What's absolutely necessary is that you take on a job as a junior faculty in the right environment. Often these people get the right training but then they start in an environment where no one is a clinician-scientist and no one has ever done anything academic and the hospital staff are unaware of the needs and requirements of a clinician-scientist and so they tell the junior staff to take a full clinical load, and if you want to do research then that's what nights and weekends are for. That's why I think 60%-80% of clinician-scientists fail within their first 5 years." (#11)

"The early career environment is critical. If you bang your head against the wall too often, you're just going to give up. If you've been trying for a few years and are not successful, CIHR funding is next to impossible…. The success rate in applying for CIHR grants in general is pretty low and a lot of it is based on how good you've been at getting those grants in the past…. A lot of people come in with the best intentions but if you don't get that first CIHR grant right off the bat, it becomes quite depressing.(#13)

Ideal Pathway to Becoming a Clinician-Scientist

"It was a blessing I didn't get into the MD/PhD program—my friends that got in are still stuck in residency training and found it difficult to pick up where they had left off." (#1)

"CIP (Clinical Investigator Program) is a more natural, organic progression—only once you're superspecialized do you go off and do research training. The intellectual process in the MD/PhD program seems to be more disjointed… in medical school you're supposed to go out and learn this extremely broad amount of information and then you have to go off and do your PhD in an extremely focused field, etc.... It makes a lot more sense to start broadly and then gradually focus yourself over time." (#2)

"Your research is so much better if you know what you're looking for. If you've done your residency, you know what clinical problems exist and you can ask the right questions, but if you do research beforehand you don't really understand the problems that exist…. You have a very different understanding of disease when you're an established clinician." (#6)

Mentoring

"I had a mentor at every step along the way and that was vital to my success." (#4)

"Mentoring is crucial. My ideas wouldn't have gone anywhere without mentors to organize and offer a pragmatic perspective to those ideas." (#7)

Fig. 1. Main issues discussed during semi-structured interviews with 16 clinician-scientists regarding the clinician-scientist pathway. Numbers in parentheses refer to the participant identification number[26]

Source: Donath E, Filion KB, Eisenberg MJ. Improving the clinician-scientist pathway: a survey of clinician-scientists. Archives of Internal Medicine. 2009;169(13):1242-4. Epub 2009/07/15.

The authors attempted to address this issue by first finding a reproducible model for bone healing in DM. Using a known type I DM rat model, the BB Wistar rat, they characterized the early and late parameters of impaired DM fracture healing.[34] Once this model was established and published, it provided a natural progression into potential fracture healing adjuncts. The authors systematically focused on key questions regarding these novel adjuncts, such as mechanical devices (i.e. LIPUS),[35] protein growth factors (i.e. insulin, platelet rich plasma, recombinant platelet-derived growth factors,[36-38] and novel organometallic salts (i.e. insulin-mimetics).[39] The authors also continued to elucidate the underlying mechanism(s) of impaired DM bone healing.[34,40] In addition, this DM model provided another application using a similar but distinct model of segmental femoral defect, using both DM and non-DM rats.[41-43] The main point is that having a highly reproducible model with well-characterized parameters allows the clinician-scientist to pursue further interests (i.e. spin off) and therefore obtain future grants.

Clearly, the animal model concept is highly applicable to a basic science program, however those with a focus on clinical research may utilize a similar program with a well-characterized treatment and well-characterized outcome parameters to investigate their question. Once standardized and published, the orthopedic clinician-scientist may follow with new potential treatments and protocols, whether they are preoperative, intraoperative or postoperative.

MENTORSHIP

Mentorship is a relationship between a student (mentee) and a senior individual (mentor) by which the mentor commits to the advancement of the mentee in both personal and professional aspects of a career. It often gradually develops over time as the two individuals work together and build a mutual respect for one another. Talent tends to draw

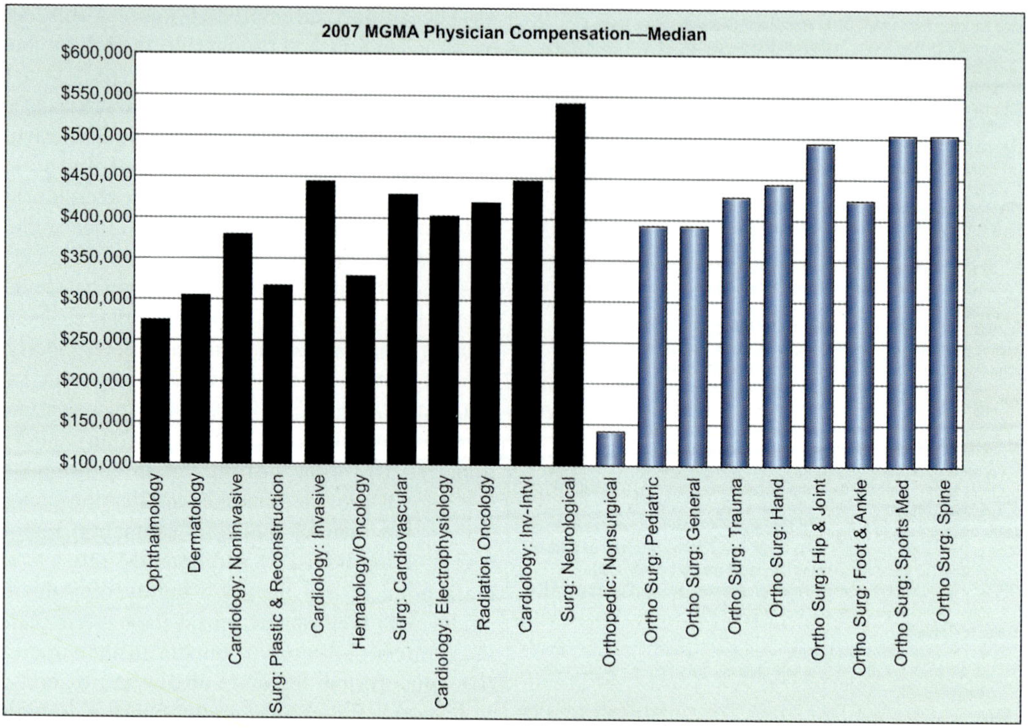

Fig. 2: Data on physician compensation from the Medical Group Management Association (MGMA) 2007 report[27]
Source: Emery SE, Waddell JP, Waddell AE, et al. Orthopaedic education—are we attracting the best and the brightest? J Bone Joint Surg Am. 2009;91(5):1253-63. Epub 2009/05/05.

the mentor, while accomplishment in a given area of interest draws the mentee to such a relationship. Clearly, a successful mentorship is dependent on a substantial time commitment from both the mentor and mentee. Given its personal nature, it also involves compatible personalities and shared career interests. An ideal mentoring relationship is one that is reciprocal and personal. It must utilize the mentor's experience and influence in a given field to acquire knowledge and directly support the mentee in regards to professional development and career advancement.

In any mentorship, the mentor serves to recognize a mentee's strengths and weaknesses, provides guidance to achieve certain established goals, and facilitates the advancement of the mentee in a chosen career path. The mentee should identify and communicate to the mentor what he/she desires to accomplish by way of the mentorship (e.g. goals to be achieved, skills/knowledge to be attained, timeline to accomplish within). Furthermore, the mentee can also serve as a resource partner, share information and provide feedback that may be valuable to both mentor and mentee. Most importantly, the mentee must always be actively involved in any opportunity to learn and develop academically. Mentoring can be extremely helpful in orthopedic surgery, for both clinical training and pursuing an academic career.[44-46] Finding a mentor that is able and willing to provide guidance can enable the young investigator to overcome many of the barriers and to succeed as a clinician-scientist.

RESEARCH FUNDING OPPORTUNITIES

Overall, there has been a decline of the so-called "medical science generalist", as witnessed by falling attendance of the annual joint meeting of the American Society for Clinical Investigation (ASCI), Association of American Physicians (AAP) and American Federation of Medical Research (AFMR).[3] Although this seems disheartening at first glance, attendance at specialty research societies has been on the rise,[3] suggesting that clinicians are interested in research, but only after reaching a highly specialized level. However, one cannot judge the success of the clinician-scientist on this alone. When looking at grant applications, the majority of successful applications belong to PhDs and not MDs—a disparity also reflected in the type of research the grants are most often awarded to: basic science. In the medical world, basic science research is commonly seen as the domain of PhDs. In this way, patient-oriented and disease-oriented research falls by the wayside, most likely due to the lack of clinical insight that can only be gained from the experience of an MD.

What does this have to do with the orthopedic clinician-scientist? The surgical residency and lifestyle in particular preclude one from keeping pace with the breakneck speed of scientific discovery, and the competition to stay ahead puts full-time researchers (i.e. PhDs) at a significant advantage over their clinically-oriented counterparts. By the time the average orthopedic surgeon has the time and begins pursuing research, although their training is highly specialized, the majority lack both the experience and the mentorship when it comes to writing successful grant proposals and securing funding for their own projects.[5] Furthermore, the financial burdens of their educational debt and family life begin to add up, putting more pressure on their clinical productivity. Essentially, they have neither the knowledge of specific resources nor the skill to obtain them, as evidenced by the dropping number of successful R01 applications by orthopedic surgeons.[12]

Of note is one particular program designed to tackle this problem head on. The American Association of Orthopedic Surgeons (AAOS), the Orthopedic Research and Education Foundation (OREF) and the Orthopedic Research Society (ORS) jointly created the Clinician Scholar Development Program, which seeks orthopedic surgeons (ranging from PGY2 through junior faculty) with an interest in becoming a clinician-scientist. Included in the program are workshops on grant writing, mentoring and general career training. As far as accrued debt, the National Institutes of Health (NIH) has a number of competitive loan repayment programs for those seriously committed to clinically-oriented research.[25] Additionally, we have ended this chapter with some general guidelines to be of help when securing funding for your own project.

- *Seek out a possible source/financier for the project.*

Clearly, your topic interests you, but does this fill a goal of a certain financier or society? For example, scientists are advised to consult the National Science Foundation for direct fellowship and scholarship opportunities along with a list of public sector sources. (See Table 1 for a list specific to Orthopedics).

Table 1: List of funding opportunities by career level

Residency	*Post-Residency*	*Early Career*	*Mid-Career and Later*
• Research Block (2–4 months) ▪ OREF Research Grants ▪ Department or Private Attending Funding • Research Year(s) ▪ Department Funding ▪ NIH K23 Award ▪ Howard Hughes Medical Institute ▪ Subspecialty Society Grants – AOFAS – OTA • Research Degree ▪ PhD, MPH, MS	• OREF Research Grants • NIH K08, K23, K22 Awards • Private Foundation Grants ▪ Aircast Foundation ▪ American Cancer Society ▪ Arthritis Foundation ▪ March of Dimes ▪ Muscular Dystrophy Association ▪ Musculoskeletal Transplant Foundation ▪ Shriner's Hospital Grants ▪ Subspecialty Society Grants	• OREF Research Grants • NIH K08, R03 Awards • Department of Defense • Private Foundation Grants	• NIH R01 Award • Department of Defense • VA Federal Grants • Private Foundation Grants

(NIH: National Institutes of Health; AOFAS: American Orthopedic Foot and Ankle Society; OTA: Orthopedic Trauma Association)
Source: Adapted from the Orthopedic Research and Education Foundation (OREF) website.

- *Develop a research proposal consistent with criteria set forth by your prospective source.*

Each agency or private source will have a different criteria or set of standards required for a proposal. Overall, it is necessary to prepare several different sets of research proposals, with each proposal being more suitable than another for a specific audience. For instance, a Small Business Innovation Research (SBIR) is more focused on the commercial applications of the research, than a proposal to the National Science Foundation or the NIH.

- *Submit your initial research proposal to qualified peers in your field for a useful critique.*

Repeat the review and editing process several times. Once your proposal has been "critiqued", repeat this step several times before submitting the final draft of the proposal to the agency or financier.

REFERENCES

1. Wyngaarden JB. The clinical investigator as an endangered species. N Engl J Med. 1979; 301: 1254-9.
2. Nabel GJ. The MD PhD physician scientist—endandered species or the next generation? Mol Med. 1995;1:369-70.
3. Goldstein JL, Brown MS. The clinical investigator: bewitched, bothered, and bewildered-but still beloved. J Clin Invest. 1997;99:2803-12.
4. Rosenberg L. Physician-scientist—endangered and essential. Science. 1999;283:331-2.
5. Hurwitz SR, Buckwalter JA. The orthopedic surgeon scientist: an endangered species? J Orthop Res. 1999;17:155-6.
6. Clark JM, Hanel DP. The contribution of MD-PhD training to academic orthopedic faculties. J Orthop Res. 2001;19:505-10.
7. Jackson DW. The orthopedic clinician-scientist. J Bone Joint Surg Am. 2001;83:131-5.
8. Clawson DK. Cultivating a valuable hybrid: the orthopedic clinician-scientist. J Bone Joint Surg Am. 2001;83:1432-3.
9. Sweeney G. The demise of the clinician-scientist matters to everyone. Clinical and investigative medicine Medecine clinique et experimentale. 2001;24:212-3.
10. Wright JG. Supporting the orthopedic clinician-scientist. J Bone Joint Surg Am. 2002;84:145-6.
11. Faxon DP. The chain of scientific discovery: the critical role of the physician-scientist. Circulation. 2002;105:1857-60.
12. Brand RA, Chaw ES, Karam MD. The number and scope of activity of orthopedic clinician-scientists in the United States. J Bone Joint Surg Am. 2003;85:374-9.
13. Schafer AI. The vanishing physician-scientist? Translational Research:The Journal of Laboratory and Clinical Medicine. 2010;155(1):1-2. Epub 2009/12/17.
14. Bradford WD, Anthony D, Chu CT, et al. Career characteristics of a graduate Medical Scientist Training Program. Acad Med. 1996;71:484-7.
15. McClellan DA, Talalay P. MD-PhD training at the Johns Hopkins University School of Medicine 1962-1991. Acad Med. 1992;67:36-41.
16. Schwatz P, Gaulton GN. Addressing the needs of basic and clinical research:analysis of graduates of the University of Pennsylvania MD-PhD program. JAMA. 1999;281:96-7.
17. Watt CD, Greeley SA, Shea JA, et al. Educational views and attitudes, and career goals of MD-PhD students at the University of Pennsyvania School of Medicine. Acad Med. 2005;80:193-8.
18. Ley TJ, Rosenberg LE. The physician-scientist career pipeline in 2005: build it, and they will come. JAMA. 2005;294(11):1343-51. Epub 2005/09/22.
19. Ahn J, Man L, Wanderer J, et al. The future of the orthopedic clinician-scientist Part I:the potential role of MD-PhD students considering orthopedic surgery. J Bone Joint Surg A. 2008;90-A(8):1794-9.
20. Atesok KI, Hurwitz SR, Egol KA, et al. Perspective: Integrating research into surgical residency education: lessons learned from orthopaedic surgery. Acad Med. 2012;87(5):592-7. Epub 2012/03/28.
21. Segal LS, Black KP, Schwentker EP, et al. An elective research year in orthopaedic residency: how does one measure its outcome and define its success? Clinical Orthopaedics and Related Research. 2006;449:89-94. Epub 2006/06/09.
22. Bernstein J, Ahn J, Iannotti JP, et al. The required research rotation in residency: the University of Pennsylvania experience, 1978-1993. Clinical Orthopaedics and Related Research. 2006;449:95-9. Epub 2006/06/01.
23. Ahn J, Donegan DJ, Lawrence TR, et al. The future of the orthopedic clinician-scientist. J Bone Joint Surg Am. 2010;92(4):1041-6.
24. Rosier RN. Institutional barriers to the orthopaedic clinician-scientist. Clinical orthopaedics and related research. 2006;449:159-64. Epub 2006/08/05.
25. Einhorn TA. Funding the mandate for the orthopaedic clinician scientist. Clinical orthopaedics and related research. 2006;449:76-80. Epub 2006/06/01.

26. Donath E, Filion KB, Eisenberg MJ. Improving the clinician-scientist pathway: a survey of clinician-scientists. Archives of Internal Medicine. 2009;169(13):1242-4. Epub 2009/07/15.
27. Emery SE, Waddell JP, Waddell AE, et al. Orthopaedic education—are we attracting the best and the brightest? J Bone Joint Surg Am. 2009;91(5):1253-63. Epub 2009/05/05.
28. Graves DT, Alblowi J, Paglia DN, et al. Impact of diabetes on fracture healing. J Exp Clin Med. 2011;3(1):3.
29. Cozen L. Does diabetes delay fracture healing? Clin Orthop. 1972;82:134-40.
30. Kagel EM, Einhorn TA. Alterations of fracture healing in the diabetic condition. Iowa Orthop J. 1996;16:147-52.
31. Papa J, Myerson M, Girard P. Salvage, with arthrodesis, in intractable diabetic neuropathic arthropathy of the foot and ankle. J Bone Joint Surg Am. 1993; 75(7):1056-66.
32. Stuart MJ, Morrey BF. Arthrodesis of the diabetic neuropathic ankle joint. Clin Orthop. 1990;253: 209-11.
33. Tisdel CL, Marcus RE, Heiple KG. Triple arthrodesis for diabetic peritalar neuroarthropathy. Foot Ankle Int. 1995;16(6):332-8.
34. Beam HA, Parsons JR, Lin SS. The effects of blood glucose control upon fracture healing in the BB Wistar rat with diabetes mellitus. J Orthop Res. 2002;20(6):1210-6.
35. Gebauer GP, Lin SS, Beam HA, et al. Low-intensity pulsed ultrasound increases the fracture callus strength in diabetic BB Wistar rats but does not affect cellular proliferation. J Orthop Res. 2002;20(3): 587-92.
36. Al-Zube L, Breitbart EA, O'Connor JP, et al. Recombinant human platelet-derived growth factor BB (rhPDGF-BB) and beta-tricalcium phosphate/ collagen matrix enhance fracture healing in a diabetic rat model. J Orthop Res; 2009.
37. Gandhi A, Beam HA, O'Connor JP, et al. The effects of local insulin delivery on diabetic fracture healing. Bone. 2005;37(4):482-90.
38. Gandhi A, Doumas C, O'Connor JP, et al. The effects of local platelet rich plasma delivery on diabetic fracture healing. Bone. 2006;38(4):540-6.
39. Paglia DN, Wey A, Park AG, et al. The effects of local vanadium treatment on angiogenesis and chondrogenesis during fracture healing. J Orthop Res. 2012;In Press.
40. Tyndall WA, Beam HA, Zarro C, et al. Decreased platelet derived growth factor expression during fracture healing in diabetic animals. Clin Orthop. 2003;408:319-30.
41. Azad V, Breitber E, O'Connor JP, et al. rhBMP-2 enhances the bone healing response in a diabetic segmental defect model. Journal of Orthopedic Trauma. 2009;23(4):267.
42. Breitber E, Azad V, Meade S, et al. Augmentation mesenchymal stem cells accelerate bone allograft incorporation in the presence of diabetes mellitus. J Orthop Res. 2010;28(7):942-9.
43. Dedania J, Breitber E, Paglia D, et al. Effect of local insulin in autograft incorporation. J Orthop Res; 2011.
44. Wilson FC. Mentoring in orthopaedics: an evolving need for nurture. J Bone Joint Surg Am. 2004; 86-A(5):1089-91. Epub 2004/05/01.
45. Flint JH, Jahangir AA, Browner BD, et al. The value of mentorship in orthopaedic surgery resident education: the residents' perspective. J Bone Joint Surg Am. 2009;91(4):1017-22. Epub 2009/04/03.
46. Pellegrini VD. Mentoring during residency education: a unique challenge for the surgeon? Clinical orthopaedics and related research. 2006;449:143-8. Epub 2006/06/09.

SECTION 2

Forefoot Problems

Chapters Outline

12

Bunions (Hallux Valgus)

Emilio Wagner, Cristian Ortiz, Pablo Wagner

INTRODUCTION

Hallux valgus (HV) is one of the most common chronic foot complaints presenting to foot and ankle specialists, occurring when the hallux deviates laterally towards the other toes, and the first metatarsal head becomes prominent medially. As well as being a major contributor to the costs of forefoot surgery, hallux valgus has been linked to functional disability, including foot pain, impaired gait patterns, poor balance, and falls in older adults. A wide range of prevalence estimates for HV has been presented in a multitude of independent reports. A recent meta-analysis of 78 papers reporting results of 76 surveys (total 496,957 participants) showed a pooled prevalence estimate for HV of 23% in adults aged 18–65 years and 35.7% in elderly people aged over 65 years. The prevalence increased with age and was higher in females (30%) compared to males (13%).[1]

ETIOLOGY AND PATHOPHYSIOLOGY

The first ray is an inherently unstable axial ray that relies on a fine balance between its static and dynamic stabilizers to maintain its alignment. In some feet there is a genetic predisposition for a nonlinear osseous alignment or a laxity of the static stabilizers that disrupts this balance. The anatomical metatarsal variants have been suggested to play an important role in hallux valgus such as a long first metatarsal, rounded joint and metatarsus primus varus. Over this genetic predisposition the extrinsic factors play a role as contributing factors, including poor footwear (high heels and narrow shoes) and excessive weight-bearing. Once the metatarsal head starts to escape the ligamentous and muscular control, the extrinsic tendons become a deforming force. The deep transverse ligament and the adductor muscle hold the phalanx in place, while the incompetent medial metatarsosesamoid ligament and medial collateral ligament allow the metatarsal head to drift into varus.[2]

Although the authors agree with Coughlin that first cuneometatarsal instability is secondary to deformity and is corrected after surgery,[3] they consider that a few patients maintain instability after proper correction and might need this problem to be addressed primarily by a Lapidus arthrodesis. There is no preoperative indicator that can predict which patients have a tarsometatarsal (TMT) instability as a contributing factor that has to be addressed, but our threshold to perform arthrodesis at this level has lowered, specifically when treating older patients with severe hallux valgus and poor bone quality, and when mediolateral radiologic first TMT instability is detected on preoperative weight bearing X-rays.

DIAGNOSIS

The patient must have a painful medial prominence for adequate diagnosis. If there is a dorsal bunion a hallux rigidus must be ruled out as a source of pain. A few patients may have both and an appropriate treatment must be planned for both. A complete clinical analysis must be performed, considering associated general pathology that could force us to change the best method of treatment, such as rheumatoid arthritis, vascular insufficiency or diabetes. All other painful deformities should be treated at the same time including flat foot, hammer toes, cross-over toes, Morton's neuroma, etc.

CLASSIFICATION

When correcting a hallux valgus deformity, the technique chosen should depend on the deformity to be corrected and the individual correction power a particular technique possesses. Although the classic

Table 1: Classification of hallux valgus depending on the angle to be corrected

Severity Grading	*Angle to be Corrected (Degrees)*
Mild	< 5
Moderate	5–9
Severe	> 10

intermetatarsal (IMT) angle value is < 9° there are individual variations in the angular measurements and not every hallux valgus is the same. We should try to achieve the alignment and therefore correction more "normal" to each patient individually. In order to do so, as it has been shown that in hallux valgus the deformity comes from a medial deviation of the metatarsal bone, where the sesamoids mark the "original" position where the metatarsal head was located.[4] The ideal position for the metatarsal head should be on top of the sesamoid complex. Indeed, it has been shown that an incomplete postoperative reduction of the sesamoids constitutes a risk factor for recurrence of the deformity.[5] Following this line of thinking, the authors currently use a new angular measurement to choose their osteotomy to correct the intermetatarsal angle, which is the "angle to be corrected". This angle is obtained drawing a line through the first metatarsal axis and then drawing a second line from the same starting point on the base of the first metatarsal but going distally through the middle of the sesamoid complex. This angle represents the amount of degrees one has to move the metatarsal in order to center the head over the sesamoids.[6] After defining the correction power of each technique, the surgeon can choose correctly the proper surgical procedure, using three basically different techniques, mainly the distal 90° Chevron, the diaphyseal rotational scarf osteotomy and the proximal oblique slide closing wedge (POSCOW) osteotomy. Depending on their correction capacity, we can correct three different sets of deformities. The correction capacity of these techniques has been defined previously.[7] This has allowed us to classify hallux valgus into three groups (Table 1).

TREATMENT

Treatment should always begin with a recommendation of conservative treatment with special attention to shoe fit. It must be considered that feet change in width with aging, as well as with weight gain and pregnancy. For some patients there is no suitable off-the-shelf solution and they may require a custom shoe. The proper shoe must include: rounded toe box, seamless in the bunion area, low heel, soft and expandable upper cover, and potentially create a "bunion pocket" with a ball-ring stretcher in the painful area. There are some other conservative options that provide minor levels of relief including toe separators and shoe inserts.[8]

For patients who do not respond to conservative treatment and have a symptomatic hallux valgus, or have overload symptoms of the second ray such as metatarsalgia or a secondary cross-over toe, a surgical option is selected among more than 150 procedures described in literature. It must always be considered that some patients may have "hindfoot driven forefoot symptoms" (like in a flat foot) or may have associated deformities that may require surgery at the same procedure, such as symptomatic flat foot, metatarsalgia, hammer toes, crossover toes, bunionette, Morton's neuroma, etc. On the contrary, nonsymptomatic conditions, such as mild cavo varus feet, flexible asymptomatic flatfeet, mild metatarsus adductus, brachymetatarsia within others, do not need specific treatment. The authors do consider hallux valgus deformities in the aforementioned conditions more difficult to treat, and sometimes change their surgical technique to the next more powerful one in their protocol of treatment.

When the authors recommend surgery, they advise their patients as follows:

- Success rate is about 90%
- A popliteal block is done to control postoperative pain
- Pain, swelling and difficulties for shoe wear last approximately one year
- Complication rate is 10–50%.

The authors advise their patients concerning the following complications: mild issues such as temporary neuritis, self resolving wound problems; and more severe issues which might require a new surgery including symptomatic hardware, partial or complete deformity correction loss, arthritis, avascular necrosis, nonunion or malunion.

Table 2: Surgical technique decision depending on the preoperative deformity

Severity Grading	*Surgical Technique*
Mild	Chevron
Moderate	Rotational scarf
Severe	POSCOW, Lapidus or MTP arthrodesis

SURGICAL TECHNIQUES

Once the surgical treatment is selected, the authors totally agree with Trnka and many others that despite the fact that different forms of soft tissue procedures are still in use, they should be abandoned. And although there is no level one evidence to guide us as to which surgical treatment is the best, there is sufficient information to consider that nowadays a thoughtful selection of an osteotomy is the gold standard treatment for hallux valgus.[9]

Although the minimally invasive surgical techniques may have benefits in a specific group of patients, the authors disagree with the recommendation of one single procedure for every patient and they totally agree with the recently published conclusion about these techniques, which states that data is lacking to allow definitive conclusions on the use of minimally invasive techniques for routine management of patients with hallux valgus.[10]

Special Considerations

The authors carefully analyze their patients, considering their age, bone stock, metatarsophalangeal deformity, intermetatarsal deformity, distal metatarsal articular angle, presence of secondary pathologies such as metatarsalgia or claw toes, and then they select one of the procedures depending on their classification based on "the angle to be corrected" (Table 2). It is to be noted however, that any classification has its limitations, as every hallux valgus is unique and they may share an angular deformity, but they may have different other factors that will change the decision. Also, angular measurements have limitations, as it has been shown that although interobserver reliability is high for HV angle and intermetatarsal angle,[11] the same is not true for distal metatarsal articular angle where variation is high and many times dependent on, for example, metatarsal rotation.[12]

Age

Regarding age, in juvenile and adolescent patients, the surgical decision is harder to make, as other factors come into play, as open physes, cosmetic issues, reliability of the procedure, possible future side effects, and patient's familiar environment. When there are still open physes present, the authors try their best to insist on conservative approaches before considering a surgical approach. Every aspect is discussed with the family, and many visits are planned, so as to really determine what will be the best option for that particular case, not only focusing on the angular deformity. If a surgical option is taken, the authors do not trust partial epiphysiodesis of the first metatarsal as it has been shown not to be reliable and capable of small corrections.[13] As a general rule, if the patient still has open physes, for mild deformities, the authors prefer distal procedures as the Chevron and possibly Akin osteotomies. When the deformity is severe, the authors prefer medially opening wedge techniques over the medial cuneiform, adding, if needed, a distal Chevron osteotomy and/or an Akin osteotomy. When the authors treat adolescent patients with little or no growth potentially, they use their general rule depending on the angle to be corrected (Table 2). Good results have been published in adolescents using the traditional scarf osteotomy,[14] but results are scarce relative to other osteotomies. It has been the authors' experience that POSCOW osteotomy is the best surgical treatment for adolescent severe hallux valgus in an attempt to avoid a Lapidus in this young age population. Young patients are indeed very good candidates when a proximal osteotomy is indicated, as they have great healing potential, and thus should have a very good outcome.

In older patients, when osteoporosis is present, for mild and moderate deformities the authors use the protocol already mentioned (Tables 1 and 2). When arthritic changes are present, they generally debride and perform microdrilling of the chondral lesions. Dorsal osteophytes are also removed from the metatarsal and from the proximal phalangeal base. For severe deformities, the authors change their technique and instead of performing a proximal osteotomy, they perform a Lapidus arthrodesis, using two crossed screws or one screw and a medial plate as fixation. The authors consider the healing potential of a cuneometatarsal fusion better than the healing potential of the POSCOW osteotomy, as most of their failures when performing proximal osteotomies have occurred in the older population.

Metatarsophalangeal (MTP) Deformity

Metatarsophalangeal angular values are taken into consideration preoperatively and intraoperatively after the intermetatarsal deformity is corrected. Preoperatively, if the intermetatarsal deformity shows a moderate angle to be corrected (between 5° and 9°), but the metatarsophalangeal angle (HV angle) is greater than 35°, the authors choose the next surgical technique in their protocol (a POSCOW technique), because empirically the correction power of the metatarsal osteotomy may not be enough in such a deformity because of failure of soft tissue balance and long standing metatarsophalangeal deformity. Intraoperatively, if there is still a need to correct the subluxation of the extensor hallucis longus tendon, or there is a hallux valgus interphalangeus, the authors add an Akin osteotomy.

Distal Metatarsal Articular Angle (DMAA)

It has been said already that this measurement is not reliable between observers and it can be altered just by metatarsal rotation. However, the authors believe that as it can alter the surgical result, it has to be taken into account. When performing displacement osteotomies, as the distal Chevron, no alteration in the DMAA results, as translational osteotomies do not alter this angle. Rotational osteotomies do alter the DMAA value, and thus care has to be taken when performing diaphyseal osteotomies or proximal osteotomies with rotational components. For mild deformities with an altered DMAA, the authors utilize biplanar Chevron osteotomies, removing generally a wedge of 2 mm in order to correct the DMAA. As the authors' scarf is a rotational one and the POSCOW osteotomy includes rotation as a way to improve their correction power, they limit their use to normal DMAA values. As an example, when a hallux valgus with an angle to be corrected of 12° also is combined with an altered DMAA (greater than 6°), a consideration to add a distal metatarsal osteotomy to the proximal osteotomy is taken. The final decision is taken intraoperatively.

Metatarsalgia

When considering metatarsalgia over the lesser metatarsal bones, if present, the authors generally do not rely on the power of the first metatarsal osteotomy to normalize the first metatarsal function which should, at least theoretically, regain its push off power and unload the lesser metatarsal heads and thus relieve pain. If pain is present the authors consider that there is some damage to the plantar plate of the corresponding metatarsal head, and they add a modified Weil osteotomy to elevate the metatarsal head. Having said this, they strive to add a plantar displacement effect over the first metatarsal after whichever technique was chosen, i.e. on the rotational scarf or on the POSCOW or with the Lapidus. For the scarf osteotomy, the authors perform the osteotomy cuts in a slight cephalocaudal direction in order to produce a plantar displacement of the bone when displacing it laterally. For the POSCOW osteotomy they remove a thin wafer of bone from the plantar aspect of the osteotomy, and for the Lapidus, they plantarly displace the metatarsal base 3–4 mm in relation to the medial cuneiform.

In summary, the surgical technique chosen can be modified by any of the previously mentioned factors. The authors' most commonly performed procedures in young and healthy patients are the Chevron, rotational scarf and POSCOW osteotomy.

MILD DEFORMITIES: DISTAL CHEVRON OSTEOTOMY

These osteotomies are inherently displacement osteotomies, and as such, they are limited by the width of the metatarsal bone. Classically, 5 mm of lateral displacement for this osteotomy has been performed, and it is well known that it corrects 1° of intermetatarsal angle (IMTA) per mm of lateral displacement. Increasing the angle between the arms of the osteotomy has been suggested as a way to increase compressive forces between the fragments, and therefore increase mechanical bonding.[15] The 90° Chevron is currently the authors' choice when performing a Chevron osteotomy for mild deformities when the angle to be corrected is 5° or less (Fig. 1). Another advantage of this modification is that it gives more room for fixation, a 2.0 minifragment screw is used in preference to a pin, and does not require later removal.

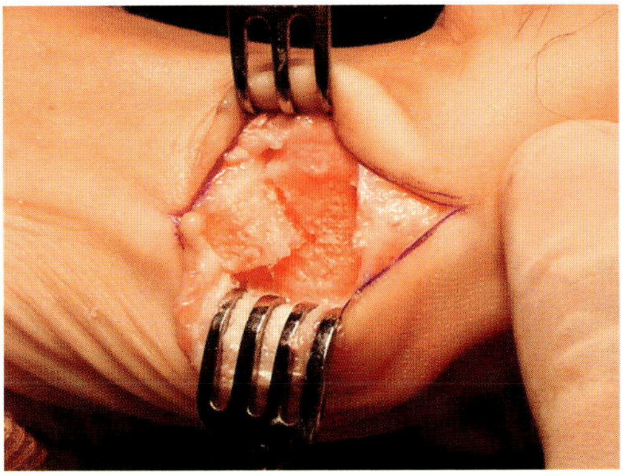

Fig. 1: A typical Chevron osteotomy is shown. The osteotomy is fixed with a 2.0 minifragment screw

MODERATE DEFORMITIES

Diaphyseal Scarf Osteotomy

The most well-known diaphyseal displacement osteotomy is the scarf osteotomy, which has been well described in the literature.[16,17] Its major theoretical advantage compared to a distal Chevron osteotomy is a bigger area of bone contact,[18] which allows a greater displacement, therefore achieving a better correction of the deformity. It can correct up to 6° of intermetatarsal angle, limited by the width of the metatarsal bone.[19] Modifications such as short straight osteotomy arms instead of a 60° inclination apparently reduce the risk of troughing, a complication which occurs 35% of the time.[17] Regarding fixation, classically a two point fixation has been recommended, using Barouk cannulated or minifragment screws.[20] Structural failures are most commonly seen at the most proximal fixation site, i.e. the proximal screw where the osteotomy runs longitudinally from plantar proximal to distal dorsal.[21] To avoid this type of failure, care has to be taken in order to leave as thick as possible a dorsal shelf of bone at the proximal apex of the osteotomy.

Rotational Scarf

In an effort to improve the correction power of the scarf osteotomy, rotation was added to it, using two of the more commonly used concepts in osteotomy execution, displacement and rotation. Described in 1992, the rotational scarf uses rotation in relation to the most proximal lateral aspect of the metatarsal bone, keeping the general shape of the scarf osteotomy. This maintains a broad bone contact between the fragments. In this way, better angular corrections with more than 50% of lateralization of the distal fragment can be achieved keeping at least 50% bone contact.[22] Recent clinical articles suggest that the rotational scarf decreases the risk of troughing[23] and the need of an Akin osteotomy.[24] The literature, however, does not actually confirm this statement, as the rotational component is not consistent in the various articles.

Geometrically it has been shown that the rotational scarf osteotomy can achieve correction through a proximal center of rotation, and has the power of correcting up to 9° of intermetatarsal angle maintaining bone contact in 50%.[6] The authors currently prefer three points of fixation; i.e., three screws as this theoretically should decrease the failure rate noted which they have seen when fixing with just two screws.

Surgical Technique

A medial longitudinal incision over the first metatarsophalangeal joint is performed. An inverted "L" capsulotomy is performed, exposing the metatarsal bone. The first metatarsal is exposed and dissected subperiosteally, leaving the lateral and plantar distal area intact to preserve circulation. A diaphyseal osteotomy is performed, starting from plantar proximal to distal dorsal, with two arms oriented 90° to the main osteotomy line exiting through the plantar and dorsal cortex correspondingly. The proximal extent of the osteotomy has to be done with care, as enough dorsal bone has to be left when performing the diaphyseal cut. Soft tissue protectors have to be used in the plantar side of the skin as in this area the saw blade might damage the skin. The osteotomy is performed as long as possible, normally measuring 4 cm in length (Fig. 2). Then, a translation and rotation around a proximally situated center of rotation is performed, leaving approximately two thirds of the width of the bone in contact proximally and one third of contact between the two fragments distally, which corresponds approximately to 4 mm of displacement proximally and 11 mm of displacement distally (Fig. 3). This amount of displacement, as it is unequal in both bone ends, will produce a lateral displacement and a rotation of the distal fragment, achieving a correction of approximately 8–9° of intermetatarsal angle. The authors have observed that when treating deformities close to the maximum correction capacity of this technique, due to small intraoperative changes,

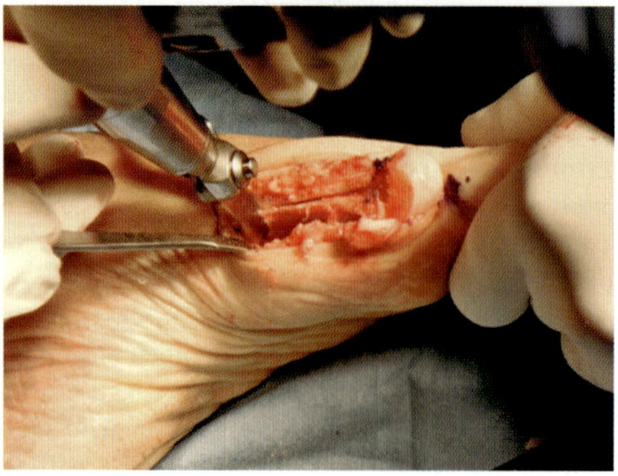

Fig. 2: Intraoperative photograph of a rotational scarf osteotomy. Note the length of the osteotomy, with vertical arms distally and proximally. Care has to be taken when performing the proximal vertical arm, as in this area skin damage may occur

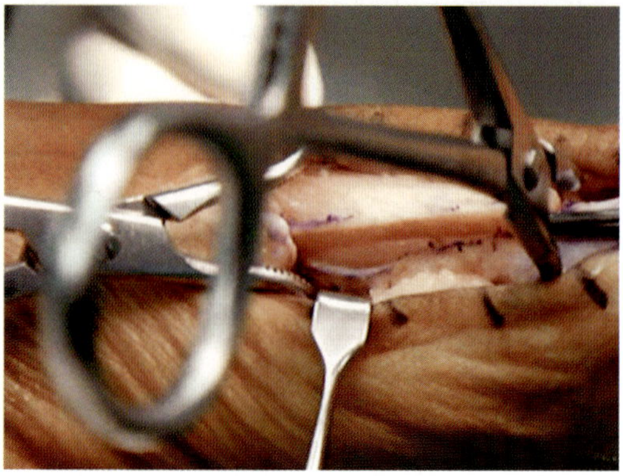

Fig. 3: Intraoperative photograph of a rotational scarf osteotomy where the displacement is shown. The plantar fragment is laterally displaced

internal fixation and postoperative bone remodeling, a higher displacement is needed to achieve an adequate correction, and in these cases the authors currently displace distally near to 90% of the width of the metatarsal head, and proximally 30% of the width of the metatarsal base. Both fragments are held temporally with a K-wire and a bone clamp and fixed with three 2.0-mm screws. The authors use three 2.0-mm screws from the compact foot set (Synthes, Switzerland), from the dorsal to the plantar aspect of the bone, unevenly spaced from proximal to distal (Fig. 4). The overhanging bone is resected, and a traditional closure of the periosteum and capsule is performed. Depending on the metatarsophalangeal balance after the metatarsal correction, a decision is made regarding the need of performing an Akin osteotomy (Figs 5 and 6). The subcutaneous and skin layers are closed with reabsorbable sutures. A postoperative dressing is applied, and a postoperative shoe is used.

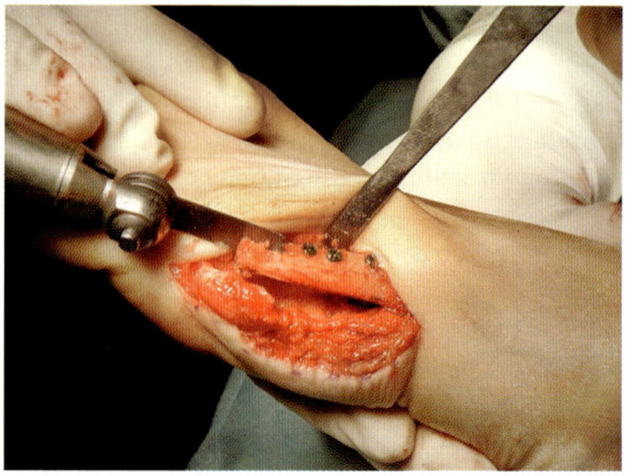

Fig. 4: Fixation of a rotational scarf osteotomy with three 2.0 mm screws. The medial overhanging bone is resected

SEVERE DEFORMITIES

Proximal Osteotomies and Opening Wedge with Current Specialized Plates

The basilar opening wedge was described in 1923, but difficulty with fixation and potential nonunions limited its popularity.[25] This osteotomy corrects the intermetatarsal angle through lateral rotation of the metatarsal bone with the addition of medial wedges of different sizes. It can lengthen the bone and increase the distal metatarsal articular angle as all the correction is achieved through angular correction without displacement. This lengthening may not be beneficial as it may distract soft tissues around the MTP joint, making joint reduction more difficult and possibly creating postoperative pain. New fixation options have appeared in the last few years. A medical locking plate is effective fixation, and compares favorably with Ludloff constructs, at least in initial cyclic loading in a cadaveric study.[26] Clinical outcomes show excellent results, with hallux valgus angle improvements of 14.7° and intermetatarsal angle improvement

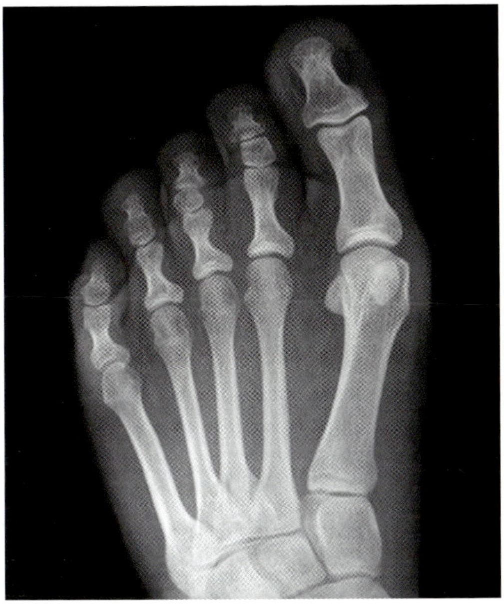

Fig. 5: Preoperative X-ray of a patient with hallux valgus deformity with an angle to be corrected of 8°

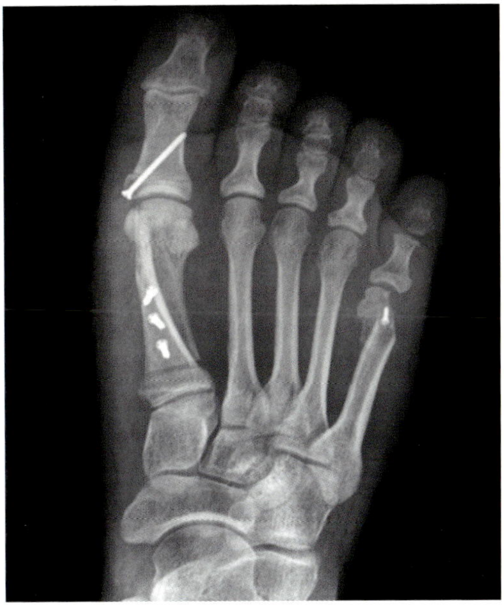

Fig. 6: Postoperative X-ray of the same patient shown in Figure 5. A rotational scarf osteotomy and an Akin osteotomy were performed. Also a bunionette was corrected. Note the differential displacement of the scarf osteotomy proximal versus distal. A greater displacement is done distally than proximally, achieving a rotational effect

of 6.4°. The mean increase in metatarsal length was 2.3 mm, which could not be associated to any symptom related to tightening of soft tissues such as decreased MTP range of motion[27] or predisposition to jamming of the metatarsophalangeal joint.[28]

Efforts to improve its correction power have been essentially increasing the medial wedge without violating the integrity of the lateral cortex. A linear relation appears to exist between the size of the medial wedge and the correction achieved, with a maximum using the 6 mm opening wedge plate.[28] The largest correction of intermetatarsal angle published is 10° and concern still remains regarding the possible effect of the MTP pressure.[27-29]

Proximal Oblique Slide Closing Wedge (POSCOW) Osteotomy

In an effort to combine the advantage of proximal displacement osteotomies with the maintenance of length without altering the distal metatarsal articular angle, and the correction power of angular osteotomies, a modification of a closing wedge technique was designed and named a proximal oblique sliding closing wedge osteotomy (POSCOW).[30] The authors' first cases were fixed with dorsal mini fragment plates, and over the last years they changed to mini fragment locked medial plates. Using medial fixation improves the stiffness of the construct over dorsal plates by 158% if using titanium locked plates and 228% when using steel nonlocked plates (JSOA, in press). Geometrically, it was determined that a lateral proximal displacement of 5 mm would correct 4° of intermetatarsal angle, and that for 1° of additional intermetatarsal angle correction, a bone wedge with a lateral base of 0.4 mm had to be resected. As the osteotomy is performed perpendicular in both planes (transverse and sagittal) to the metatarsal bone, its plane is oblique in relation to the second metatarsal bone, going proximal medial to lateral distal. Thus, with the lateral displacement, a slight lengthening of the bone is achieved. This lengthening will partially compensate for the expected shortening any closing wedge osteotomy produces.

Surgical Technique

A medial longitudinal incision over the first metatarsophalangeal joint is performed. An inverted "L" capsulotomy is performed, exposing the MTP joint. The first metatarsal is exposed and dissected subperiosteally, leaving the lateral and plantar distal

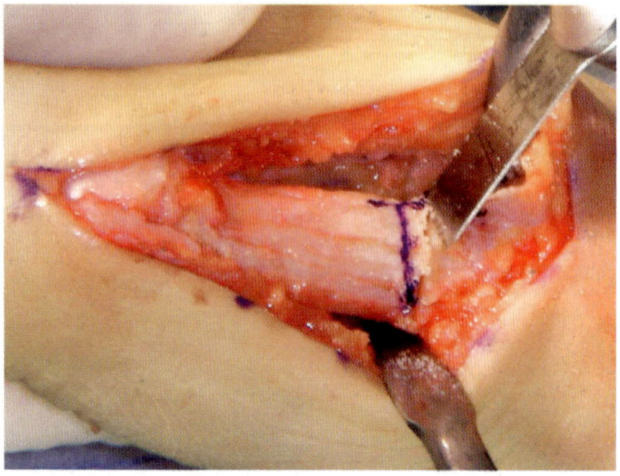

Fig. 7: Intraoperative photograph of a POSCOW osteotomy. A vertical osteotomy is performed, 15 mm distal to the cuneiform-metatarsal joint. Depending on the preoperative planning, a lateral base wedge is resected thereby achieving a complete correction of the intermetatarsal deformity

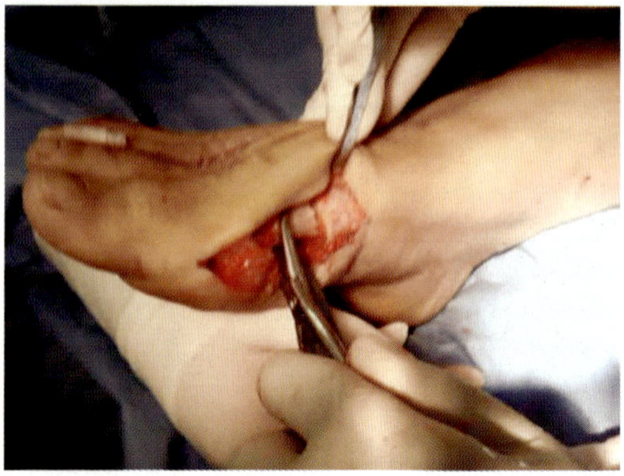

Fig. 8: The lateral displacement of the distal fragment of the metatarsal bone after performing a POSCOW osteotomy is shown. Up to 5 mm of lateral displacement can be achieved with a bone clamp, fixing it temporarily with two K-wires until definitive fixation is achieved

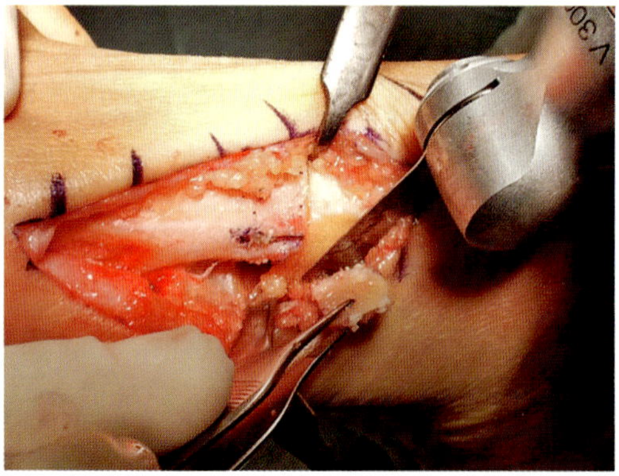

Fig. 9: The overhanging bone of the base of the metatarsal bone, left after lateral displacement of the metatarsal is resected with a saw. This helps to create a flat surface where to apply the definitive plate

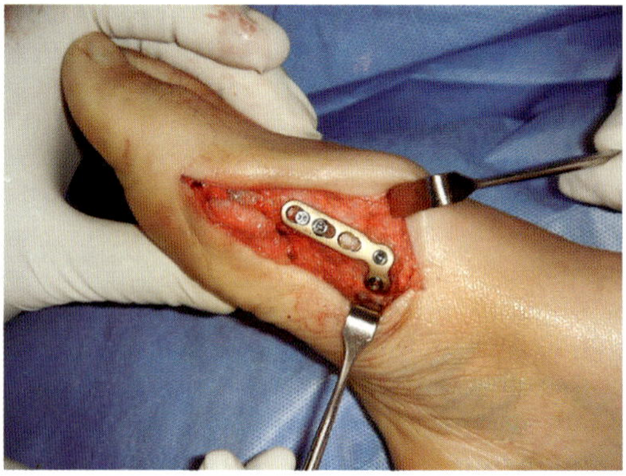

Fig. 10: Definitive locked plate is shown, applied over the medial surface of the metatarsal bone. Two locked screws are used in the distal and proximal aspects of the plate respectively

area intact to preserve circulation. A careful resection of the bunion is performed following the medial cortex of the metatarsal bone. Then a proximal metatarsal osteotomy is performed, with a straight cut from the dorsal to the plantar aspect of the metatarsal bone 15 mm distal to the base of the bone and perpendicular to the long axis of the metatarsal bone. Depending on the angular correction needed, a laterally-based wedge of bone is removed from the proximal aspect of the distal fragment as determined in the preoperative planning (Fig. 7). A lateral displacement of 5 mm is performed, moving laterally the base of the metatarsal bone (Fig. 8). The prominent bone of the base of the metatarsal is removed (Fig. 9) and fixation is performed with a medially placed angular stable plate with two locking screws distally and two locked screws proximally (Fig. 10). Radiographs are taken at this moment to ensure that parallelism is achieved between the first and second metatarsal bones. Depending on the metatarsophalangeal balance after the metatarsal correction, a decision is made regarding the need of performing an Akin osteotomy. The capsule, subcutaneous and skin layers are closed with reabsorbable sutures. A postoperative dressing is applied, and a postoperative shoe is used. Preoperative and postoperative X-rays of a POSCOW osteotomy are shown in Figures 11 and 12.

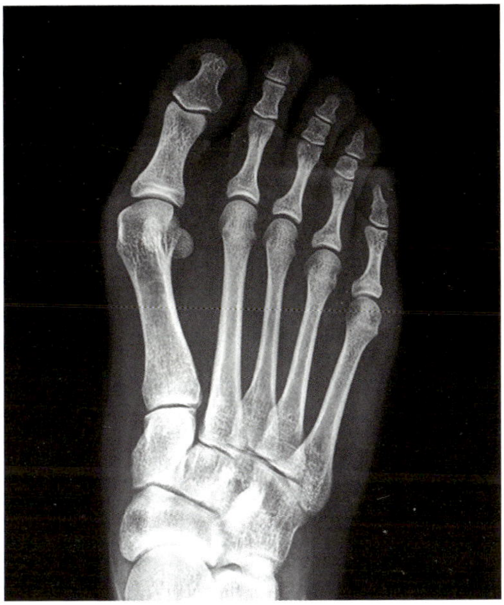

Fig. 11: Preoperative X-ray of a patient with hallux valgus deformity showing an angle to be corrected over 10°

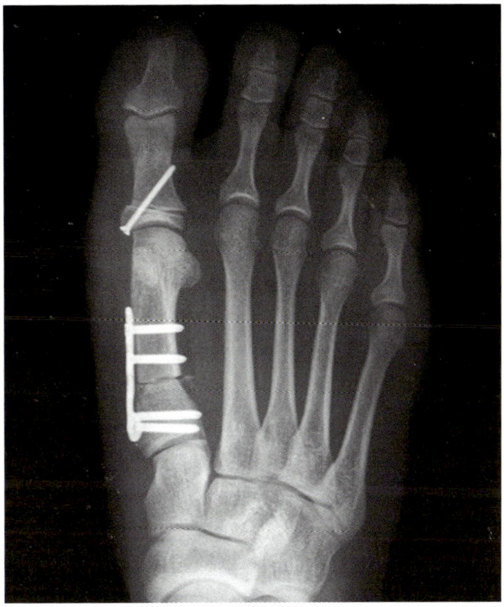

Fig. 12: Postoperative X-ray showing a POSCOW osteotomy and an Akin osteotomy performed on the patient shown in Figure 9. Complete axial correction is achieved

POSTOPERATIVE CARE

Stitches and dressing are normally removed at about 2 weeks. The authors keep patients in a postoperative shoe, weightbearing as tolerated, and they are usually able to go back to restricted normal activities after 1 month depending on the chosen surgical technique; the Chevron heals in 4–6 weeks, while the POSCOW takes from 6–8 weeks.

COMPLICATIONS

The complication rate in hallux valgus surgery ranges from 10% to 55%[31] and include recurrence (the most common one), hallux varus, arthritis, avascular necrosis, skin sloughs, infection, etc.

Commonly, neuropathic pain can be present around the area of inflammation. These neuropathic problems are diminished with careful surgical technique including the use of surgical loupes and if they occur, they are self-limited and easily treated with physical therapy and topical pain relievers.

The authors' experience with wound sloughs in hallux valgus surgery has been that most of these patients have self-limited skin problems that in rare cases require more than 8 weeks of local wound care to resolve. Very infrequently do they need surgical debridement or soft tissue covering procedures.

Hallux varus is rare after Chevron or scarf osteotomies; it is more common after proximal osteotomies. If there is a negative intermetatarsal angle, it must be corrected by redoing the initial osteotomy or performing a simpler one like a reverse Chevron. If the intermetatarsal angle is neutral, a soft tissue procedure alone could be attempted as has been recommended by Myerson. The extensor hallucis brevis is detached distally, rerouted under the intermetatarsal ligament, and fixed to the proximal phalanx under proper tension.

Recurrence is the most common significant complication. Many factors need to be considered when evaluating a recurrent hallux valgus deformity. Recurrence after certain procedures can be generated by the surgery itself (extensive soft tissue scarring), by the patient (not following general recommendations) and when hallux valgus component factors are not fully addressed. As a general rule, we face this complication by choosing the procedure we would have chosen primarily after calculating the angle to be corrected. Patients treated with a Chevron osteotomy for a larger than expected deformity can be treated with a Scarf osteotomy, if the angle to be corrected indicates that the technique will have the power enough. If the recurrence is partial, and mainly due to metatarsophalangeal imbalance, we can correct it just with an Akin osteotomy.

SUMMARY

The goal of hallux valgus surgery is to correct a painful deformity and recover a functional foot able to go back to normal shoe wear. Since the most common significant complication after surgical treatment is recurrence, a strict protocol is recommended to decrease the incidence of this complication. The authors recommend using the "angle to be corrected" to choose the best surgical procedure. The best surgical treatment will be the one which achieves the best result with the simplest procedure which will be rediable over time. One has to consider that hallux valgus is a deformity which results from many different factors, some of them still unknown, and every effort should be made to correct all components of the deformity. If distal or diaphyseal osteotomies are not enough, more powerful corrective techniques such as the proximal osteotomies and arthrodesis must be chosen. With this strategy in mind, patients will be offered the best surgical treatment with the least complication rate possible.

REFERENCES

1. Nix S, Smith M, Vicenzino B. Prevalence of hallux valgus in the general population: a systematic review and metaanalysis. Journal of Foot and Ankle Research. 2010;3:21.
2. Perera AM, Mason L, Stephens MM. Current Concepts Review. The pathogenesis of hallux valgus. Bone Joint Surg Am. 2011;93:1650-61.
3. Coughlin MJ, Jones CP. Hallux valgus and first ray mobility: a prospective study. J Bone Joint Surg Am. 2007;89(9):1887-98.
4. Tanaka Y, Takakura Y. Precise anatomic configuration changes in the first ray of the hallux valgus foot. Foot Ankle Int. 2000;21:651-6.
5. Okuda R, Kinoshita M, Yasuda T, et al. Postoperative incomplete reduction of the sesamoids as a risk factor for recurrence of hallux valgus. J Bone Joint Surg Am. 2009;91(7):1637-45.
6. Wagner E, Ortiz C, Keller A. Modified diaphyseal osteotomy with a proximal center of rotation for moderate to severe hallux valgus. Techniques in Foot and Ankle Surgery. 2007;6(2):113-7.
7. Wagner E, Ortiz C. Osteotomy considerations in hallux valgus treatment: improving the correction power. Foot Ankle Clin. 2012;17(3):481-98.
8. Sanders M, Hagemeire K. Conservative treatment and shoewear options for hallux valgus. Foot Ankle Clin. 1997;2(4):639-53.
9. Trnka HJ. Osteotomies for hallux valgus correction. Foot Ankle Clin. 2005;10(1):15-33.
10. Maffulli N, Longo UG, Marinozzi A, et al. Hallux valgus: effectiveness and safety of minimally invasive surgery: a systematic review. Br Med Bull. 2011;97:149-6.
11. Smith B, Coughlin M. Treatment of hallux valgus with increased distal metatarsal articular angle: use of double and triple osteotomies. Foot Ankle Clin N Am. 2009; 14:369-82.
12. Coughlin MJ, Freund E. The reliability of angular measurements in hallux valgus deformities. Foot Ankle Int. 2001;22(5):369-79.
13. Davids JR, McBrayer D, Blackhurst DW. Juvenile hallux valgus deformity: surgical management by lateral hemiepiphyseodesis of the great toe metatarsal. J Pediatr Orthop. 2007;27(7):826-30.
14. John S, Weil L Jr, Weil LS Sr, et al. Scarf osteotomy for the correction of adolescent hallux valgus. Foot Ankle Spec. 2010;3(1):10-4.
15. Matzaroglou C, Bougas P, Panagiotopoulos E, et al. Ninety-degree Chevron osteotomy for correction of hallux valgus deformity: clinical data and finite element analysis. Open Orthop J. 2010;22(4):152-6.
16. Barouk LS. Scarf osteotomy for hallux valgus correction. Local anatomy, surgical technique, and combination with other forefoot procedures. Foot Ankle Clin. 2000;5(1):525-58.
17. Coetzee JC, Rippstein P. Surgical strategies: scarf osteotomy for hallux valgus. Foot Ankle Int. 28(4): 529-35.
18. Vienne P, Favre P, Meyer D, et al. Comparative mechanical testing of different geometric designs of distal first metatarsal osteotomies. Foot Ankle Int. 2007;28(2):232-6.
19. Dereymaeker G. Scarf osteotomy for correction of hallux valgus. Surgical technique and results as compared to distal Chevron osteotomy. Foot Ankle Clinics. 2000;5(3):513-24.
20. Gupta S, Fazal MA, Williams L. Minifragment screw fixation of the scarf osteotomy. Foot Ankle Int. 2008;29(4):385-9.
21. Favre P, Farine M, Snedeker JG, et al. Biomechanical consequences of first metatarsal osteotomy in treating hallux valgus. Clinical Biomechanics. 2010; 25:721-7.
22. Duke HF. Rotational scarf (Z) osteotomybunionectomy for correction of high intermetatarsal angles. Journal Am Pod Med Assoc. 1992;82(7):352-60.

23. Murawski CD, Egan CJ, Kennedy JG. A rotational scarf osteotomy decreases troughing when treating hallux valgus. Clin Orthop Relat Res. 2011;469(3):847-53.
24. Adam SP, Choung SC, Gu Y, et al. Outcomes after scarf osteotomy for treatment of adult hallux valgus deformity. Clin Orthop Relat Res. 2011;469(3):854-9.
25. Easley ME, Trnka HJ. Current concepts review. Hallux valgus Part II:Operative treatment. Foot Ankle Int. 2007;28(6):748-58.
26. Hofstaetter SG, Glisson RR, Alitz CJ, et al. Biomechanical comparison of screws and plates for hallux valgus opening-wedge and Ludloff osteotomies. Clin Biomech. 2008;23(1):101-8.
27. Shurnas PS, Watson TS, Crislip TW. Proximal first metatarsal opening wedge osteotomy with a low profile plate. Foot Ankle Int. 2009;30(9):865-72.
28. Saragas NP. Proximal opening-wedge osteotomy of the first metatarsal for hallux valgus using a low profile plate. Foot Ankle Int. 2009;30(10):976-80.
29. Smith WB, Hyer CF, DeCarbo WT, et al. Opening wedge osteotomies for correction of hallux valgus: a review of wedge plate fixation. Foot Ankle Spec. 2009; 2:277-82.
30. Wagner E, Ortiz C, Keller A. Proximal oblique slide closing wedge metatarsal osteotomy with plate fixation for severe hallux valgus deformities. Techniques Foot Ankle Surg. 2007;6(4):270-4.
31. Duan X, Kadakia AR. Salvage of recurrence after failed surgical treatment of hallux valgus. Arch Orthop Trauma Surg. 2012;132:477-85.

13 Hallux Rigidus and Arthritis of the First Metatarsophalangeal Joint

John S Gould

INTRODUCTION

Hallux rigidus is basically "stiffness" of the metatarsophalangeal joint of the great toe. The etiology is usually unknown with the literature replete with theories related to the length, shape and position of the first metatarsal. In some cases, there may be a traumatic origin, often related to a hyperextension injury of the joint ("turf toe") experienced particularly by athletes.[1]

The condition is classified by three types: Type 1 characterized by lack of dorsiflexion with dorsal spurring of the joint and first noted during adolescence; Type 2 has lack of dorsiflexion without apparent spur formation; Type 3 demonstrates generalized arthritis. Type 1 is the classic entity, is clearly a developmental condition which typifies the designation, "hallux rigidus". Type 2 may be developmental, but seems to be a form of arthrofibrosis, more likely related to a ligamentous injury to the joint. Type 3 may be of primary origin, traumatic, or associated with misalignments such as hallux valgus. It is really a separate entity and, surgically, should be treated as such.

Pain is frequently associated with the condition and is what usually causes the patient to seek medical care. In Type 1, the dorsal spur is frequently visible as a bulge under the skin with erythema and tenderness at the site (Fig. 1). In Type 3, the swelling and redness may be all around the joint and there may be aching at rest. Associated compensatory hyperextension may be noted at the interphalangeal joint. In addition to the loss of motion range in the joint, pain may be elicited in Type 1 with attempts to "plantar flex" the joint passively. To differentiate Types 1 and 3, pushing the joint surfaces together with the "grind test" should not elicit pain to any great extent in neutral or slight plantar flexion in Type 1 with increased pain in the dorsiflexed position. In Type 3, the "grind test" is positive in all positions of the joint. In Type 2, other than lack of motion, the "grind test", when positive, suggests joint surface damage.[2]

Plain X-rays of the metatarsophalangeal joint in the anteroposterior (AP) and lateral positions should further clarify the extent of the disease (Fig. 2). Sesamoid views are important to determine if there

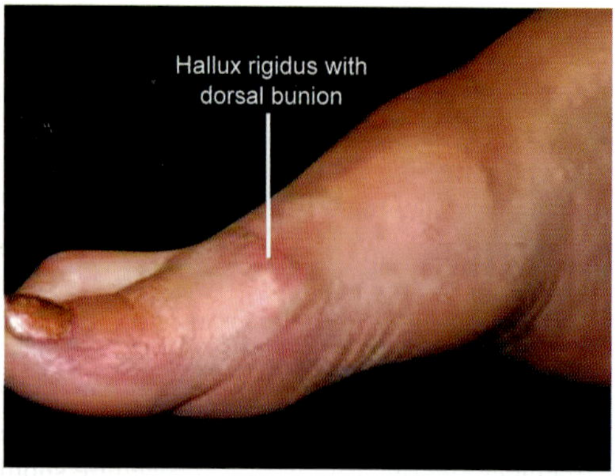

Fig. 1: Hallux rigidus with bony prominence visible at the joint

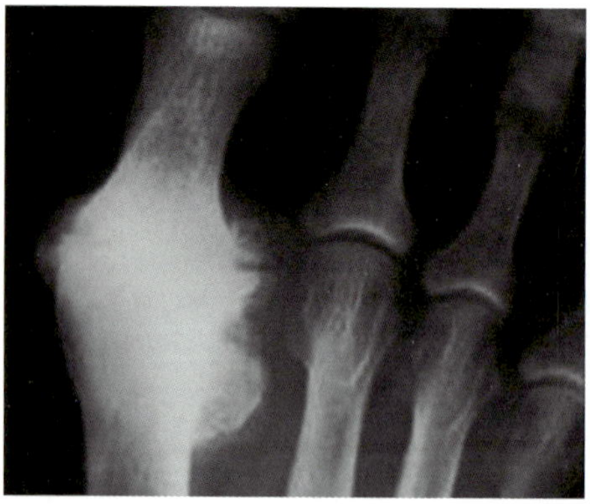

Fig. 2: Extensive arthritic changes are noted in Type 3 hallux rigidus

is disease between these structures and the overlying metatarsal surface. A computed tomography (CT) scan of the great toe joint has a place in subtle cases and in potential surgical reconstructive decisions.

With the history not suggestive of systemic disease and the physical findings, and X-ray compatible with a localized process, further diagnostic testing is not indicated. When multiple metatarsophalangeal (MTP) joints are involved, further testing particularly for collagen disorders is indicated. The great toe MTP joint, alone, can be the site of an acute gouty attack, but without a personal, or family history, evidence of tophi, gouty crystals, and periarticular erosions on X-ray; and with typical dorsal spurring, or changes of osteoarthritis, gout or pseudogout are very unlikely. It is not unusual, however, to have patients referred with typical hallux rigidus who have already undergone medical therapy for these crystalline deposit conditions without proper supporting evidence.

CONSERVATIVE MANAGEMENT

The decision to treat a patient conservatively is essentially based on patient preference and functional needs, as well as proper expectations from surgical intervention. Functional incapacity also includes the type of shoewear the patient uses or wishes to use, the extent of incapacity, and a thorough knowledge of what a conservative approach can realistically be expected to provide as well.

Short-term care with an oral anti-inflammatory medication and/or the use of a topical anti-inflammatory agent can be helpful in acute flare situations, but does not usually provide a satisfactory solution alone for the long term. Splinting of the joint can be accomplished in several ways: a stiff rocker sole available in running or walking shoes; the addition of such by a pedorthist or shoemaker on a standard shoe; the insertion of a rigid but flexible extended steel or carbon fiber shank placed between the out and midsole of a shoe (Fig. 3), loose under the sock liner or insert for a shoe; or built into a shoe insert (orthotic device). A variation of this approach, when only the great toe is involved as opposed to multiple MTP joint disease, is to use a "Morton's extension" where an extended steel or carbon fiber shank is narrowed just proximal to the MTP joints to continue distally just under the great toe. This allows some flexibility in the other toes with toe off. However, the key to using these stiffening devices and approaches is to have a forward rocker sole on the shoe. Without it, the toes will attend to extend with toe off with resultant pain and walking is clumsy (as noted when one attempts to walk with cycling shoes or downhill ski boots). In fact, the forward rocker sole design, alone, can be helpful in some patients without using a stiffening maneuver as well. The author typically starts patients who have opted for this approach with over-the-counter stiff sole rocker sole walking shoes and the use of a topical anti-inflammatory. Other modifications can be used for dress shoes. In fact, there are "faux" high heel shoes, a type of wedge, which some women find satisfactory for more formal wear.

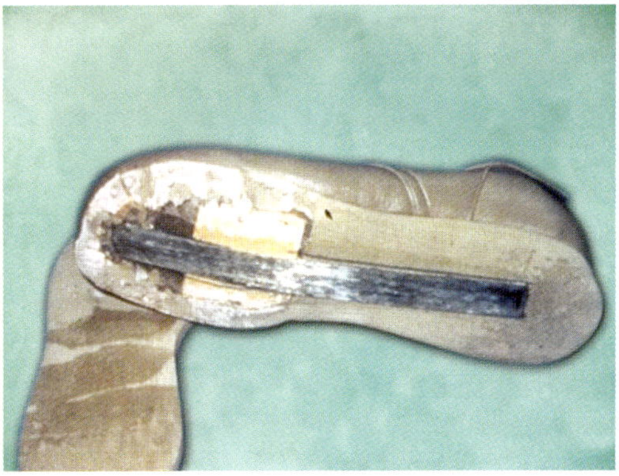

Fig. 3: Steel shank applied between mid and out sole of shoe

SURGICAL APPROACHES

The extent of the disease determines, for the most part, the appropriate options for surgical intervention. The patient's complaints and functional issues are also factors which weigh in the decision.

Type 1 Disease

Although it may have been determined that only the dorsal part of the joint is involved, in middle age patients and in the course of the procedure, one may find that the disease is more extensive. The CT scan can be helpful, but even with this and an MRI, denuded areas of cartilage in the plantar aspects of the joint may be found. The extent of the disease will affect the ultimate outcome. It is agreed in the literature that the procedure of choice is a "cheilectomy".[2,3] However, there is no agreement on how extensive the procedure should be or anticipated outcomes.

Cheilectomy

The author's standard approach for a cheilectomy is through a medial sagittal incision which allows adequate exposure for removal of dorsal and even lateral osteophytes and improved visualization of the plantar aspects of the joint. It also avoids the dorsal capsule damage to and scarring around the medial cutaneous nerve of the foot (branch of the superficial peroneal) which can be a source of postoperative pain or hypersensitivity. Finally, by not disturbing the extensor hallucis longus, one avoids postoperative scarring or adherence with loss of motion.

The medial eminence is removed with a microsagittal saw along with the dorsal osteophyte (Fig. 4). If the incision medially is taken to the midpoint of the length of the first metatarsal and distally to just proximal to the interphalangeal joint, the exposure is adequate for removal of the lateral spurring from the metatarsal with a curved rongeur and from around the base of the proximal phalanx, if needed. The question is: "how much of the metatarsal head should be removed?" As a rule of thumb, one typically takes the upper third of the joint. The cut is beveled proximally. If there is a loss of cartilage a little more plantar, the osteotomy may be carried more plantar to include this area; otherwise, drilling with a small pin (e.g. 0.062) of areas denuded of cartilage is done along with a synovectomy. In older patients, erosion on the medial sesamoid is often found and is easily visualized. The lateral sesamoid is a bit harder to see, but is less often involved. A freer is used under the plantar metatarsal to clear adhesions and strip the proximal end of the plantar plate to allow more dorsiflexion. One hopes to achieve at least 75° of passive dorsiflexion with the procedure. The capsule is then repaired with size 0 dissolving suture. If the periosteum continuity to the capsule is disrupted, which the author tries to avoid, it is reattached with small bone anchors. A bulky dressing is applied postoperatively and the patient allowed to weight bear as tolerated in a postoperative wedge bunion shoe. Sutures are removed at two weeks and the patient mobilized with active assistive range of motion exercises. Physical therapy may be enlisted to assist with this in selected patients. Dynamic splinting is also an option.

An alternative approach is to do the procedure arthroscopically with portals on either side of the extensor hallucis and using a 1.9-mm arthroscope and small shaver.[4] Plantar visibility is poor and it is difficult to improve passive range of motion beyond what is achieved with removal of the dorsal spur. A plantar portal carries the risk of damage to neurovascular structures. The author has little experience with this method beyond the laboratory.

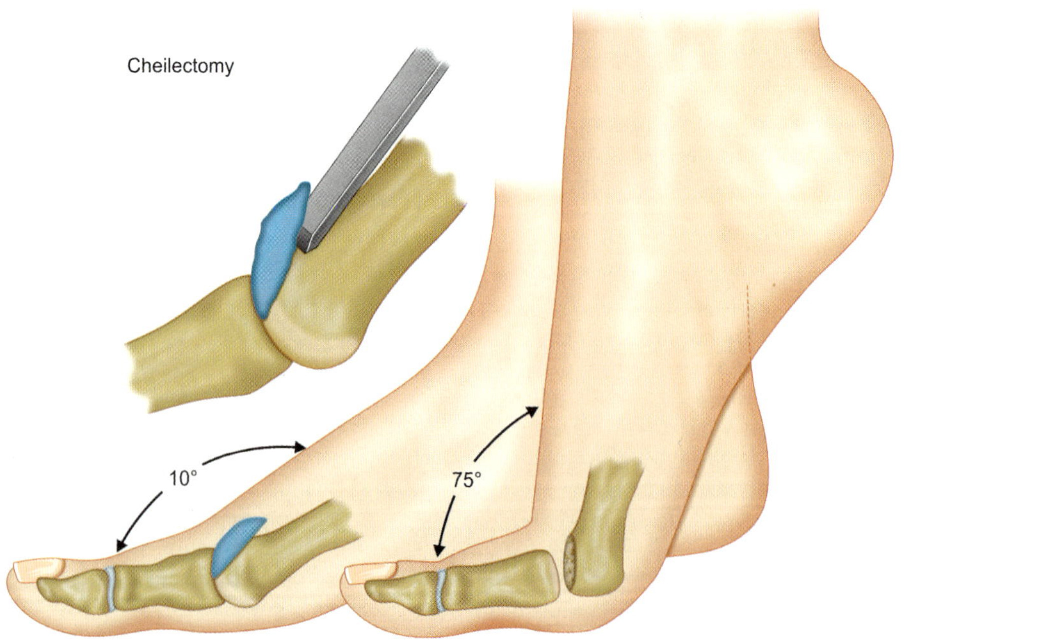

Fig. 4: Cheilectomy for hallux rigidus

The reports on outcomes with "cheilectomy" are all favorable for significant pain relief, particularly when the dorsal osteophyte alone is the main finding. Improvement is achieved for up to 1 year postoperative. Range-of-motion improvement has various outcomes with the best outcomes occurring with less disease. With minimal disease, dorsal osteophyte primarily, the durability of the outcome appears also to be longstanding. The arthroscopic approach may therefore be applicable in such cases of less disease as in younger patients. It is worthy to note, however, that even when there has been more extensive disease which required microfracture, a significant degree of pain relief was achieved, although the gain in motion ultimately was minimal, in the author's experience. Consequently, it is very important to know what the goal of the procedure is in selecting the procedure of choice. *If pain relief without concern for the amount of motion gained is the goal, simple cheilectomy may be sufficient.*[2,3]

Alternative Procedures in Type 1 and 2 Diseases

Functional improvement in dorsiflexion can be achieved with a dorsally based osteotomy of the base of the proximal phalanx at the time of the cheilectomy (Fig. 5). The "Moberg osteotomy"[5] has been advocated in various case reports as a useful adjunct which moves the arc of motion of the joint to a more dorsal starting point without significant net increase in range, other than that gained by the cheilectomy. The author's experience with the technique is limited but favorable. The procedure seems to have a place when passive range gain is limited after the cheilectomy. Type 2 disease may be a primary indication. Less motion after joint debridement is typically achieved in these cases. The procedure is done with a microsagittal saw and fixation with one or two 0.062" or 0.045" (1.4 or 1.6 mm) K-wires. Staples have been designed as well for this procedure (as well as for the medially based Akin osteotomy for hallux valgus interphalangeus) which require initially drilling through a template followed by insertion of a staple which also provides compression. When using such a device, it is ideal to have the staple tines cross the lateral cortex as well the medial and to place the staple above the dorsal/plantar midline to close the osteotomy. The advantage of the staple is that, unlike the pin(s), they do not require removal after healing.

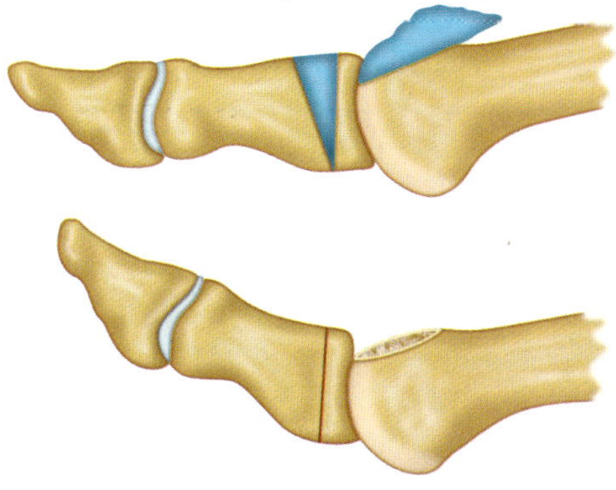

Fig. 5: The "Moberg osteotomy" added to the cheilectomy

Type 3 Disease

This is generalized arthritis of the joint and, when operated, requires a salvage procedure. On the occasional patient who is willing to chance the possibility/probability that further surgery may be needed and, in whom, increased motion is not required or particularly desired; a cheilectomy with microfracture may be a consideration. The options for stage 3 are: "arthrodesis" or "arthroplasty".

Arthrodesis

This procedure is the "gold standard", at this point in time, for stage 3 hallux rigidus. It provides pain relief, placing the joint in a fixed functional position and is a durable procedure. Many patients are already accustomed to minimal motion in the joint and pain relief is very welcome. In many patients, compensatory hyperextension of the interphalangeal joint has occurred and functional limitations are minimal. Some patients, particularly younger women, do not want loss of motion which would further limit shoe heel height options, and opt for an arthroplasty.

The surgical technique: The joint is approached through a medial sagittal incision from the midpoint of the first metatarsal to the interphalangeal joint. A subperiosteal dissection exposes the head of the metatarsal and base of the proximal phalanx. The medial approach rather than the dorsal is chosen to avoid damage or scarring around the medial cutaneous nerve and adherence postoperatively of the extensor hallucis longus which would limit interphalangeal joint motion, adding to the potential decreased function of the toe. A cone in cup preparation of the surfaces is provided with concave and convex reamers. The distal convex surface and the medial eminence are initially removed with a microsagittal saw prior to use of the cannulated

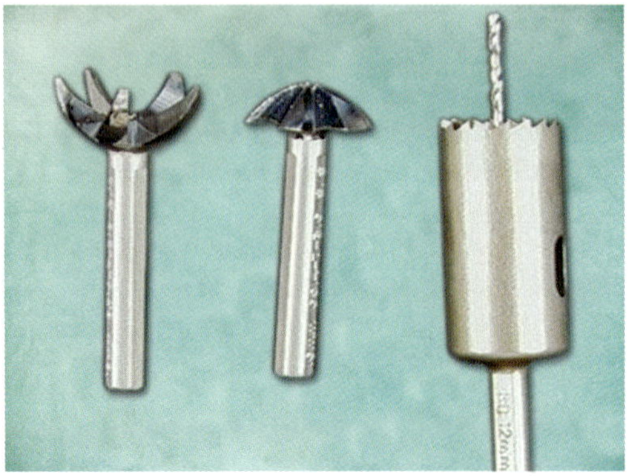

Fig. 6: Reamers used for arthrodesis

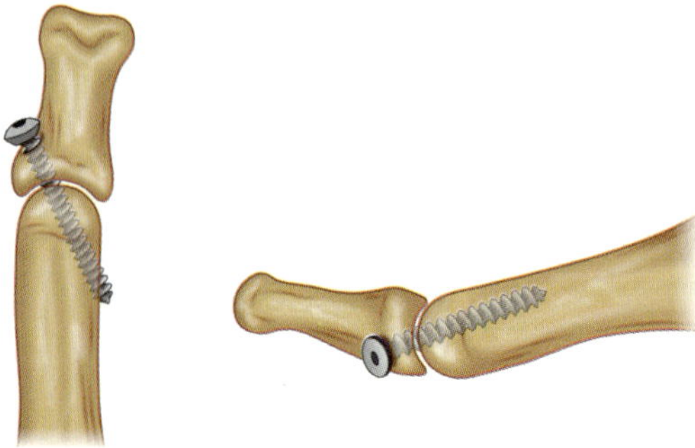

Fig. 7: Initial fixation with interfragmentary lag screw (artist rendition). Note that compression allows metatarsal head to invaginate within the proximal phalanx concave surface for maximal bone contact

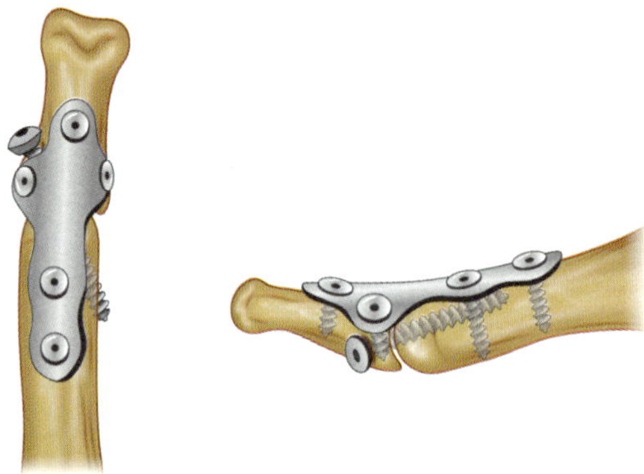

Fig. 8: Final fixation with neutralization plate

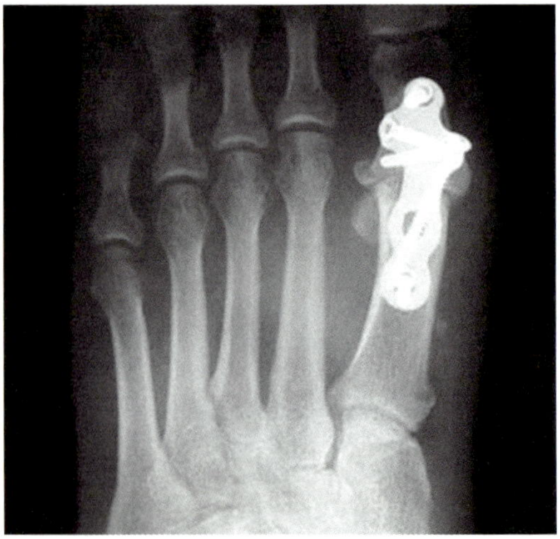

Fig. 9: X-ray of great toe arthrodesis

power reamers. Multiple companies now provide reamers and plates for this procedure (Fig. 6). Most surgeons place the joint in about 15° of dorsiflexion in neutral varus/valgus. The author uses a plate angled at 15° of dorsiflexion for reference and places a 1.6-mm fixation pin obliquely across the dorsal joint usually from distal medial to proximal lateral to hold the position (Plates are available at various angles: 0°, 10° and 15°). A fluoroscopy image is obtained to check the position of the pin (across all cortices) and the reduction of the cone in cup articulation. Adjustments can be made, if necessary, including redirection of the pin from proximal to distal. It is also essential to visualize the toe position clinically from dorsal and plantar aspects relative to the second toe and to check rotation by looking at the toe, end on. Finally, an equipment tray cover or other flat surface is placed on the plantar aspect of the foot to assure that the interphalangeal (IP) joint will allow the pad of the great toe to flex to this surface so that later the patient's toe will make contact with the floor.

At this point, the author uses a 3.5-mm cortical screw using lag technique for initial fixation, placing the screw plantar and parallel to the initial pin from distal to proximal (Fig. 7). This provides compression of the surfaces, and with the temporary pin still in place while this is done, maintains the desired joint positioning. Another half turn may be taken on the screw after this pin is removed. Both fluoroscopic and clinical assessment is again performed. A dorsal neutralization plate is then applied (Figs 8 and 9). An alternative technique using dorsal compression plating has been described, but the risk of loss of initial desired position with opening of the plantar aspect of bone contact is a risk with this approach. A bulky dressing is applied in the operating room. At 2 weeks, the sutures are removed and the patient allowed ambulating with the orthopedic wedge bunion shoe. Full mobilization is usually permitted at 6 weeks. Failure of fusion is rare and complications minimal with this approach. In unpublished data from the author's institution, 33/34 patients (97%) went onto primary fusion with this technique as compared to 18/22 (82%) with various other plate and screw techniques.

Arthroplasty

There are two basic arthroplasty types: "biologic" and "prosthetic". Of the "biologic", there are pure resection arthroplasties and resections with interposition of various biological materials ranging from capsule to tendon and fascia. Some materials are local, others from a more remote site. Allograft interpositional materials have also been used. Of the prosthetic arthroplasties, resurfacing of the metatarsal head alone, the base of the proximal phalanx alone, and both surfaces with articulated and nonarticulated designs have been described and are available commercially. Silicone, metal, metal hinge and metal polyethylene materials have all been used. When conducting a "hemiarthroplasty", minimal to no disease should be present on the opposing surface or it is insignificant enough for simple debridement. The goal of arthroplasty is to relieve pain and provide functional motion. The concern with arthroplasty techniques and devices has been failure to provide dependable pain relief, predictable range of motion, and durability of the device, as well as complications of subluxation or dislocation of the device and the effects on the host bone (e.g. silicone synovitis).[6] For these reasons, arthroplasty has not generally found much favor among orthopedic surgeons, although there are still advocates and new designs and techniques attempted. The desire to find an acceptable arthroplasty continues for a number of valid reasons: patients want the motion preserved or regained for more ease in crouching, tip toeing, and these requirements in various occupations; sports; and shoewear. Women, in particular, do not like a stiff great toe metatarsophalangeal (MTP) joint. In addition, patients with multiple joint stiffening diseases, such as rheumatoids, particularly need and desire motion where possible. When there is arthritis in adjacent, particularly in longitudinally adjacent joints, such as the interphalangeal (IP) and tarsometatarsal (TMT) joints, maintaining a mobile segment in this area is desirable for function. As neither the IP nor the TMT joints have an arthroplasty option, attention continues to focus on the MTP.

Resection and Interpositional Arthroplasties

Resection arthroplasty is the classic option to fusion for pain relief. The fundamental disadvantage of the procedure is that it disturbs the normal biomechanics of gait. In normal toe off, the first metatarsal head is pushed into a plantar position by the combined action of the plantar fascia, short flexors, and plantar plate with the intact fulcrum of the metatarsal and proximal phalanx. With this action, the first metatarsal assumes 50% of the weight with the lesser metatarsals sharing the remainder.[7] With loss of this mechanism, the weight shifts laterally with the majority borne by the more rigid 2nd and 3rd metatarsals. This results in transfer metatarsalgia, with a minimum of increased plantar callusing under the 2nd or 3rd or both metatarsal heads, plantar bursal formation, intermetatarsal neuritis, and possibly stress fractures. As normal biomechanics are also disturbed by loss of motion in the first metatarsophalangeal joint secondary to arthritis, in selected patients, including those with less demand, such as the elderly or those with collagen disorders, resection of the joint relieves pain without a significant loss of existing function. Loss of alignment of the joint with secondary varus/valgus, or even hyperextension, however, can be problematic.

Simple resection of the base of the proximal phalanx (the "Keller arthroplasty") (Figs 10A and B),[8] with or without temporary pinning for 6 weeks; or of the first metatarsal head (the "Mayo arthroplasty")[9] is still practiced in the low demand patient and in the rheumatoid. Various modifications of the basic technique attempt to stabilize the joint in an attempt to prevent malalignment. A technique in which the base of the proximal phalanx is preserved while resecting the rest of the surface obliquely from distal dorsal to plantar proximal and using interpositional tendon has gained some favor in an attempt to also preserve the fulcrum of the joint and resultant biomechanical action.[10]

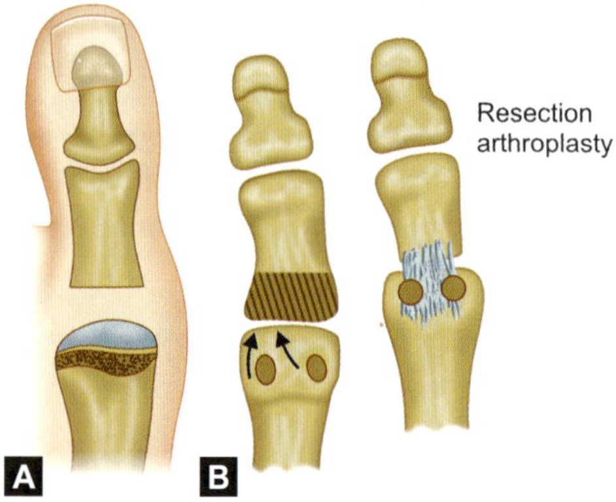

Figs 10A and B: (A) Simple resection of the base of the proximal phalanx; (B) A modified Keller with reattachment of the plantar plate

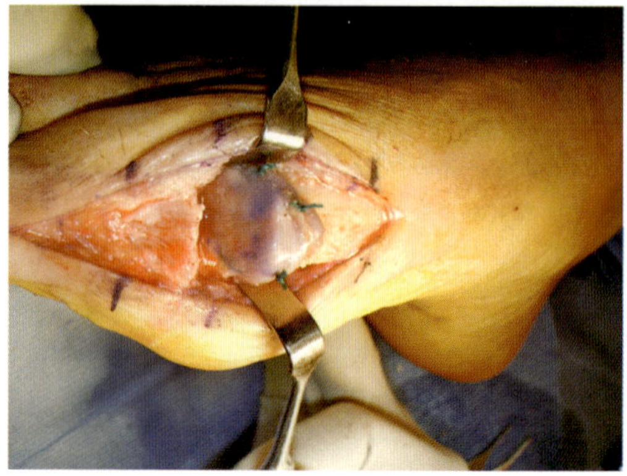

Fig. 11: Myofascia applied to the debrided and shaped metatarsal head type of interpositional arthroplasty

Biological interpositional arthroplasty has also been an attempt to add stability, and, in some cases, maintain the fulcrum. Infolded medial capsule and dorsal extensor hallucis brevis have both been used for this purpose.[11] Resurfacing with free myofascia and other materials, both auto- and allograft, have been attempted with various optimistic short-term results.[12] In the author's experience, none of these efforts have been durable with wearing away of the interposing tissues, recurrent bone on bone articulation, with pain and loss of motion. A notable attempt, in the author's experience, was to drape myofascia from the gastrocnemius over a smooth reshaped metatarsal head, holding the material in position with small bone anchors. The results were excellent for 12–18 months, after which all deteriorated (Fig. 11).

The most successful technique using interpositional material has been the use of autogenous fascia lata graft after complete resection of the joint. This has provided pain relief, flexibility, allowing the use of various dress shoe heel heights, maintained joint alignment, and been durable. Toe flexion power is decreased and some degree of transfer metatarsal callusing has occurred, but patient satisfaction has been high. It appears to be an alternative to fusion in selected patients. In a recent study at the author's institution, 20 patients (18 females, 2 males), ages 35–75 (mean of age 55), underwent a primary procedure for advanced hallux rigidus with a minimal follow-up of 1 year and a mean of 28 months, American Orthopedic Foot and Ankle Society (AOFAS) scores went from 32 to 90. Pain scores averaged 7/10 preoperatively and 1/10 postoperatively. Dorsiflexion averaged 10° preoperatively and 25° postoperatively; plantar flexion 10°–23°. Most importantly for many women, over 80% could now wear what they considered satisfactory fashion shoes, where none could do so preoperatively. This procedure was also done following removal of a prosthetic implant or for a takedown of a fusion. This subgroup was excluded from this study. Nonetheless, they achieved similar motion and minimal pain.

Technique of Fascia Lata Interpositional Arthroplasty

The leg is prepped from the toes to the iliac crest with draping to the groin. A linear incision is made just distal to the greater trochanter along the lateral thigh. A sheet of fascia lata, typically measuring 12 cm × 25 cm is taken after the fascia is bluntly separated from the muscle. Meticulous hemostasis is achieved. The deep and superficial subcutaneous are closed with dissolving suture and the skin is closed with a running subcuticular prolene. Steristrips are added to the closure. A sterile tourniquet is applied to the high thigh. The fascia is folded over and over to form an "anchovy" slightly oval in shape and sutured together with 4-0 absorbable suture. The great toe is approached through a midsagittal incision from the IP joint to the mid first metatarsal level. A subperiosteal dissection is made after a midlongitudinal incision through the periosteum and medial joint capsule. The medial eminence is excised as well as the spurs from the metatarsal head and base of the proximal phalanx. The convexity of the metatarsal head is removed with a microsagittal saw. After inserting a centralizing pin into the end of the metatarsal and later the proximal phalanx, a convex reamer is used to create two opposing concave surfaces. The interposing "anchovy" is fairly tightly packed between the opposing surfaces and the capsule is closed with 0 absorbable sutures (Figs 12A to C). Flexion and extension is tested to assure no bone contact between the components. A bulky dressing is applied and the patient placed in an orthopedic wedge postoperative bunion shoe. Immediate ambulation is allowed. After suture removal at 2 weeks, full mobilization is allowed and encouraged (Figs 13A and B).

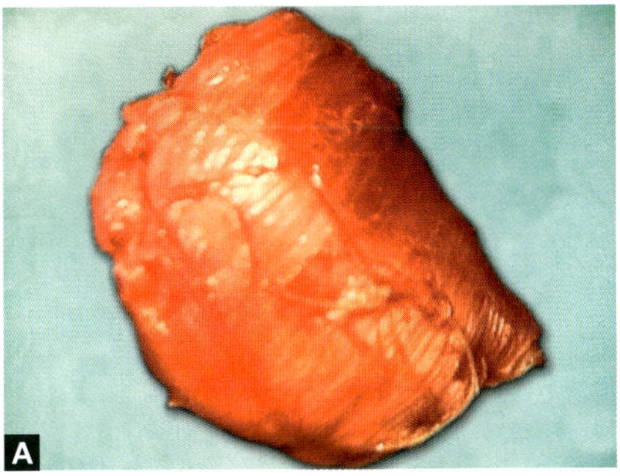
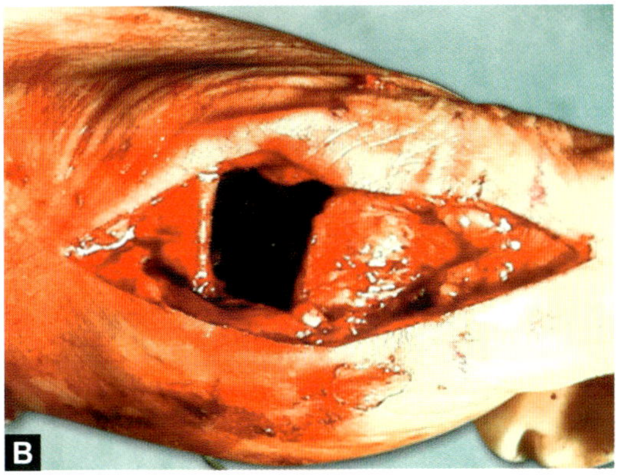
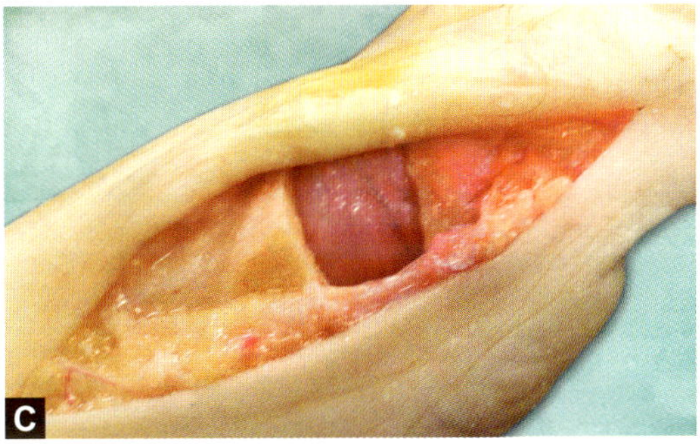

Figs 12A to C: (A) The folded fascia lata "anchovy"; (B) The resection gap; (C) Interpositional arthroplasty

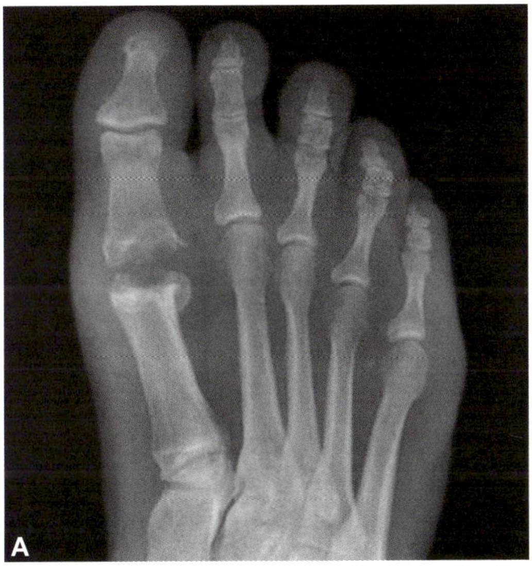
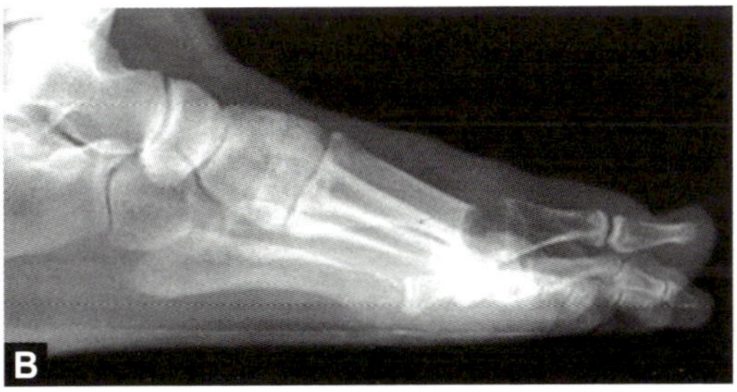

Figs 13A and B: Postoperative X-rays of the interpositional arthroplasty

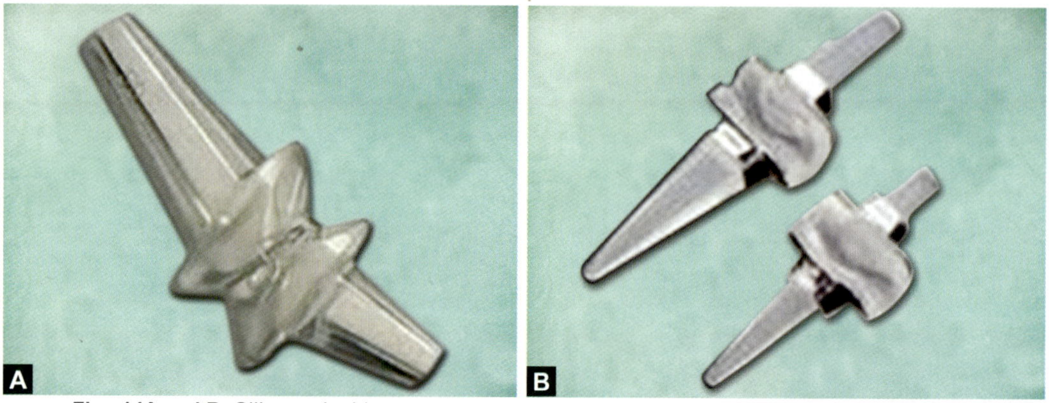

Figs 14A and B: Silicone double stem prostheses—(A) Without grommets; (B) With grommets

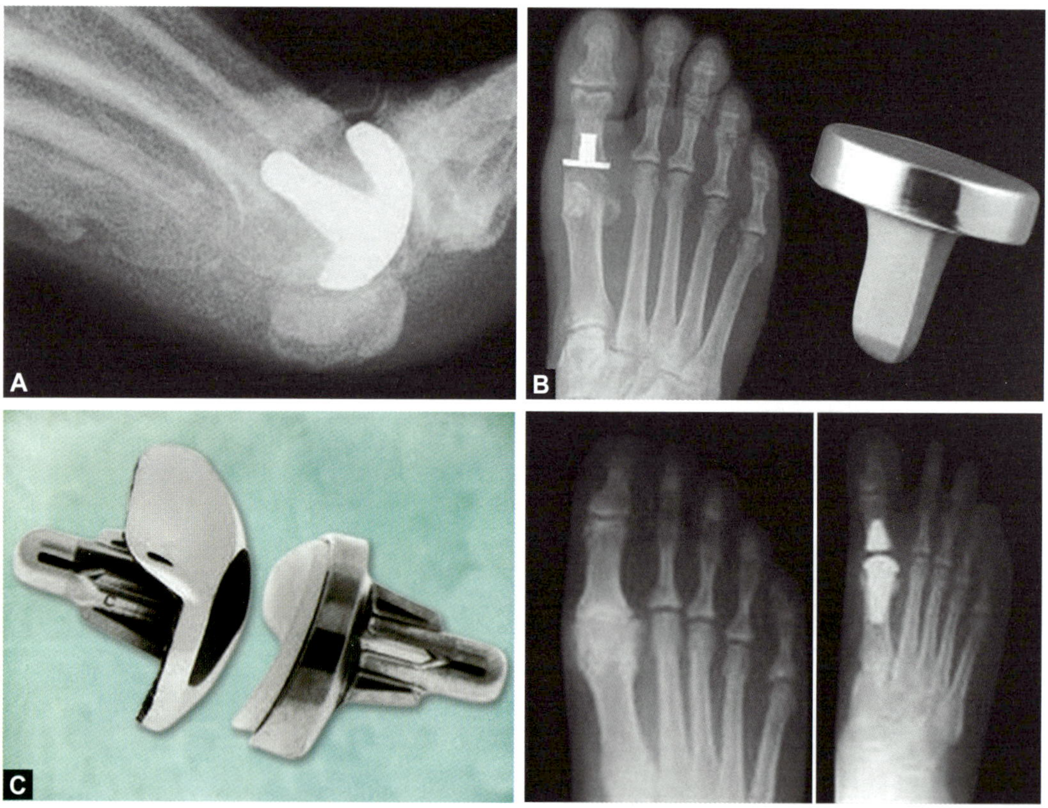

Figs 15A to C: Prosthetic replacements for the (A) metatarsal articular surface; (B) proximal phalanx surface; and (C) "total toe"

Prosthetic Arthroplasty

Prosthetic arthroplasty was a highly popular technique in the 1970s at the peak of silicone prosthetic use in the hand, wrist and feet. At the great toe, silicone replacements for the base of the proximal phalanx and later for the entire joint with stems extending up to the medullary canals of both the phalanx and metatarsal. With fractures noted at the bases of the double stem prostheses, metal grommets were placed around the base of each stem as reinforcement (Figs 14A and B).

These failed to prevent the problem. Single stem devices led to a high incidence of reaction around the stems and into adjacent bones, known as "silicone synovitis".[6,13] Today, numerous devices (Figs 15A to C) are available for both sides of the joint; the most popular of which are the "total toe" with a metal polyethylene articulation and resurfacing of the metatarsal head alone. There are no long-term studies to assure the efficacy of their use to date. Early results have had mixed reports of success.

REFERENCES

1. Yee G, Lau J. Current concepts review: Hallux rigidus. Foot Ankle Int. 2008;29(6):637-46.
2. Coughlin MJ, Shurnas PS. Hallux rigidus. J Bone Joint Surg Am. 2004;86-A Suppl 1(Pt 2):119-30.
3. Gould N. Hallux rigidus: cheilectomy or implant? Foot Ankle. 1981;1(6):315-20.
4. van Dijk CN, Veenstra KM, Nuesch BC. Arthroscopic surgery of the metatarsophalangeal first joint. Arthroscopy. 1998;14(8):851-5.
5. Moberg E. A simple operation for hallux rigidus. Clin Orthop Relat Res. 1979;142:55-6.
6. Esway JE, Conti SF. Joint replacement in the hallux metatarsophalangeal joint. Foot Ankle Clin. 2005;10(1):97-115.
7. Frimenko RE, Lievers W, Coughlin MJ, et al. Etiology and biomechanics of first metatarsophalangeal joint sprains (turf toe) in athletes. Crit Rev Biomed Eng. 2012;40(1):43-61.
8. Keller WL. The surgical treatment of bunions and hallux valgus. New York Med J. 1904;80:741-2.
9. Grondal L, Broström E, Wretenberg P, et al. Arthrodesis versus Mayo resection: the management of the first metatarsophalangeal joint in reconstruction of the rheumatoid forefoot. J Bone Joint Surg Br. 2006; 88(7):914-9.
10. Thordarson DB, Hahn MP, Gerhardt BS. Medial capsular interpositional arthroplasty for severe hallux rigidus. Foot Ankle Int. 2009;30(6):494-9.
11. Hamilton WG, OMalley MJ, Thompson FM, et al. Capsular interposition arthroplasty for severe hallux rigidus. Foot Ankle. 1997;18(2):68-70.
12. Berlet GC, Hyer CF, Lee TH, et al. Interpositional arthroplasty of the first MTP joint using a regenerative tissue matrix for the treatment of advanced hallux rigidus. Foot Ankle Int. 2008;29(1):10-21.
13. Gould JS. Salvage of failed silicone implants. Operative Foot Surgery. Philadelphia: WB Saunders Co; 1994 pp.131-40.

14

Second Hammer Toe and Cross-over Toe

John S Gould

INTRODUCTION

With the rare exception of a traumatic origin, the etiology of a second hammer toe is unknown. The cause of the crossing over, or "cross-over toe", typically over the great toe, is also unknown and the pathophysiology is described as an idiopathic synovitis. In the aligned hammer toe, there is apparently a disruption of the second plantar plate, with shifting of the intrinsic dorsally, resulting in hyperextension of the metatarsophalangeal (MTP) joint and flexion of the proximal interphalangeal (PIP) joint. The dorsal interphalangeal (DIP) joint is usually in neutral and may lose flexion (Fig. 1). In the crossover variety, the "blowout" plantarly includes the fibular collateral ligament, resulting in the tibial deviation. The natural history is increased hyperextension of the MTP joint and, in the malaligned type, more deviation and crossing over of the second toe of the great toe. The flexion deformity of the PIP joint becomes fixed. With time, the vertical motion at the MTP joint increases and the joint dislocates, leaving the base of the proximal phalanx resting on the dorsal neck of the second metatarsal. Erosion of the dorsal portion of the metatarsal articular surface also occurs, leaving the joint even more unstable after an attempted reduction (Fig. 2).

The patient's symptomatology is primarily related to parts of the anatomy of the second toe. The symptoms are accentuated in a closed shoe and patients may resort to wearing only sandals or cutting holes in the dorsum of the toe box of the shoe. Irritation occurs over the dorsum of the

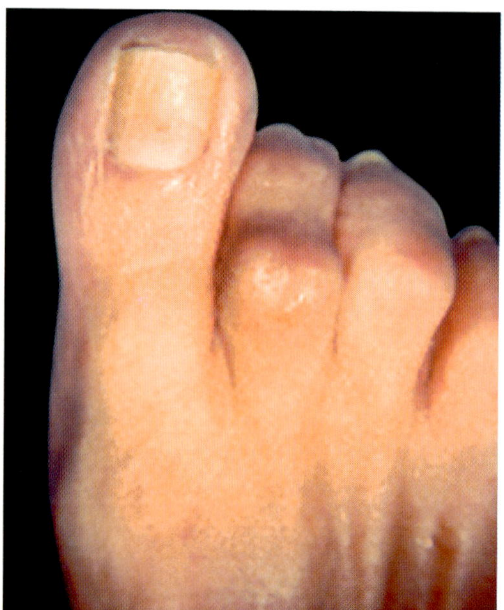

Fig. 1: The hammer toe

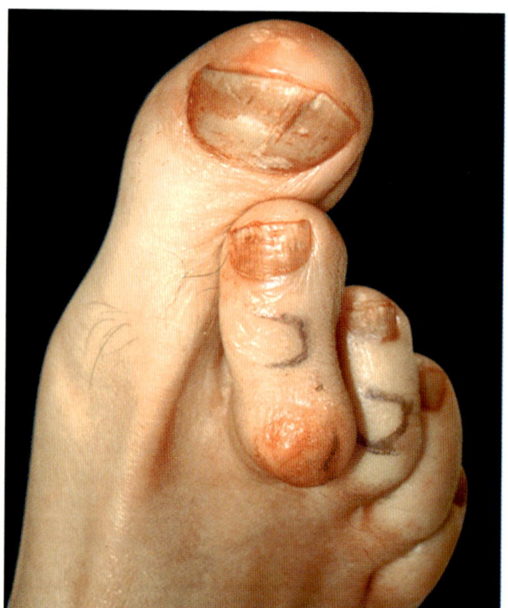

Fig. 2: The cross-over hammer toe

PIP joint of the second toe, and later callusing, the formation of a hard "corn". A "soft corn" or "clavus" may form in the web between the great and second toes. With the hyperextension of the MTP joint, the second metatarsal head will not elevate in normal gait, and pain and callusing may occur plantar to the head (Figs 3A and B). With the eccentric positioning of the head and MTP joint, the intermetatarsal ligament may be canted with intermetatarsal nerve irritation or neuritis. All in all, the primary complaints are pain and appearance. The diagnosis is clear from the history and physical examination. The hypermobility of the second MTP joint is demonstrated by the so-called positive "shuck test", as the proximal phalanx can be passively moved up and down abnormally at the joint.[1]

The conservative treatment includes shoe wear modification, including the use of sandals or spandex elastic toe boxes on special shoes. Toe spacers of various designs are helpful for the painful corns between the toes. A metatarsal pad placed just proximal to the metatarsal head will help decrease the symptoms of metatarsalgia. An orthotic device can include this metatarsal pad, a relief area under the metatarsal head filled with a viscoelastic polymer, with an extra depth shoe and relief in the toe box over the second toe PIP joint, either with spandex, deerskin, or stretching of the leather with a shoemaker's wand. In early stages of the hammer toe, a "Budin splint" is a device which can be placed on the toe which provides a pad under the metatarsal and an elastic band which fits over the proximal phalanx just proximal to the PIP joint which decreases the MTP hyperextension and PIP flexion (Fig. 4). While the deformity is flexible and the MTP not dislocated, this device may be useful. *Conservative treatment is applicable in patients with minor deformities, low demand and elderly patients, and in patients in whom the circulation to the toe is potentially inadequate to provide healing of a surgical procedure.*

SURGICAL TREATMENT

The concept behind most efforts to reverse the biomechanics of the hammer toe has been to reroute the extrinsic flexor, the flexor digitorum tendon to the toe, from plantar to dorsal to replace the failed intrinsic and have the new tendon flex the MTP and extend the PIP joints (Figs 5A to C).[2,3] Two factors thwart the success of the procedure: the capsular contractures at the joints and the critical positioning of the transferred tendon to actually carry out the desired action, particularly the PIP extension. Since digital joint motion is so critical *in hand function*, every effort is made to release the contractures and place the insertion site of the transferred tendon distally on the dorsum of the proximal phalanx. *In the foot*, digital motion, particularly at the PIP joint is not critical, so that either fusion or resections of the PIP are the standard approaches to deal with the joint contracture. At the MTP joint, these two maneuvers are not options and releases for the hyperextension contracture are a significant focus. The dorsal contracture problem becomes further accentuated when the joint is dislocated dorsally and even deviated as in the crossover problem.

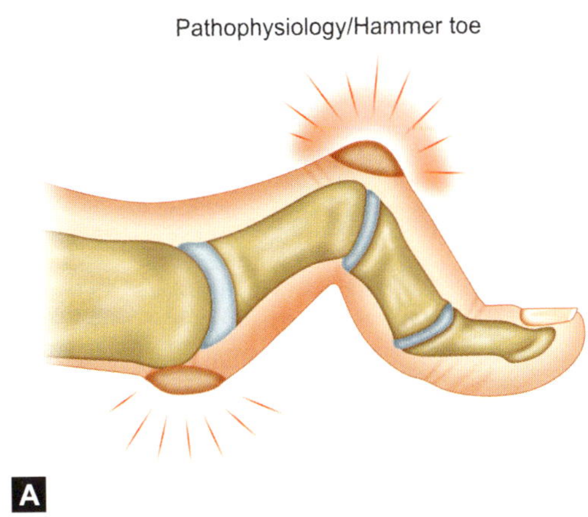

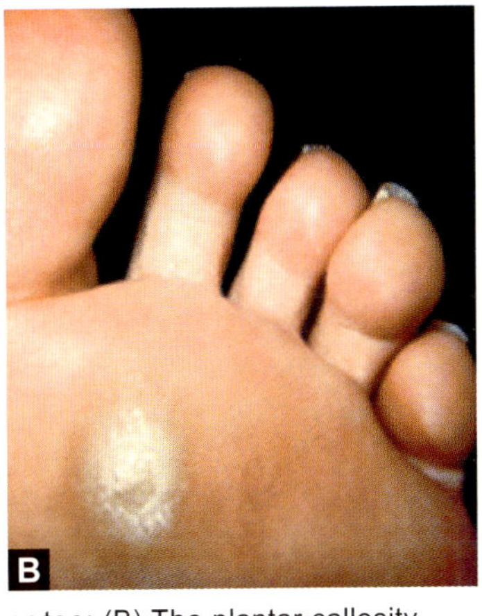

Figs 3A and B: (A) The symptomatic hammer toe; (B) The plantar callosity

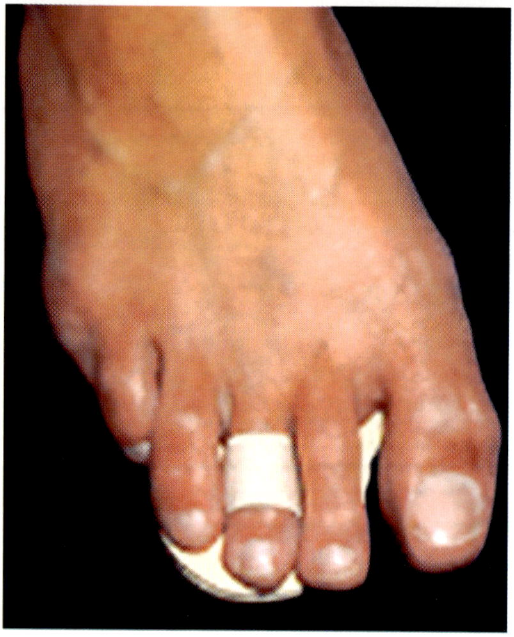

Fig. 4: The Budin splint

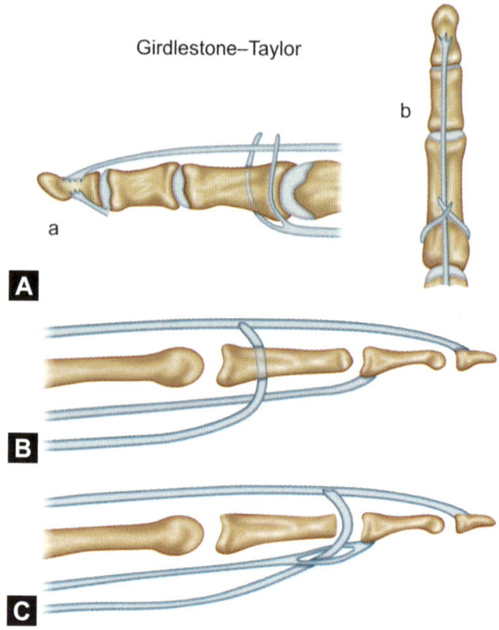

Figs 5A to C: Flexor to extensor transfer around either side of the bone (A); through the proximal phalanx (B) and; through a resection arthroplasty of the PIP joint (C)

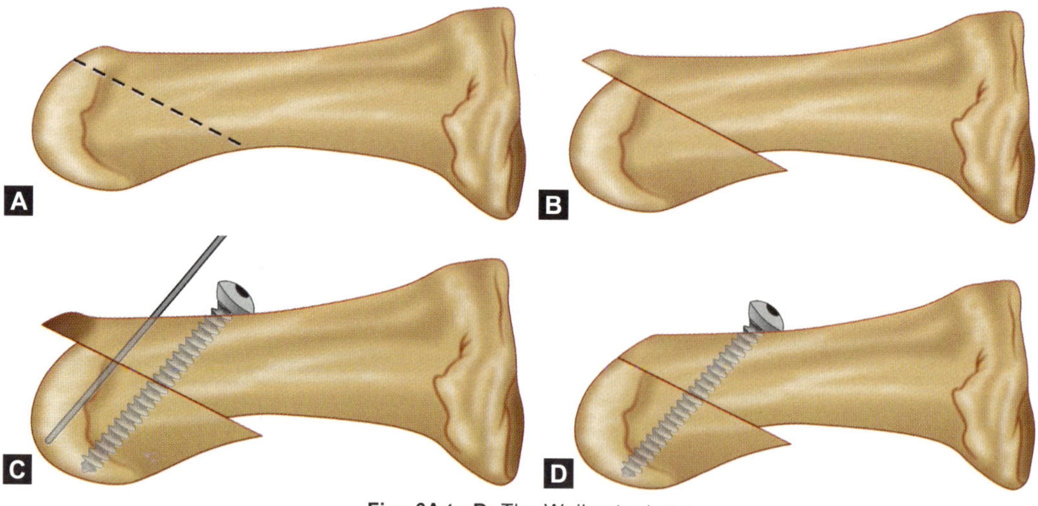

Figs 6A to D: The Weil osteotomy

A useful adjunct to the approaches to the tight dorsal joint has been shortening of the second metatarsal, decreasing the tension at the joint. The Weil osteotomy (Figs 6A to D)[4] is one method which can successfully accomplish this goal. However, overshortening can alter the intrinsic alignment at the MTP joint leading to the inability to actively flex the joint, resulting in the "floating toe" and plantar positioning of the metatarsal head. This can lead to an increased prominence and a painful callus under the head.[5]

The author's approach to the second hammer toe is as follows: The incision is via a dorsal zigzag from the distal shaft of the metatarsal onto the dorsum of the proximal phalanx. The zigzag (Bruner)[6] incision is used to prevent a later linear contracture dorsally and to allow immediate easier closure. An alternative is to use a Z-plasty type incision and this is done in salvage cases or when the dorsal contracture is particularly tight. A long Z-lengthening is done of the extensor mechanism including the retinaculum and long and short extensors. When there is a cross over tibially, the long proximal limb on the Z-incision for the tendon is left on the fibular side. The dorsal capsule of the joint is cut transversally at the joint level and longitudinally over the head and neck of the metatarsal. If there is no deviation at the joint and the soft tissue release seems to be sufficient, the author then moves onto the PIP contracture. However, if the joint is deviated, tight, or not fully reduced, the Weil osteotomy is then performed.

With the metatarsal head well exposed, using a micro-oscillating or sagittal saw, the osteotomy is begun at the junction of the middle and upper third of the articular surface and directed plantarward at an angle parallel to the sole of the foot. The saw blade exits just behind the plantar condyle of the metatarsal head. One notes immediate shortening of the plantar side of the osteotomy. In order to prevent too much plantar positioning of the head, the saw cut is made with two stacked identical blades. Consequently, the kerf, or width of the bone cut is twice as thick and, after fixation of the osteotomy, even with plantar shifting of the condyle, it is not too prominent. The shortening of the metatarsal is maintained less than 3 mm, which seems to be the limit for preventing the intrinsic dorsal shift which causes the “floating toe”. After the shortening maneuver, the tendency for the toe to deviate is usually resolved. If not, a further tibial side capsule and also intrinsic release can be carried out. If this is insufficient, the plantar condyle of the metatarsal can be rotated into alignment prior to fixation. Fixation of the osteotomy can be done is two ways. If one has sufficient help, the surgeon can maneuver the osteotomy position and close the gap between the components by applying pressure with a freer elevator when the assistant inserts a temporary pin (1.2 mm) from dorsal to plantar to hold the position. Final fixation is carried out by drilling a hole centrally with a 1.5-mm drill and inserting a proper depth 2.0-mm cortical screw. The author chooses to not penetrate the plantar cortex. After trimming the dorsal component overhanging bone with a rongeur to a flush surface, the provisional pin is removed. One must take care not to pull apart the osteotomy with the rongeur by taking bites of the bone “head on” rather than sideways with the rongeur and not pulling on the rongeur rather than completing the “bite”. There are now easier ways to hold and fix the osteotomy. Today, the author uses a special osteotomy holding clamp and twist off screw. The lower tines on the clamp fit under the plantar condyle component and the upper U-shaped tine grasps the dorsum, after which the clamp ratchet is engaged. The osteotomy position is adjusted as needed for rotation and the amount of shortening. Once the position is achieved, fixation can be done by the surgeon himself with the hand held twist off 1.5 or 2.0-mm screw. The proper length of the screw can be read off the holding clamp after it is properly engaged. After the overhang of bone is removed, the capsule is not closed, but the Z-lengthened tendon and retinaculum is repaired with 4-0 absorbable suture.

The contracted PIP joint is treated with a resection arthroplasty. An ellipse incision is made over the joint from the midsagittal position on either side of the joint. The extensor tendon is divided over the proximal phalanx head. Both collateral ligaments are divided and the head delivered. The head is grasped end on by a multitoothed (Brown-Adson) forceps. The depth of the forceps grip is to the end of the plantar condyle. A microsagittal saw is used to excise the head and directed perpendicular to the end of the forceps and directed dorsal to plantar. The joint, now resected on the proximal side only, is reduced to neutral flexion and maintained in this position by imbrication of the overlying tendon. The “vest over pants” repair is done with 4-0 absorbable suture and a small needle, bringing the proximal edge of the tendon under and to the insertion of the dorsal component. The initial stitch is placed exactly in the center so that the joint is properly aligned. Two, sometimes three sutures are placed on each side of center in a like manner and a second layer reinforces the repair. No longitudinal pin is used, unless this is a secondary salvage procedure and the soft tissues are insufficient. A postoperative bunion shoe is used for 6 weeks after the surgery. In many patients, sutures are removed at 2 weeks and a stiff soled sandal or standard postoperative shoe is used at 4 weeks for an additional 2 weeks. The author believes that although motion at the PIP joint resection site is minimal after surgery, it is preferable for most patients to a fusion of the joint. The potential complication of a poorly done resection arthroplasty is recurrent flexion at the site or angular deviation from a misaligned osteotomy, inappropriate suturing position, or failure to correct a pre-existing malpositioned joint. If one pins the joint prior to suturing, deformity may occur after the pin is removed. Hence, the author prefers to not use a pin and clinically review the toe position during the procedure. Fusion does have a place for salvage of a misaligned joint and is used readily for this. Fusion techniques vary from straight cuts to interdigitating bone cut techniques (using cone in cup or V cut configurations). The author prefers V cuts with K-wire fixation-crossed 1.2–1.4 pins. Currently, several intramedullary devices are advertised for this procedure with no studies to support their advocacy.

The flexor to extensor transfer technique is no longer used routinely. On occasion with a recurrent deviation, a tibial soft tissue release and a flexor to extensor transfer to the fibular side may be employed.

In a scenario where recurrent subluxation is encountered or, when the initial dislocation is so severe that the now standard soft tissue release and 3 mm metatarsal shortening will not be sufficient (the soft tissue component was done and the surgeon can readily see that the prospective shortening will be insufficient), a more drastic approach is needed for a satisfactory outcome. The author's approach has been to resect the base of the proximal phalanx rather than the metatarsal head. This leaves an unstable toe, despite the joint reduction, which could potentially deviate in any direction. In order to prevent this possibility, it is essential to syndactylize the second toe to the third in a very specific way. Prior to the base resection, a skin marker is used to mark the plantar side of the web commissure from the midpoint of the web between the toes to the level of the PIP joint. The second toe is then pressed against the third in as close to the reduced position as possible. This marks the exact position desired for the second toe to remain after resection of the bone and repair of the web. The incision for the webbing is made following the mark and the edges mobilized. A single skin hook is placed initially in the center of the plantar flap and the two sides repaired from the apex at the hook with 4-0 absorbable sutures to the PIP level on each toe. The dorsal flap is managed in the same manner, sewing from the midpoint of the flap to the dorsal edge of the PIP joint. The points of the flaps are invaginated so that from the dorsal aspect there appears to be a cleavage between the toes rather that a web. No skin is removed. As a result of this maneuver, the second toe remains in position.

Two further points need to be made: patients do not really like webbing of the toes in most cases, but it is not cosmetically unattractive, and is superior to the subluxated toe position which can be both unattractive and allow continued shoewear problems. Secondly, patients are advised to clean between the toes with an alcohol and cotton tipped applicator routinely along with usual nail care. It is essential, therefore, to forewarn patients when you are planning this approach or in the event that it could be a possibility. Most patients will concede that syndactylization is not a bad option, particularly considering the alternatives.

REFERENCES

1. Shirzad K, Kiesau CD, DeOrio JK, et al. Lesser toe deformities. J Am Acad Orthop Surg. 2011;19(8): 505-14.
2. Taylor RG. The treatment of claw toes by multiple transfers of flexor into extensor tendons. J Bone Joint Surg Br. 1951;33:539-42.
3. Boyer ML, DeOrio JK. Transfer of the flexor digitorum longus for the correction of lesser-toe deformities. Foot Ankle Int. 2007;28(4):422-30.
4. Weil LS. Weil head-neck oblique osteotomy: technique and fixation. Presented at Techniques of Osteotomies on the Forefoot; 1994 October 20-22; Bordeaux, France.
5. Migues A, Slullitel G, Bilbao F, et al. Floating-toe deformity as a complication of the Weil osteotomy. Foot Ankle Int. 2004;25(9):609-13.
6. Bruner JM. The zig-zag volar-digital incision for flexor-tendon surgery. Plast Reconstr Surg. 1967; 40(6):571-4.

15

Other Lesser Toe Problems

John S Gould

CLAW TOES

Claw toes and hammer toes are very much the same, except that the distal interphalangeal (DIP) joint is usually flexed as well as the proximal interphalangeal (PIP) joint, multiple toes may be involved, and the etiology for the claw toes or its association with other known conditions may not be obscure (Fig. 1). For example, the claw toes are frequently associated with cavus feet,[1] which will be discussed later. The cavus foot, of course, has multiple etiologies ranging from the idiopathic to various neurogenic causes. Claw toes may also be seen in collagen disorders associated with bone, cartilage and soft tissue effects. Claw toes may also develop in neuropathy, which may affect the intrinsic tendons; and following ischemic insults to the small muscles of the foot as in compartment syndromes of the foot. It may even occur from local trauma and iatrogenic sources.[1] Whatever the cause, shoewear problems may ensue.

Increasing the depth of the shoe toe box and the use of various devices from inserts with relief wells under the metatarsals and pads proximal to the metatarsal heads to Budin splints, as described earlier, may be considered for nonoperative solutions.

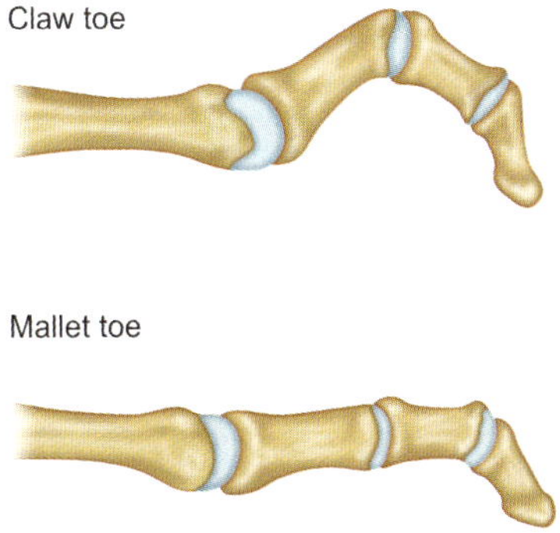

Fig.1: The claw and mallet toes

Surgical options will be described under the cavus foot discussion. However, the first issue is to determine if the deformity is passively correctible. If it is, it is also important to know if the condition is progressive or static. If progressive as in forms of cerebral palsy, Charcot-Marie-Tooth, and in resolving stroke patients, it is often best to await a static state prior to surgical intervention. Flexor to extensor transfers should be considered in static conditions in which the toes have remained flexible, but are dynamically clawed.

There are multiple variations of the flexor to extensor transfer in the literature (See illustration in Chapter 14). In all, the flexor digitorum longus to the toe is released at the distal toe flexor crease and retrieved through the divided flexor pulley at the plantar base of the toe. The distal tendon is then split longitudinally to create two limbs. An incision is made over the dorsum of the toe, or on either side, and one or both slips delivered dorsally. The hemostat is tunneled from distal to proximal, from dorsal to plantar below the level of the intermetatarsal ligament, following the lateral band of the intrinsic along the retinaculum. The tendon is then sutured into the extensor tendon. There are three important issues here: the tunneling by the hemostat must hug the bone, staying inside of the neurovascular bundle to avoid entrapping it as the tendon is passed from plantar to dorsal; the attachment into the extensor tendon should be placed just proximal to the PIP joint for optimal function; and the tension of the transfer must be such that with the ankle in neutral the toe sits with the metatarsophalangeal (MTP) in neutral and the PIP also in neutral. One should note that if you use a slip of tendon on either side of the toe, balance will be lost if the two slips are not of equal tension and double neurovascular entrapment can result in a painful ischemic toe, even necrosis. Finally, if the

PIP joint is fixed and a plantar plate and accessory collateral ligament release is insufficient to easily gain full extension in the joint, then a resection arthroplasty is needed. In this case, the flexor to extensor transfer can be brought between the slips of the flexor digitorum brevis for centering purposes and through the resection site and sutured to the tendon over the proximal phalanx.[2,3]

A "curly toe" is a congenital contracture of a toe, often the third or fourth, which is seen in infancy and early childhood. There is no successful conservative approach. When the deformity is problematic, at least in the eyes of the parent, a simple flexor tenotomy is the permanent solution.[4] A careful transverse incision is made at the level of the middle toe crease. It should be done with magnifying loupes to avoid damage to the neurovascular bundles. The sheath is opened and the flexor digitorum released. Usually the flexor brevis is left intact. Absorbable sutures are used and the toe and foot mobilized immediately.

FREIBERG'S INFRACTION

Strictly speaking, an "infraction" is a partial fracture of the bone. This entity was described by radiologist, Joseph Freiberg (Figs 2 and 3).[5] The etiology is unknown but the entity is an avascular necrosis of the metatarsal head, usually the second but sometimes the third. It usually occurs primarily in young women, though sometimes men, and manifests as swelling and pain of the MTP joint. Stiffness of the joint is routine. Revascularization does occur in many people with enlargement and deformity of the joint. In some patients, it is noted only on X-ray, incidentally, and is not the reason for the patient visit. When a patient presents with pain and swelling, as the diagnosis is made, immobilization with a stiff soled shoe, a postoperative shoe, or even a boot walker in some cases is the procedure of choice. When conservative treatment is not successful after 6–12 weeks of treatment, a synovectomy and debridement of the joint, removing fragments of avascular bone and cartilage, is the standard procedure.[6] When this approach fails to work, and it occasionally does fail, there is no consensus on the salvage approach.[7] No one really wants to remove a solitary metatarsal head, but this has been recommended. When this is done, the toe tends to displace proximally and dorsally, which is undesirable cosmetically and can result in shoewear problems. The problem existing when simple debridement fails to work is that the residual metatarsal head has lost its articular cartilage. The author has used interpositional extensor tendon after debridement, as a solution, but the typical solution used has been the resection of the base of the proximal phalanx with syndactylization of the second toe to the third, as described above in the difficult hammer toe situation. This has provided pain relief, toe alignment and good appearance. Gait is not adversely affected.

MALLET TOE

A mallet toe is a flexion contracture of the distal interphalangeal joint (Fig. 1). When flexible, this can be treated with a flexor tenotomy through the distal toe crease. When the contracture is fixed, a resection arthroplasty is done through a dorsal transverse incision. The distal condyle of the middle phalanx is excised in the same manner

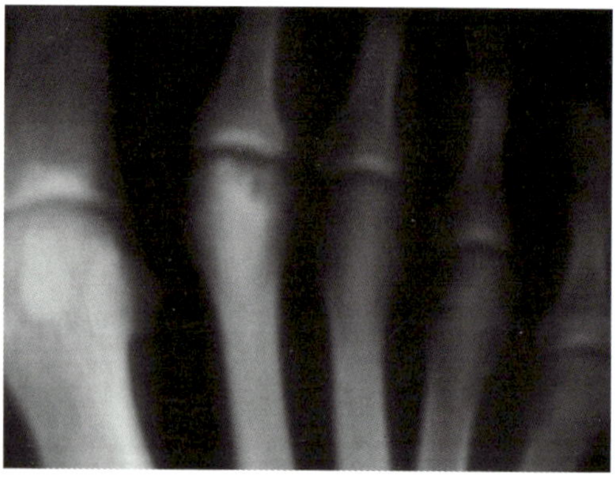

Fig. 2: Freiberg's infraction of the second metatarsal head

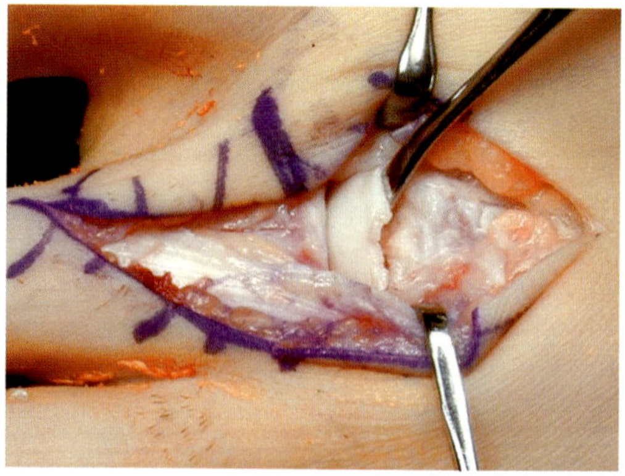

Fig. 3: Desquamation of the articular cartilage in Freiberg's infraction

as the procedure described earlier for the PIP joint. Although the extensor mechanism is also repaired in a like manner, the joint is pinned with a longitudinal K-wire, due to the strong action of the flexor digitorum longus. The pin is run retrograde out through the end of the toe and then advanced proximally to the base of the middle phalanx attempting to do this with one pass and not violating the PIP joint. The single pass with the pin proximally usually prevents the pin from "working out" in the postoperative period. A pin ball is placed over the end of the pin and it is left in place for 6 weeks. A recurrence is treated with a more formal joint fusion.

ANGULAR DEFORMITY OF THE TOE, INCLUDING THE FIFTH TOE

The angular deformities of the toes tend to occur at the PIP joint level, with typical deviation tibially, and are secondary to a developmental abnormal growth of the middle phalanx. On occasion, they occur directly through the PIP joint, and this can be post-traumatic and associated with or without an arthritic joint. When the deformity is asymptomatic, the patient is encouraged to ignore it. When the deformity is symptomatic, causing pain, callusing, or corn formation between the toes, realignment surgically may be indicated. *When the complaint is primarily based on appearance, the patient will also not be happy with a shortened toe, which should lead the surgeon to either make sure the patient understands this possibility and accepts it, to take a photograph of the toe position to use as a reminder if the patient is unhappy with the outcome, or for the surgeon to forego doing the procedure entirely.*

Other than shoewear modifications, such as the use of a wider size or different style of shoe, and the use of toe spacers, there is little to offer the patient as conservative treatment. Surgically, a corrective osteotomy is done as close to the site of the deformity as possible. If the deformity is based at the PIP joint, the corrective osteotomy is done through the joint and a fusion is done. The osteotomy through the proximal or middle phalanx is usually a wedge and is fixed with K-wires. The author usually uses 1.4–1.6 sized wires. Two crossed wires are used to control rotation. The first wire is inserted and manual compression of the osteotomy is done prior to inserting the second. Both nonunion and malunion can occur as a result of the procedure, with a rotational deformity the most common problem. Despite the fact that this is "only a toe", very unhappy patients may result when this procedure is not done well or there is any complication. Salvage is to redo the procedure with further risks of complication.

COCK-UP FIFTH TOES

These are difficult congenital or developmental deformities which include contracture of the dorsal skin, extensor mechanism, joint capsule, with hyperextension of the MTP joint, and flexion deformity of the PIP joint. There is also an external rotation deformity of the toe, making the dorsum of the PIP joint particularly vulnerable to formation of a "corn". The only conservative measures are a wider and higher toe box, change in shoe style and protective "corn pads". Classic corrective procedures include proximal phalangectomy with plantar resection of skin and transfer of the extensor communis tendon after detachment proximally, under the intermetatarsal ligament and resuture to the extensor dorsally to derotate the toe. (This is actually a tenodesis rather than a tendon transfer, as the distal tendon is used). An alternative to the classic approach is to Z-plasty the dorsal skin, extensor mechanism, and do a PIP joint resection arthroplasty. The resultant instability of the PIP joint makes it prone to injury when walking barefoot, so that syndactylization of the 5th toe to the 4th is also needed.

BUNIONETTES (TAILOR'S BUNION)

Prominence of the lateral eminence of the 5th metatarsal with overlying bursal formation secondary to shoewear is a common source of pain. This is a developmental phenomenon and present with three types. The first type, which occurs in young and middle-aged people, particularly in women wearing stylish shoes with a narrow toe box, is simple external rotation of the metatarsal which makes the lateral side and sometimes the plantar condyle more prominent. The second type of bunionette presents with flaring of the 5th metatarsal; and the third presents with flaring or splaying of the entire 5th metatarsal. The toe, distal to the 5th MTP joint is typically angled toward the 4th toe. The bone underlying the lateral prominence may be either the base of the proximal phalanx of the 5th toe, the 5th metatarsal lateral eminence, or both.

The diagnosis is made by the history and the physical examination as evidenced by observation, tenderness over the anatomic parts, and often erythema over this area. Plain X-rays provide detail of the specific anatomy and aids in surgical planning.

Conservative treatment includes modification of shoewear with a wider toe box, appropriate sandals, and various padding schemes. Systemic and topical anti-inflammatories are helpful when the symptoms are acute.

When the condition becomes recalcitrant to conservative care, surgical intervention can be considered. As with all small bone surgery, appropriate skilled technique is imperative for a good result. *The admonition that "there is no condition that cannot be made worse with surgery" applies here, as this is a really benign condition which can have painful complications.*

With Type 1 bunionettes, a simple ostectomy of the lateral eminence and sometimes the plantar prominence of the condyle can be curative (Fig. 4). It is important to review the anatomy carefully with inspection and palpation and with fluoroscopy to be certain that the correct bony prominence and the correct amount is taken. A prominent base of the 5th proximal phalanx may be left inappropriately. Also, the 5th metatarsal head is small and too generous an ostectomy may leave the patient prone to a stress fracture. As a simple ostectomy may not really be sufficient here, a distal Chevron osteotomy is an attractive alternative. This is also the appropriate procedure for a Type 2 bunionette, and even, at times, for the Type 3.[8]

Technique for the 5th metatarsal distal Chevron osteotomy (Fig. 5) is as follows: The lateral eminence is approached through a lateral sagittal incision, with the lateral periosteum and capsule of the 5th MTP opened in a similar line. Dorsal to this point is the dorsal branch of the sural nerve and plantar, the plantar branch of the same nerve. Under the abductor digiti quinti muscle lies the lateral digital neurovascular bundle to the fifth toe. It is important to understand this anatomy because blind percutaneous ostectomies can damage these structures with subsequent recalcitrant postoperative pain.

A minimal ostectomy of the lateral eminence is done with a micro-oscillating or microsagittal saw from dorsal to plantar to create a flat surface and demonstrate the oval shape of the 5th head. Using a 1.6 pin, the author drills a hole through the center of this surface from lateral to medial. If the plantar condyle is too prominent, the drill hole slants slightly dorsal from lateral to medial; otherwise it is perpendicular to the surface. Using the small saw indicated above, the chevron cuts are made at a 60° angle from the center hole proximally; one exiting dorsally, the other plantarward. The soft tissue above and below the metatarsal are protected with small Hohmann type retractors. Every effort is made not to crisscross the cuts through the center or apex hole and create a stress riser. When the surgeon is certain that all cuts have been completed, traction is placed on the toe with one hand, with the thumb placed on the distal metatarsal head, and a small towel clip or tenaculum is placed on the shaft of the fifth metatarsal. The shaft is pulled outward and the thumb on the head gently pressed medially. The distal component should overlap the proximal by at least 50%. Fixation is done with a 1.4–1.6 K-wire driven from plantar proximal to central distal dorsal in the head. Once the K-wire is engaged, the author advances it under fluoroscopy to the subchondral bone. He tries not to have to adjust it which will make it more prone to "work out" in the postoperative period. The author cuts the pin off in the subcutaneous tissue and removes

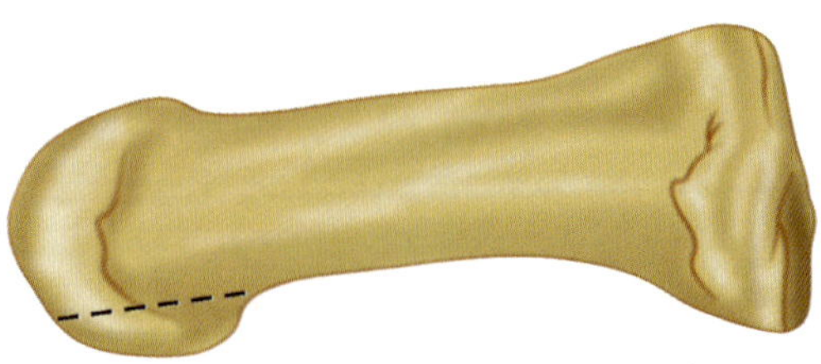

Fig. 4: Simple ostectomy of the lateral eminence and plantar condylectomy, if needed for a Type 1 bunionette

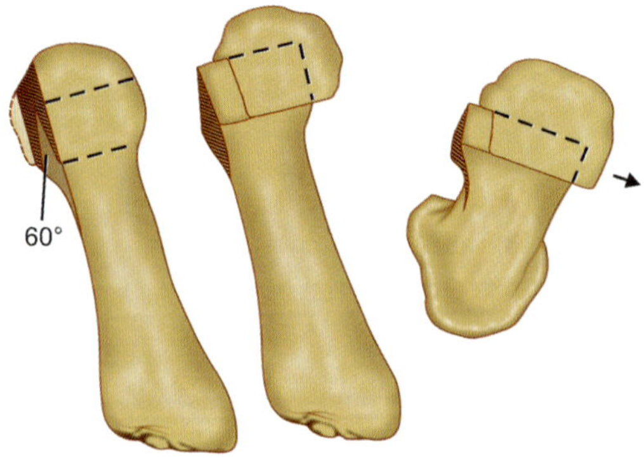

Fig. 5: Chevron osteotomy for a Type 2 bunionette, and many Type 1 and 3's

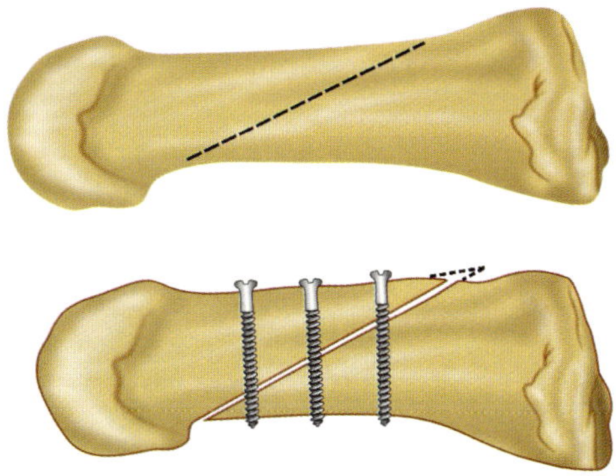

Fig. 6: Diaphyseal osteotomy for Type 3 bunionettes

it sometime after 6 weeks, as necessary. Other forms of fixation are available, including screws and absorbable pins and screws. Working with small bones, the author prefers to keep it as simple as possible, although other surgeons have their preferences. The metaphyseal osteotomy heals readily. A postoperative soft dressing and bunion wedge shoe are used for 6 weeks.

In Type 3 bunionettes, the problem is to realign the entire 5th metatarsal. Basilar osteotomies of any type, i.e. concentric, wedge, or chevron are all prone to nonunions as are fractures in this region of the bone. If the amount of splay is not too great, and there is no specific formula, the distal chevron may be sufficient. If not, a diaphyseal osteotomy will be needed (Fig. 6). This can be done with either a Ludloff type of long oblique procedure or a scarf osteotomy similar to that done on the first metatarsal. The only caveat is that use of a small plate and screws is superior fixation to screws alone.

Complications of these procedures include nerve injuries, nonunions and incomplete corrections. Excision of the fifth head leads to instability of the fifth toe alignment and balance issues in some patients. Salvage of the nerve issues including neuromas and painful nerves in continuity will be discussed in the section on "nerves". Instability of the fifth toe is managed with syndactylization of the fifth toe to the fourth. Inadequate resection requires either a further resection, or occasionally the Chevron procedure. Nonunions are treated with imaginative fixation devices, typically compression plates and screws, and bone grafting.

REFERENCES

1. Myerson MS, Shereff MJ. The pathological anatomy of claw and hammer toes. J Bone Joint Surg Am. 1989;71(1):45-9.
2. Coughlin MJ. Subluxation and dislocation of the second metatarsophalangeal joint. Orthop Clin North Am. 1989;20:535-51.
3. Boyer ML, DeOrio JK. Transfer of the flexor digitorum longus for the correction of lesser-toe deformities. Foot Ankle Int. 2007;28(4):422-30.
4. Hamer AJ, Stanley D, Smith TW. Surgery for curly toe deformity: a double-blind, randomised, prospective trial. J Bone Joint Surg Br. 1993;75(4):662-3.
5. Freiberg AH. The so called infracture of the second metatarsal bone. J Bone Joint Surg. 1926;8:257.
6. Carmont MR, Rees RJ, Blundell CM. Current concepts review: Freiberg's disease. Foot Ankle Int. 2009;30(2):167-76.
7. Frieberg AA, Freiberg RA. Core decompression as a novel treatment for early Freiberg's infraction of the second metatarsal head. Orthopedics. 1995; 18(12):1177-8.
8. Weil L Jr, Weil LS Sr. Osteotomies for bunionette deformity. Foot Ankle Clin. 2011 ;16(4):689-712.

16

Great Toe Sesamoid Problems

John S Gould

SESAMOIDITIS

When a callus and tenderness is located over a sesamoid of the great toe, sesamoiditis is a possible diagnosis. There is often a history of overuse, as with increased mileage or speed in running and a change in the type of shoewear being worn. A change in the routine and in shoewear may ameliorate the condition. The diagnosis and offending underlying bone prominence can be identified both from the surface anatomy and by placing a small pellet marker over the lesion and obtaining a plain X-ray.

When a skin lesion does not fall over a bony prominence, another diagnosis, such as a herpetic lesion (plantar wart), should be considered. Side to side exquisite tenderness and paring of the lesion to produce bleeding points should make this diagnosis obvious. The medial sesamoid is larger than the lateral and may be more prominent in some patients; a condition which becomes apparent with an increase in activity level, as in running sports.

Irritation and callus formation under the great toe sesamoids are usually managed easily with an orthotic device which provides relief under the callus area filled with a viscoelastic polymer and other substances, with posting placed just proximal to the lesion. Oral and topical anti-inflammatories can be helpful adjuncts.

When conservative measures fail to relieve the problem, shaving of the plantar aspect of the sesamoid can be curative. A low midsagittal incision is made at the metatarsophalangeal (MTP) joint level and just proximal. The medial neurovascular bundle is protected, and the capsule and periosteum of the medial and plantar medial sesamoid is raised. The ostectomy is done with a small microsagittal saw, making certain that the ostectomy is horizontal and level, without beveling from medial to plantar. The periosteum is closed along with the subcutaneous and skin. A postoperative shoe is used for two weeks or until the patient can return to comfortable shoes. Isolated lateral sesamoiditis is not usually seen except after great toe fusions. In these situations, the author has carried out other approaches, as will be described below, under "Complications".

STRESS FRACTURES, NONUNIONS AND AVASCULAR NECROSIS

The above diagnoses are all seen in running and jumping athletes, particularly in track, football, basketball, and dance. The diagnosis can often be made by the history, location of tenderness and plain X-rays. The tangential view of the great toe, or "sesamoid view", is useful along with the lateral and oblique views of the great toe joint area (Fig. 1). A CT scan makes the diagnosis of fracture fairly easy. Both feet should be X-rayed and scanned to differentiate a fracture from a bipartite sesamoid. If the separation is jagged, and the two components of the fracture are not larger than the expected size of one bone, the diagnosis is that of fracture (Fig. 2). An oversize component sum

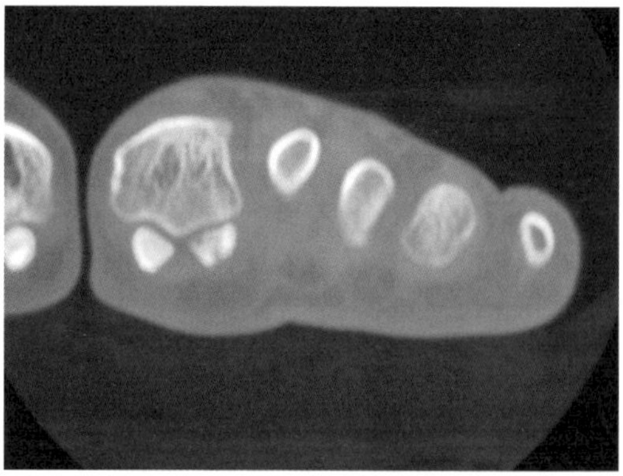

Fig. 1: Sesamoid view showing changes in the lateral sesamoid suggestive of avascular necrosis

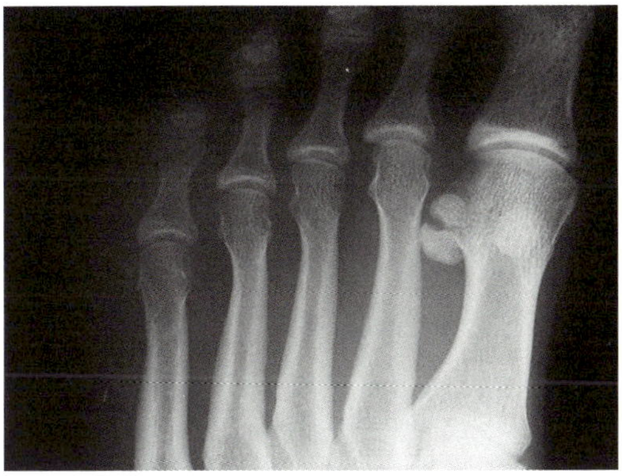

Fig. 2: Fracture of the lateral sesamoid

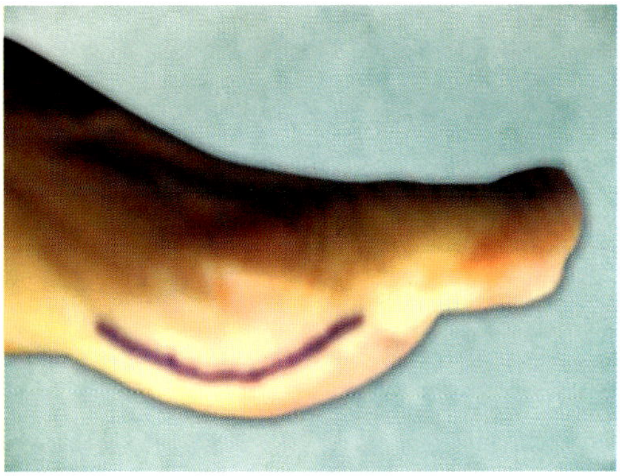

Fig. 3: Incision for medial sesamoidectomy

and smooth line between the components usually indicates the bipartite structure. A diagnosis of fracture through this cartilaginous seam can be made by comparing the bilateral films or scans. The diagnosis of avascular necrosis can be suggested by the longevity of the symptoms and the density of the bone on X-ray. An MRI, showing signal change, is the key to the diagnosis. When these findings are equivocal, and surgery is done, the diagnosis is finally confirmed from the pathological specimen.

Sesamoids do not heal particularly readily, and this is even truer when the fracture is comminuted. Certainly, when there is a single fracture line, the patient should be given the opportunity for conservative care. Immobilization in a cast or boot would be the treatment of choice, but the atrophy resulting in the muscles in an athlete makes this very problematic. An orthopedic wedge shoe which off loads the forefoot, is the usual treatment of choice. Toe taping and bandaging to prevent extension at the MTP joint is used along with an orthotic device providing a relief well under the sesamoid, posting proximal to the bone, and a stiff rocker sole shoe.[1]

There are reports of successful bone grafting of nonunions and delayed unions of the sesamoids, and admonitions not to consider excisions. As the sesamoids provide a fulcrum for the short flexors to the toe, provide dynamic balance of the toe and protect the adjacent neurovascular bundles, these warnings should be considered and often heeded.[2] Nevertheless, persistence of pain and dysfunction cannot be ignored. With this in mind, efforts to preserve at least a part of a sesamoid is usually made and except under extraordinary circumstances, only one of the sesamoids is ever removed. When a sesamoid is avascular, however, the entire structure is removed and the flexor hallucis brevis tendon repaired/reconstructed.[3]

MEDIAL SESAMOIDECTOMY (PARTIAL AND COMPLETE)

The medial sesamoid is approached through a low midsagittal incision, centered on the MTP joint, with emphasis on the proximal end of the incision, where the sesamoid components are located (Fig. 3). If a partial removal is intended, it is important to determine the larger segment and, using fluoroscopy, know where the fracture line is when it is encountered. The dissection is carried dorsally (or superiorly) to the articulation between the medial metatarsal condyle and the medial sesamoid. It is then carried plantar, carefully dissecting off the plantar component of the medial flexor hallucis brevis. The incision needs to be carried proximal to the proximal end of the condyle and the dissection must stay on the bone to avoid damage to the medial neurovascular bundle. Fluoroscopy is used, and copies retained, to verify that either all of the sesamoid was removed or that the appropriate portion was retained and the remainder removed. Clearly, this documentation is necessary for both the desired outcome and medical-legal purposes. After the portion of the sesamoid, or all of it, if this is warranted, is removed, the redundant splayed out flexor hallucis brevis is gathered and imbricated from medial to lateral, tightening the structure (Figs 4A and B). Each pass of the absorbable suture is made deliberately under direct vision to avoid damage to the nerve and artery. Gentle passive motion of the MTP joint begins with the first dressing change, with sutures

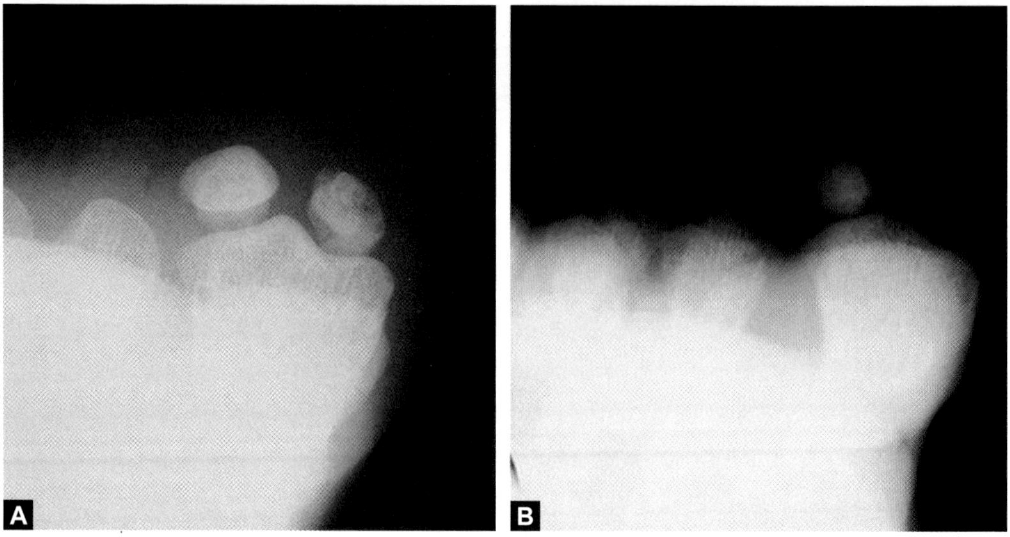

Figs 4A and B: (A) Medial sesamoid disease; (B) Sesamoidectomy

removed at 2 weeks and a protective stiff sole postoperative shoe worn for 6 weeks.

LATERAL SESAMOIDECTOMY (PARTIAL OR COMPLETE)

Probably one of the most difficult procedures in foot surgery is to attempt to remove the lateral sesamoid through a dorsal incision, although this was recommended for many years to avoid a plantar incision and damage to the neurovascular bundle. As plantar incisions, closed properly, and seeing the neurovascular structures and protecting them is far superior to a blind dissection, the rationale of using the dorsal approach defies logic. Consequently, the lateral sesamoid is approached plantarly following the semicircular skin line longitudinally just lateral to the sesamoid (Fig. 5). The plantar fascia is divided longitudinally and, using loupe magnification, the lateral hallucal (digital) bundle is found and dissected from the surrounding structures. It is retracted laterally and the plantar aspect of the investing lateral flexor hallucis brevis is dissected from the dorsally lying sesamoid. The whole or portion of the sesamoid to be removed is dissected free and removed (Figs 6A and B). The maneuver is verified by fluoroscopy, and copies saved. The tendon is repaired with 2-0 absorbable suture. The plantar fascia is not repaired; and the author does not close the subcutaneous on the plantar incisions, avoiding the possibility of reactive sutures in this area. The skin is closed usually with 3-0 nylon everting suture technique. (Typically, a locking horizontal mattress suture is used which everts the incision, while the locking strand crosses the incision line to maintain its precise and near anatomic closure). Motion is begun with the first dressing change; sutures removed at 2 weeks; and a stiff sole postoperative shoe used for 6 weeks.

COMPLICATIONS

Theoretically, metatarsalgia may occur after removal of one sesamoid from excessive pressure on the other. Weakness of toe-off is also a theoretical possibility.[4] Neither has been observed in the author's series, even in high performance athletes. Hypertrophic scar formation does not occur with the technique described and the lateral sesamoid excision scar essentially disappears. Plantar scar problems can occur with other techniques and can be problematic. Revisions with the use of Z-plasty can resolve most, but not all cases. Postoperative varus or valgus is not a problem if the great toe began well aligned. If there has been malalignment, preoperatively, a worsening of the condition can occur and may require a great toe MTP fusion as salvage. Damage to a neurovascular, and particularly to a hallucal nerve, can be very problematic. Neurolysis may be attempted, but

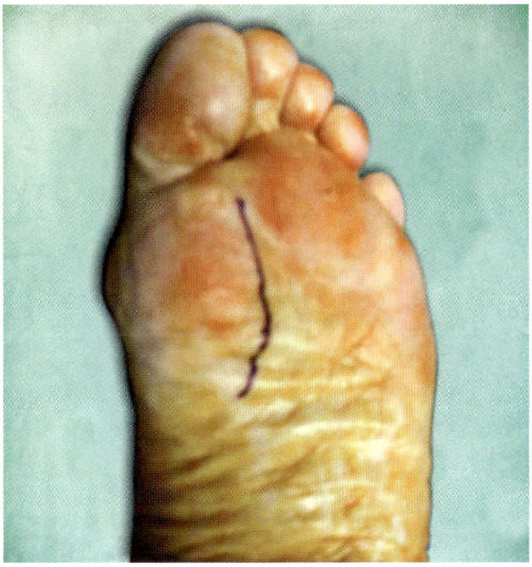

Fig. 5: Incision for lateral sesamoidectomy

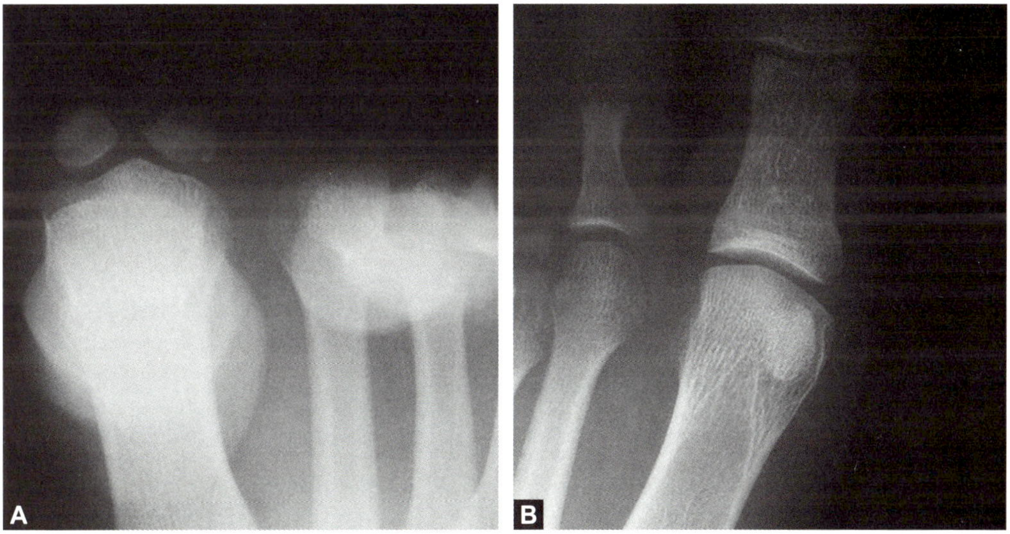

Figs 6A and B: (A) Lateral sesamoid disease; (B) Sesamoidectomy

frequently does not succeed. Wrapping, or isolation barrier techniques, as described by the author for painful nerves in continuity (Chapter 21) has not been successful for digital and hallucal nerves. A neuroma of a hallucal nerve, particularly the medial, notoriously does not respond to simple resection. The author has found that resection of the neuromas with the use of a vein or collagen conduit, as described in Chapter 43 is the best option.

Sesamoid pain after a metatarsophalangeal joint arthrodesis is extremely problematic.[5] The sesamoids retract and there is a pressure problem directly over them. At times, there is minimal retraction and they are still painful. If one sesamoid is removed, the other may become symptomatic. Removing both may be curative, but neuritic pain may ensue. Although various types and combinations of excisions have been used, some successful and some not, there is no predictable outcome with these approaches. In a small series, successful pain relief has occurred with takedown of the fusion joint and use of an interpositional arthroplasty, as described in Chapter 13. This has also been successful when there has been sesamoid pain and interphalangeal joint arthritis pain. Arthrodesis of the interphalangeal (IP) joint and interpositional arthroplasty of the MTP has resolved the symptoms.

REFERENCES

1. Gould JS, Ford D. Orthoses and insert management of common foot and ankle problems. In: Porter DA, Schon LC (Eds). Baxter's The Foot and Ankle in Sport. 2nd edn. Philadelphia: Mosby Elsevier; 2008.
2. Mann RA, Wapner KL. Tibial sesamoid shaving for treatment of intractable plantar keratosis. Foot Ankle. 1992;13(4):196-8.
3. Bichara DA, Henn RF, Theodore GH. Sesamoidectomy for hallux sesamoid fractures. Foot Ankle Int. 2012; 33(9):704-6.
4. Aper RL, Saltzman CL, Brown TD. The effect of hallux sesamoid excision on the flexor hallucis longus moment arm. Clin Orthop Relat Res. 1996; 325:209-17.
5. Tan J, Lau JT. Metatarso-sesamoid osteoarthritis as a cause of pain after first metatarsophalangeal joint fusion: case report. Foot Ankle Int. 2011;32(8): 822-5.

SECTION 3

Midfoot Problems

Chapters Outline

17

Tarsometatarsal and Midtarsal Joint Arthritis

Bruce Cohen

INTRODUCTION

The midfoot is a complex region that consists of the tarsometatarsal articulations, intertarsal articulations and extends into the naviculocuneiform region. The midfoot stability is derived from both the bony architecture and the interosseous ligaments. The bony architecture consists of both a longitudinal arch as well as a rigid arch in the coronal plane.

From a functional standpoint, the midfoot is divided into three columns. The medial column consists of the 1st metatarsal and the medial cuneiform. The middle column consists of the 2nd and 3rd metatarsals and the middle and lateral cuneiforms. The 2nd metatarsal serves as the rigid keystone of the arch. The lateral column consists of the 4th and 5th metatarsals and the cuboid. The middle and medial columns are fairly rigid in normal gait while the lateral column is flexible and is critical for function and accommodating for uneven ground.[1]

TARSOMETATARSAL (TMT) JOINT ARTHRITIS

Description

There are many etiologies of midfoot arthritis. These include: traumatic, degenerative arthritis, inflammatory arthropathy and neuroarthropathy. Significant gastrocnemius tightness or contracture can contribute to the development of midfoot arthritis and potential collapse.

Medial column instability and collapse will lead to axial subluxation of the medial midfoot joints, abduction deformity of the midfoot and forefoot and fixed forefoot varus with an elevated first ray. Severe collapse may result in a rocker bottom deformity, valgus of the hindfoot and rotational collapse of the medial cuneiform. In the latter stages of collapse and deformity, lateral column involvement will occur which will be discussed later.

Diagnosis

The diagnosis is typically made based on clinical examination. Localized tenderness, swelling and bony prominence are the hallmarks of midfoot arthritis. With more severe cases, the foot alignment is affected with abduction, loss of longitudinal arch height and can present with significant pes planovalgus. This can frequently be mistaken for posterior tibial tendon insufficiency (Figs 1A and B).

Weight-bearing radiographs with oblique views are important components of the work-up. Further diagnostic studies such as CT scans are helpful in evaluating which joints are involved.

OPTIONS OF MANAGEMENT

Conservative Treatment

Conservative management should always be the initial treatment for these disorders. The goals of conservative management are to reduce pain, enhance function and prevent progression of deformity. This consists of accommodative shoewear and orthotic devices which support the longitudinal arch. The use of fluoroscopic-guided injections can be beneficial from both a therapeutic and diagnostic standpoint. Confirmation of the joints causing the majority of symptoms can be accomplished with these injections.

The chance of success of nonoperative treatment is variable with some patients experiencing long-term reduction of symptoms while some continue to have progression of symptoms and functional limitations.

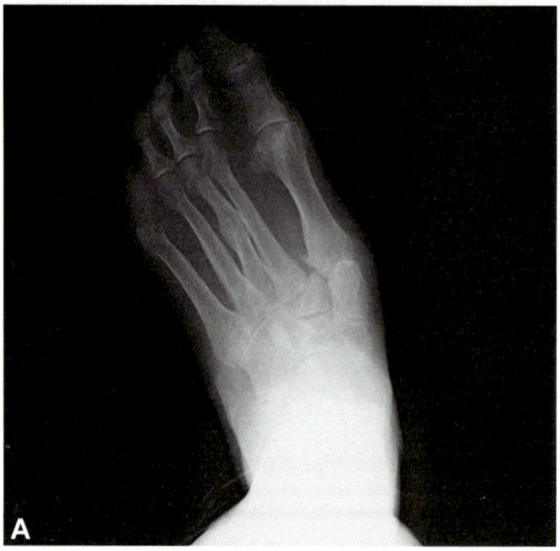

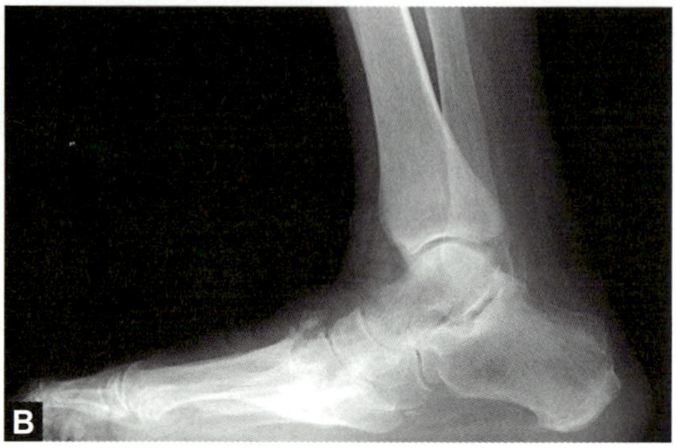

Figs 1A and B: Standing anteroposterior (AP) and lateral radiograph of foot demonstrating significant midfoot collapse with loss of longitudinal arch height and abduction through the midfoot

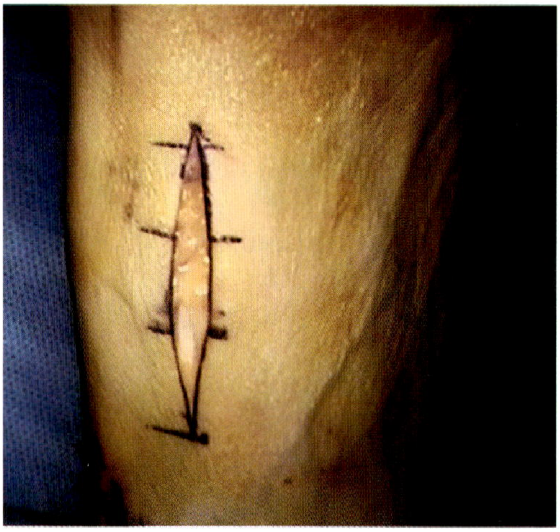

Fig. 2: Dorsal incision for midfoot arthrodesis

When is it time for Surgery?

When the symptoms increase and function is increasingly limited, then surgical reconstruction needs to be considered. These symptoms would be pain, shoewear limitations and activity restriction.

What do you tell the patient?

Typically the patient is told that "they will know when it is time for surgery." When the pain interferes significantly with daily activities, it is time to consider operative treatment. The patient is informed that the surgery will improve their pain and function with a fairly minimal loss of motion. They are also informed of the risks of infection, wound healing problems, nonunion and need for further surgical procedures.

Operative Treatment

Goals—Pain relief, deformity correction and prevention of progression.

Procedure—For medial and middle column symptomatic arthritis, the treatment of choice is arthrodesis. The arthrodesis is typically limited to the symptomatic joints. The location is often confirmed preoperatively with injections under fluoroscopy.

Midfoot Arthrodesis

Anesthesia: Regional anesthesia: ankle or popliteal block.

Incision: A longitudinal incision is used for a single joint; multiple incisions are needed for medial and dorsal locations. Care is taken to protect the dorsal neurovascular bundle (Fig. 2).

Joint preparation: Exposure of tarsometatarsal and intercuneiform joints is shown in Figure 3.

Remove all dorsal osteophytes:

- Remove all remaining cartilage
- Drill or feather the subchondral bone
- Do not leave gaps
- Consider bone graft or substitute.

Deformity correction:

- Consider gastrocnemius recession vs tendo-achilles lengthening
- Mobilize involved joints.

Stabilize sequentially:

- Proximal to distal
- Medial to lateral.

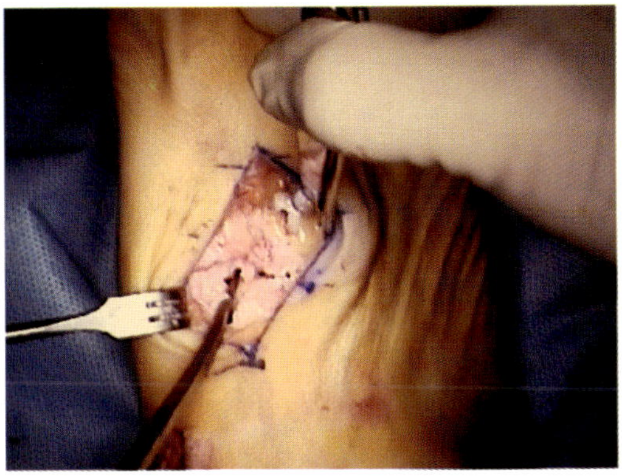

Fig. 3: Exposure of tarsometatarsal and intercuneiform joints

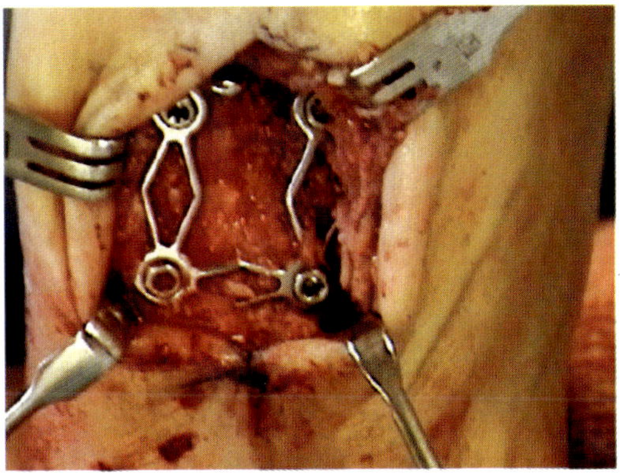

Fig. 4: Arthrodesis of medial midfoot joints with fixation in place

Must also address nonmidfoot deformities:
- Hindfoot valgus
- Hallux valgus
- Lesser toes.

Internal Fixation:
- Need two points of fixation
  - Screws—avoid breaking out dorsal cortex by countersinking or using a burr at the insertion site
  - Plates—buttress plates or compression plates (Fig. 4)
  - Avoid using dorsal compression plates alone, which may cause excessive dorsiflexion.

Postoperatively: splint for 2 weeks; cast for 4 weeks non-weight bearing; walking boot from 6 weeks interval for an additional 6 weeks.

COMPLICATIONS AND SALVAGE

The most significant complication of midfoot arthrodesis is nonunion. The rate of nonunion ranges from 8% to 22%. Many of these patients have asymptomatic nonunions or successful fusions of some of the multiple joints fused.[2-6] Infection and wound healing issues can occur, especially with dorsal incisions which can also heal very slowly. Salvage procedures used include revision arthrodesis with more robust internal fixation or fine wire external fixators in instances of previous infections. Interpositional arthrodesis with autograft or allograft can be performed in situations with significant bone loss or severe deformity.[7]

The issues of complications and salvage procedures are accentuated in the neuropathic patient. Medial column plating with multiple points of fixation and prolonged period of immobilization is critical in these challenging patients. For severe deformities, multiplanar osteotomies/arthrodesis techniques are utilized.

REFERENCES

1. Trevino SG, Licht N. Degenerative problems of the midtarsal joints. In: Gould JS (Ed). Operative Foot Surgery. Philadelphia: WB Saunders;1994.p.163.
2. Mann RA, Prieskorn D, Sobel M. Mid-tarsal and tarsometatarsal arthrodesis for primary degenerative osteoarthritis or osteoarthrosis after trauma. J Bone Joint Surg. 1996;78A:1376-85.
3. Sangeorzan BJ, Veith RG, Hansen ST. Salvage of Lisfranc's tarsometatarsal joint by arthrodesis. Foot Ankle. 1990;10:193-200.
4. Nemec SA, Habbu RA, Anderson JG, et al. Outcomes following midfoot arthrodesis for primary arthritis. Foot Ankle Int. 2011;32(4):355-61.
5. Bibbo C, Anderson RB, Davis WH. Complications of midfoot and hindfoot arthrodesis. Clin Orthop Relat Res. 2001;(391):45-58.
6. Filippi J, Myerson MS, Scioli MW, et al. Midfoot arthrodesis following multi-joint stabilization with a novel plating system. Foot Ankle Int. 2012; 33(3):220-5.
7. Horton GA, Olney BW. Deformity correction and arthrodesis of the midfoot with a medial plate. Foot Ankle. 1993;14:493-9.

18

Fourth and Fifth Tarsometatarsal Arthritis

Bruce Cohen

DESCRIPTION

The etiology of arthritis of the lateral column is the same as that of the medial and middle columns. With increased abduction through the medial column, the lateral column involvement and potential for increased symptoms is worsened. Fractures of the cuboid can also lead to significant post-traumatic arthritis of these joints. Lateral column joint pain may improve with realignment arthrodesis of the medial column, thus consideration of addressing the medial column deformity alone and assessing the improvement laterally is an option. The lateral column joints are described as essential joints due to their function in accommodating for uneven surfaces.

DIAGNOSIS

As with arthritis of the medial and middle columns, weight-bearing radiographs are critical. Further evaluation with CT scans can be beneficial. Clinical examination can identify the deformity, pinpoint areas of swelling and tenderness and note other abnormalities. It is important to remember that the radiographic appearance of arthritis does not always correlate with the amount of symptoms. The radiographs often look worse than the current clinical picture (Fig. 1).

OPTIONS OF MANAGEMENT

Conservative Treatment

Conservative treatment of lateral column arthritis is usually in combination with symptomatic medial column degeneration with or without collapse. Orthotic management is the hallmark of this treatment as well as fluoroscopic-guided corticosteroid injections (Fig. 2). In the uncommon instance of the isolated 4th and 5th tarsometatarsal involvement, the orthotic devices are prescribed with lateral posting to support the involved joints.

The chance of success of nonoperative treatment is variable, with some patients experiencing long-term reduction of symptoms while some continue to have progression of symptoms and functional limitations.

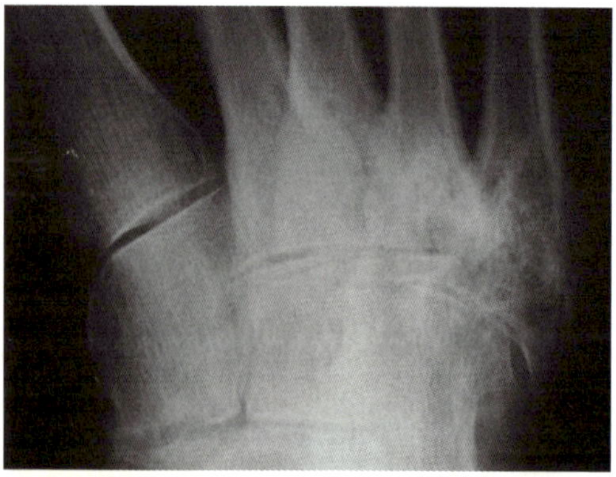

Fig. 1: Degenerative arthritis involving lateral tarsometatarsal joints demonstrated on radiograph

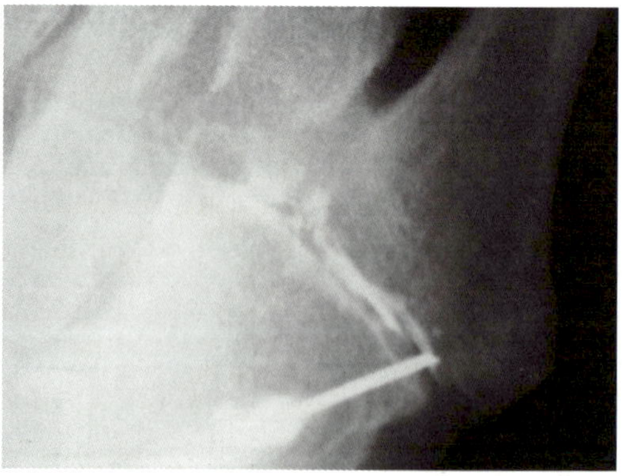

Fig. 2: Radiograph of selective injection in the fourth and fifth tarsometatarsal joints

When is it time for Surgery?

When the symptoms increase and function is increasingly limited, then surgical reconstruction needs to be considered. These symptoms would be pain, shoewear limitations and activity restriction.

What do you tell the Patient?

Typically, the patient is told that "they will know when it is time." When it interferes significantly with daily activities, it is often time to consider operative treatment. The patient is told that the surgery will improve their pain and improve their function with no significant loss of motion. They are also explained the risks of infection, wound healing problems, nonunion and need for further surgical procedures.

Operative Treatment

Goals—Pain relief and maintenance of lateral column motion.
Procedure—The options for treatment include arthroplasty procedures of the 4th and 5th tarsometatarsal joints. Arthrodesis of the joints should be avoided due to loss of compensatory motion and significant risk of nonunion. The types of arthroplasty procedure include tendon interpositional procedures and spherical interposition with ceramic implants. The author's preferred technique is the spherical implant arthroplasty.

Interpositional Arthroplasty of the 4th and 5th Tarsometatarsal Joints

Anesthesia: Regional anesthesia with ankle block or popliteal block.

Incision: A dorsal incision is made over lateral cuboid in line with 4th and 5th metatarsals.

Joint preparation:
- Exposure of lateral joints after debridement of osteophytes (Fig. 3)
- Burr is used to create a spherical defect in the central portion of the opposing tarsometatarsal (TMT) joints (Fig. 4)
- Semicircular finishing burr enlarges the recess on each side of the joint(s) (Fig. 5)
- Sizing guides are used to confirm the size of the implant. The most common size is 11 mm.

Implant insertion:
- Plantar flexion across the TMT joints allows insertion of the implant(s) (Fig. 6)
- Avoid placing definitive fixation in the medial column prior to implant insertion due to risk of disrupting fixation with this plantar flexion.

Postoperatively:
- Depends on concomitant procedures such as medial column arthrodesis
- If isolated, transition to full weight bearing and boot at 2 weeks
- Transition to accommodative shoe with arch support at 6–8 weeks.

COMPLICATIONS/SALVAGE

The results of spherical interpositional arthroplasty were reported in 13 patients with an average of 20 months follow-up. There was noted an 83% improvement in the American Orthopedic Foot and Ankle Society (AOFAS) scores and a significant improvement in the pain scores.

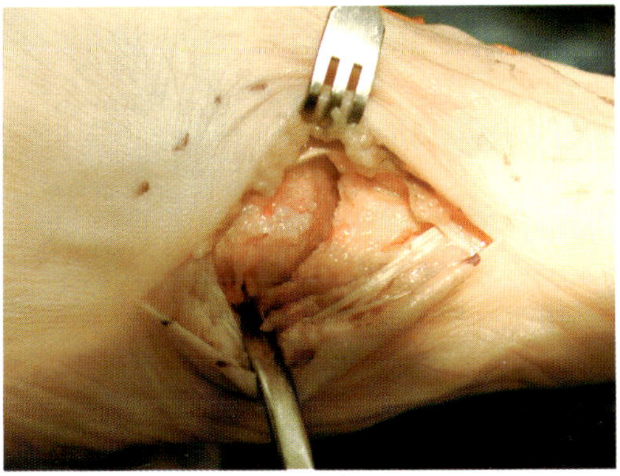

Fig. 3: Dorsal exposure of degenerative fourth and fifth tarsometatarsal joints

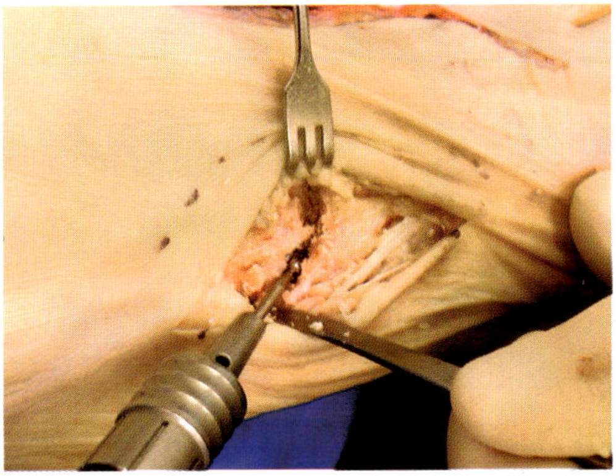

Fig. 4: Entry burr used to create defect for interpositional arthroplasty

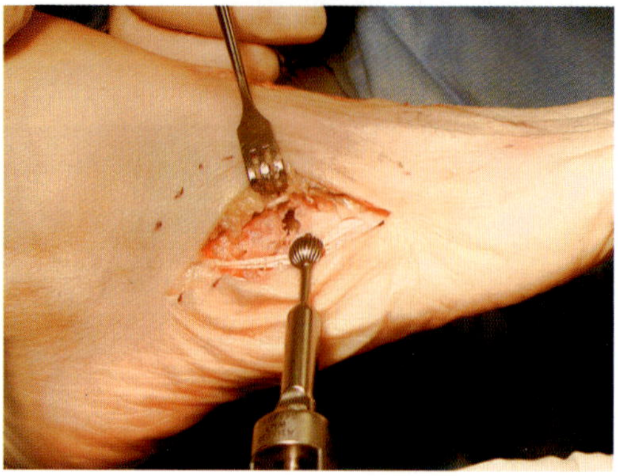

Fig. 5: Semicircular rasp used to fashion space for ceramic implant

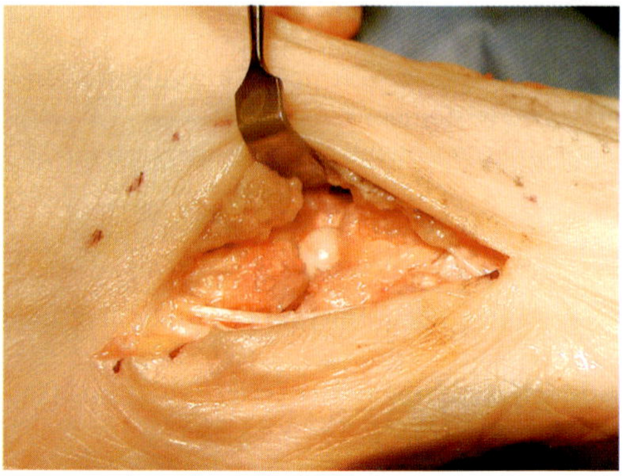

Fig. 6: Final position of ceramic interpositional arthroplasty

There were no revisions or major complications. The most dramatic improvement was in patients with concomitant medial column arthrodesis.[1] Interpositional tendon arthroplasty has also been reported. The results of this series reported less improvement in the AOFAS score postoperatively and a 35% improvement in the pain scores.[2] While the interpositional tendon arthroplasty is believed to be a reasonable salvage procedure, the results of the ceramic arthroplasty appear to be more promising. No randomized trial has been conducted comparing these two procedures.

Arthrodesis of the lateral column joints has been shown to significantly increase the contact pressures of the lateral column and the calcaneocuboid joint.[3] The nonunion rates can be significant with failure of fixation commonly seen. To avoid significant pressure increases in the hindfoot and forefoot in a non-neuropathic patient, arthrodesis of these joints should be avoided.[3,4]

REFERENCES

1. Shawen SB, Anderson RB, Cohen BE, et al. Spherical ceramic interpositional arthroplasty for basal fourth and fifth tarsometatarsal arthritis. Foot Ankle Int. 2007;28(8):896-901.
2. Berlet GC, Anderson RB, Davis WH. Tendon arthroplasty for basal 4th and 5th metatarsal arthritis. Foot Ankle. 2002;23:440-6.
3. Nadaud JP, Parks BG, Schon LC. Plantar and calcaneocuboid joint pressure after isolated medial column fusion versus medial and lateral column fusion: a biomechanical study. Foot Ankle Int. 2011;32(11):1069-74.
4. Raikin SM, Schon LC. Arthrodesis of the fourth and fifth tarsometatarsal joints of the midfoot. Foot Ankle. 2003;24:584-90.

19 Stress Fractures of the Tarsal Navicular

Bruce Cohen

ETIOLOGY

Stress fractures of the navicular have been receiving an increased amount of attention in the media. The incidence ranges from 14% to 35% of all foot stress fractures.[1-5] The incidence of these fractures continues to rise due to increased recognition, better diagnostic evaluation and advanced imaging modalities.

PATHOPHYSIOLOGY

The navicular articulates with the three cuneiforms distally and the head of the talus proximally. The distal surface has three separate articular facets with minimal motion in this region. The talonavicular joint is critical for hindfoot motion of inversion and eversion. The navicular has a unique vascular supply that contributes to the occurrence of navicular stress fractures. The vascular supply arises from small branches of the posterior tibial and dorsalis pedis arteries. These vessels enter at the posterior tibialis tendon insertion medially and plantarly; and laterally from the dorsalis pedis. This results in a relative avascular area in the central one third of the navicular.[6] This is consistent with the location of most navicular stress fractures being in the central one third.

The exact foot mechanics that contribute to navicular stress fractures have not been determined. It is thought that the greatest contact stresses in the navicular occur in the central third with axial loading.[7] There may be a relationship to athletes with cavus or cavovarus alignment with some degree of metatarsus adductus.[8]

DIAGNOSIS

The clinical presentation of navicular stress fractures can be varied. The onset of symptoms are often slow and insidious. The clinical complaints are of vague anterior ankle pain that is worse with activity, particularly running and jumping. This can often be misdiagnosed as anterior impingement of the ankle, a midfoot sprain, and posterior or anterior tibial tendonitis. Khan et al.[2,9] described a dorsal location of tenderness directly over the central portion of the navicular termed the "n-spot".

Radiographic evaluation includes weight-bearing plain radiographs. Khan et al.[9] found that only 24% of incomplete fractures and 81% of complete fractures were adequately diagnosed with plain radiographs. A CT scan is preferable in diagnosing a navicular stress fracture and provides important information about the location of the fracture, whether it is complete or incomplete as well as the direction of the plane of the fracture. The fracture typically begins on the dorsal surface and courses to the plantar surface in an oblique direction. Magnetic resonance imaging (MRI) has become popular in the initial diagnosis of these injuries. It can detect early stress fractures, stress reaction and incomplete stress fractures; however, MRI cannot differentiate a stress fracture from avascular necrosis (Figs 1A and B).[10,11]

OPTIONS OF MANAGEMENT

Conservative Treatment

Conservative treatment is a reasonable option in most incomplete or nondisplaced complete fractures. This consists of a 6-week course in a non-weight-bearing cast. Khan et al. reported that 86% of patients returned to activity at 5.6 months following 6-week treatment in a non-weight-bearing cast. The results significantly declined with weight bearing in the cast.[9] The fracture type or the presence or absence of displacement was not described.

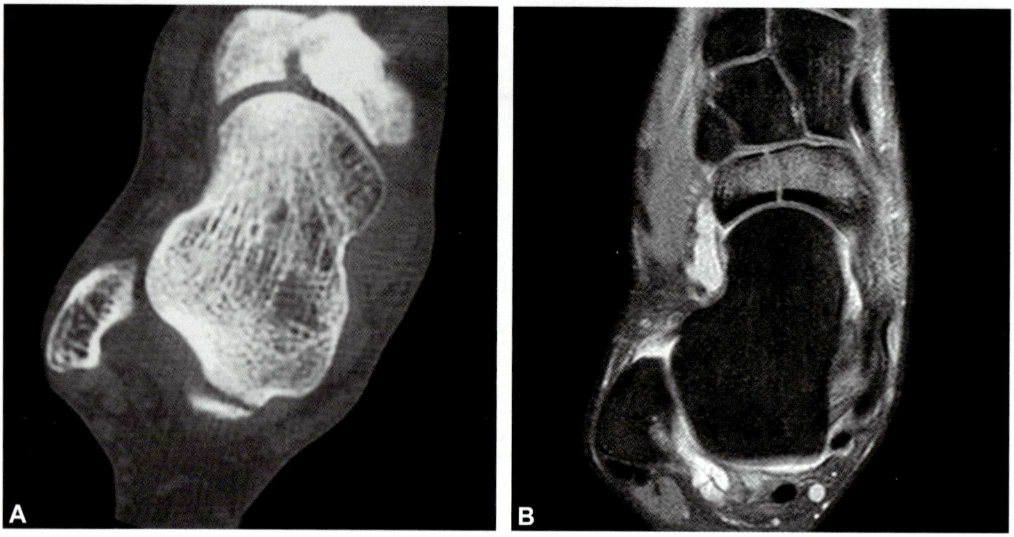

Figs 1A and B: Magnetic resonance imaging (MRI) demonstrating complete stress fracture of navicular

When is it time for Surgery?

For displaced fractures, nondisplaced fractures with sclerotic edges and high level athletes who cannot be out of activity for a prolonged amount of time, these fractures are typically treated operatively. Failure of nonoperative treatment is also an indication for surgical intervention. It should be noted that navicular stress fractures may take up to 6–8 months to completely heal with conservative treatment.[12-14]

What do you tell the Patient?

The patient is given options for treatment depending on the fracture type and the presence or absence of displacement. Radiographic appearance of chronicity such as sclerosis of the fracture margins may indicate an increased chance of a failure of conservative treatment. The other important fact to discuss with the patient is that even though Khan et al. reported 86% success rate with nonoperative treatment, the average time to return to activity was 5.6 months vs 3.8 months for operatively treated fractures.[11,15,16] Depending on the patient's occupation, sport or general activity level, they are informed of these risks of nonunion and restriction of activity.

Operative Treatment

Goals—Achieve union, prevent further displacement and return to activity.

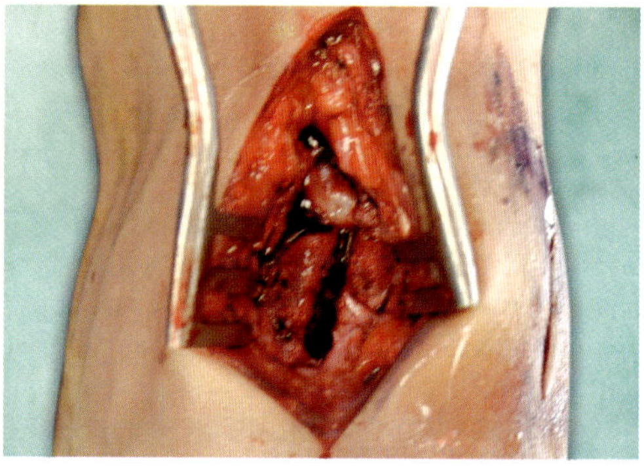

Fig. 2: Defect in tarsal navicular with displacement after bone preparation

Procedure: Operative Technique

Anesthesia: Regional or general anesthesia is used for percutaneous screw fixation of incomplete or complete nondisplaced fractures or for open reduction and internal fixation, when indicated.

Incision/Exposure: A longitudinal incision on the dorsum of the foot overlying the navicular fracture is made. Intraoperative imaging assists in localizing the fracture line. The neurovascular structures are identified and retracted medially while the extensor tendons are retracted laterally. It is frequently necessary to open the talonavicular joint capsule in order to identify the location of the fracture and visualize the degree of involvement, as well as to remove any dorsal loose bodies or debris. A dorsal defect is developed along the fracture line with care taken to preserve the articular joint surfaces.

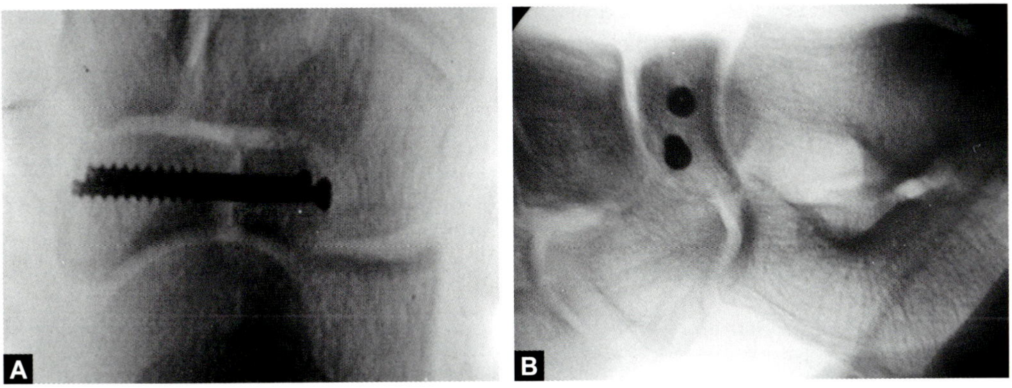

Figs 3A and B: Intraoperative anteroposterior (AP) and lateral radiograph of fixation of navicular stress fracture. Screws are inserted from lateral to medial

This defect can then be filled with autogenous or allogenic bone graft (Fig. 2).

Fixation: Two 4.0–4.5 mm partially threaded screws are placed across the fracture, perpendicular to it. As the fracture is typically in the lateral one third of the navicular, it is preferable to place the screws lateral to medial in order to obtain maximal thread purchase in the larger medial fragment. Care must be undertaken not to place an excessively long screw that may impinge on either the anterior or posterior tibial tendon medially (Figs 3A and B).

Postoperative: The patient is immobilized initially in postoperative splint. Strict non-weight bearing is recommended for the first 6 weeks. In a compliant patient, they are allowed to transition to a boot at 2 weeks but are still non-weight bearing. Immobilization is discontinued at 12 weeks. Impact activities and sport are not allowed until follow-up CT scan documents solid union.

COMPLICATIONS/SALVAGE

Delayed union or nonunion is the most significant complication of the treatment of navicular stress fractures. The diagnosis is made by complaints of continued pain with activity and is typically confirmed by CT scan. Operative intervention involves the usual risks of infection, neurovascular injury and nonunion or delayed union. The development of talonavicular arthrosis is a serious potential outcome of operative and nonoperative management of these patients. The management of this complication can be approached with an isolated talonavicular arthrodesis. Revision of failed screw fixation requires opening the fracture site, curetting the sclerotic bone, drilling the fracture surfaces and bone grafting the fracture/nonunion site. With associated deformities such as cavus and hindfoot varus, osteotomies of the hindfoot (calcaneus) or the forefoot (metatarsals) to alter the weight-bearing stresses within the foot need to be considered. Most often these osteotomies will consist of a valgus-producing calcaneal osteotomy, a dorsiflexion-first metatarsal osteotomy, or both.[8]

REFERENCES

1. Ha K, Hahn S, Chung M, et al. A clinical study of stress fractures in sports activities. Orthopedics. 1991;15:1089-95.
2. Khan K, Brukner P, Kearney C, et al. Tarsal navicular stress fracture in athletes. Sports Med. 1994;17: 65-76.
3. Hunter L. Stress fracture of the tarsal navicular: more frequent than we realize? Am J Sports Med. 1981;9:217-9.
4. Towne L, Blazina M, Cozen L. Fatigue fracture of the tarsal navicular. J Bone Joint Surg. 1970;52A(2): 376-8.
5. Matheson G, Clements D, McKenzie D, et al. Stress fractures in athletes: a study of 320 cases. Am J Sports Med. 1987;15:46-58.
6. Torg J, Pavlov H, Cooley L, et al. Stress fractures of the tarsal navicular: a retrospective review of twenty-one cases. J Bone Joint Surg. 1982;64A:700-12.
7. Kitaoka H, Luo Z, An K. Contact features of the talonavicular joint of the foot. Clin Orthop Relat Res. 1996;325:290-5.
8. Anderson RB, Cohen BE. Stress fractures of the foot and ankle. In: Coughlin M, Mann R, Saltzman C (Eds). Surgery of the Foot and Ankle. 8th ed. Vol II. Philadelphia: Elsevier; 2007. pp.1565-601.

9. Khan K, Fuller P, Brukner P, et al. Outcome of conservative and surgical management of navicular stress fracture in athletes: 86 cases proven with computerized tomography. Am J Sports Med. 1992; 20(6):657-66.
10. Pavlov H, Torg J, Freiberger R. Tarsal navicular stress fractures: radiographic evaluation. Radiology. 1983;148(3):641-5.
11. Kiss Z, Khan K, Fuller P. Stress fractures of the tarsal navicular bone: CT findings in 55 cases. Am J Roentgenol. 1993;160(1):111-5.
12. Saxena A, Fullem B, Hannaford D. Results of treatment of 22 navicular stress fractures and a new proposed radiographic classification system. J Foot Ankle Surg. 2000;39(2):96-103.
13. Fitch K, Blackwell J, Gilmour W. Operation for the non-union of stress fracture of the tarsal navicular. J Bone Joint Surg.1989;71B:105-10.
14. Ting A, King W, Yocum L, et al. Stress fractures of the tarsal navicular in long-distance runners. Clin Sports Med. 1988;7(1):89-101.
15. Goergen T, Venn-Watson E, Rossman D, et al. Tarsal navicular stress fractures in runners. Am J Roentgenol.1981;136:201-3.
16. Coughlin M. Tarsal navicular stress fractures. Techn Foot Ankle Surg. 2002;1(2):112-22.

20 Avascular Necrosis of the Tarsal Navicular

Bruce Cohen

ETIOLOGY

Avascular necrosis of the navicular can occur from different etiologies. The most common etiology is following trauma. This can be high-energy trauma where the typical location of the injury is in the central portion of the navicular often associated with significant comminution. This is the same location where stress fractures of the navicular occur.[1]

Spontaneous osteonecrosis of the navicular can occur and is called Mueller-Weiss disease in adults and Kohler's disease in children. Kohler's disease is typically unilateral and is predominantly seen in males. It is frequently self-limited and rarely requires surgical intervention. Mueller-Weiss disease occurs predominantly in females and is usually bilateral. This uncommon disorder has been classified into five stages: Stage 1—changes seen only on MRI or bone scan; Stage 2—mild compression seen on navicular side; Stage 3—bone fragmentation and arch collapse; Stage 4—increased fragmentation of the navicular with further arch collapse; Stage 5—complete extrusion of the navicular.[2-4]

PATHOPHYSIOLOGY

The central portion of the navicular has poor blood supply which contributes to the risk for osteonecrosis. The vascular supply predominantly arises from small branches of the dorsalis pedis and posterior tibial arteries which well supply the lateral and medial portions respectively. This leaves the central portion in a vascular watershed area.[1]

DIAGNOSIS

The diagnosis of these disorders is similar to that described for navicular stress fractures. The plain radiographs are typically unremarkable in the early stages and the late findings include fragmentation and collapse of the navicular with eventual dorsal extrusion of the navicular with collapse of the longitudinal arch. In the earlier stages, MRI currently is the most useful diagnostic test, while technetium bone scan was historically used. Computed tomography (CT) scans can be helpful in the later stages in evaluating the adjacent joints and the bony fragments and assist in planning arthrodesis procedures.[1,3]

OPTIONS OF MANAGEMENT

Conservative Treatment

In the early stages of the disorder, conservative management consists of rest, immobilization and NSAIDs. This treatment is more symptomatic and may halt or delay progression of the disease. In the more advanced stages of osteonecrosis with nonunited fragments and collapse, conservative management would be reserved for patients who are poor surgical candidates.

When is it time for Surgery?

Surgical treatment is indicated in cases with deformity, loss of longitudinal arch height, collapse of the navicular and significant pain.

What do you tell the Patient?

The patient is informed that this is a progressive deformity. Without proper support of the navicular, the arch will collapse and there will be progressive painful degeneration of the talonavicular and naviculocuneiform joints. For these reasons, surgical intervention should be considered. The patient is also informed of the significant risk of nonunion and need for further surgical procedures with these procedures.

Operative Treatment

Goals—Stabilization of the longitudinal arch, successful union/consolidation of the navicular in early stages, prevention of further deformity and pain.

Procedures

There have been different surgical procedures recommended for the treatment of osteonecrosis of the navicular. In the early stages, treatment has been open bone grafting with internal fixation of the fragments.

Fishman et al. recently described a technique using vascularized pedicle bone grafting for nonunions of the navicular including those with avascular necrosis. A vascularized graft from the cuneiform was used to provide additional vascularized bone to this area. This was used both in addition to fixation of nonunion as well as an adjunct to arthrodesis of the talonavicular joint.[1]

A recent report in the literature describes percutaneous decompression of the navicular for Mueller-Weiss disease. This is a single case report of using techniques similar to core decompression for early stages of femoral head avascular necrosis. This would only be considered for early stage Mueller-Weiss disease without any collapse or significant joint involvement. It should be cautioned that this is an anecdotal report.[5]

Other surgical options that have been described in the literature are primarily arthrodesis procedures. The most commonly described is an arthrodesis of the talonavicular with additional arthrodesis of the naviculocuneiform joint. This is performed with the use a tricortical structural bone graft. The collapsed avascular bone is removed and the region is replaced with a structural graft. Attention is taken to restore the longitudinal arch height and position as well as the medial column length. Fixation options include dorsal plate placement with or without concomitant screw fixation.

COMPLICATIONS

The complications of the treatment of this challenging problem are primarily related to achieving successful bony union. The use of autogenous graft or even the consideration of vascularized grafting can improve union rates. For late cases with deformity, it is critical to restore the foot position, the longitudinal arch height and medial column length to successfully treat this problem. Isolated talonavicular arthrodesis does not address the incongruence at the naviculocuneiform joint and does not provide adequate stability for successful arthrodesis and can lead to pseudoarthrosis. Salvage of failed fixation of the navicular is most reliably addressed with a perinavicular arthrodesis.[3,4]

REFERENCES

1. Fishman FG, Adams SB, Easley ME, et al. Vascularized pedicle bone grafting for nonunions of the tarsal navicular. Foot Ankle Int. 2012;33(9):734-9.
2. Tosun B, Al F, Tosun A. Spontaneous osteonecrosis of the tarsal navicular in an adult: Mueller-Weiss syndrome. J Foot Ankle Surg. 2011;50(2):221-4.
3. Cao HH, Tang KL, Xu JZ. Peri-navicular arthrodesis for the Stage III Muller-Weiss disease. Foot Ankle Int. 2012;33(6):475-8.
4. Yu G, Zhao Y, Zhou J, et al. Fusion of talonavicular and naviculocuneiform joints for the treatment of Mueller-Weiss disease. J Foot Ankle Surg. 2012; 51(4):415-9.
5. Janositz G, Sisak K, Toth K. Percutaneous decompression for the treatment of Mueller-Weiss syndrome. Knee Surg Sports Traumatol Arthorsc. 2011;19:688-90.

SECTION 4

Hindfoot Problems

Chapters Outline

21 Heel Pain Syndrome and Plantar Fasciitis

John S Gould

INTRODUCTION

Plantar heel pain is an extremely common complaint in a general orthopedic practice; however, this condition may have a variety of etiologies. Plantar heel pain occurs primarily in adults but includes all age groups, genders, the active athletic types, and the more sedentary patients. The etiology may include a contusion ("stone bruise"), foreign body, or an infection of the soft tissues or bone, usually from a penetrating wound or even a stress fracture. One of the most frequent diagnoses is plantar fasciitis, an enthesiopathy involving the origin of the plantar fascia. The probable origin of this reaction is minor tears of the ligament at its origin brought on typically from an increase in walking, running, or other activity which places the fascia on stretch.

The presentation is pain on the plantar aspect of the heel at the medial tubercle attachment of the fascia on the medial tubercle of the calcaneus. The pain typically manifests with the first step from bed in the morning or upon arising from a resting position during the day. The pain is momentary and recedes rapidly with further steps. The natural course of the condition is for it to spontaneously remit after a period of about 6 weeks. Recurrences are not infrequent. Various events may lead to a chronic state particularly frank rupture or even attenuation of the ligamentous structure.[1]

The diagnosis is primarily based on the typical history, clinical presentation, and the physical finding of tenderness over the medial tubercle of the calcaneus (Fig. 1). The X-ray is negative for soft tissue or bony changes. The history and the absence of X-ray findings should rule out most other etiologies. An MRI often will show a signal change at the medial tubercle, typical of an enthesiopathy, while aiding in the exclusion of infection or a stress fracture. If the location of the signal change is atypical, a CT scan may be helpful to confirm or deny the fracture. It is important to point out that the origin of the flexor digitorum brevis is a broad bony shelf on the anterior plantar calcaneus which is actually flat on its plantar surface but projects on a lateral X-ray so prominently in some patients that this has been known as a "heel spur". This structure, historically, has been implicated as the "obvious" etiology of the pain and the condition is referred to as the "heel spur syndrome",[2] a flagrantly notorious misnomer for this condition.

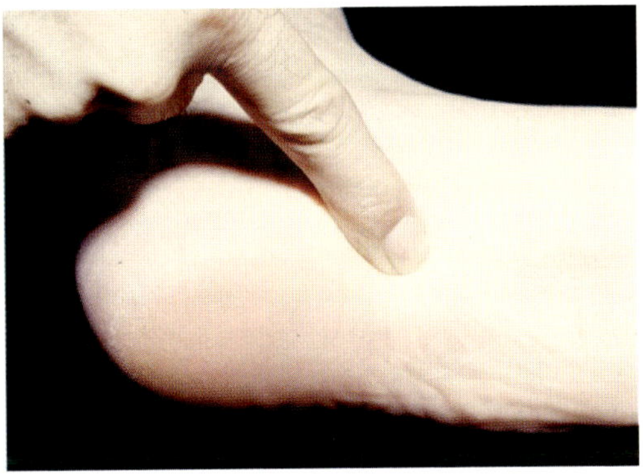

Fig. 1: Location of tenderness over the medial tubercle of the calcaneus

The differential diagnosis should include frank rupture of the plantar fascia and a variety of presentations of the tarsal tunnel syndrome involving the tibial nerve and its branches.[3] This will be discussed in detail in Chapter 44, but it is important to note that prior to the appreciation of a neuritic etiology, pain in the central heel pad, lateral border of the heel, and more distally along the plantar fascia was interpreted as a variation of plantar fasciitis. In addition, these conditions were treated unsuccessfully for plantar fasciitis. An additional issue is that plantar fasciitis can evolve into a chronic state due to attenuation of the plantar fascia, either spontaneously or after steroid injections into it. When this occurs, the history and physical findings change as will be noted in the later section. However, pain in the plantar fascia also occurs and may become unremitting. In the physical examination of the plantar fascia, the ankle is dorsiflexed along with the great toe, and the medial edge of the fascia is palpated and compared to the uninvolved contralateral side. A distinct medial border of the fascia is the norm from the plantar aspect of the great toe metatarsophalangeal joint essentially to the calcaneus. Defects may be palpated along with an indistinct edge with rupture and attenuation.

CONSERVATIVE MANAGEMENT

Plantar fascia stretching exercises are the hallmark of treatment. This can be accomplished in several ways, including standing with the involved foot more posteriorly, the heel on the floor, and leaning forward with the arms extended to a wall. Baumhauer, DiGiovanni, et al. demonstrated that anatomy specific stretching of the fascia by the patient in a seated position, crossing the legs, and dorsiflexing the great toe and ankle while massaging the plantar fascia on stretch was particularly effective.[4] Heel cups, over-the-counter orthotic devices, and oral anti-inflammatories are also routine treatment modalities. Taping of the foot, binding the fascia, and the use of ice has also been recommended. Injection of the plantar fascia origin with steroid preparations has been a standard of care by many practitioners. It is such a common practice in the United States that it is difficult to condemn it. While it is effective in relieving the initial episode, the incidence of fascial rupture and the development of a chronic state, while undocumented, are frequently seen among orthopedic foot and ankle specialists causing the author to recommend against its use. Iontophoresis and phonophoresis, physical therapy modalities in which steroids on the plantar surface are transmitted to the target fascia using electrolysis or ultrasound, seem to have a far lower incidence of rupture.

OPERATIVE TREATMENT

As a rule, the author tends to avoid surgical treatment of pure plantar fasciitis. The customary treatment is to release the plantar fascia origin through a small medial incision. As the release of the plantar fascia is associated with dorsal arch and lateral border pain with immediate ambulation, most authors recommend release only of the medial band of the fascia. In addition, there is an endoscopic technique in which the fascia is released through a very small medial portal. The author's objection to these approaches is the significant incidence of chronic pain mimicking symptoms after a frank incomplete rupture, or the development of neuropathic pain due to traction on the tibial nerve and branches. Consequently, the release carried out, and described in Chapter 44, is a complete release of the plantar fascia and the distal tarsal tunnel. The outcome of such releases approaches 95% complete relief without recurrence.[3]

COMPLICATIONS

The primary complication of treatment of plantar fasciitis is failure to relieve the condition and /or the development of a chronic neuritic condition. Ruptured plantar fascia responds to complete release, but the possibility of developing traction neuritis requires the distal tarsal tunnel release be done as well.

REFERENCES

1. Gould JS. Chronic plantar fasciitis. Am J Orth. 2003;32(1):11-3.
2. Johal KS, Milner SA. Plantar fasciitis and the calcaneal spur: fact or fiction? Foot Ankle Surg. 2012;18(1):39-41.
3. Labib SA, Gould JS, Rodriguez del Rio FA, et al. Heel pain triad: the combination of plantar fasciitis, posterior tibial tendon dysfunction, and tarsal tunnel syndrome. Foot Ankle Int. 2002;23(11):1054.
4. DiGiovanni BF, Nawoczenski DA, Lintal ME, et al. Tissue-specific plantar fascia-stretching exercise enhances outcomes in patients with chronic heel pain: a prospective, randomized study. J Bone Joint Surg Am. 2003;85-A(7):1270-7.

22

Subtalar and Transverse Tarsal Arthritis

John S Gould

INTRODUCTION

Hindfoot and apparent "ankle pain" may originate in the subtalar and transverse tarsal joints. While a dislocation or fracture involving these joints may be an etiology for the arthritis, particularly with calcaneal fractures and the subtalar joint, the spontaneous development of arthritis in these areas is by far the most common. Tarsal coalitions may account for a few, and avascular necrosis of the tarsal navicular, either spontaneous or traumatic, may be the source of a few more. Ankle, actually subtalar, instability due to trauma especially with frequent sprains may account for a few more. Both posterior tibial tendon dysfunction with the valgus foot and the cavus foot with multiple etiologies may account for arthritic changes in this joint complex. The presentation is pain in this area especially with attempted walking on uneven ground.

The diagnosis is suspected by the history of the presentation and the physical examination with tenderness over the talonavicular and calcaneocuboid joints and in the sinus tarsi over the posterior facet of the subtalar joint. Inversion/eversion and adduction/abduction (also known as supination/pronation of the foot) may show limited motion and pain when carried out passively. X-rays may show narrowing and osteophyte formation at the joint(s) and CT scans are definitive. The findings include narrowing of the joint, osteophytes, and subchondral cysts. An MRI will demonstrate signal changes indicative of bone edema adjacent to the joints.

CONSERVATIVE TREATMENT

The UCBL (University of California Berkeley Laboratories) orthotic device is designed to control motion in the hindfoot (Fig. 1). Using this device in a shoe with a good heel counter is the conservative treatment of choice. Although there are multiple more restrictive braces, including those which restrict the ankle, if the prescription is properly filled and fitted with a good shoe, this approach should be as good or better than any other option.[1] When this approach is unsuccessful, the adjacent ankle is uninvolved, and the patient has been compliant, surgery may be the next option.

SURGICAL TREATMENT

The primary option for relief of pain in these arthritic joints is arthrodesis. There is some controversy concerning which joints may be amenable to a successful solo fusion and there are a plethora of techniques described, both currently and historically, in the literature.[2]

Most authors concede that a solitary arthrodesis of the subtalar joint may be appropriate; some will do a solitary talonavicular fusion; and few attempt to do a solitary calcaneocuboid fusion,[3] citing the high incidence of nonunion when this is attempted. It is also important to know that subtalar fusions are more likely to fail when there is an adjacent

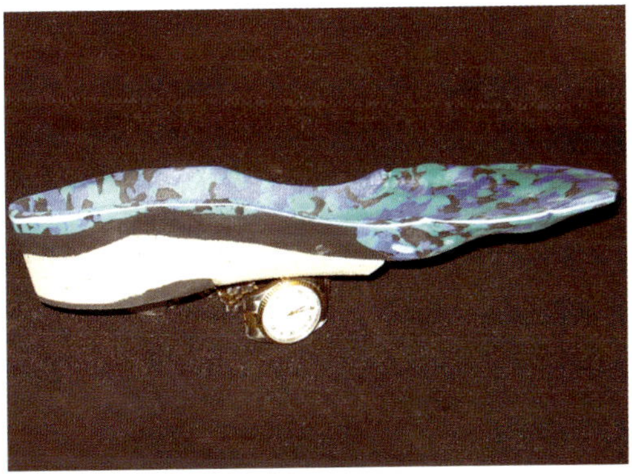

Fig. 1: The UCBL (University of California Berkeley Laboratories) insert (orthotic device) to control hindfoot motion

ankle fusion or a subtalar coalition; and that when attempting to fuse the talonavicular and the adjacent naviculocuneiform joints simultaneously, there are more failures at one site or another. Obtaining fusion is also more problematic when there are metabolic, vascular, and neuropathic factors in play, as in collagen disorder patients on steroids, avascular necrosis, and diabetic neuropathy.[4] These situations require variations in technique, use of adjunctive measures, and a change in postoperative care from the usual. These will be discussed in the relevant chapters.

Arthrodesis may be done in situ when the joint is anatomically aligned in neutral but has lost its normal articular surface. Often times restoration of alignment is required with possible use of wedges and/or osteotomies. These adjuncts are particularly important in posterior tibial tendon dysfunction, cavus, and post-traumatic cases. The variations and adjuncts will be described with the surgical corrections for these diagnoses. Positioning for the surgery and the hardware used for fixation will vary according to the requirements for each correction.

The fundamental axioms for a successful arthrodesis are careful, thorough preparation of the joint surfaces and strong compression hardware fixation. The use of adjuncts to stimulate bone formation with bone autograft as the "gold standard"[5] is usually recommended for these joints. It is always important to remember that earlier attempts for fusion of these joints involved only the preparation of the surfaces, without hardware, without adjuncts, and using casts postoperatively. Although malalignment and nonunions were frequent, many went on to successful fusion.[6] The point for emphasis is that the fixation and adjuncts have provided a more predictable outcome.

SUBTALAR ARTHRODESIS

The patient is supine with a sizable bump under the affected side hip. The hip and knee are flexed and a roll placed against the popliteal space to maintain the knee flexion. A curvilinear incision is made over the sinus tarsi beginning just below the tip of the fibula, extending obliquely across the sinus tarsi, and curving back plantar at the upper distal corner of the sinus (Fig. 2). The deep incision is made just above the peroneal tendons along the anterior process of the calcaneus, extending posteriorly and falling into the floor of the sinus tarsi (Fig. 3). The deep knife continues to the back wall of the sinus, meeting the lateral process of the talus where it sweeps dorsally dividing fat pad attachments. The extensor digitorum brevis is lifted off the anterior process of the calcaneus and the fat pad, still attached to the proximal origin of the muscle, is swept out of the sinus tarsi. At the closure, the muscle and still attached fat pad may be laid back in place, eliminating any dead space. The posterior facet of the subtalar joint is now exposed anteriorly and the sinus tarsi almost fully exposed. Small amounts of remaining fat pad remnants are removed with a rongeur. The posterior facet is opened to denude the articular surfaces. This may be accomplished with a narrow osteotome, elevator, laminar spreader, or Hintermann distracter. The author uses a sharp curved osteotome to essentially peel or scrape remaining cartilage and fibrous tissue from the bony surfaces. It is important to remove this soft tissue from both the upper and lower facets and particularly from the rims. When this is done properly and the distraction released, the facet should fall together. The subchondral surfaces

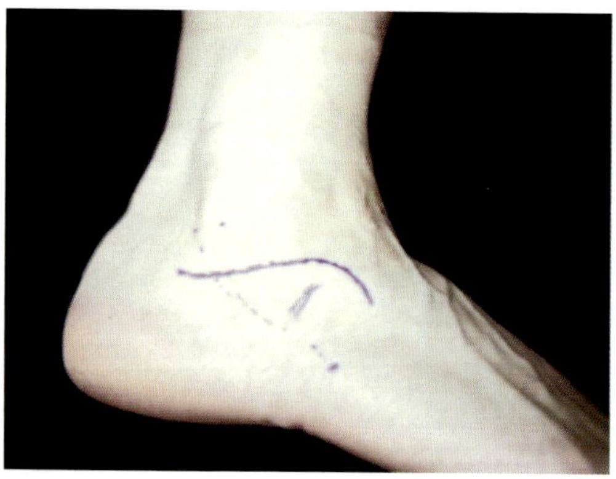

Fig. 2: The sinus tarsi incision for the subtalar fusion

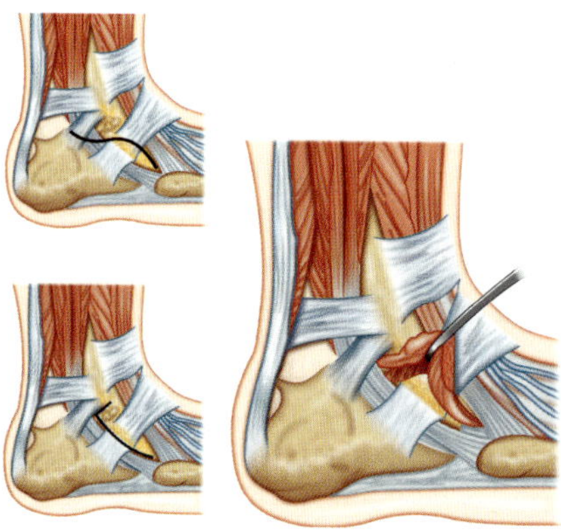

Fig. 3: The deep incision parallel to the peroneal tendons into the sinus tarsi, elevating the extensor digitorum brevis and fat pad

should be broached with the osteotome, a punch, or by drilling with a K-wire. The middle facet is visualized by placing a laminar spreader into the sinus tarsi. The facet is cleared of cartilage with curettes (Fig. 4). No effort is made to prepare the anterior facet except in tarsal subtalar coalitions and this will be discussed later. Many surgeons prepare only the posterior facet and may do so through an even more limited exposure. Bone graft or bone graft substitute is then placed in the facets and sinus tarsi.

The bump is removed from the hip and roll from the knee and the patient returned to a full supine position. A second incision is made anteromedially to expose the neck of the talus. The incision is made between the anterior tibial tendon and the extensor hallucis longus, centered over the talar neck (Fig. 5). This point is determined by drawing a line from the tip of the medial malleolus anteriorly and dorsally to where it meets the line between the tendons anteromedially. The deep incision divides the extensor retinaculum and continues to the bone staying directly anterior/posterior and avoiding the neurovascular structures under the extensor hallucis longus. Only a few crossing veins are encountered in the path to the bone. The heel is elevated with towels and the fluoroscope is draped and brought into the field to obtain a sagittal view of the talus and calcaneus. The surgeon stands at the foot of the table facing the video monitor while the assistant retracts. A guidewire for a 7.3 mm or similar sized cannulated cancellous screw is placed on the fovea in the medial/lateral midline in the neck of the talus, just distal to the articular surface, directed toward the posterior-inferior portion of the tubercle of the calcaneus. The pin in the power driver is held in the dominant hand while the heel is placed in a few degrees of valgus with the opposite hand (Fig. 6). The midpoint of the heel is held in the midpalm of the surgeon. The pin is driven across the subtalar joint, toward the midpoint of the surgeon's palm. (Intuitively, if the point of the heel is in the mid palm, the pin will be directly pointed to the correct spot). The position of the pin is confirmed with fluoroscopy. If the direction of the pin is correct, the hip is flexed farther and the valgus position of the heel verified by noting its position relative to the leg from the posterior view. A Saltzman[7] view, which is a tangential view of the heel, includes the distal tibia and will demonstrate the heel position and confirm the desired valgus. If the foot position and pin are correct, the pin is advanced to the inner plantar cortex. A tangential view is obtained by fluoroscopy. If the pin is well aligned, the depth gauge is used to determine screw length, the pin is overdrilled at least across the subtalar joint and farther if the bone is particularly hard, tapped if desired, and the permanent screw inserted and compressed. Screw position is assessed again with both views and the images are saved. The author

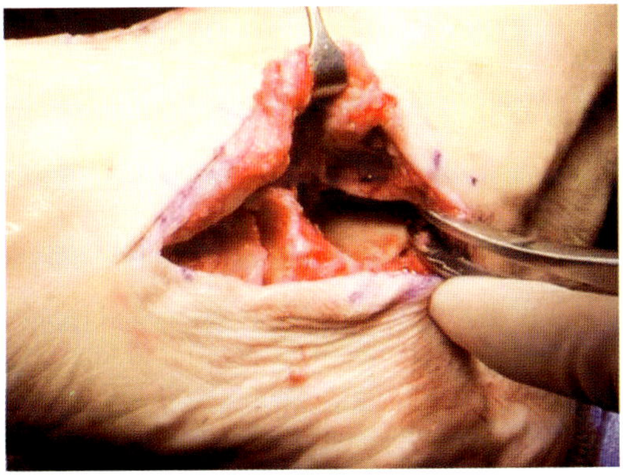

Fig. 4: The posterior facet of the subtalar joint is prepared and the calcaneocuboid joint when a triple arthrodesis is also being done

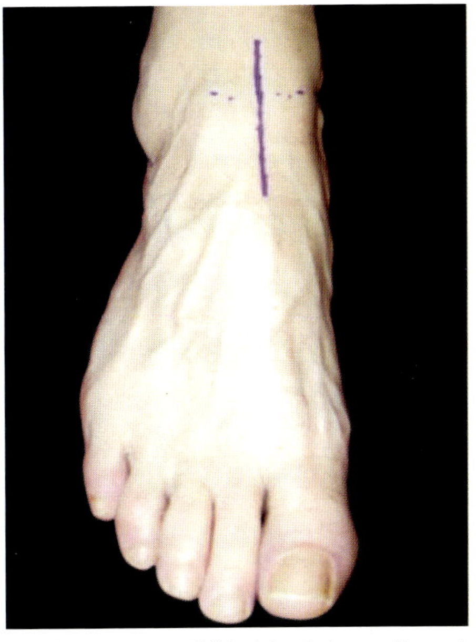

Fig. 5: The anteromedial incision between the anterior tibial tendon and the extensor hallucis longus, centered over the line made anteriorly from the tip of the medial malleolus

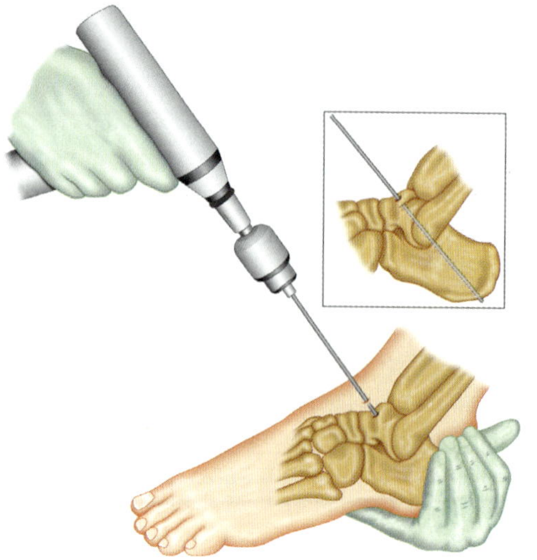

Fig. 6: Technique for placing the guidepin through the neck of the talus, using the special technique of directing the pin toward the midpalm of the nondominant hand

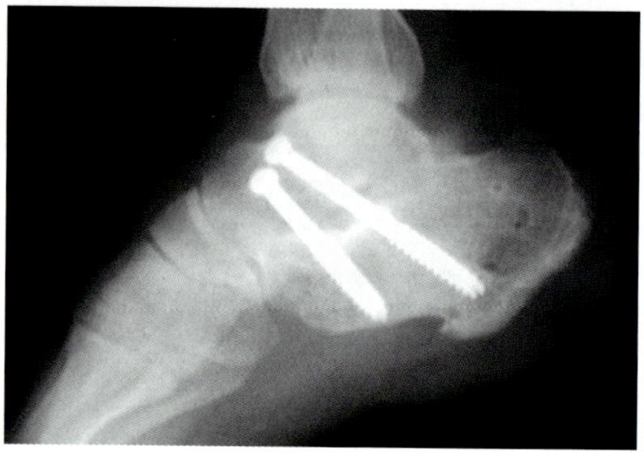

Fig. 7: Subtalar fusion with screws placed from neck of talus

uses a second screw starting more medially and distally, aiming more laterally and vertically into the anterior process of the calcaneus (Fig. 7). The more proximal screw must be flush with the cortex to assure that it does not impinge on the tibia with dorsiflexion of the ankle.

Another option for fixation of the subtalar joint is to insert the screws in a parallel fashion from the heel across the subtalar joint into the body and neck of the talus.[8] Insertion into the heel with the patient in the supine position is awkward, so if this method of fixation is preferred, it is far easier to place the patient in the lateral decubitus position with the operative site superior and the lower opposite knee flexed. The exposure of the joint and the insertion of the screws can be done from the seated position. For the screw insertion, the surgeon is seated facing the monitor, and the fluoroscopy camera is placed in the anterior/posterior position to obtain the sagittal view. The tangential view is a little more difficult to obtain and can be obtained either by X-raying the heel when the hip is markedly externally rotated, or more usually by placing the camera for a lateral view and aiming obliquely across the heel from proximal to distal. Pull out studies in our laboratories have confirmed that the strength of fixation of the screws are essentially the same whether they are inserted from the neck or the heel. In the next section, the use of a calcaneal osteotomy concomitant with the subtalar fusion will be discussed. In this situation, the insertion from the heel is required. Another indication for the heel insertion would be the threat of avascular necrosis of the talus with a dorsal approach after a subtalar dislocation has occurred and is the etiology of the subtalar arthritis. The disadvantages of the heel insertion is the potential prominence of the screw heads and need for later removal, an issue which can be avoided by the use of headless screws and other heads which can be buried in the plantar bone. The arguments to go dorsal or plantar are unresolved, and it becomes "surgeon preference" unless there is a specific indication to go one way or another as indicated.

The closure is completed and the patient placed in a bulky dressing with a fiberglass shell which is bivalved in the operating room. It should be noted that the author uses a tourniquet, inflated after the skin is marked and releases it following application of the bulky dressing and prior to application of the fiberglass. The sutures are removed at 2 weeks with application of a short leg non-weight-bearing cast. X-rays are taken in the clinic at 2 and 6 weeks. At 6 weeks, a walking cast is applied with X-rays 2 weeks later. If all is well, a removable boot is provided to be worn for 4 more weeks and the patient mobilized at 3 months postoperatively.

TALONAVICULAR ARTHRODESIS

This fusion is done using the anteromedial incision described above between the anterior tibial tendon and the extensor hallucis longus with an extension more distally to the naviculocuneiform joint level. The patient is supine and a tourniquet is again used. Although the appearance of the neck of the talus is usually adequate for orientation, it is always wise for the less experienced surgeon or any surgeon when the anatomy is distorted by trauma or extensive disease to confirm the location of the joints with fluoroscopy prior to proceeding with preparation of the joint for fusion. Although the convex/concave shape of the talonavicular joint is relatively easy to identify, dorsal spurs and bone bridges can be confusing and the surgeon can find himself/herself too distal at the naviculocuneiform level. Consequently, the advice above should be heeded. The joint is distracted and the preparation begun with a curved osteotome followed by curettes and breaching of the subchondral bone with the osteotome, a bone punch, or K-wire. Bone graft or substitute is inserted and fixation achieved. Several fixation options can be considered. Longitudinally placed 4.5 screws begun at the naviculocuneiform level is one option. A notchplasty is carried out at the distal edge of the navicular bone and a half threaded screw is placed over a guidepin after using the depth gauge and drill. In this fusion, it is essential to position the joint in neutral abduction/adduction and pronation/supination. This is assessed with the perspective of looking at the foot from the toes proximally. An anterior/posterior X-ray of the foot helps with the adduction/abduction, but the clinical perspective is essential. The first and fifth metatarsal heads and bases should be in an equally prominent position on the plantar foot. The author also prefers to place Hintermann compression pins and forceps across the joint to obtain the compression prior to insertion of the first screw. If correction of alignment was needed, a temporary pin may be used to hold the position prior to fixation. A second fully threaded pin is inserted across the joint to control rotation. If necessary, a third screw can be placed percutaneously from the prominent medial navicular across the joint.

The author prefers, particularly in soft bone, to use a plate across the talonavicular joint rather than screws. Several are available which provide compression, locking and nonlocking screws, and the like. Using Hintermann compression initially, the author prefers a plate which provides the ability to be compressed against the bone and has variable angle locking screw holes. These seem to provide control of rotational forces and excellent fixation. At the completion of the procedure, the same dressing is used as with the subtalar fusion and the same postoperative regimen.

TALONAVICULAR AND CALCANEOCUBOID ARTHRODESIS

The talonavicular joint is exposed as described above. The calcaneocuboid joint is exposed through a curvilinear incision which could be an extension of the subtalar incision if one were doing a triple arthrodesis. It crosses the joint with equal arms over the calcaneal anterior process and the cuboid. Following distraction and preparation of the joint, fixation is carried out. While longitudinal screw fixation is an option, plate and screw fixation is superior in this relatively soft bone. After joint preparation, alignment is the first concern. In addition, it is essential not to remove more bone from either joint or one of the two will not come together. Essentially, no bone is removed, the surfaces are prepared, the subchondral bone is breached, and the bones fixed after adding adjunct graft. The author provides fixation of the talonavicular joint first and then the calcaneocuboid joint. Frequently, when there has been realignment, the two surfaces of the calcaneus and cuboid are not flush. This is corrected with a burr and then the compression and plate are placed. The preferred plate is the same as the one used with the talonavicular joint. If a bone wedge is needed in the calcaneocuboid joint, it is placed prior to the fixation. The postoperative management for this fusion is the same as that used in the above fusions.

TRIPLE ARTHRODESIS

With a triple arthrodesis, all three joints are fused. The curvilinear incision across the sinus tarsi is extended to include the calcaneocuboid joint (see Fig. 4), and the approach anteromedially between the anterior tibial and extensor hallucis longus is extended to the naviculocuneiform level. The subtalar joint and the calcaneocuboid joints are exposed and prepared and the adjunct placed. The bump is removed from the hip and the patient returned to the supine position. The anteromedial approach is completed and the talonavicular joint prepared. The subtalar joint is fixed initially, followed by the talonavicular and the calcaneocuboid. As indicated above, in subtalar fixation, correction of varus/valgus is the critical point; while the transverse tarsal fixation is done with correction of adduction/

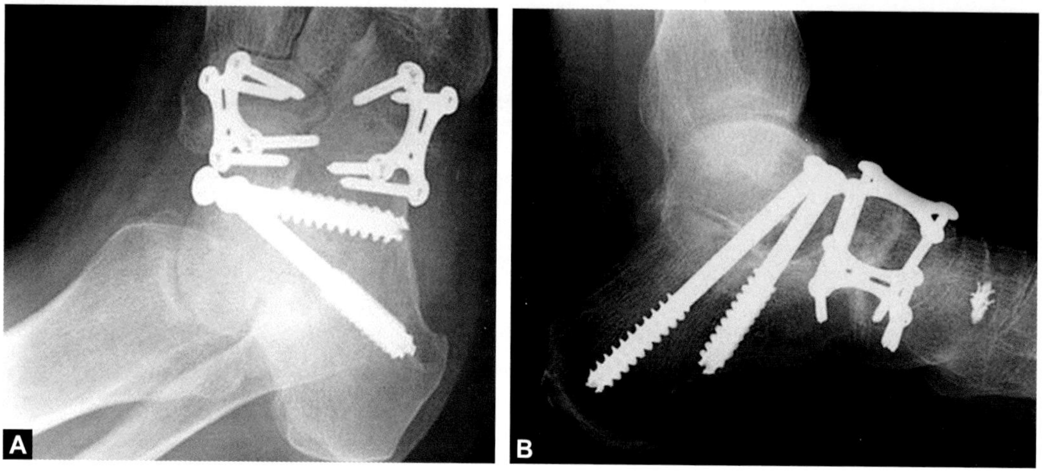

Figs 8A and B: Triple arthrodesis with compression plating of the transverse tarsal joints, (A) Anterior/posterior view of the foot; (B) Sagittal view

abduction and pronation/supination (Figs 8A and B). The postoperative regimen is identical to the previous three.

COMPLICATIONS AND SALVAGE

Malunion and nonunion are the typical complications.[9,10] Inadequate pronation of the foot distal to the transverse tarsal joints is the most common problem. The patient complains of pressure under the base of the fifth metatarsal. Although shaving of the base of the fifth metatarsal is an option, a takedown of the transverse tarsal joint is the best solution with proper pronation of the joints achieved.

Alternatively, the base of the fifth metatarsal is not a problem, but the patient complains that the great toe metatarsal does not take enough pressure and the head of the fifth metatarsal is too prominent. The Cotton plantar flexion osteotomy of the medial cuneiform, as discussed in Chapter 23, will bring the first metatarsal into alignment. The same osteotomy through the base of the first metatarsal is an alternative, although this leaves the medial dorsal surface of the foot a little too prominent.

Nonunions are relatively uncommon if the techniques described above are used. If only one screw was used for the subtalar joint, repreparation, bone graft, and two screws will probably be successful.[8] The use of plates, compression, better preparation, and bone graft should resolve nonunions in the transverse tarsal joints. On occasion, double plates may be used for talonavicular nonunions. Bone marrow concentrate may be used as an adjunct when operating on nonunions along with the use of bone stimulators in the postoperative period. A variety of bone stimulation techniques are available.

REFERENCES

1. Scranton PE. An overview of ankle arthrodesis. Clin Orthop. 1991;268:96-101.
2. Mann RA, Van Manen JW, Wapner K, et al. Ankle fusion. Clin Orthop. 1991;268:49-55.
3. Deland JT, Otis JC, Lee KT, et al. Lateral column lengthening with calcaneocuboid fusion: range of motion in the triple joint complex. Foot Ankle. 1995;16:729-33.
4. Frey C, Halikus NM, Vu-Rose T, et al. A review of ankle arthrodesis: predisposing factors to nonunion. Foot Ankle Int. 1994;15:581-4.
5. Davies MB, Rosenfeld PF, Stavrou P, et al. A comprehensive review of subtalar arthrodesis. Foot Ankle Int. 2007;28(3):295-7.
6. Angus PD, Cowell HR. Triple arthrodesis: a critical long-term review. J Bone Joint Surg Br. 1986; 68(2):260-5.
7. Saltzman CL, el-Khoury GY. The hindfoot alignment view. Foot Ankle Int. 1995 ;16(9):572-6.
8. Chuckpaiwong B, Easley ME, Glisson RR. Screw placement in subtalar arthrodesis: a biomechanical study. Foot Ankle Int. 2009;30(2):133-41.
9. Scranton PE. Results of arthrodesis of the tarsus: talocalcaneal, midtarsal, and subtalar joints. Foot Ankle. 1991;12:156-64.
10. Sangeorzan BJ, Smith D, Veith R, et al. Triple arthrodesis using internal fixation in treatment of adult foot disorders. Clin Orthop Relat Res. 1993; 294:299-307.

23

Posterior Tibial Tendon Dysfunction

John S Gould

INTRODUCTION

The development of a unilateral flat foot with collapse of the medial arch, hindfoot and midfoot, occurring primarily in middle age women, is a complex process and far more involved anatomically than the term "posterior tibial tendon dysfunction" implies. The classic description of this disorder begins with a tenosynovitis of the posterior tibial tendon, followed by tendinosis, and finally rupture of the structure. In the meantime, the other supporting structures of the posteromedial foot and ankle deteriorate, attenuate, and eventually give way. Johnson's classic stages included an inflammatory reaction of the posterior tibial tendon in Stage 1; collapse of the arch which was passively correctible in Stage 2; and a fixed deformity in Stage 3 (Fig. 1).[1] The more current classifications provide more detail and suggest remedial surgery based on the failed anatomic structures.[2,3] Biomechanically, the heel falls into valgus while the transverse tarsal joint becomes abducted, translated laterally, and supinated. The collapsed medial foot deformities in rheumatoid arthritis and the neuropathic foot are similar, but the effects on the anatomy are far more destructive and will be discussed in those sections.

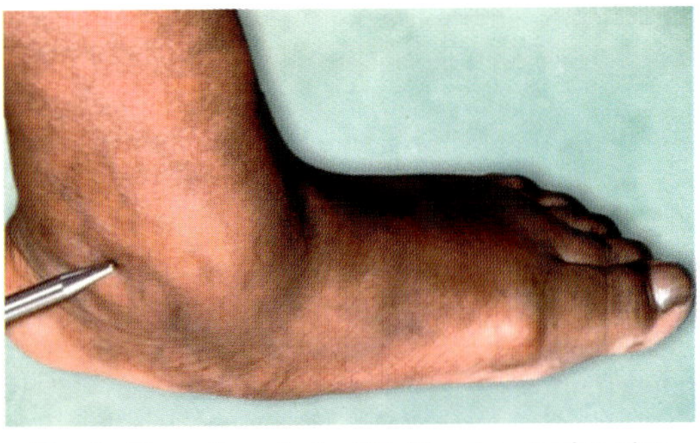

Fig. 1: Stage 3 posterior tibial tendon dysfunction

The physical findings will be discussed at each stage of the progressive condition. Palpation for tenderness at the subtalar and transverse tarsal joints will suggest joint inflammation and possible arthritis. Standard X-rays of the foot including a tangential view of the calcaneus and the Saltzman view as discussed earlier are essential. A CT scan is also essential in stages 2, 3 and 4. As the deformity worsens, a three-dimensional CT will help demonstrate the exact position of the anatomy, including subfibular impingement.

STAGE 1

The patient complains of posteromedial ankle pain, which begins insidiously, and a fullness and swelling behind the medial malleolus extending to the medial prominence of the tarsal navicular. The symptoms are continuous and increased by activity. The diagnosis may be made on history and physical examination. Tenderness, fullness and crepitus are noted on palpation of the posterior tibial tendon. The single leg toe-up test is used to further confirm the impression. Observed from behind, the patient is asked to stand on one leg and to proceed to a tip toe position on this foot. In the normal patient, with a little support by the examiner for balance, patients can perform this toe up and the heel is noted to invert simultaneously. In the pathologic state, due to pain and weakness, the patient is unable to toe up; or, if he/she can go up on tip toe, the heel does not invert. It is important not to allow the patient to lean forward on his/her hands, which allows spurious simulation of the desired maneuver.

Typically, many patients respond to a brief period of immobilization, followed by the use of a well-padded UCBL (University of California Berkeley Laboratories) insert for the shoe. The author typically has the patient begin to use the orthotic device as soon as it has been fabricated.[4,5]

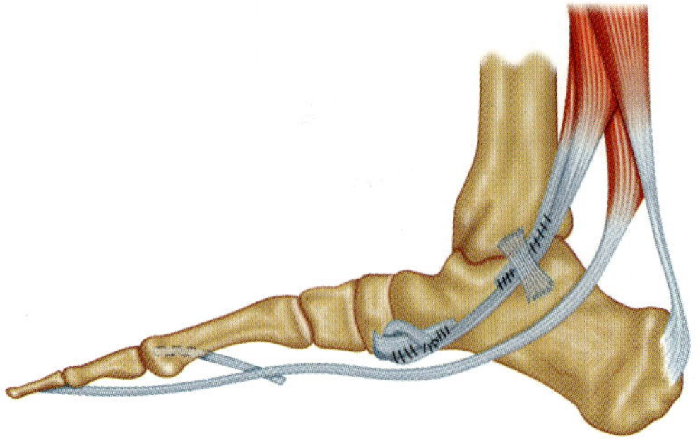

Fig. 2: Flexor digitorum longus transfer for deficient posterior tibial tendon dysfunction. Note that the author typically places the tendon through a drill hole from plantar to dorsal in the medial tubercle of the tarsal navicular. This procedure is done in conjunction with a medial displacement osteotomy of the calcaneus or a subtalar fusion

When the patient fails to respond, or the plateau reached is not satisfactory, surgery is indicated.

Through a posteromedial incision which follows the distal tendon (from the tip of the medial malleolus to the insertion on the medial navicular), the tendon sheath is opened and the tendon debrided. As the author has never found this maneuver alone to be sufficient, he also carries out procedures which are indicated for Early Stage 2 patients: the transfer of the flexor digitorum communis tendon into the tarsal navicular (Fig. 2) and the medial displacement osteotomy of the calcaneus, which are described below.

STAGE 2 (EARLY)

Patients at this level have the symptoms and signs of patients at Stage 1, but also have collapse of the arch or medial sag with abduction of the foot. The deformity is flexible and normal shape resumes with non-weight bearing. Viewed from behind, the patient's weight-bearing foot demonstrates the "too many toes sign", noted by Johnson.[1] A patient who has contraindications to or refuses surgery at this stage, can be treated with the UCBL orthosis. Otherwise, this is a surgical condition.

Medial Displacement Calcaneal Osteotomy and Flexor Digitorum Communis Transfer into the Tarsal Navicular

The patient is placed in the lateral decubitus position exposing the lateral calcaneus on the superior leg. A "beanbag" positioner is used to maintain the lateral alignment of the patient. A tourniquet is placed on the thigh and the fluoroscope camera is positioned in the anterior/posterior position for sagittal views. Using fluoroscopic control and a 7.3 mm cannulated screw guidepin, the osteotomy line is marked on the skin with a marking pencil. The line across the calcaneus is made parallel to the peroneal tendons and midway between the subtalar joint and the posterior edge of the calcaneal tubercle. The direction for the parallel screws, which will be used for fixation, is also marked on the skin. It is essential that the heel is absolutely flat on the operating table cushion in order that the fluoroscopic views are not distorted.

The incision is made to the bone and a subperiosteal exposure is made which allows a small Hohmann retractor to be placed around the plantar and superior borders of the bone in the line of the intended osteotomy. Using a wide osteotome, the alignment of the osteotomy is again checked with fluoroscopy, and the bone cortex is subsequently grooved with the osteotome. The osteotomy is then made with a microsagittal saw to the depth of the inner medial cortex. The osteotomy is completed with small osteotomes, being careful not to "plunge" into the medial structures including the neurovascular anatomy.

Laminar spreaders are used to open the osteotomy, in order to complete any undivided medial, dorsal, or plantar cortex and finally to gently stretch the medial soft tissues. Without this maneuver, the medial shift is very difficult to accomplish. The plantar fragment is then displaced medially by the operator's thumb and fingers. The overlap of the fragments should be in the range of 5–10 mm. Fixation is achieved with two parallel 7.3 mm cannulated cancellous screws, using standard technique. The pins are inserted through the heel with the operator seated, facing the fluoroscope monitor. After the two pins are placed, while the reduction is maintained (by the surgeon or his assistant) and is satisfactory on the sagittal view, a tangential view is obtained to view the placement of the pins and the displacement achieved. The amount of displacement can also be measured directly in the wound. If not satisfactory, the pins or displacement are adjusted. The first pin length is assessed, overdrilled, and the screw inserted and compressed. The same steps are carried out for the second pin. The second pin should not be overdrilled until the first screw is placed, as the displacement achieved may be lost by carrying out this maneuver for both pins simultaneously. The lateral wound is closed in layers.

The "beanbag" is released, the patient rolled to the supine position and the tendon transfer performed.

Through a posteromedial incision, the posterior tibial tendon is debrided, but usually not discarded. The sheath of the flexor digitorum communis (FDC), located plantar and deep to the posterior tibial, is opened to the level of the naviculocuneiform joint. The FDC is divided after the foot is inverted and the toes flexed to obtain maximum length. The FDC is moved into the residual sheath of the posterior tibial tendon. The dorsal surface of the medial tubercle of the tarsal navicular is exposed and a drill hole made from dorsal to plantar and, from the proximal/distal midpoint of the bone, from distal to proximal. The anatomy of the talonavicular joint should be noted to avoid entering the joint in the dorsal to plantar pass of the small drill. Fluoroscopic guidance is advised. The hole is enlarged with increasingly larger drills. A Hewson suture passer is placed from dorsal to plantar and a "whip" stitch is taken through the end of the FDC tendon. The suture ends are placed through the passer and the device withdrawn dorsally, pulling the tendon through the bone. While the foot is placed into inversion, significant tension is placed on the tendon and it is secured in place by suturing the FDC to the tendon of the posterior tibial with 2-0 or 3-0 permanent suture just proximal to the plantar entrance of the FDC into the bone. The dorsal FDC tendon is sutured into the periosteum. While standard tendon tensioning is done by placing the foot in neutral and setting the tendon at about 60% of its elastic excursion when applying first zero pull and then 100% pull on the structure,[6] experience has shown that in this transfer and often elsewhere in the foot, the tension should be somewhat greater. When the tension has been set and the foot relaxed, it should remain slightly inverted. Bone anchors and interference screws are alternative means of fixation. Postoperatively, immobilization for these procedures should be for 6 weeks and then the patient should wear a UCBL orthosis for about 9 months.

STAGE 2 (MID-RANGE)

Many of these patients are less flexible and do not fully return to a neutral arch position with non-weight bearing. They are frequently post-menopausal women and many are overweight. For this population, the author finds that a subtalar fusion (described in Chapter 22) rather than a medial displacement osteotomy of the calcaneus, along with the FDC transfer is more successful.

STAGE 2 (LATE)

In these patients, the heel remains flexible, but the midfoot has some fixed supination. This is most notable when the heel is passively brought back to neutral. This supination is a compensatory position secondary to the heel valgus.[7] In these cases, the author performs the subtalar fusion, the tendon transfer, and a dorsal wedge medial cuneiform osteotomy (Cotton).

Cotton Osteotomy

The medial cuneiform is exposed either straight dorsally or medial. The author prefers the dorsal approach. The locations of the naviculocuneiform and cuneiform-first metatarsal joints are identified clinically, as well as the joint between the medial and middle cuneiforms. Fluoroscopic control is helpful. The osteotomy is performed with a microsagittal saw, dorsal to plantar transversely across the midpoint of the cuneiform. The plantar cortex is creased by the saw and wedged open from the dorsum with a laminar spreader. The plantar soft tissues are not disturbed. The goal is to wedge down the distal-first metatarsal to the level of the fifth metatarsal head. There are several commercially available wedge plates used for this purpose with varying wedge width. There are also wedges available in various synthetic materials including tantalum for this procedure as well. Traditionally, the author has used a triangular wedge of either autogenous or more recently allograft bone taken from a segment of iliac crest. Fixation is achieved with a small plate and screws or an oblique 3.5 mm screw (Fig. 3).

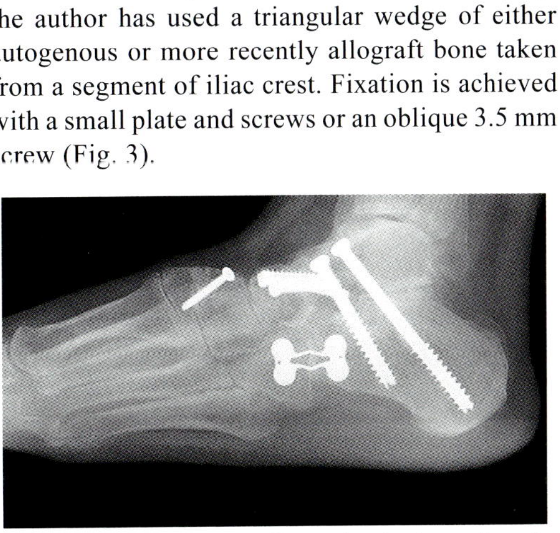

Fig. 3: Medial cuneiform (Cotton) osteotomy done in conjunction with a triple arthrodesis

STAGE 3

In this stage, the deformities are fixed, with the heel in valgus, the foot distal to the transverse tarsal joints abducted and supinated. There may be subfibular impingement between the valgus calcaneus and the tip of the fibula. The required surgery is a triple arthrodesis; however, the goal of surgery is to restore, as well as possible, the normal alignment of the anatomy. A fusion in situ is not satisfactory. The deformity, at this stage, appears like that in the rheumatoid foot, the neuropathic Charcot foot, and in the flatfoot conditions in childhood and adolescence. These are different, however, and the techniques used for them vary according to special needs. In the child with an immature foot, for example, every effort is made to preserve joints; whereas in this condition, the joints are usually arthritic and when procedures intended for the adolescent are done alone, without accounting for the concomitant joint pathology, there is persistent pain. The essence of the surgery is to use fusion with realignment, including wedging and osteotomies to achieve the goal.

Correcting the Subtalar Joint

In the severely valgus subtalar joint, the anterior process of the calcaneus abuts the lateral process of the talus, totally obliterating a view of the sinus tarsi. "Booking open" the posterior facet with a wedge is not the appropriate maneuver. The sinus tarsi should be opened transversely, increasing the distance between the anterior process and the lateral process of the talus. This moves the talus back up the inclined plane of the facet and reorients the heel. This is the natural movement of the talus and calcaneus in the normal foot as the subtalar joint moves from valgus to varus. This maneuver can be accomplished with a laminar spreader between the aforementioned structures. Preparation of the fusion surfaces, use of the laminar spreader, temporary fixation, use of a bone wedge (commonly an allograft) and permanent fixation is the typical approach. In some very advanced feet with soft tissue contracture in the periarticular tissues, full correction cannot be achieved. In such patients, a medial displacement osteotomy of the calcaneus is carried out at this time as well. When this combination is needed, the lateral decubitus position is utilized and the subtalar joint prepared. The sinus tarsi is wedged open as much as possible and temporary fixation applied across the posterior facet with a 0.062" or 1.6 or 2.0 mm fixation pin. With the medial displacement osteotomy of the calcaneus completed, but not fixed, a wedge of iliac crest allograft is placed in the interval between the lateral process of the talus and the anterior process of the calcaneus after squaring off the base of the anterior process. Fixation of both the osteotomy and the subtalar joint is then done with two parallel 7.3 mm cannulated cancellous screws inserted through the heel. For the author, the easiest way to carry out this fixation is to hold the distal fragment of the heel between the thumb and fingers of the non-dominant hand, and place the guide pin exactly in the center of the bone midway between medial and lateral, following the direction of the skin directional markings. The reduction of the osteotomy is then maintained and the pin driven across this site. Fluoroscopic help is used. The pin is then passed across the subtalar joint which has already been temporarily fixed. One pin is placed into the body of the talus and the other into the neck. After one is satisfied with the pin positions in the sagittal plane, the position is checked for the osteotomy with a tangential view. Finally, the pin position in the talus is checked with an AP view of the ankle. If the position of the pins need adjusting, one pin is left in the original position, while the other is changed. This maintains the osteotomy correction. Final fixation is done with the 7.3 cannulated screws.

Correcting the Abducted, Supinated Mid- and Forefoot

To correct the transverse tarsal joint, the navicular (and the foot distal to this bone) must be pronated, adducted and subsequently fixed in the corrected position. When this reduction is attempted, there may be a gap at the calcaneocuboid (C-C) joint and the articular surfaces may or may not be congruently aligned. In the adolescent, an anterior process of the calcaneus osteotomy (the Dillwyn-Evans) aides the correction. In the adult, as the fusion of the calcaneocuboid joint is needed, a wedge is placed here, rather than proximally, to gain the correction.

Initially, the talonavicular (T-N) reduction is attempted. If it is sufficient clinically and the talonavicular-first metatarsal alignment on the anterior/posterior view of the foot is corrected, temporary and then permanent fixation is applied. If the calcaneocuboid joint comes together but the levels of the lateral borders of the bones are incongruent, they are shaved with a burr prior to application of the plate and screws.

If the C-C joint tends to gap, an allograft wedge from iliac crest bone is applied with the cancellous sides of the wedge against the native articular surfaces. If the T-N joint cannot be brought around, even with a laminar spreader attempting to wedge open the C-C joint, more bone is taken off the talar articular surface to allow the reduction and then it is fixed with a wedge also placed in the C-C joint. If adduction to neutral is corrected by these maneuvers but the pronation is not quite sufficient, the Cotton osteotomy (medial cuneiform dorsal opening wedge), described above, is done to level the first and fifth metatarsal heads.

While the patient is under anesthesia following correction of the deformities, the alignment should be checked with fluoroscopy to include the AP and lateral views of the foot and the tangential view which shows the tibial-calcaneal alignment. One should also note that the fibular tip clears the calcaneus. Finally, a bimalleolar view of the ankle stressing the deltoid should be done to rule out laxity in this structure (the Stage 4 deformity).

STAGE 4

The most involved stage of this deformity includes all the issues noted above and adds laxity of the medial ankle ligaments, the deltoid. This issue results in deformity and pain with weight bearing and eventually arthritis of the ankle. Correction is required at this level. This is not an easy accomplishment and investigations are in progress at this time to find the best approach. Several soft tissue reconstructions and various osteotomies of the medial malleolus to shorten or advance this bone have been proposed. These procedures are usually performed at the same operation as the triple arthrodesis and Cotton osteotomies making the entire reconstruction a formidable undertaking.

Reconstructing the Deltoid Ligament for Medial Laxity at the Ankle

In a somewhat complex procedure described by Deland,[8,9] the peroneus longus is divided proximally well above the ankle, and then through an incision in the distal sinus tarsi, directed through an oblique drill hole across the neck of the talus in the direction of the medial malleolus. It is then brought through a drill hole which is almost transverse of the medial malleolus (reproducing the direction of the deep deltoid). Another drill hole is made from lateral to medial across the tibia and the tendon brought through it and secured. The ankle is held in a reduced position and the tension maximized on the tendon. The intent is to reproduce a ligament, and is not a tendon transfer, as the distal tendon is being used.

The author prefers to use an advancement of the deltoid and periosteum due to its simplicity, reserving the above approach as a salvage procedure. A linear incision is made from the tip of the medial malleolus to above the medial apex of the ankle plafond. An incision is made through the periosteum transversely from the anterior edge of the plafond to the posterior apex, taking care not to damage the tendons in either area. A subperiosteal dissection peals the periosteum and subsequently the superficial deltoid from the malleolus. The soft tissue is taken off the tip of the malleolus and inside the malleolus, on the lateral side, the attachment of the deep deltoid is also released. The periosteum above the incision line is also elevated. The surface of the malleolus is gently burred to stimulate healing to the repositioned periosteum and ligament. Two large bone anchors with #0 or #2 permanent suture attached are placed in the tibia above the plafond; one is more posterior, and one more anterior. With the ankle reduced, maximum tension is placed on the sleeve, advancing it proximally, and it is then anchored with the sutures from the anchors. The superior component of the periosteum is then lapped over the anchored lower section and sutured with 2-0 dissolvable suture, covering the knots from the anchors and reinforcing the repair.

When patients have already reached the stage where the ankle is arthritic and symptomatic, a CT scan confirms the changes and further reconstruction is needed at this joint as well. Classically, these patients were considered for a pantalar fusion, adding the ankle to the procedures indicated above.[10] As the deltoid reconstruction would not be done in that case, the ankle fusion might have been done simultaneously or, more likely done later as a staged procedure. This procedure, as well as the tibiotalocalcaneal (TTC) and tibiocalcaneal (TC) fusions will be discussed in a later chapter.

Today, there is a far greater tendency to carry out a total ankle replacement after the triple arthrodesis, as a staged procedure. The deltoid reconstruction would be done concomitant to that operation.

REFERENCES

1. Johnson KA, Strom DE. Tibialis posterior dysfunction. Clin Orthop Relat Res. 1989;236:196-206.
2. Raikin SM, Winters BS, Daniel JN. The RAM classification: a novel, systematic approach to the adult-acquired flatfoot. Foot Ankle Clin. 2012; 17(2):169-81.
3. Bluman EM, Myerson MS. Stage IV posterior tibial tendon rupture. Foot Ankle Clin. 2007;12(2):341-62.
4. Alvarez RG, Marini A, Schmitt C, et al. Stage I and II posteriortibial tendon dysfunction treated by a structured non-operative management protocol: an orthosis and exercise program. Foot Ankle Int. 2006;27:2-8.
5. Wapner KL, Chao W. Nonoperative treatment of posterior tibial tendon dysfunction. Clin Orthop Relat Res. 1999;365:39-45.
6. Myerson MS, Badekas A, Schon LC. Treatment of stage II posterior tibial tendon deficiency with flexor digitorum longus tendon transfer and calcaneal osteotomy. Foot Ankle Int. 2004;25:445-50.
7. Hirose CB, Johnson JE. Plantar flexion opening wedge medial cuneiform osteotomy for correction of fixed forefoot varus associated with flatfoot deformity. Foot Ankle Int. 2004;25:568-74.
8. Deland JT, de Asla RJ, Segal A. Reconstruction of the chronically failed deltoid ligament: a new technique. Foot Ankle Int. 2004;25:795-9.
9. Ellis SJ, Williams BR, Wagshul AD, et al. Deltoid ligament reconstruction with peroneus longus autograft in flatfoot deformity. Foot Ankle Int. 2010;31(9):781-9.
10. Russotti GM, Johnson KA, Cass JR. Tibiotalocalcaneal arthrodesis for arthritis and deformity of the hind part of the foot. J Bone Joint Surg. 1988;70A: 1304-7.

24

Flexible Flat Foot in Children and Adolescents

Joseph G Khoury

PRESENTATION

The diagnosis of "flat foot" is controversial in orthopedics. Many argue that the flat foot is simply a variation of normal and rarely, if ever, produces symptoms in isolation. Most babies have, or appear to have, a flat foot at birth. The arch has been shown to slowly appear, in most children, during the first several years of life as the fatty foot matures and strength improves.[1] By the time a child reaches the age of 5, the final adult alignment and shape of the foot is achieved. Approximately 15% of adults retain the flat foot phenotype. The majority of children presenting to the orthopedist with flat foot are accompanied by concerned parents and often grandparents who fear a future of pain and disability rather than any current complaint from the patient. Often, there is a hope that appropriate and timely use of orthotics and/or "orthopedic shoes" will gradually correct the deformity and prevent future problems. In slightly older children, complaints of pain and accelerated shoe wear become more frequent. Symptoms usually consist of pain along the medial midfoot and ankle, exacerbated by activity and fatigue. Concerns about the appearance of the foot and clumsiness are common. Symptoms may be relieved somewhat in supportive shoes. Most frequently, the presence of symptoms correlates with an Achilles contracture in the setting of a flexible flat foot.

DIAGNOSIS

The diagnosis is generally obvious. By definition, a flexible flat foot is present when standing but not while sitting. In the standing position, the longitudinal arch is depressed, the midfoot is abducted and the heel is in valgus. The hindfoot and midfoot have normal range of motion. Dorsiflexion of the great toe either manually or by having the patient stand on his toes improves foot alignment by tightening of the plantar fascia (the windlass mechanism) and inversion of the hindfoot. It is important to recognize that flattening of the longitudinal arch is only part of the overall pathoanatomy. The deformity is characterized by a depressed longitudinal arch, abduction of the midfoot and hindfoot valgus. This position may cause strain on the medial ligamentous complex, overuse symptoms of the posterior tibialis, lateral impingement of the fibula and calcaneus and pain related to the prominence of the medial midfoot. The medial counter of the shoe may be stretched and the heel may be unevenly worn. In the symptomatic patient, an Achilles contracture is often present.[2] The foot must be inverted and the knee extended in order to accurately assess ankle dorsiflexion in these patients (Figs 1A to C). Radiography serves to rule out related or similar conditions such as vertical talus and tarsal coalition. Radiographic measurements of the flat foot include Meary's angle, calcaneal pitch and talo-first metatarsal angle (Figs 2A and B). Meary's angle is drawn along the long axis of the talus and first metatarsal; normal is 0° ± 10°. The calcaneal pitch is drawn between the floor and base of the calcaneus and should measure over 20°. The talo-first metatarsal angle is drawn on the AP view and should be between 0° and 20°.

TREATMENT

Nonoperative Treatment

For asymptomatic patients with normal ankle dorsiflexion, reassurance is all that is required. There is abundant evidence that this variation is compatible with a normal functioning, pain free foot for life.[3] Families must be persuaded to believe the studies demonstrating no benefit from special orthotics, footwear or exercises on the ultimate

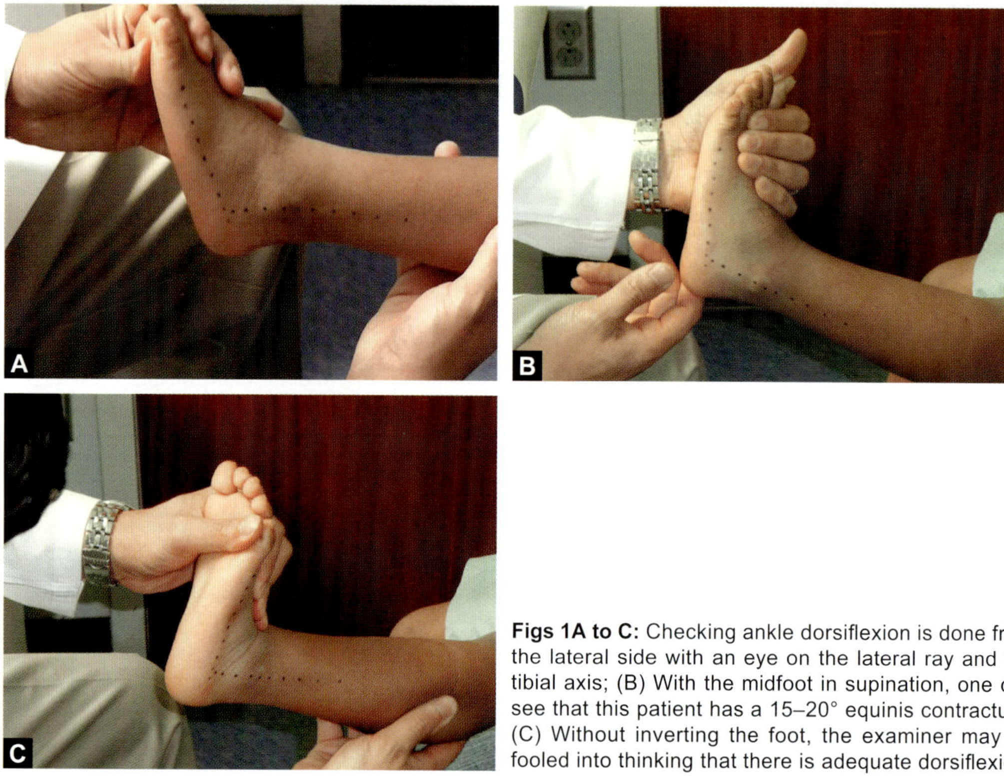

Figs 1A to C: Checking ankle dorsiflexion is done from the lateral side with an eye on the lateral ray and the tibial axis; (B) With the midfoot in supination, one can see that this patient has a 15–20° equinis contracture; (C) Without inverting the foot, the examiner may be fooled into thinking that there is adequate dorsiflexion

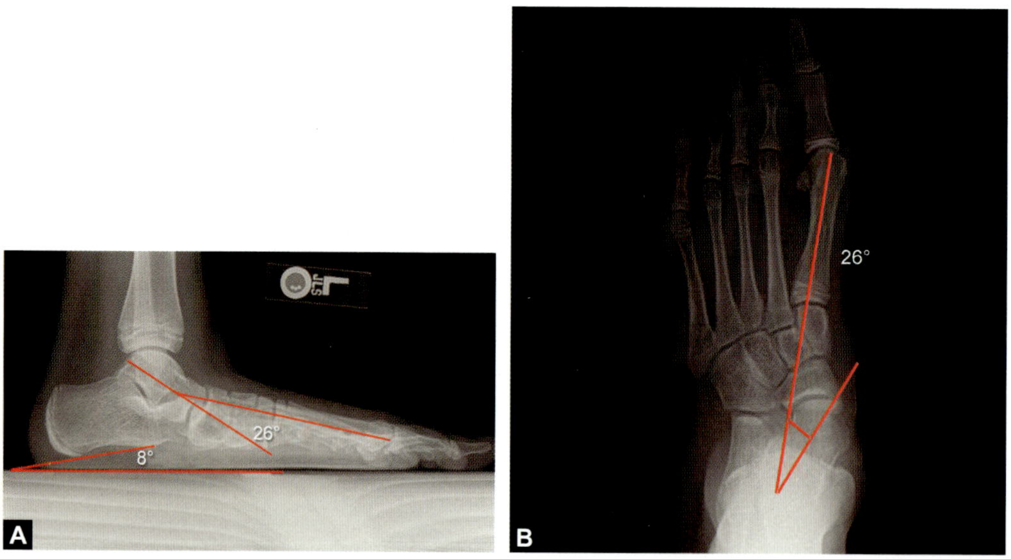

Figs 2A and B: Lateral standing radiograph of a planovalgus foot demonstrating calcaneal pitch and Meary's angle; (B) A standing AP radiograph demonstrating the talo-first metatarsal angle. Note the significant midfoot abduction and uncovered talar head medially

shape of the foot.[4] For symptomatic patients with normal ankle dorsiflexion, stabilization of the hindfoot to prevent valgus tilt is highly successful. Options include so called "motion control" running

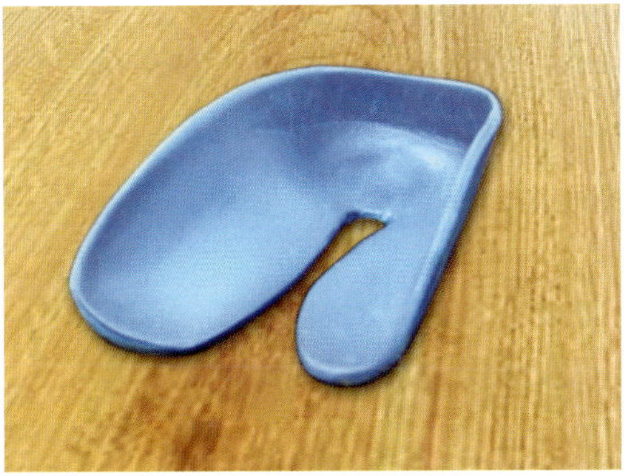

Fig. 3: A simple over-the-counter "heel stabilization" orthotic helps prevent the hindfoot from tipping into valgus

shoes with a rigid and long medial counter, hind foot stabilization orthotics (Fig. 3) or UCBL type orthotics. Arch supports, such as those available over-the-counter, or from non-medical healthcare providers place a rigid plastic support under the arch and are often counterproductive and may increase symptoms. In the presence of an Achilles contracture, nonoperative treatment is likely to be ineffective without a concerted effort to stretch the Achilles, with the hindfoot locked in inversion in order to prevent exacerbation of the midfoot break.

Operative Treatment

Symptomatic patients, who fail nonoperative intervention are candidates for operative intervention. In a busy pediatric orthopedic practice, these should be few and far between. The goal of surgery is to produce improved alignment of the hindfoot and midfoot while preserving motion and growth of the foot. Operative treatment is almost always accompanied by lengthening of the gastrocnemius-solcus complex. Options include open Z-lengthening, percutaneous lengthening or gastrocnemius recessions of some sort. Each technique has its advocates, but in the child with no neuromuscular conditions, the author prefers the percutaneous technique. He has not found overlengthening or weakness to be a problem in this population and the technique is quick and adds little morbidity to the overall procedure. The author prefers the triple cut technique of Hoke or the double cut technique of White.[5,6] Treatment of the flat foot generally involves an osteotomy of the calcaneus, itself, with or without osteotomy of other tarsal bones.

Lateral Column Lengthening

The decision to use a lateral column lengthening versus calcaneal slide hinges on the primary deformity. If the primary component of the deformity is midfoot abduction, the calcaneal lengthening is preferred. If the primary component is hindfoot valgus, the calcaneal slide is preferred with or without midfoot osteotomies, depending on the degree of midfoot deformity also present.

The lateral column (or calcaneal) lengthening is currently the most popular procedure for correction of flexible flat foot in children. Originally described by Evans as a way to salvage an over-corrected club foot, it was popularized by Mosca in the mid 1990s for flat foot correction.[7] Results have been excellent. The osteotomy is performed from the lateral side between the middle and anterior facets of the calcaneus, preserving the joints and physes. Correction is achieved by reducing midfoot abduction and secondarily by improving hindfoot valgus. A lateral incision 4 cm in length is made just proximal to the calcaneocuboid joint. Care is taken to identify and protect the sural nerve. The peroneal tendons are removed from their sheaths and retracted behind a Hohmann retractor placed over the dorsal neck of the calcaneus. Plantarly, the fascia overlying the abductor digiti quinti is divided as well as the lateral fibers of the plantar fascia. This step is essential in order to achieve uniform lengthening. The periosteum is incised in the location confirmed by fluoroscopy to be between the anterior and middle facets of the calcaneus. This is generally 1 cm behind the calcaneocuboid joint. The osteotomy is performed with a small saw and completed with an osteotome. The author finds it easiest to open the osteotomy by using two Kirchner wires (5/64th inch in diameter) in each fragment and a specially designed retractor over the wires. The osteotomy is opened enough to correct the midfoot abduction deformity and a piece of tricortical wedge allograft is cut to match the opening. The AP fluoroscopic view is used to confirm reduction of the navicular over the talar head. The author has not found autograft to be required as heeling is generally robust in the pediatric age group. The wedge averages 1 cm in length on the lateral side and 7–8 mm on the medial side for most children. The author has not found it necessary to stabilize the graft with a pin or other fixation. Some recommend stabilization of the calcaneocuboid joint before opening the osteotomy to prevent subluxation, but the author has found that this subluxation does not persist once full recovery has occurred and prefers not to joint cross the joint with a rather large pin. It is essential to evaluate the alignment of the midfoot and forefoot before completion of the procedure. Occasionally, in a longstanding deformity, the forefoot develops a compensatory supination deformity with respect to the hindfoot and midfoot. Once the osteotomy is complete, this deformity becomes uncovered and manifests as elevation of the medial ray. A firm plate must be applied to the bottom surface of the foot to demonstrate equal three-point contact of the tripod. If the first ray is elevated, a medial cuneiform plantarflexion osteotomy (Cotton osteotomy) must be performed to bring the first ray down. The first metatarsal is also an option but is farther from the apex of the deformity and the proximally located physis must also be avoided.

Postoperatively, the patient remains in a non-weight-bearing cast for 6 weeks. If X-rays show satisfactory heeling, the patient moves to a walking cast or boot for the next 4–6 weeks.

Medial Calcaneal Slide Osteotomy

The medial slide calcaneal osteotomy popularized in the early 1970s by Koutsogiannis is an extremely valuable tool in the armamentarium of the surgeon.[8] The author uses this operation in combination with a tendo-Achilles lengthening (TAL) for nearly half of his patients with flexible flat foot deformity. The ideal patient has a primary hindfoot valgus component to the deformity with secondary midfoot abduction. The calcaneus slides medially which corrects the hindfoot, but it is important to remember that the plantar fascia and intrinsic foot musculature are attached to the tuberosity fragment. As the heel slides medially, the midfoot and forefoot move medially as well. A lateral incision is made obliquely following the peroneal tendons. The sural nerve is protected. The peroneal tendons remain within their sheaths. The periosteum is incised just posterior to the tendons, proceeding from dorsally, between the Achilles and subtalar joint, to plantarly, 1.5 cm proximal to the calcaneocuboid joint. The bone is incised, perpendicular to its surface, with a saw. Care is taken to avoid penetrating the medial side. The osteotomy is taken further with a broad osteotome until it can be wedged open. At this point, a Kerrison rongeur is used to remove the medial cortex and periosteum until the tuberosity fragment is free. The fragment can then be slid medially, approximately 50% of its width, and secured with two Kirchner wires from the heel. One or two offset staples are another fixation option. An intraoperative Harris heel view is essential to confirm proper wire placement. At this point, it is important to assess the foot clinically and fluoroscopically in simulated weight bearing against a firm surface. If significant midfoot or forefoot deformity remains, additional osteotomies will be required, as discussed below.

This osteotomy heals very quickly due to the large cancellous bone apposition. Four weeks in a non-weight-bearing cast is followed by a pin removal and 4 more weeks in a walking cast or boot.

Calcaneocuboidcuneiform Osteotomy

The triple "C" osteotomy was popularized by Rathjen and Mubarak.[9] This involves medial slide calcaneal osteotomy as described above in combination with cuboid opening wedge osteotomy and medial cuneiform closing wedge osteotomy. The medial cuneiform osteotomy can be fashioned to both medialize and plantar flex the medial column. The author does not often find that the midfoot osteotomies are necessary once the calcaneal osteotomy has been performed and an "a la carte approach" is undertaken. If insufficient midfoot and forefoot correction are noted after the calcaneal slide, the author moves to the cuboid. The cuboid is exposed through an extension of the original incision. The approach moves dorsal to the peroneal tendons. Care is taken to avoid exposing the joints on either side. A sagittal saw is used to begin the osteotomy. Fluoroscopy is used to ensure appropriate depth. The osteotomy is completed with an osteotome until the bone can be wedged open. Kirchner wires are used as joysticks to aid in opening the osteotomy while a piece of tricortical wedge allograft is fashioned to fit snugly. Fixation is rarely required. Again, the foot is assessed clinically and fluoroscopically in a simulated weight-bearing position and a decision is made whether or not to approach the medial side. If additional medial column shortening is required, or if forefoot supination exists such that the tripod is not level, the medial cuneiform is approached. A medial incision is made, 3–4 cm in length centered on the medial cuneiform. Fluoroscopy must be used to guide the approach. The medial cuneiform is a very tall bone from dorsal to plantar and the incision must be centered. The posterior tibial tendon can be removed for later shortening and reattachment or it can be split. A medial and plantar-based wedge is removed. One common error is to remove too large a wedge so as to not be able to close the osteotomy. The author plans to leave enough bone on either side to accommodate one or two memory staples which help to achieve compression.

Other Procedures

Medial imbrication procedures in isolation are rarely performed. While previously very common, the initial correction tends to stretch out with time especially if not combined with bony reconstructions. Several variations exist involving shortening of the posterior tibial tendon, imbrication of the talonavicular capsule, advancement of osteoperiosteal flaps and shortening of medial ligaments. The author has generally only performed medial reefing procedures if he is coming to the medial side of the foot for other reasons, such as to perform a medial cuneiform osteotomy.

Occasionally, subtalar arthrodesis or arthroeresis is used in a child over 12 years old with a very severe deformity not amendable to other treatments. Arthrodesis is generally reserved for the very stiff and severe deformity in an older child or adolescent who will place high demands on the reconstruction. Arthrodesis can involve the subtalar joint, talonavicular joint, calcaneocuboid joint or any combination of the three depending on the nature of the deformity. The resulting stiffness corresponds to the number of joints involved and over years of use results in premature degeneration of neighboring joints. Arthrodesis should be reserved for extreme circumstances and as a last resort. Arthroeresis is reserved for older children with lower demands and high-grade deformity either in isolation or as an adjunct to the standard reconstruction. This involves jacking open the subtalar joint from the lateral side and insertion of a spacer of some kind. Currently, plastic spacers of various sizes are most commonly used. Common complications include displacement of the spacer, subsidence or particulate synovitis. This practice should be discouraged in most children. The author's preference is to use the arthroeresis in the relatively fragile child with low functional demand who requires a quick operation with little or no down time.

REFERENCES

1. Staheli LT, Chew DE, Corbett M. The longitudinal arch: a survey of eight hundred and eighty-two feet in normal children and adults. J Bone Joint Surg Am. 1987;69:426-28.
2. Harris R, Beath T. Hypermobile flatfoot with short Achilles tendon. J Bone Joint Surg Am. 1948;30: 116-50.
3. Harris R, Beath T. Army Foot Survey: An Investigation of Foot Ailments in Canadian Soldiers.Ottawa: National Research Council of Canada;1947:1-268.
4. Wenger DR, Mauldin D, Speck G. Corrective shoes and inserts as treatment for flexible flatfoot in infants and children. J Bone Joint Surg Am. 1989;71:800-10.
5. Hoke M. An operation for stabilizing paralytic feet. J Orthop Surg. 1921;3:494-507.
6. White JW. Torsion of the Achilles tendon. Arch Surg. 1943;46:784-7.
7. Mosca V. Calcaneal lengthening for valgus deformity of the hindfoot: results in children who had severe, symptomatic flatfoot and skewfoot. J Bone Joint Surg Am. 1995;77:500-12.
8. Koutsogiannis E. Treatment of mobile flat foot by displacement osteotomy of the calcaneus. J Bone Joint Surg Br. 1971;53:96-100.
9. Rathjen KE, Mubarak SJ. Calcaneal-cuboid-cuneiform osteotomy for the correction of valgus foot deformities in children. J Pediatr Orthop. 1998; 18(6):775-82.

25

Rigid Flat Foot in Children and Adolescents

Joseph G Khoury

PRESENTATION

The rigid flat foot in a child or adolescent represents a very small cohort of all flat feet. These patients present with many of the same complaints as those with flexible flat feet with the exception that there is very often associated pain and disability. The history may include a once normal foot that gradually began to assume an out-turned position or a flat foot that has become worse over time or recently painful. There may be a history of difficulty walking across uneven ground, such as a field or in the woods. Patients often have a history of frequent ankle sprains. Both of these symptoms are related to the loss of motion through the subtalar and Chopart joints. The most frequent cause of rigid flat foot is a tarsal coalition. Less frequent is subtalar joint inflammatory arthritis or some other source of hindfoot inflammation such as infection or tumor. The term "peroneal spastic flat foot" has been used, historically to describe the rigid flat foot but has fallen out of favor because peroneal spasm is not a consistent finding in these conditions.

DIAGNOSIS

Tarsal Coalition

The definition of a rigid flat foot is one which does not correct passively; or, when the patient stands on tip toe, also does not dynamically correct. In the case of a tarsal coalition, the most common joints involved are the calcaneonavicular and talocalcaneal joints in roughly equal proportions. The incidence is between 0.1% and 1% in the general population and many remain asymptomatic throughout life.[1] The most common age of presentation is 12–16 years. Tarsal coalitions are thought to be caused by failure of segmentation of the cartilaginous anlage of the hindfoot into separate bones. It is important to remember that asymptomatic coalitions are common and the painful foot cannot be attributed immediately to the coalition. The source and location of the pain may also vary. In some cases, the coalition itself may be painful due to micro motion through a fibrocartilagenous coalition or a stress fracture through a bony coalition. The pain may be remote due to stress transfer to neighboring joints. The examination may also reveal tightness or spasm of the peroneal musculature. With the patient in the seated position, the examiner may note reduced hindfoot motion or midfoot motion. However, approximately 50% of patients have a coalition on the other side and comparison is not always helpful. Many patients find it impossible to walk on the lateral border of the foot.

A coalition may be bony, fibrous, cartilaginous or some combination of the three. A coalition that is not bony may not always be apparent on plain radiography. The oblique view of the foot tends to be the best for visualizing the calcaneonavicular coalition (Fig. 1), while the Harris heel view is often useful for visualizing the talocalcaneal condition. There are other clues on the radiograph which may be helpful. On the lateral radiograph, the "C" sign is a clue to a talocalcaneal coalition (Fig. 2). Talar beaking may also be seen which is felt to be due to excessive anterior ankle joint capsular traction because of limited motion at the subtalar.[2] In almost all cases, especially when surgical treatment is considered, a computed tomography (CT) scan is required (Fig. 3). A CT is very helpful for fully elucidating the anatomy, for more clearly visualizing a nonbony coalition and for the discovery of a second coalition which may be present in 1–2% of cases. As the quality of CT has improved, it has become less common to need an MRI for the diagnosis of a purely fibrous or cartilaginous coalition but it can still be helpful

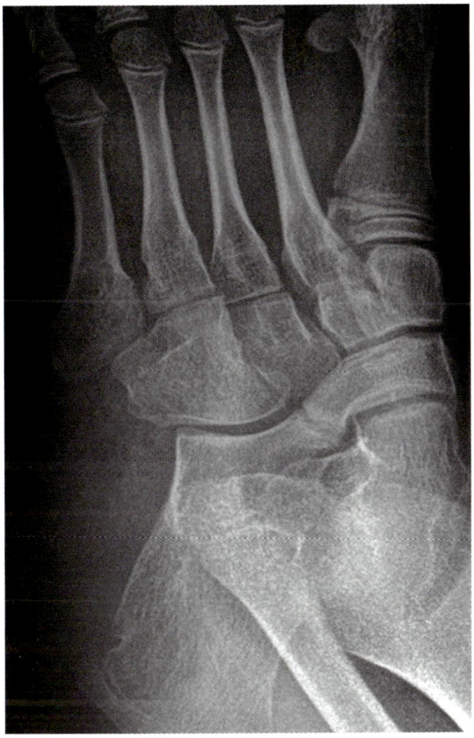

Fig. 1: Oblique view radiograph demonstrating nearly complete bony calcaneonavicular coalition

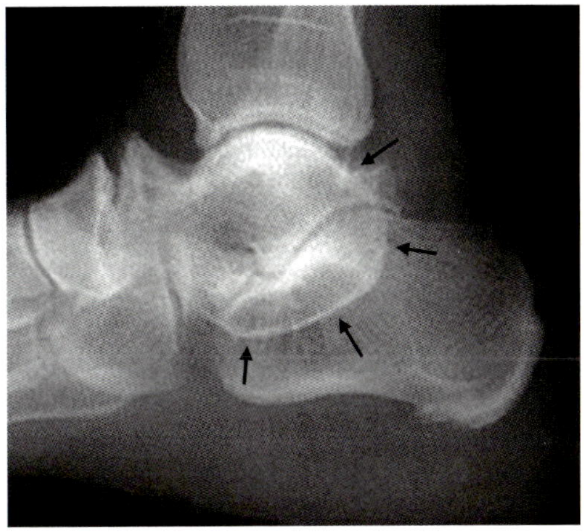

Fig. 2: The C sign, and talar breaking, seen with a subtalar coalition and early degenerative changes at the talonavicular joint

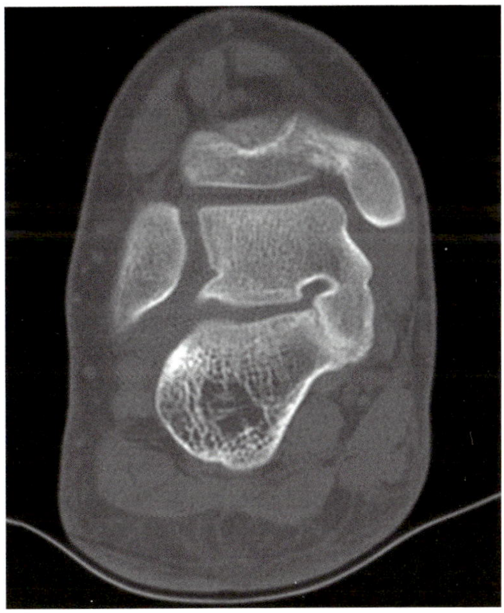

Fig. 3: A coronal plane computed tomography (CT) image demonstrating a talocalcaneal coalition involving the middle facet

in difficult cases. When imaging fails to reveal a coalition, remember that subtalar arthritis is another possible cause for rigid flat foot.

Subtalar Joint Inflammatory Arthritis

In the child, subtalar arthritis is less common and frequently forgotton as a cause of a rigid flat foot. It is frequently involved in pauciarticular juvenile arthritis and may be the first joint involved. These patients typically present several years before those with coalition. The pathoanatomy involves synovitis and pannus formation at the subtalar joint which causes stiffness of the joint itself as well as inflammation in the tenosynovium of the nearby peroneal tendon sheaths. The history may mirror those with classic inflammatory arthritis symptoms with morning stiffness lasting 30 minutes, or more gradually improving later in the morning with pain returning after activities in the afternoon or evening. Stiffness and pain may return after periods of prolonged relative rest (gelling). It is important to ask about symptoms in other joints, rash or visual problems. The examination is similar to those with coalitions. There may be tenderness medially at the subtalar joint or in the sinus tarsi, and warmth or bogginess around the joint. Synovial thickening or effusions should be elucidated in other joints.

If inflammatory arthritis of the subtalar joint is suspected, the work-up should include laboratory studies including complete blood cell count (CBC) with differential, antinuclear antibody, erythrocyte sedimentation rate (ESR), C reactive protein (CRP) and possibly a fluid aspiration of the subtalar joint.

An MRI should be obtained to rule out other causes of subtalar joint inflammation including tumor and infection. A rheumatology consult should also be obtained.

TREATMENT

Nonoperative Treatment

Nonoperative treatment of the subtalar coalition should always be the first line of treatment and in the author's experience has a 30–50% chance of relieving symptoms sufficiently to avoid surgical management. The author's preference is for orthotic management. The goal is to reduce hindfoot and midfoot motion. A UCBL (University of California Berkeley Laboratories) orthotic or supramalleolar orthosis (SMO) work well. Some prefer a short period of time in a short leg walking cast with or without transition to an orthosis.

Nonoperative management of inflammatory arthritis of the subtalar joint is the mainstay of treatment. Treatment is generally medical and managed by the rheumatologist. The orthopedist may assist by providing an orthosis to limit motion or injection of the joint with corticosteroids. This generally requires an arthrogram to confirm proper positioning of the needle and is usually done under a general anesthetic.

Operative Management of the Calcaneonavicular Coalition

If nonoperative management has failed, it is reasonable to move on to surgical management, if symptoms warrant. A preoperative CT is required. Resection of the coalition with interposition is the mainstay of treatment. Recurrence of the coalition is the most common complication and is reported to be as common as 15% of cases. In many instances, the culprit may be an incomplete resection rather than a recurrence.

The patient is positioned supine with a bump under the ipsilateral buttock to turn the foot slightly inward at rest. An Ollier approach is made extending from the peroneus tertius to the peroneus brevis. The lateral cutaneous nerves are protected. The origin of the extensor digitorum brevis is sharply incised and the entire muscle is reflected dorsally and distally until the coalition can be seen. It is important to dissect medially enough to identify the talonavicular joint and laterally enough to identify the calcaneocuboid joint without unnecessarily disturbing these joints. Mini Hohmann retractors are placed on either side of the coalition. A one-fourth inch straight osteotome is used to excise the coalition. It is important to realize how deep the coalition goes and to prevent the tendency for the osteotome cuts to converge as they move more plantarly. A rongeur is used to remove the coalition. The gap must be carefully inspected for any residual connection deep in the foot. A small rongeur such as a Kerrison can be very helpful in removing these small connections. Once the coalition is completely resected, there should be an appreciable increase in the range of motion.

Equally important to a complete resection is prevention of recurrence. The most common method is interposition of the extensor digitorum brevis muscle belly. First, the cut edges of bone are covered with bone wax. The cavity is thoroughly irrigated to remove any bony debris. Two strong sutures are placed into the origin of the extensor digitorum brevis (EDB) and threaded onto Keith needles. These are passed through the gap and arch of the foot. The sutures are tied over a plastic button and felt pad. The author's preference is fat interposition instead of the EDB and the results have been excellent.[3] The graft can be harvested through a separate incision in the inferior gluteal fold but the author has found that with careful dissection, there is more than enough fat in the sinus tarsi to accomplish the task. The fat graft is harvested before reflecting the EDB distally and stored in saline until the end of the case. After covering the bone with wax, the graft is gently inserted. After either type of interposition, the wound is closed and a short leg cast or splint is applied.

Early range of motion is important in preventing recurrence as well. The cast is removed in two weeks (3–4 with EDB interposition) after giving the wound enough time to begin healing and range of motion exercises are started. Immobilization beyond this is counterproductive. The author uses the so called "alphabet" exercises encouraging the patient to draw out the letters of the alphabet as large as they can with the big toe, while keeping the knee still. These should be completed twice each day and the patient encouraged to walk and resume normal activities as quickly as possible.

If, in addition to the coalition, the patient also has a severe planovalgus deformity, it should be managed at the same setting, if possible with a short period of immobilization. In this situation, the author prefers the calcaneal slide osteotomy, because it heals faster. The author will transition to a removable splint or boot faster in this scenario so that he can initiate range of motion exercises not later than 4 weeks after surgery. A concurrent contracture of the triceps surae should also be managed.

Operative Management of the Talocalcaneal Coalition

The talocalcaneal or subtalar coalition presents a unique set of challenges. The CT scan is critical for preoperative planning. If the coalition involves greater than 33–50% of the subtalar joint surface, resection should not be attempted.[2,4] It is important to examine the CT carefully. In many cases, while the coalition may only involve 30% of the surface area, the posterior facet of the subtalar joint may appear narrowed and dystrophic in comparison to the other side. This is likely due to a lifetime of limited motion. In the author's opinion, it is not reasonable to expect a joint like this to function normally once it has been freed. Similarly, those with severe hindfoot valgus should not have a resection. In this scenario, the coalition is the only thing keeping the hindfoot from falling into even more valgus and once resected, will leave the patient with a severely symptomatic valgus deformity. The preoperative planning is critical.

The ideal patient for a resection has a coalition involving less than 30% of the total subtalar joint surface area with a normal appearance to the rest of the joint on CT. In addition, the hindfoot is well aligned. The patient is positioned supine and a medial transverse approach below the tip of the medial malleolus is made. It is very important to identify and protect the neurovascular bundle. It should be mobilized so that it can be moved freely and protected behind a vessel loop or small penrose drain. The coalition is very hard to find clinically. The author starts by identifying the flexor hallucis longus (FHL) tendon. The sustentaculum is just above. A small 3–4 mm cutting burr is then gently swept across the middle of the sustentaculum until a thin white line is identified. Fluoroscopy can be very helpful. Once this is identified, the resection continues anteriorly and posteriorly until a normal joint surface is encountered. The author places the blunt end of a freer elevator into the posterior facet and gently attempts to book the joint open while the resection is proceeding, and until there is a sudden pop and restoration of motion.

As with the calcaneonavicular coalition, prevention of recurrence is equally as important as a complete resection. The author's preference is to transpose the entire FHL tendon into the gap through the sustentaculum tali. Many use a split FHL transfer. The wound is closed and the patient is placed in a cast. The author encourages the patient to actively and passively move the great toe through full range of motion almost constantly for 4–6 weeks after surgery. This will help prevent a recurrence. The cast can be removed in 2 weeks and weight bearing is as tolerated. The author encourages the patient to resume normal activities as quickly as possible in order to keep the joint moving and prevent recurrence.

In the case of a larger coalition, an unhealthy appearing residual subtalar joint or significant underlying hindfoot valgus, the treatment is completely different. In these cases, there are two choices: (1) realign the foot ignoring the coalition or (2) complete the coalition with realignment of the foot, if needed. If the patient has good hindfoot and midfoot alignment and pain is attributed to the coalition, all that is needed is to complete the coalition. The author generally approaches the posterior facet of the subtalar joint through the sinus tarsi and burrs the remaining cartilaginous surfaces. Bone graft is inserted and a screw is used to stabilize the joint. The use of internal fixation is not absolutely required as the coalition provides much of the stability needed in most cases. An extra-articular arthrodesis is also a perfectly reasonable alternative. In adolescents, there is a higher incidence of failure of the posterior facet fusion than with fusions for the arthritic joint. Consequently, some authors advocate using both a lateral and medial approach. The posterior facet is prepared through the lateral; and through the medial, as described above, the coalition is taken down, the anterior and medial facets prepared, and internal fixation (7.3 mm screws) used. If the patient has hindfoot valgus, the author adds a medial slide calcaneal osteotomy to the procedure.

TECHNIQUE

Completion Subtalar Arthrodesis with Calcaneal Slide Osteotomy

The patient is positioned supine with a bump under the ipsilateral buttocks to tip the foot inward slightly. A percutaneous tendo-Achilles lengthening

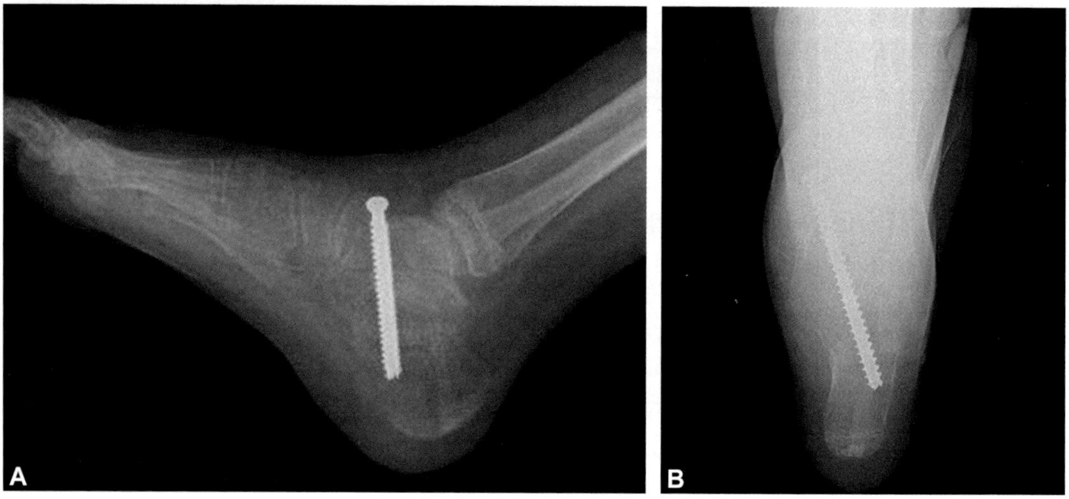

Figs 4A and B: Three-month postoperative lateral and Harris heel view radiographs of a patient after completion of a subtalar fusion and medial slide calcaneal osteotomy

is perform, if indicated. An extended Ollier incision is made to gain access to the sinus tarsi and lateral side of the calcaneus. The origin of the extensor digitorum brevis is reflected distally. The posterior facet of the subtalar joint is entered with a 4 mm cutting burr and the cartilage and subchondral bone is removed. Bone graft is packed into the void. At this point, the lateral side of the calcaneus is approached. The sural nerve is protected. The peroneal tendons remain within their sheaths. The periosteum is incised just posterior to the tendons proceeding from dorsally between the Achilles tendon and subtalar joint to plantarly 1.5 cm proximal to the calcaneocuboid joint. The bone is incised, perpendicular to its surface, with a saw. Care is taken to avoid penetrating the medial side. The osteotomy is taken further with a broad osteotome until it can be wedged open. At this point, a Kerrison rongeur is used to remove the medial cortex and periosteum until the tuberosity fragment is free. Two well spaced laminar spreaders are inserted, gently opened to stretch the soft tissues, and fragment can then be slid medially, approximately 50% of its width, and secured with two Kirchner wires from the heel. One or two offset staples are another fixation option. An intraoperative Harris heel view is essential to confirm proper wire placement. The wires can be sent across the subtalar joint as well. The author prefers to use one wire and place a screw. A small incision is made over the dorsal neck of the talus. After blunt dissection, a guidewire from the 7.3 mm cannulated screw set is sent across both the subtalar joint and the calcaneal osteotomy. This requires careful aim and a Harris heel view. The path is drilled and a fully threaded screw is placed (Figs 4A and B). Screws can also be inserted through the heel. Guide pins are inserted into the plantar fragment, the osteotomy displaced, the pins advanced, and after properly positioning the subtalar joint in a bit of valgus, advanced across the subtalar joint into the body and neck of the talus. Appropriate sized cannulated screws for the size of the bones, are used. An AP view of the ankle confirms proper positioning of the screws or pins in the talus.

REFERENCES

1. Shands Jr AR, Wentz IJ. Congenital anomalies, accessory bones, and osteochondritis in the feet of 850 children. Surg Clin North Am. 1953;97:1643-66.
2. Wilde PH, Torode IP, Dickens DR, et al. Resection for symptomatic talocalcaneal coalition. J Bone Joint Surg Br. 1994;76:797-801.
3. Mubarak SJ, Patel PN, Upasani VV, et al. Calcaneonavicular coalition: treatment by excision and fat graft. J Pediatr Orthop. 2009;29(5):418-26.
4. Comfort TK, Johnson LO. Resection for symptomatic talocalcaneal coalition. J Pediatr Orthop. 1998;18: 283-88.

26

Cavus Foot in Adolescents and Adults

Joseph G Khoury, John S Gould

PRESENTATION

In the pediatric patient, the presentation of cavus foot is often associated with a known neurologic condition. If the patient presents with a cavus foot and no associated neurologic diagnosis, a full neurologic work-up is indicated. The most common associated neurologic diagnoses are Charcot-Marie-Tooth (CMT) or a form of spinal dysraphism. Other possibilities include: poliomyelitis, sciatic nerve injury, compartment syndrome, peroneal tendon laceration and others.

Patients can present as early as a few years of age. In the case of myelodysplasia, the underlying diagnosis is obvious. In these patients, the specific form of cavus is often calcaneocavus resulting from weakness of the triceps surae while some dorsiflexion power remains. The calcaneal pitch is increased with associated intrinsic muscular contracture leading to a "pistol grip" deformity. Without treatment, heel ulceration is common. In patients with CMT, there may be a positive family history. These patients may also present within the first few years of life with the earliest signs of deformity. Patients with CMT most often present with cavovarus. The etiology is muscle imbalance. This neuropathy causes weakness of distal musculature first. The tibialis posterior and peroneus longus remain strong while the tibialis anterior and peroneus brevis begin to weaken. This imbalance leads to a plantarflexion moment on the first ray. Pronation of the forefoot upsets the tripod forcing the heel to swing into varus to allow the fifth ray to reach the floor. Eventually, the heel may become fixed in varus. In addition, contracture of the intrinsic musculature further serves to elevate the arch. In addition, the long toe extensors are working to help dorsiflex the foot which, in combination with arch elevation, leads to metatarsophalangeal (MTP) joint hyperextension. Metatarsophalangeal joint hyperextension leads to toe flexor tightness resulting in claw toe deformities.

Patients may present because of frequent ankle sprains. Varus hindfoot alignment and a weak triceps surae predisposes to ankle instability. Others may complain of pain and callusing under the base of the fifth metatarsal or metatarsal heads. Claw toes may lead to complaints regarding the appearance of the toes or callusing, blistering or shoe discomfort.

EXAMINATION

This portion of the chapter will focus on patients with CMT. The vast majority of patients with CMT have a cavovarus foot of variable stiffness. The foot is evaluated for calluses, tendon and joint contracture, strength and sensation. Vibratory sensation is often the first to be lost. The legs and feet are inspected for muscular atrophy. The patient's spine is examined for evidence of spinal dysraphism. The patient is asked to stand and walk. The hindfoot alignment in stance is noted as well as forefoot position. The toes are observed and the degree of clawing noted (Figs 1 to 3). Drop foot during gait is noted.

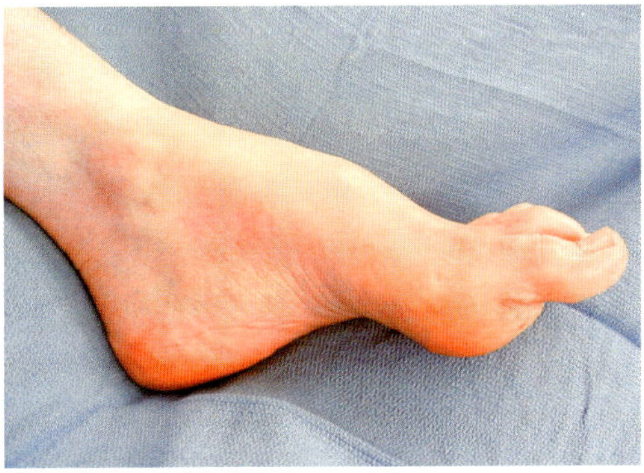

Fig. 1: Cavus foot: medial perspective

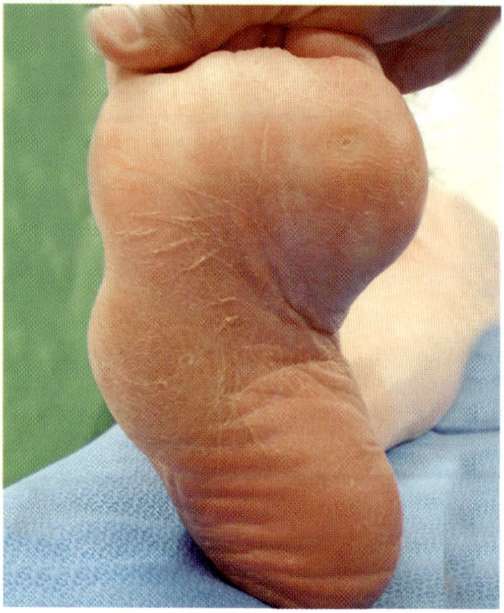

Fig. 2: Cavus foot: plantar perspective

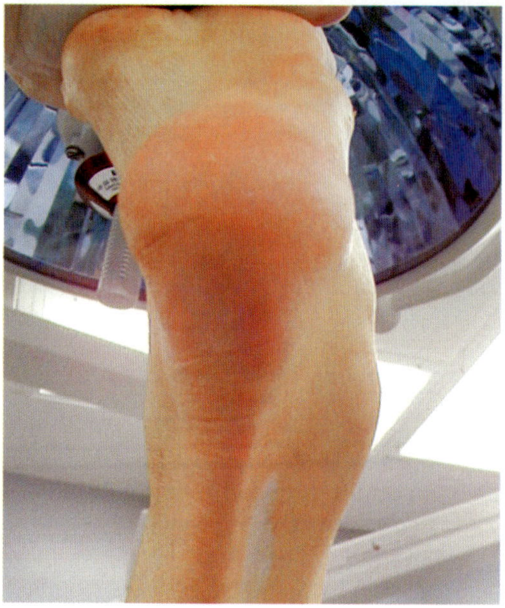

Fig. 3: Cavus foot heel varus noted from posterior perspective

Treatment decisions in the pediatric patient hinge on hindfoot flexibility. In other words, has the hindfoot varus deformity become fixed or is it merely compensatory to forefoot pronation? The Block test described by Coleman is the classic method to distinguish the two.[1] The patient is asked to stand on a wooden block 1–2 cm in height with the heel and lateral forefoot on the block. The first ray is allowed to contact the floor. The hindfoot is viewed from the rear and the alignment noted. If the heel remains in varus, the deformity is fixed, if the heel moves into valgus, the deformity is flexible (Figs 4 and 5). The authors' prefer to test the hindfoot flexibility or rigidity with the patient in the prone position and the knee flexed.[2]

Radiographic evaluation includes standing AP and lateral radiographs of the foot (Fig. 6). Even though patients with CMT often walk on their toes, the calcaneus is often noted to be in dorsiflexion. This can be noted by measuring the angle between the floor and the undersurface of the calcaneus (calcaneal pitch) which averages, normally, 15–25°. Meary's angle can also be measured between the long axis of the talus and the first ray. Meary's angle is normally 0° ± 10. Measurements above 10° are considered to be cavus (Fig. 7). An MRI of the spine may be indicated if there is no obvious cause of the deformity and there is no family history.

TREATMENT

Nonoperative Treatment

In CMT, the deformity is usually progressive. There is little role for nonoperative treatment. The authors always tell families that surgical treatment is usually inevitable. Even though nonoperative treatment may delay surgery, stretching of contracted tendons and joints may be of use in the younger child. Orthotics designed to relieve pressure on prominent metatarsal heads or assistance with dorsiflexion can be helpful. A lateral heel wedge or shoe flare may help prevent inversion sprains.

Operative Treatment

Surgical treatment of the cavovarus foot is divided into soft tissue releases, tendon transfers, osteotomies and arthrodesis. As mentioned previously, decision making hinges on the flexibility of hindfoot varus. If the hindfoot is flexible, all that is needed is to realign the forefoot and the hindfoot will revert to its proper position. If the hindfoot varus is fixed, osteotomy or arthrodesis is also required.

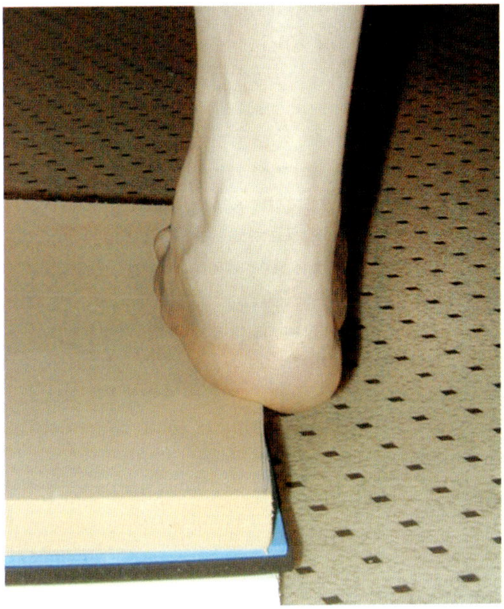

Fig. 4: Coleman block test.Heel remains fixed in varus

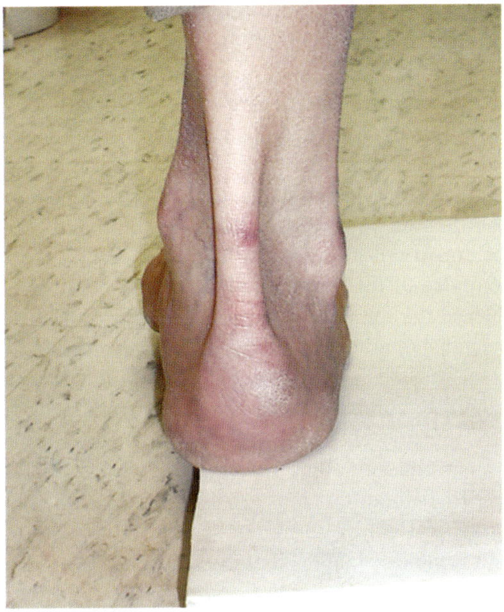

Fig. 5: Coleman block test. Heel corrects to valgus indicating that it is a forefoot driven varus

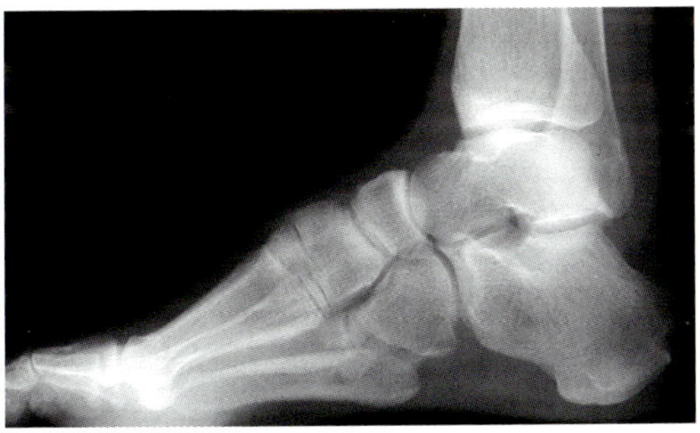

Fig. 6: Lateral X-ray of the cavus foot. Note the full lateral view of the posterior, anterior and middle facets of the subtalar joint with the varus hindfoot

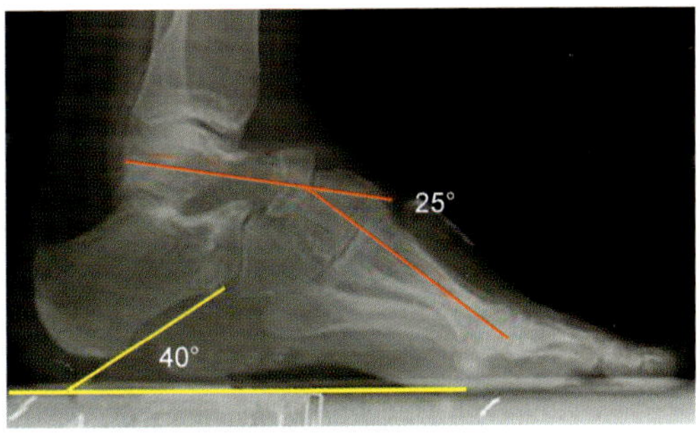

Fig. 7: Standing lateral radiograph of the foot of a patient with Charcot-Marie-Tooth. Note the increased calcaneal pitch and Meary's angle

In a very young child, soft tissue surgery is often sufficient. Plantar release is the cornerstone of treatment. This can consist of a simple division of the plantar fascia or a more thorough release of plantar structures as described by Steindler.[3] A medial incision is made; the tibial nerve is traced to its branching into medial and lateral plantar nerves. The origin of the abductor hallucis is divided. The plantar fascia is divided. The origin of the intrinsic plantar-flexor musculature is subperiosteally released from its origin on the calcaneal tuberosity. This may result in complete correction of the deformity. At times, serial casting is required to complete the correction. While most patients with CMT do not have an equinus contracture, in those rare cases where it exists, it is important to defer an Achilles tendon lengthening until another setting. After plantar release, it is important to have an intact Achilles tendon to "push against" while stretching the plantar structures.

Other soft tissue procedures are performed with the plantar release as indicated. Peroneus longus to brevis transfer is frequently employed. This transfer removes some of the plantarflexor moment from the first ray while preserving eversion power. The tibialis posterior can be lengthened, sectioned or transferred anteriorly through the interosseous membrane to assist with ankle dorsiflexion, if needed. If significant claw deformity exists, this may need to be addressed at a separate surgical procedure. The authors find claw toe deformity requires treatment in 30–50% of young patients with CMT. The authors' preference is for transfer of the long toe extensors to the metatarsal necks (Jones Procedure).[4] The transfer removes the deforming force leading to claw toes and may also aid in correcting the cavus whilst preserving some dorsiflexion power. In addition, the authors release the dorsal capsule of the MTP joint, resect the distal condyles of the proximal phalanx at the PIP joint, release the toe flexors and pin the entire toe from distal phalanx to metatarsal for 8 weeks. For the great toe, an interphalangeal (IP) joint fusion is generally combined with the Jones transfer. This procedure is extensive and cannot be performed concurrent with other procedures.

When hindfoot varus is fixed, soft tissue surgery alone will not be sufficient. The tibialis posterior and peroneus longus should still be addressed as these are the primary deforming forces. Arthrosis is generally not a factor and, therefore, osteotomy is preferred over arthrodesis in older children and adolescents. The plantar release is performed first or may be skipped altogether. Correction of cavus can be achieved through the metatarsal bases or through the midfoot. The medial column may be addressed in isolation or the entire foot, depending on the character of the cavus. The authors' preference is for midfoot correction. A dorsally based closing wedge osteotomy through the naviculocuneiform joints and cuboid provides excellent correction. Medial and lateral incisions are made centered over the cuboid and naviculocuneiform joints. The incisions are connected subperiosteally on the dorsal and plantar side in order to protect the neurovascular and tendinous structures. Two 0.045 inch diameter Kirschner wires are inserted under fluoroscopic guidance to subtend a dorsally based closing wedge through the naviculocuneiform joints and cuboid. An osteotome is used to remove the wedge of bone and the osteotomy is closed. Kirschner wires or staples can be used for fixation. If only the medial column needs to be addressed, the authors prefer a dorsal closing wedge osteotomy of the proximal first metatarsal. Care must be taken to preserve the proximal physis. While many advocate performing this at the medial cuneiform, the authors have found it difficult to close due to the capsular attachments to the middle cuneiform.

All that remains is to address the hindfoot varus. The authors perform a laterally based closing wedge osteotomy of the calcaneus with lateral translation similar to the Dwyer osteotomy.[5] An oblique lateral incision is made over the calcaneus. The sural nerve is protected. A 1 cm wide swath of bone is exposed just plantar to the peroneal sheath from just anterior to the Achilles insertion to 1.5 cm behind the calcaneocuboid joint. A laterally-based closing wedge osteotomy of the calcaneus is performed leaving the medial cortex intact. A lamina spreader is used to open the osteotomy while a Kerrison rongeur is used to remove the medial cortex and periosteum. The distal fragment is then slid laterally 30–50% of its width while the wedge is closed down. The osteotomy is secured with either Kirschner wires or offset staples.

CAVUS FOOT IN ADULTS

The cavus foot in adult patients retains no flexibility and adds the factor of arthritic changes in the subtalar and transverse tarsal joints. These patients become particularly symptomatic after an increase in activity and with multiple lateral ankle sprains. Even in the more subtle cavus feet, peroneal subluxation and tears become a problem, as well as stress fractures of the fifth metatarsal.[6]

On examination, the patients must be viewed from both the frontal and posterior perspectives. The valgus heel should be noted from the posterior, and the "peek-a-boo heel" sign, coined by Manoli,[7] is visible from the front. The high, inflexible arch on weight bearing is visible from the medial perspective. It is important for the examiner to palpate for tenderness in the sinus tarsi over the posterior facet of the subtalar joint, as well as medially and laterally over the talonavicular and calcaneocuboid joints. Positive findings would suggest arthritic changes in these joints. The peroneal tendons should be palpated for tenderness, crepitus, and bogginess suggesting tenosynovitis and/or a tear in these structures. Patients also complain of dorsal arch pain, dorsal pressure in shoes on the mid arch and often clawed toes; and, metatarsalgia with pressure calluses under the first and fifth metatarsal heads and the heel. Some patients have calluses as well under the base of the fifth metatarsal. A CT scan is an essential study which would confirm an impression of arthritis in the joints or rule it out. If there are positive findings over the peroneals, an MRI can confirm pathology here and at the deltoid ligament of the ankle. An ultrasound study is ideal to confirm peroneal subluxation and show a tear in the tendons, if the MRI is equivocal.

Conservative Treatment

These patients require various elements of shoe modification and custom orthotic devices. Short of this, modifications of shoe lacing and over-the-counter cushioned orthoses can be helpful. The ideal prescription includes an extra depth shoe to deal with the dorsal pressure in the midfoot and toes, and to accommodate the placement of an insert thicker than the standard sock liner. Adding a lateral flare to the heel decreases the likelihood of turning the ankle and having a lateral sprain. A rocker sole with the apex behind the metatarsal heads facilitates the toe off component of gait and off loads the metatarsal heads. Interposing SACH cushioning material within the heel of the shoe provides shock absorbency as well, as the cavus arch fails to provide this element in normal gait.

A well cushioned full length total contact insert of the UCBL (University of California Berkeley Laboratories) design, well molded to fill the arch, also helps with the dorsal pain and stabilizes the hind- and midfoot. Relief wells are placed under the heel and the metatarsal heads and these are filled with a resilient viscoelastic polymer.

Surgical Treatment in Adults

The surgical approach, of course, depends on the extent of the findings. If there are multiple problems, including the ankle and the toes, staging of the procedures may be necessary, choosing the most essential problems to be corrected, initially. The hind- and midfoot take precedence, as failure to correct these may lead to failure of the subordinate procedures if there is residual varus in the hindfoot. It is essential to explain carefully to the patient "what and why the surgeon is doing the procedures in stages?" If, for example, the patient complains mostly about the peroneal tendons and the surgeon is not planning to correct these, even if it is a subordinate procedure, in the initial stage, the patient will be disappointed with the outcome. Consequently, it is important not only to do the essential procedure, but also not to ignore the patient's chief complaint.

If there is a varus heel and inverted mid- and forefoot, but no arthritis, the surgeon can avoid fusions and correct the deformities with osteotomies and soft tissue procedures as in the adolescent. From the lateral "beanbag" position, the authors perform, under fluoroscopy control, a lateral displacement, valgus wedge osteotomy of the calcaneus (Figs 8 and 9). As with the medial displacement osteotomy done for the valgus heel, the approach is the same, but the plantar segment is moved laterally and a wedge of bone is removed from the lateral side. The site of the osteotomy and direction of the guidepins for fixation are indicated with a marking pencil. In contrast to the osteotomy done for valgus conditions, the cavus heel has a higher calcaneal

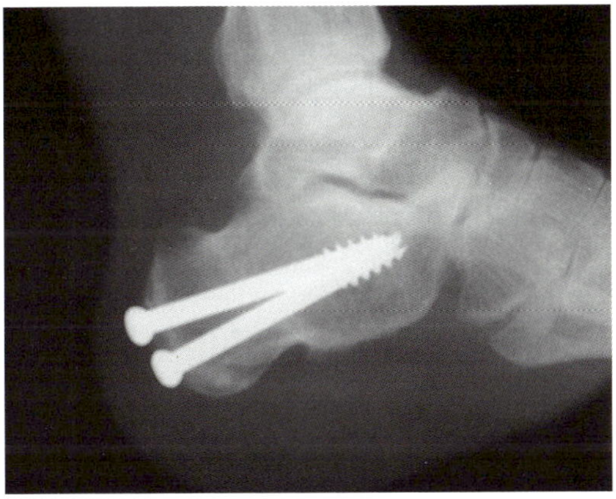

Fig. 8: Lateral displacement osteotomy of the calcaneus: sagittal view

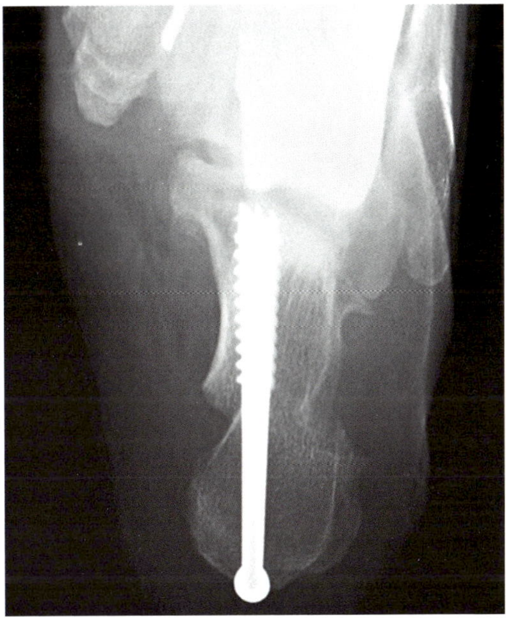

Fig. 9: Lateral displacement osteotomy of the calcaneus: tangential view

pitch and the line of the osteotomy is more vertical rather than parallel to the direction of the peroneals. This allows the more posterior fragment to slide dorsally, as well as laterally, decreasing the height of the arch. The guidepins are inserted through the heel while the displacement of the posterior segment of 5–10 mm while the dorsal shift, and closure of the osteotomy are maintained. The tangential views of the calcaneus are taken and also those which include the tibia (Saltzman view) to assure the correction of all these aspects. The admonition to only over drill one guidepin and to insert the screw while the other pin is untouched also applies in this osteotomy. (See the detailed description of the medial calcaneus osteotomy in Chapter 23). The patient is then rolled back to the supine position and the medial surgery performed. A posteromedial incision is used, started midway between the posterior border of the tibia and the medial border of the tendo-Achilles. It begins well above the medial malleolus and extends distally over the course of the neurovascular bundle, crossing over the "soft spot" on the medial border of the heel (Fig. 10), where these structures enter the foot (Fig. 11). The incision then continues transversely across the heel just distal to the pad. The laciniate ligament (flexor retinaculum) is divided, exposing the N-V bundle. The abductor hallucis muscle and its superficial and deep fascia are divided (using the cutting cautery on the muscle), while protecting the underlying critical structures. The plantar fascia is fully divided, along with the underlying flexor digitorum brevis. These maneuvers lower the arch and unwind the adducted forefoot. Proximally, the posterior tibial and flexor digitorum longus tendons are Z-lengthened above the posterior malleolar sheaths. As the flexor hallucis tendinous component is very short behind the ankle, this structure is lengthened in its subcutaneous fatty bed in the longitudinal arch. The incision is made under the abductor hallucis muscle here and the tendon is palpated by flexing and extending the great toe IP joint. The medial plantar nerve is encountered

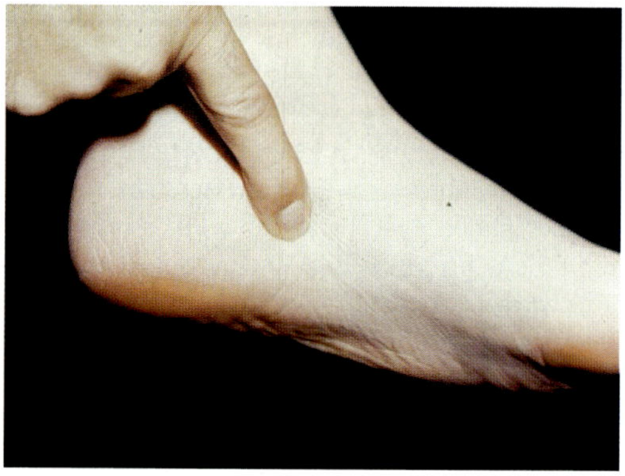

Fig. 10: The posteromedial "soft spot" on medial heel where tibial nerve and artery enter the foot

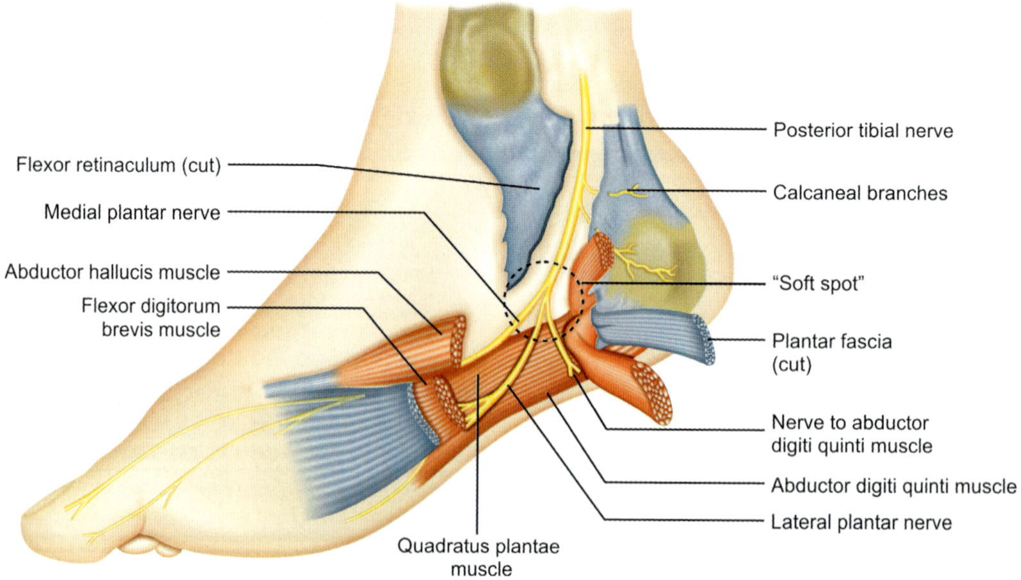

Fig. 11: Posteromedial neurovascular structures

initially and is protected. The oval flexor hallucis is differentiated from the flexor digitorum and then Z-lengthened. This posteromedial release and the calcaneal osteotomy may be sufficient to correct the foot. The first metatarsal may still be plantar flexed, however. If this is the case, it is elevated at the base with an osteotomy. A dorsal based wedge is the easiest technique; although a concentric osteotomy done from dorsal to plantar, with the convexity pointed distally allows one to dial in the exact correction. Fixation is carried out with a dorsal plate and screws or crossed K-wires or screws. The authors use the small plate and screws with compression. Healing in this metaphyseal bone is typically not a problem.

Tendon Transfers

During the lateral approach, a Z-lengthening is carried out for the peroneus longus (this eliminates the plantar flexion action of the muscle on the first ray). On the medial side, the medial portion of the anterior tibial which inserts on the medial side of the first metatarsal is elevated and repositioned on the lateral side of the remaining lateral portion of the tendon on the dorsum of the metatarsal, sewing it into the periosteum and lateral side of the lateral slip (in the manner of the Goldthwaite transfer of the patellar tendon done for the subluxing patella in years past).

Transfer of the Posterior Tibial Tendon

If there is definitely foot drop as in the CMT condition, the posterior tibial tendon is not lengthened, but rather is released from its insertion on the medial tarsal navicular and transferred to the middle of the foot. Although this may be done as a transfer through the interosseous membrane between the tibia and fibula, an alternative is a subcutaneous transfer to the middle cuneiform. This is done with the patient in the supine position. The tendon is released at the insertion and withdrawn though the posteromedial incision proximally enough to allow a fairly direct line of pull dorsally from the origin to the insertion. The middle cuneiform is exposed subperiosteally and a drill hole is made with fluoroscopic control from dorsal to plantar. The hole is enlarged with a 7.3 mm screw drill. Two bone anchors are placed inside the hole; one directed medially, the other, laterally. Large anchors with #2 suture is used. A whip stitch with 0 nylon or prolene is taken through the end of the beveled tendon of the posterior tibial. A large tendon passer (a large Kelly or uterine packing forceps) is used to burrow from the insertion point to the proximal wound in which the transfer tendon lies. The space is enlarged by spreading the forceps. The suture is grasped and the tendon brought to the insertion point. A Keith needle is placed on the two suture ends and the needle is driven through the drill hole and through the bottom of the foot. The ankle is placed in neutral to 15° of dorsiflexion and the tendon is pulled well into the drill hole. It is secured with the two pairs of sutures from the anchor. Strong tension is applied to the transfer tendon. At the completion of the repair, the foot should rest in neutral flexion/ extension. The nylon suture is withdrawn through the plantar foot.

If the subtalar and transverse tarsal joints are arthritic, a triple arthrodesis has to be done as well (Fig. 12).When joint fusions need to be added to deal with the pain component, some correction of the cavus deformity can be achieved through the joints. It is rarely possible, however, to gain full correction; and consequently, both the fusions and the osteotomies, as well as the soft tissue releases are usually necessary. The important point is to plan well and mark out the proposed incisions prior to actually carrying out the surgery in order to avoid creating a skin slough. The sinus tarsi incision to expose the subtalar posterior facet is a short oblique to avoid a narrow skin bridge with the calcaneal osteotomy incision. Fixation is achieved with 7.3 mm screws across both the osteotomy and the subtalar joint.

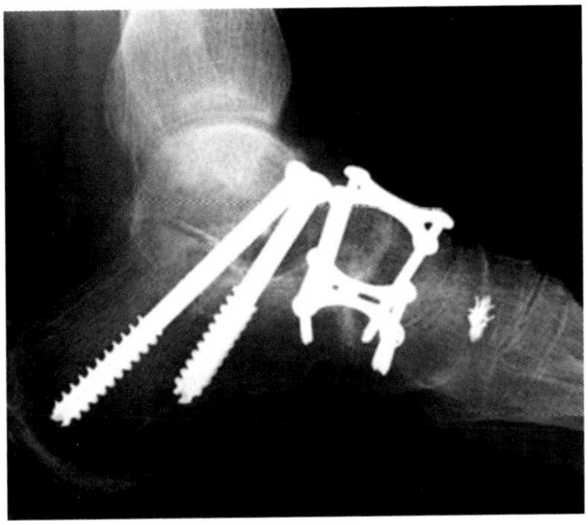

Fig. 12: Transfer of the posterior tibial into the midfoot in conjunction with a triple arthrodesis. Note that suture anchors in cuneiforms to anchor the tendon transfer to the midfoot

If surgery is needed for the peroneal tendons, this is done while the patient is in the lateral "beanbag" position. *If there is lateral ankle ligament instability,* the lateral ligament reconstruction, may be done at this time, as well, with the same incision.

If there is also clawing of the toes, this is usually staged if everything else, which takes precedence, is needed. While a simple flexor tenotomy and clasis of the PIP joint may be considered as a quick and easy procedure for the more elderly patient, a more formal and appropriate approach takes time, which may not be available during the initial procedure. Here, to do the procedure properly with fixed proximal interphalangeal (PIP) joint contractures and MTP hyperextension, a skin Z-plasty incision or at least a zigzag incision, followed by Z-lengthening of the extensor mechanism, dorsal capsulotomy of the MTP joint and a possible Weil osteotomy (see Chapter 14) may be needed. In addition, a resection arthroplasty of the PIP joint may be added as described earlier.

COMPLICATIONS AND SALVAGE OF THE CAVUS FOOT SURGERY

The primary concerns are inadequate corrections and nonunions of the bony procedures. The usual salvage is to redo the procedure which has failed, using better fixation and adjuncts such as iliac crest bone graft or high powered adjunctive bone substitute materials. It is essential that if one has to repeat a procedure that one has a plan to improve on the technique which also improves the odds that one will have success. Postoperative use of bone stimulators should also be considered in these situations. Preoperative planning and the use of staging are important. Procedures must be done in a timely manner, and the surgeon must have a realistic expectation for the time that each step will take. The tourniquet must be used judiciously and there must be an understanding of appropriate ischemic time, necessary reperfusion time, and the consequences of prolonged ischemia and multiple reapplications of the tourniquet, relative to postoperative swelling, edema, and wound problems.

REFERENCES

1. Coleman SS, Chesnut WJ. A simple test for hindfoot flexibility in the cavovarus foot. Clin Orthop Relat Res. 1977;123:60-62.
2. Price BD, Price CT. A simple demonstration of hindfoot flexibility in the cavovarus foot. J Pediatr Orthop. 1997;17:18-19.
3. Steindler A. Stripping of the os calcis. J Orthop Surg. 1920;2:8-12.
4. Jones R. The soldier›s foot and the treatment of common deformities of the foot. Part II. Claw-foot. BMJ. 1968;1:749-53.
5. Dwyer FC. Osteotomy of the calcaneum for pes cavus. J Bone Joint Surg Br. 1959;41:80-86.
6. Chilvers M, Manoli A. The subtle cavus foot and association with ankle instability and lateral foot overload. Foot Ankle Clin. 2008;13(2):315-24.
7. Manoli A, Smith DG, Hansen ST. Scarred muscle excision for the treatment of established ischemic contracture of the lower extremity. Clin Orthop. 1993;292:309-14.

27 Subtalar Arthroscopy, Hindfoot Endoscopy and Tendoscopy

Shana N Miskovsky

INTRODUCTION

This chapter will serve as an overview of arthroscopic, endoscopic and tendoscopic techniques successfully employed in the treatment of disorders of the posterior ankle, subtalar joint and hindfoot. As the technology improves and further indications for arthroscopic or endoscopic treatments evolve, it is important for the surgeon to be familiar with the indications, portal anatomy, complications and outcomes of these techniques. Compared with open procedures, these minimally invasive techniques have been associated with greater accuracy in the diagnosis and treatment of pathological conditions of the subtalar joint, less postsurgical morbidity, better cosmesis and faster recovery in the current published studies.[1-5]

SUBTALAR ARTHROSCOPY

In this section, subtalar arthroscopy will be discussed in detail including indications, complications, anatomy and step-by-step surgical technique. Then, an overview of the conditions treated via subtalar arthroscopy will be reviewed along with surgical technique pearls, outcomes and postoperative rehabilitation details, where appropriate.

In the literature, reported indications for subtalar arthroscopy include the treatment of loose bodies, synovitis, arthrofibrosis, osteochondral defects and symptomatic os trigonum.[6] Additionally, arthroscopic-assisted techniques such as calcaneal fracture reduction and fixation,[7] and subtalar joint arthrodesis[8] have been developed. Arthroscopic subtalar joint fusion has been successfully used to treat patients with painful arthritic subtalar joint or adults with a painful talocalcaneal coalition. This procedure is contraindicated in cases of severe degenerative arthrosis with significant deformity, soft tissue infection, large amount of edema or if there is concern for significant peripheral vascular disease. Lastly, subtalar arthroscopy can be performed in the supine, lateral decubitus or prone positions, depending on surgeon preference and concomitant procedures planned for one operative setting. Distraction of the joint can be performed via a noninvasive distractor or applied manually by a surgical assistant.

Outcomes after subtalar arthroscopy are reported to be in the range of 86–94% good to excellent results.[9,10] The consensus in these studies was that subtalar arthroscopy enabled the diagnosis of articular pathology better than the radiological studies available. However, its utility in the treatment of degenerative joint disease was minimal. With respect to complications, the overall rate was 10%.[10] But, most complications were related to transient neuropraxia.

Portal Options and Anatomy

The subtalar joint is divided by the tarsal canal into an anterior compartment (talocalcaneonavicular articulation) and a posterior compartment (talocalcaneal articulation). The sinus tarsi represent the lateral extension of the tarsal canal. The tarsal canal and sinus tarsi contain the interosseous talocalcaneal ligament, inferior extensor retinaculum (medial and intermediate roots) and cervical ligament. The anterior compartment is not accessible during arthroscopy due to the large interosseous ligament complex that prevents a connection forming in between the anterior and posterior compartments of the subtalar joint. A synovial lining about the posterior subtalar joint exists along with lateral, medial and anterior recesses which are accessible arthroscopically.

The ligaments which stabilize the subtalar joint include the lateral talocalcaneal ligament, posterior talocalcaneal ligament, lateral root of inferior extensor retinaculum and calcaneofibular ligament.

The anterolateral portal is located 1 cm inferior to the distal fibular tip and approximately 2 cm anterior to the distal fibular tip. The superficial peroneal nerve with its dorsal intermediate cutaneous branch is at risk.

The middle or central lateral portal is placed just inferior and anterior to the distal fibular tip. It is anterior to the calcaneofibular ligament and enters the joint at the level of the sinus tarsi. There are no neurovascular structures at risk with this portal.[10]

The posterolateral portal is located in line with the distal fibular tip just along the lateral border of the Achilles tendon. The sural nerve and lesser saphenous vein are at risk and so careful technique is required to prevent complications.[10] Inadvertent entry into the peroneal tendon sheath also is a possibility.

Accessory anterolateral and posterolateral portals (located alongside the primary portals) can be used for instrumentation in certain situations such as loose body removal.

Subtalar Arthroscopy: Step-by-Step Technique

Anesthesia

The procedure is performed under general anesthetic and a popliteal block is placed by anesthesia service to help with postoperative pain control.

Tourniquet

A well-padded tourniquet is placed on the upper thigh of the operative extremity after adequate padding has been placed. Tourniquet is elevated to 280 mm Hg for a maximum of 2 hours.

Equipment Notes

- 1.9-mm 30° arthroscope, double port (one for inflow, one for suction)
- 2.7-mm 30° arthroscope, double port (one for inflow, one for suction) to aid in visualization and negates need for additional fluid inflow portal
- Small joint arthroscopy set with curved and straight punches, graspers, ring and closed curettes, probe (with 1 mm hatchmarks to aid in measurements), osteotome probe, tissue elevators
- Sterile noninvasive distractor system with disposable sterile ankle stirrup sling
- Small joint oscillating shaver (short handle) 2.5-mm full radius shaver (less aggressive)
  - Small joint burr (short handle) 3.0-mm hooded burr
  - Micro Vector guide (Smith and Nephew, Andover MA) with K-wire guides for 0.045" (1.1 mm), 0.062" (1.6 mm), 0.125" (3.2 mm) or use an ACL targeting guide to assist for aiming for retrograde drilling of osteochondral defect (OCD) or for placing guidewires for arthroscopic fusion procedures.
  - Subchondral picks (45°or more acute angles are most useful)
- 18-gauge spinal needle for help with portal localization
- 10-cc syringe and connector tubing to attach to spinal needle for joint insufflation
- # 11-blade, small mosquito hemostats
- Arthroscopy pump with pressure set at 30 mm Hg
- Basic foot instrument tray with small retractors, osteotomes, curettes, etc.

Patient Positioning

The patient is positioned supine on the operating table, with the patient's knees at the same level as the break in the table that allows for lower leg and foot elevation or depression. Then, a bump, consisting of a 3 L bag of saline with towel secured around it, is placed underneath the ipsilateral hip so that the lower leg is rotated properly and the ankle is oriented straight up and down, not externally rotated during the procedure. While the hip is flexed at least 45° and held by an assistant, a foam-padded leg holder is placed approximately 4 fingerbreadths proximal to the popliteal crease to protect the neurovascular bundle, support the thigh and provide a stable base on which to apply traction to the ankle. For ease of positioning, the longer metal arm of the leg holder should be kept vertical. Holder position is then secured by the use of a clamp which attaches to the bed and is tightened with an interlocking teeth mechanism. The medial-to-lateral location of the foam pad support of the thigh can be adjusted with sliding the apparatus on the shorter metallic arm of the leg holder.

Patient positioning is essentially the same as that already described for ankle arthroscopy as presented in Chapter 30. However, the surgeon should place the ankle stirrup low enough on the posterior heel to allow for placement of a posterolateral portal.

But, the strap's position has to be secure enough around the posterior tuberosity of the calcaneus so that traction can be applied without stirrup slippage.

Step-by-Step Surgical Technique

1. After sterile prepping and draping, the noninvasive, sterile ankle distractor clamp is attached over the last sterile extremity sheet to the operating table and slid until the end of the table's rail. While draping, it is important not to have multiple layers of sheets over the rail where the clamp is applied and slid into position as the drapes bunch up and prevent the surgeon from advancing the table clamp to the end of the table rail and could limit the amount of traction that can be applied. The hinged distal portion of the clamp is oriented superiorly so that the clamp can be easily tightened and secured to the table. The L-shaped support bar is temporarily secured to the table clamp. The distractor's excursion ring is twisted and set to allow for maximum flexibility in the amount of traction applied and the distractor is attached to the support bar.
2. A sterile ankle stirrup sling is placed on the operative ankle with the posterior heel pad placed just above the posterior tuberosity of the calcaneus, and the dorsal foot pad to protect the dorsalis pedis neurovascular bundle. The portion of the ankle stirrup with a clip to attach to the distractor comes out plantar to the foot, making sure that the straps that run alongside the foot are not twisted. It is important not to get the foot and ankle or the ankle stirrup wet as they may slip off as traction is applied. A Coban wrap can be helpful to avoid this occurrence. The support bar is secured in the table clamp in a position that has the maximum height from the operating room (OR) table to allow for enough room for use of instruments in posterior portals.
3. Once the traction is set to the desired amount, landmarks are marked out with a sterile skin marker as shown in Figure 1 and include the distal fibula, medial malleolus, lateral and medial borders of the Achilles tendon, posterior facet area, sinus tarsi, and calcaneofibular ligament.
4. Localization of the anterolateral portal is done with an 18-gauge spinal needle directed towards the posterior joint and away from the sinus tarsi. The anterolateral portal then is approximately 1 cm distal and 2 cm anterior to the distal tip of the fibula. A spinal needle is used to establish the proper portal position, and sterile saline is injected into the subtalar joint with excellent backflow confirming intra-articular position. A # 11-blade is used to nick the skin only and the portal is created by using a blunt curved hemostat.
5. After the blunt trocar and sleeve are positioned, a double port 2.7-mm 30° arthroscope is introduced into the subtalar joint. Fluid inflow is set at 30 mm Hg or less.
6. Under direct visualization, the posterolateral portal is localized with a spinal needle first. The portal is at the level of the distal fibular tip and just along the lateral border of the Achilles tendon. The incision is made and blunt dissection with the hemostat establishes the portal. An arthroscopic picture is shown in Figure 2.

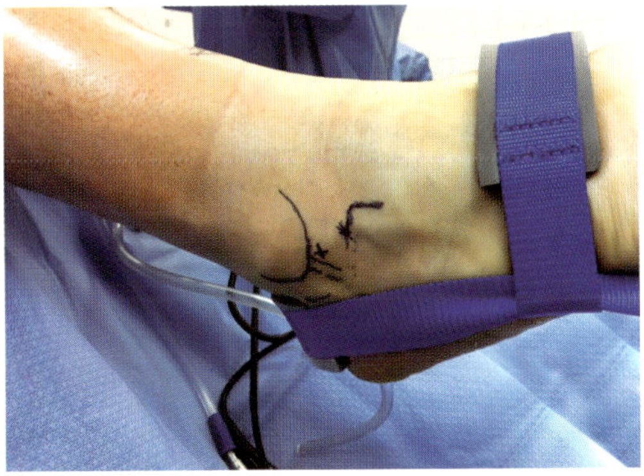

Fig. 1: Subtalar arthroscopy: Landmarks of the distal fibula, midportion of the tip of the distal fibula (vertical parallel lines), anterior process of calcaneus, sinus tarsi and posterior facet are drawn. Proposed locations of the anterolateral, middle and posterolateral portals are marked with an "x"

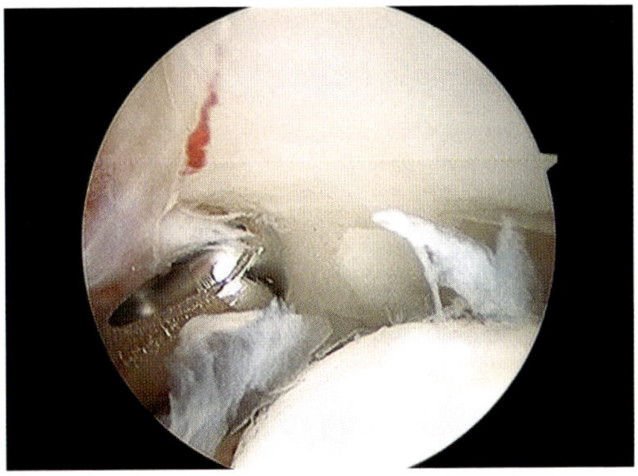

Fig. 2: Subtalar arthroscopy: The posterolateral portal is established under direct visualization from the anterolateral portal. An arthroscopic shaver is pictured entering the joint from the posterolateral portal

7. A thorough examination of the subtalar joint commences as has been described by Ferkel as a 13-point examination.[11] The arthroscope in the anterolateral portal is now used to evaluate the anterior portion of the posterior subtalar joint as shown in Figures 3A to C which includes: deep interosseous talocalcaneal ligament, superficial interosseous talocalcaneal ligament, anterior portion of the talocalcaneal joint, anterolateral corner of talocalcaneal joint, lateral gutter with the talocalcaneal ligament, reflection of calcaneofibular ligament in posterolateral aspect of the lateral gutter. In order to see the cartilage surfaces well and to minimize iatrogenic cartilage injury, the surgeon's hand should minimally move the scope side to side or up and down, as rotation of the light cord can yield an extensive view of the subtalar joint. Initially, to help with orientation upon entry into the joint, determine the location of the deep interosseous ligament which is located medially in the sinus tarsi. Then, the scope can be carefully retreated and rotated to see the anterior portion of the talocalcaneal joint or the anterior process area of the calcaneus.
8. The arthroscope is now switched to the posterior portal as seen in Figures 4A to C and the posterior aspect of the subtalar joint is evaluated systematically from laterally to medially. Important structures to identify include the lateral gutter, lateral talocalcaneal ligament reflection, calcaneofibular ligament reflection, talocalcaneal articulation, posterolateral gutter and posteromedial recess.
9. For additional access and visualization, a direct lateral or middle portal can be created just inferior and anterior to the distal tip of the fibula.
10. After completion of the procedure, the portals are closed with 4-0 nylon. To supplement the block and provide postoperative pain relief, a ropivacaine and morphine mixture is injected into the joint (5 cc total) and 0.5% marcaine without epinephrine is injected only into the skin incisions. A drain is not routinely placed, but, if needed, a 7 French round drain with Jackson-Pratt attachment can be placed into the joint under arthroscopic visualization by use of a small mosquito clamp.
11. A dressing is applied and the patient is then placed in a well-padded short leg splint. A few

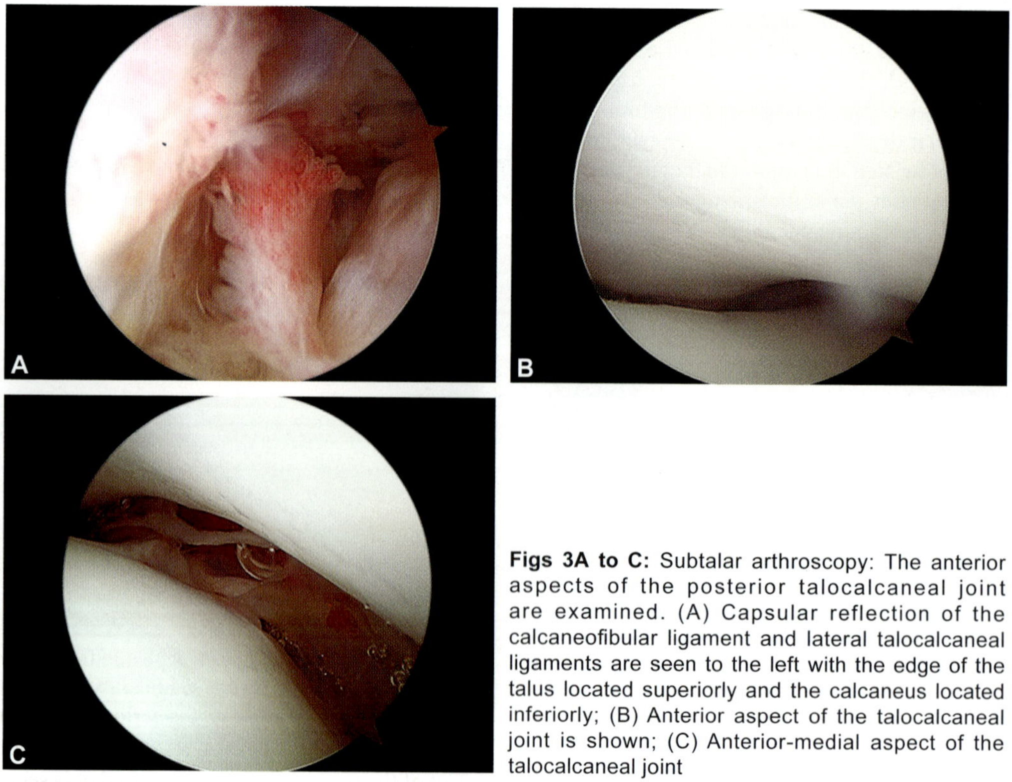

Figs 3A to C: Subtalar arthroscopy: The anterior aspects of the posterior talocalcaneal joint are examined. (A) Capsular reflection of the calcaneofibular ligament and lateral talocalcaneal ligaments are seen to the left with the edge of the talus located superiorly and the calcaneus located inferiorly; (B) Anterior aspect of the talocalcaneal joint is shown; (C) Anterior-medial aspect of the talocalcaneal joint

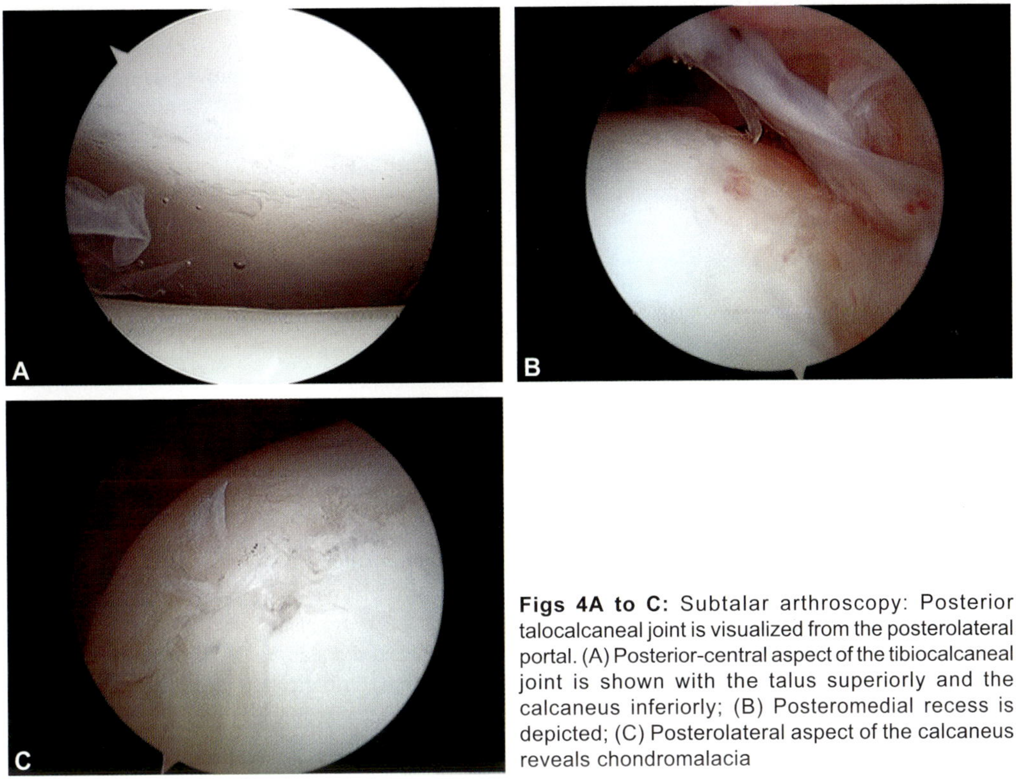

Figs 4A to C: Subtalar arthroscopy: Posterior talocalcaneal joint is visualized from the posterolateral portal. (A) Posterior-central aspect of the tibiocalcaneal joint is shown with the talus superiorly and the calcaneus inferiorly; (B) Posteromedial recess is depicted; (C) Posterolateral aspect of the calcaneus reveals chondromalacia

days postoperatively, the patient is transitioned into a CAM walker boot brace and physical therapy is begun depending on the exact procedure performed.

Overview of Subtalar Joint Conditions Treated Arthroscopically

This section will serve as a short review of clinical conditions affecting the subtalar joint for which arthroscopic treatment has been successful. The discussion will also include surgical technique pearls, presentation of assorted pathological pictures and rehabilitation guidelines, where appropriate.

Loose Bodies

Loose bodies within the subtalar joint can be accessed and removed with subtalar joint arthroscopy. Due to the constrained nature of this joint, arthroscopic management leads to better visualization than an open incision. Accessory portals can also be utilized in order to temporarily stabilize the fragment with a spinal needle while a grasper is brought in through the portal with the best trajectory. Fluid inflow can also be temporarily turned off while the grasper is maneuvered and placed around the loose fragment. If the loose body is located in the sinus tarsi, then the arthroscope should be placed in the anterolateral portal and instrumentation through the middle portal.

Osteochondral Defect of the Calcaneus

The surgeon has to keep in mind the size and location of the osteochondral defect (OCD). Most lesions can be accessed arthroscopically. Instrumentation through the posterolateral portal can be used to access very posterior lesions and can be used to access anterior lesions of the posterior half of the facet with the arthroscope placed in the anterolateral portal. When preparing a stable rim of cartilage around the OCD, the surgeon can switch portals to access different portions of the lesion with ring or closed curettes and prepare a perpendicular edge around the defect. A middle (or straight lateral) portal can also be created just anterior to the distal fibular tip and is used to assess an osteochondral defect of the posteromedial calcaneus that is seen in

Figure 5A while viewing through the posterolateral portal. The prepared OCD defect is shown in Figure 5B . The most angled of the subchondral picks available is chosen and carefully placed through the portal following the curve of the instrument for easy joint entry. The pick is positioned as perpendicular as possible with respect to the surface of the lesion as seen in Figure 5C. Gentle tapping with a mallet under direct visualization is performed to ensure that the pick does not skid across the surface and lose position. Each drill hole should be spaced apart by a few millimeters. Once finished with the microfracture procedure, the fluid to the scope is temporarily stopped to determine whether adequate bleeding occurs at the OCD site. The joint is then copiously irrigated, the arthroscopic equipment is removed, portals are closed, and a dressing and posterior splint are applied.

Postoperatively, the patients are non-weight bearing and released to home the same day if they fulfill discharge criteria. Patients are seen in the office within a week and changed to a tall CAM walker boot. A continuous passive motion machine protocol is then started for 4–6 hours a day for 4–6 weeks. Physical therapy is started. Patients then progress to weight bearing as tolerated in a CAM boot brace usually at week 6 postoperatively. Impact activities and running are initiated after 12 weeks. Sports return takes at least 4–6 months. Unfortunately, there is limited information available concerning OCD lesions of the calcaneus or undersurface of the talus at this time with respect to locations, outcomes, prognosis and optimal treatment.

Subtalar Joint Arthritis

Significant subtalar joint arthritis (post-traumatic or inflammatory) can be treated via an arthroscopic approach for arthrodesis.[12] As opposed to the supine position, arthroscopic fusion is more readily done in the prone position as hindfoot alignment can be more accurately evaluated.[13] A two or three portal technique has been described. The patient is positioned prone and a triangularly-shaped cushion is placed underneath the lower leg to elevate the operative foot and ankle, allow for circumferential access, and enable free motion of the ankle and subtalar joint during surgery. A thigh post is positioned to buttress the ipsilateral thigh and the bed is tilted towards the operative extremity so that leg rotation is neutral and foot is oriented vertically.

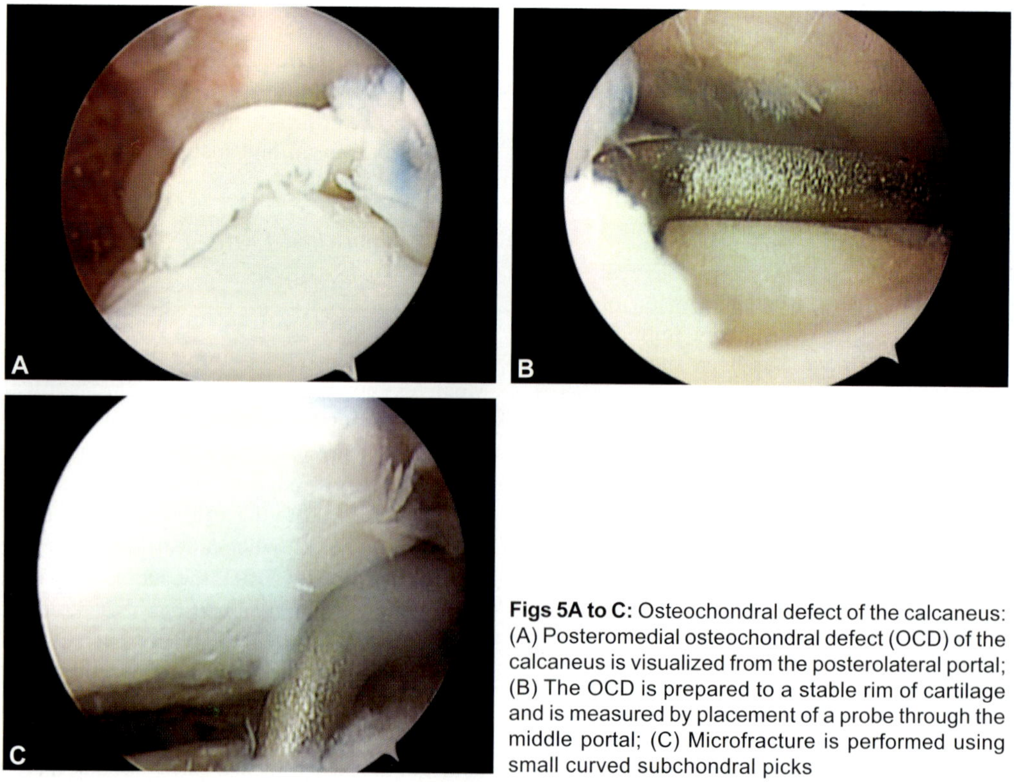

Figs 5A to C: Osteochondral defect of the calcaneus: (A) Posteromedial osteochondral defect (OCD) of the calcaneus is visualized from the posterolateral portal; (B) The OCD is prepared to a stable rim of cartilage and is measured by placement of a probe through the middle portal; (C) Microfracture is performed using small curved subchondral picks

Arthroscopic Subtalar Arthrodesis: Step-by-Step

1. A posterolateral portal is established similarly as to that for hindfoot endoscopy, as described in the next section of this chapter, just lateral to the Achilles tendon border at the level of the distal fibular tip. A posteromedial portal then is created just medial to the medial border of the Achilles at the level of the distal fibular tip. The extra-articular adipose tissue, crural fascia and posterior capsule of the subtalar joint are debrided under direct visualization with an oscillating shaver. The posterior talus and calcaneus now can be identified and to improve visualization of the posterior compartment of the subtalar joint, the soft tissue and retinacular attachments around the posteromedial talar process are released and, in the process, the flexor hallucis longus (FHL) is located and protected.
2. The posterior aspects of the talocalcaneal articulation are prepared with curettes (open and ring type) and burr. The underlying contour of the talus and calcaneus is preserved as debridement extends down to the bleeding subchondral bone.
3. The subtalar joint has limited distractibility and use of posterior portals alone does not generally allow the surgeon to prepare the anterior aspects of the posterior facet of the calcaneus for fusion. An accessory sinus tarsi portal has been utilized to prepare that anterior portion of the posterior facet, serve as a way to provide joint opening by carefully levering with a blunt trocar to increase the working space for the posteriorly placed instruments. The accessory sinus tarsi portal is localized with a spinal needle placed in the sinus tarsi aiming towards the distal fibular tip. The large diameter blunt trocar is introduced and moved in a medial-to-lateral fashion only while applying distraction of the subtalar (ST) joint in order not to cause iatrogenic grooving of the subchondral bone. Another option is to place an additional accessory posterolateral hindfoot portal for the distraction trocar but it may decrease posterior working space for joint preparation.[14]
4. Preparation of the joint surfaces posterior to the interosseous ligament are then completed after changing portals and using a burr to create vascular channels in the subchondral bone.
5. The hindfoot is positioned appropriately in 5° of valgus. Guidepins for 6.5 mm or 7.3 mm cannulated screws for fixation of the subtalar joint fusion are introduced through a posterior incision(s) on the heel. An aiming guide such as that used for a cruciate reconstruction can also be used. The scope can be positioned to check that pin placement is appropriate and joint surfaces are flush prior to full advancement of the guidepins.
6. Fluoroscopy is used to confirm proper location and trajectory of the guidepins on lateral and Harris axial views. Cannulated screws are placed in sequence after preparing with an opening reamer.
7. Skin incisions are closed and patients are placed in a well-padded non-weight bearing plaster splint.

At 10–14 days postoperatively, a short leg cast is placed. At 4–6 weeks, the patients begin weight bearing on the operative extremity in a tall CAM walker boot. It generally takes at least 6 weeks until early fusion healing is noted on X-rays. Physical therapy can be started as patients work on flexibility, strength, gait training and eventual weaning out of the boot over a few weeks. Outcomes in several studies show average fusion time to be 6–8.9 weeks.[13,15,16]

HINDFOOT ENDOSCOPY

In this section, hindfoot endoscopy will be discussed in detail including indications, complications, anatomy and step-by-step surgical technique. Then, an overview of the conditions treated via hindfoot endoscopy will be reviewed.

Overview and Indications

Initial hindfoot endoscopy techniques utilized supine positioning and three portals (anteromedial, anterolateral and posterolateral). There were reports of complications from the posteromedial portal including tibial nerve, posterior tibial artery and tendinous injuries.[17] The prone position affords easy access and less potential risks of neurovascular injury. This technique of posterior ankle and hindfoot endoscopy, utilizing posterolateral and posteromedial portals with the patient in the prone position, also is versatile and can be used to evaluate and treat disorders in the posterior ankle, subtalar joint and retrocalcaneal space. Reportedly, conditions successfully treated with this approach include those that are intra-articular (loose bodies, posterior osteochondral defects, subtalar joint arthritis, synovitis, and calcaneal fractures) and those that are extra-articular (avulsion fracture fragments, nonunions of posterior talar process, os trigonum, Haglund deformities, retrocalcaneal bursitis, FHL tendinopathy, Achilles tendinitis).[18-20] Some authors recommend using fluoroscopy for localization purposes, particularly when direct entry into the posterior ankle joint is desired as a concomitant procedure.[20] For the most part, no distraction is needed for hindfoot endoscopy. In cases where joint distraction is needed to address a posterior talar osteochondral defect or access the ankle or subtalar joints, distraction can be accomplished via a noninvasive ankle distractor or via a calcaneal pin,[21] with no increase in complications reported with respect to the type of distraction used.[20]

Complications

Historically, there have been concerns regarding the use of posterior portals and safety of the neurovascular structures in the area. However, complications of hindfoot endoscopy have been reported to be few,[5] with one large study noting a 1.4% rate which represented patients who had persistent numbness over the posterior heel pad post surgery.[18] In another study which focused on the rate of neurological injury and risk factors associated, an overall complication rate of 8.5% was found in 189 ankle and hindfoot arthroscopy and endoscopy procedures.[20] Complications included: plantar numbness (2.1%), Achilles tendon tightness (2.1%), sural nerve dysesthesias (1.6%), postoperative infection (1.1%), complex regional pain syndrome (1.1%) and posteromedial portal cyst (0.5%). The majority of the sural nerve injuries resolved over time and were felt to be related to neuropraxia from proximity of the nerve to the posterolateral portal. Finally, Achilles tendon tightness was associated with extra-articular procedures and did resolve with a supervised physical therapy program.

Portal Options and Applied Anatomy

For the posterolateral portal, the anatomical landmarks are distal fibular tip, lateral border of the Achilles tendon and the first interdigital webspace. Draw a horizontal line with a skin marker from the distal fibular tip across the back of the foot until one gets to the Achilles tendon. The intersection point of this line and the vertical border of the lateral aspect of the Achilles tendon serves as the start point for the portal incision. Incision is made and extended superiorly from this point. When inserting the arthroscope or instruments, the surgeon aims towards the first interdigital webspace. In one study, the mean distance of sural nerve to posterolateral hindfoot portal was 13.1 mm.[22] Neutral foot position offered the best safety and other foot positions were found not to be advantageous with respect to avoiding neurological complications.

For the posteromedial portal, the same landmarks are used. The posteromedial portal is placed at the same level with respect to the fibula as the posterolateral portal, but the portal is created just medial to the medial border of the Achilles. The mean distance described from the posteromedial portal to the posterior tibial nerve was 16.5 mm.[22]

To prevent neurological complications, it is very important to use careful technique in establishing portals by cutting the skin only with the scalpel and then bluntly dissecting with a hemostat deeper to establish the portal. Additionally, as a rule of thumb, the sural nerve crosses the lateral border of the Achilles approximately 9.8 cm from the insertion point of the Achilles tendon on the calcaneus.[23] Also, identification of the FHL is important so that dissection does not proceed any further medially due to the potential risk of posterior tibial neurovascular bundle injury. There are anatomical variations of the FHL that could pose the surgeon difficulties such as the presence of the peroneocalcaneus internus muscle which can be mistaken for the FHL.[24]

Hindfoot Endoscopy: Step-by-Step Technique

The equipment used is similar to that listed for ankle arthroscopy, with the addition of small osteotomes and periosteal elevators, as needed. The patient is positioned prone on the operating table on thoracic chest rolls. Special eye protection and facial pillow is used. Neutral cervical alignment is maintained. Both arms are abducted and externally rotated on arm boards with padding to keep pressure off of the ulnar nerves. A pillow is placed beneath the knee and blankets used to support and elevate the operative leg. The surgeon should be able to easily move the ankle through a range of motion. During the case, low pump pressures generally are used (i.e. 20–30 mm Hg) or gravity inflow. A 2.7-mm 30° arthroscope or 4.0-mm arthroscope can be used depending on the surgeon's preference.

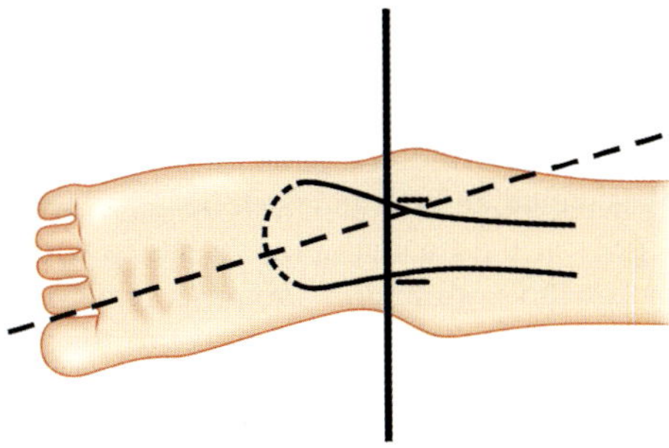

Fig. 6: Hindfoot endoscopy: Diagram of landmarks of the posterior hindfoot, including horizontal line drawn at the level of the distal tip of the fibula (solid black line) serving as a start point for the posterolateral and posteromedial portals (vertical lines). Trajectory of small hemostat entry to create the posterolateral portal is directed towards the first webspace (dotted line)

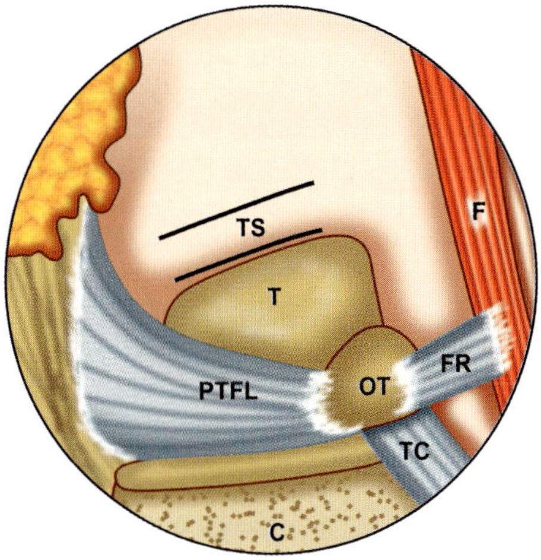

Fig. 7: Hindfoot endoscopy: Diagram of structures to be identified surrounding an os trigonum (OT) for example. Flexor hallucis longus tendon (F) serves as an important landmark medially. Other structures depicted include: flexor retinaculum (FR), posterior talocalcaneal ligament (TC), posterior calcaneus with subtalar joint surface (C), posterior talofibular ligament (PTFL), posterior talus (T), and tibial slip (TS)

1. Anatomical landmarks are identified including the tip of distal fibula and lateral edge of the Achilles tendon and a skin marker is used to mark out the portal sites as diagrammed in Figure 6.
2. A small skin incision with a # 11 blade is made approximately 5 mm proximal to the tip of the fibula just lateral to the Achilles tendon (or start portal incision at the same level of the distal fibular tip and extend incision superiorly). A small curved mosquito hemostat then creates the portal and the surgeon aims toward the landmark of the first interdigital webspace of the foot. Curved hemostat then is used to dissect down through the thick crural fascia onto the bone.
3. The arthroscope is introduced into the working space created from blunt dissection. The posteromedial portal is then localized with a spinal needle placed just medial to the Achilles tendon and at the same level as the posterolateral portal. An incision is made and a blunt trocar or hemostat creates the portal. The hemostat or trocar is aimed 90° to the shaft of the arthroscope. The hemostat is advanced down along the shaft of the scope cannula until triangulation occurs and the tip of the instrument is seen arthroscopically. This maneuver is done to prevent inadvertent damage to the posteromedial neurovascular bundle. The hemostat is utilized to bluntly dissect the extra-articular soft tissues.
4. An oscillating shaver is then introduced through posteromedial portal aiming 90° to the shaft of the scope and then followed the scope shaft all the way down to the tip of the scope as before and every time the posteromedial portal is entered with an instrument. The extensive crural fascia and thin posterior capsule of the subtalar joint is debrided to improve visualization.
5. Posterior structures then are identified as diagrammed in Figure 7. The flexor hallucis longus (FHL) then can be seen and serves as a reference point for the surgeon (stay lateral to this structure and stay out of trouble). The posterior talofibular ligament, flexor retinaculum, posterior talocalcaneal ligament, posterior process talus, tibia, posterior facet of calcaneus and FHL are visible. The posterior ankle ligaments (tibiofibular, talofibular) also can be seen more superiorly. Pathologies are addressed by the surgeon as discussed in the following sections.
6. After copious irrigation, wounds are closed with 4-0 nylon. The patient is placed in a well-padded short leg splint and kept non-weight bearing for 3–5 days for comfort and to protect the wounds. Then, patients are transitioned to a walking tall CAM boot and physical therapy is initiated for range of motion and strengthening exercises.

If the surgeon has to perform ankle arthroscopy, needing to reach anteriorly as well as posteriorly, there is a method that can be used to avoid repositioning of the patient to do the hindfoot endoscopy.[25] The patient is positioned on a beanbag in a lateral decubitus position. An axillary role is placed and neutral cervical alignment is maintained. The down leg (nonoperative leg) is padded to prevent any pressure on the common peroneal nerve area about the proximal fibular head and to prevent the heel from touching the bed. The operative leg is placed in the leg holder as usual and normally the ipsilateral hip joint has enough flexibility to allow for positioning the foot with the toes towards the ceiling. This is a similar position to that described for supine ankle arthroscopy in Chapter 30. The sterile noninvasive ankle distractor is placed on the ipsilateral side for ankle arthroscopy. At the completion of this portion of the procedure, the sterile noninvasive distractor is moved to the contralateral side of the bed and secured in place with its L-shaped arm extended upwards as much as possible to elevate the operative extremity off of the table and allow for adequate room for the surgeon to work through posterior portals. The ankle stirrup is kept in place during this transition so that fluid does not get on the interface between the skin and the foam of the stirrup (to avoid slippage of the stirrup on the foot as traction is applied). The stirrup then is attached to the distractor as usual and slight traction is applied. Now the patient's leg, foot and ankle are in the lateral position and the surgeon now can proceed with posterior hindfoot endoscopy as described above or with posterior ankle arthroscopy. If there are concomitant open procedures that also have to be done, including a lateral ankle ligament reconstruction or peroneal tendon exploration with repair, the leg then is taken out of traction, the holder is removed from underneath the drapes and sterile bumps are placed underneath the lower leg to allow for visualization of the lateral ankle structures in the lateral decubitus position.

Posterior Ankle Impingement

Posterior ankle impingement can occur from several conditions with its clinical hallmark of pain with hyperplantarflexion, particularly seen in athletes such as ballerinas and soccer players.[18] A diagnostic and therapeutic injection can be performed in the office to help differentiate the source of the patient's discomfort. Further imaging with MRI or CT scanning may be helpful. Structures that are thought to contribute to posterior ankle impingement include an os trigonum, Steida posterior process of the talus, posterioinferior tibiofibular ligament, transverse tibiofibular ligament, tibial slip and tendons including FHL and posterior tibial tendon. But, generally a traumatic injury has to occur in order for those structures to cause symptomatic impingement due to disruption of the cartilaginous synchondrosis, tearing of the ligaments leading to fibrosis or hypertrophy, or nonhealing of a fracture.

Os Trigonum

An os trigonum represents a failure of fusion of the lateral tubercle of the talus with the talar body. It is noted in 14–25% of the population, occurs bilaterally in 1.4% and articulates with the talar body through a synchondrosis.[26] Patients are painful with forceful plantarflexion of the ankle and have posterolateral palpation tenderness in the area in between the Achilles and peroneal tendons. If there is significant tethering of the FHL also present, then patients can have decreased, painful great toe extension and flexion. For diagnostic and therapeutic purposes, the clinician may elect to inject the area with lidocaine (with cortisone as indicated) with the patient positioned prone with or without the use of ultrasound. If conservative treatment does not relieve the patient's symptoms, then surgical intervention is indicated. Options for access to the os trigonum include hindfoot endoscopy, subtalar arthroscopy or posterior ankle arthroscopy technique.

Hindfoot endoscopy is generally used, due to the ease of positioning, visualization and access. Patient positioning and portal placement is as described earlier in this section. Upon removal of the crural fascia and posterior capsule, the large os trigonum is localized via fluoroscopy as in Figure 8A and is seen with the arthroscope in Figure 8B. The FHL then can be identified and serves as the medial-most border of any dissection or debridement in order to protect the tendon itself and the neurovascular bundle medial to it. The surgeon can then proceed to carefully release the soft tissues around os trigonum going from lateral to medial. The ligamentous attachments to the os trigonum have to be released including the posterior talofibular ligament (lateral attachment), flexor retinaculum (superior and medial attachment), and posterior talocalcaneal ligament (inferior-medial attachment). With a large os trigonum, it may have to be split into pieces carefully with a small curved osteotome or burr

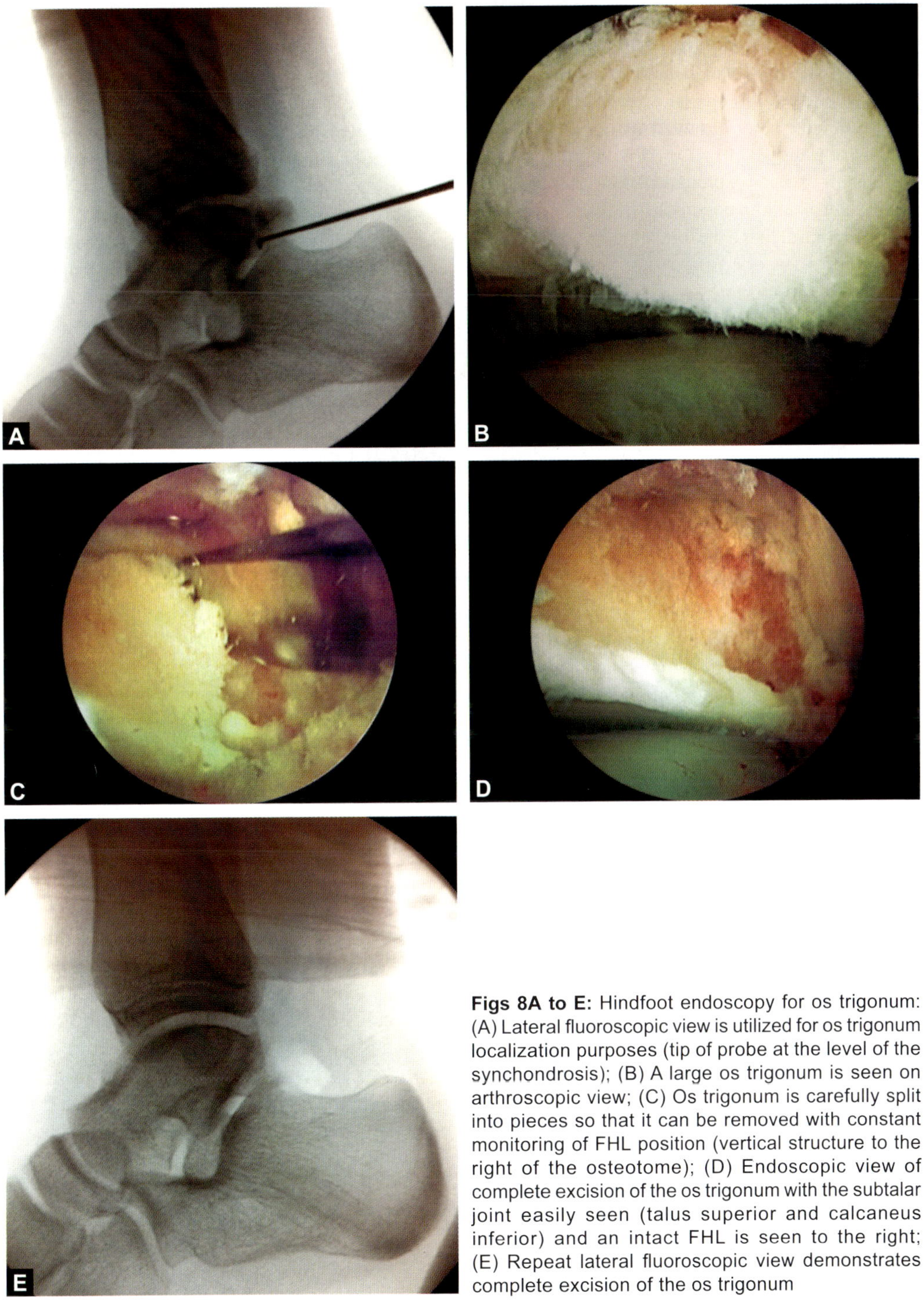

Figs 8A to E: Hindfoot endoscopy for os trigonum: (A) Lateral fluoroscopic view is utilized for os trigonum localization purposes (tip of probe at the level of the synchondrosis); (B) A large os trigonum is seen on arthroscopic view; (C) Os trigonum is carefully split into pieces so that it can be removed with constant monitoring of FHL position (vertical structure to the right of the osteotome); (D) Endoscopic view of complete excision of the os trigonum with the subtalar joint easily seen (talus superior and calcaneus inferior) and an intact FHL is seen to the right; (E) Repeat lateral fluoroscopic view demonstrates complete excision of the os trigonum

under direct visualization, aiming away from the posteromedial structures as depicted in Figure 8C. The demarcation between normal talar cartilage and where os trigonum started is noted. After complete excision of the os trigonum, the subtalar joint is seen as in Figure 8D. A final fluoroscopic view in Figure 8E confirms that the entire os trigonum has been excised. Also, while looking with the arthroscope, the ankle is hyperplantarflexed to make sure that no further impingement exists.

Outcomes of surgical treatment for posterior ankle impingement have been reported, but further investigations are needed as most are case series. One study covering surgical treatments including excision of os trigonum, excision of prominent posterior process of talus, excision of painful nonunions, FHL tenolysis, and loose body removal found the following: average time to return to work of 4 weeks, average time to return to sports 5.8 months, return to same level of sport for majority of patients, and excellent health-related quality of life scores.[5]

Retrocalcaneal Bursitis and Haglund Deformity

First described in 1928,[27] Haglund deformity and its resultant painful syndrome is thought to occur due to chronic inflammation of the retrocalcaneal space and Achilles tendon often combined with Achilles insertional tendinopathy that leads to the formation of an enlarged posterosuperior bony prominence on the calcaneus. Patients present with posterior heel lump and pain with shoewear pressing in that area, along with palpation, tenderness or swelling in the retrocalcaneal bursa and along with tenderness at the Achilles proximal to its insertion. Conservative treatment is attempted first and includes a short period of immobilization in more painful cases, a daily stretching program, shoewear modification, heel lift or orthotic inserts, nonsteroidal anti-inflammatory medications, and occasionally diagnostic and therapeutic injection into the retrocalcaneal space.

Surgical treatment is indicated in patients who failed a complete course of conservative treatment, demonstrate persistent pain to palpation over the retrocalcaneal bursa and experience mechanical impingement from a Haglund deformity. Contraindications would include patients with the following: significant insertional Achilles tendinopathy, posterior exostosis formation involving more than 50% of the Achilles tendon insertion, significant peripheral vascular disease, active infections, open wounds, and cosmetic concerns (combined with minimal pain and no functional limitations).[3,4] Open procedures have been associated with wound healing complications, Achilles tendon damage or avulsion, dysesthesias around the heel, scar sensitivity, stiffness of ankle or hindfoot, and others.[28] In comparison with open procedures, if appropriate visualization and debridement can be performed, an endoscopic procedure can provide the opportunity for a faster patient recovery and improved cosmesis, with decreased complications and with minimal risk to the surrounding neurovascular structures.[2,29]

Patient positioning for endoscopic decompression procedures can be supine[3] or prone. With the supine position, the operative extremity is moved to the side off of the table and the foot rests on the surgeon's chest. Then, both of the surgeon's hands are free to hold the arthroscope and instrumentation respectively. Use of the prone position may be more favorable as the foot rests on the table with a bump placed beneath the lower leg, allowing the surgeon access to both sides of the Achilles tendon for portal placement and instrument use.

Portal Options and Applied Anatomy

The retrocalcaneal bursa is normally a horse-shoe or disk-shaped structure which covers the posterior-superior surface of the posterior calcaneus.[30] Its thickness is normally 4 mm and its superior-to-inferior length is on average 22 mm. The Achilles does not attach on the proximal-most aspect of the posterior-superior calcaneus, as the bursa is there. The Achilles attaches more inferiorly on the calcaneus in the apophyseal area. The average height of its tendon insertion is 19.8 mm. The average width at the proximal aspect of the insertion is 23.8 mm as compared to 31.2 mm at the distal aspect. Anatomically, the safest way to do a partial excision of Achilles tendon for insertional tendinopathy is proceeding from the superior aspect of the bony prominence going distally.[31]

The lateral portal is placed alongside the lateral border of the Achilles tendon and anterior to the Achilles tendon at the level of the superior aspect of the calcaneus. The sural nerve is at risk with this portal and careful surgical technique utilizing blunt dissection is recommended.

The medial portal is placed just medial to the medial border of the Achilles tendon at the level of the superior aspect of the calcaneus. The structure at risk here is the calcaneal branch of the lateral plantar nerve.

Surgical Technique for Retrocalcaneal Endoscopy: Step-by-Step

1. The patient is positioned prone on the operating table as described previously. Extra blankets or bump is placed underneath the lower leg of the

operative extremity. The operative extremity then is slightly higher as compared to the normal side and off of the table to allow posterior access to the hindfoot. A tourniquet is placed. Sterile prepping and draping are performed.

2. The lateral portal is localized in the soft spot just lateral to the lateral border of Achilles. A small vertical incision just through skin is done with a # 11-blade. Blunt dissection with a small curved hemostat creates the portal with minimal risk to the sural nerve and opens up the retrocalcaneal space.
3. A 4.0-mm 30° arthroscope is inserted into the lateral portal. The surgeon can also use a 2.7-mm scope in patients with a smaller body habitus. The medial portal is localized with a spinal needle under direct visualization with the arthroscope. The spinal needle should be introduced just medial to the medial border of the Achilles tendon and enter the retrocalcaneal space just above the superior-medial aspect of the calcaneus. A small stab incision is made and blunt dissection with trocar establishes the medial portal.
4. Debridement begins on the scarred, inflamed retrocalcaneal bursal tissue with a 3.5-mm shaver brought in through the medial portal. A working space is created and the posterosuperior calcaneal prominence is carefully exposed with its margins identified.
5. A 4.0-mm burr or the shaver can be used to resect the bony prominence, starting from the posterior-superior aspect of the bony prominence and working inferiorly until the proximal attachment of the Achilles tendon is reached. This distance is approximately 2–4 cm depending on the size of the bony prominence. The Achilles tendon is protected throughout debridement by keeping the hood of the instrument towards the tendon.
6. As the excision proceeds, the surgeon can palpate the edges of the calcaneus and posterior calcaneus to make sure that all edges are smooth and to determine if an adequate amount of bone has been removed. Fluoroscopic evaluation also is helpful to determine the amount of bone resected. The surgeon can put the ankle through a range of dorsiflexion and plantarflexion with the arthroscope in place to visualize and confirm that there is no further bony or soft tissue impingement. Additional debridement can be performed otherwise.
7. Throughout the process, the insertion point of the Achilles is carefully identified, visualized and protected. A probe is utilized to confirm the integrity of the Achilles tendon attachment. If the anterior portion of Achilles tendon shows evidence of inflamed tissue or tendinopathy, the arthroscopic shaver can be used to carefully debride the unhealthy tendinous tissue from a superior to inferior direction. If the surgeon feels that it is necessary to further encourage tendon healing, trephination of the tendon with a spinal needle can be performed. If the tendon is severely involved with tendinopathy and more than 50% from a superior to inferior extent (or greater than about 10 mm) has to be excised,[31] then the surgeon can convert to an open procedure (Chapter 34).
8. Copious irrigation is performed and then the wounds are closed with 4-0 nylon suture. Dressings are placed and a well-padded short leg splint in slight plantarflexion is applied on the operative extremity.

Patients are made non-weight bearing postoperatively. Follow-up in the office occurs 10–14 days later where patients are switched to a tall CAM boot walker brace with a heel lift, depending on the surgical findings and the patient's comfort level. The patient begins weight bearing as tolerated on the operative extremity with crutches and the heel lift is weaned over 1–2 weeks. Physical therapy is begun and suture removal and boot weaning starts at 3–4 weeks post surgery. A graduated physical therapy protocol is continued for gait training, hip and core and leg strengthening, eccentric strengthening, cardio conditioning (first with stationary bike, then pool), proprioception, agility and finally a sports-specific program.

With respect to outcomes, there have been small studies showing promising results. In one prospective case series of 30 patients with a mean follow-up of 35 months, there were 26 excellent results reported. There was one major complication with an early, acute Achilles tendon rupture after surgery due to patient noncompliance with postoperative bracing. Another patient developed recurrent pain and swelling, requiring an open procedure. There were no reported wound complications, painful scars or neuroma formation. The average time to return to weight bearing was 4 weeks. Patients comfortably returned to shoes with a heel counter and resumed normal activities on an average of 8 weeks postoperatively. This is also the average time to return to sports.[32] It appears that endoscopic decompression offers adequate exposure and can be a viable treatment option with low morbidity and high patient satisfaction. However, further comparative studies with open procedures are needed.

TENDOSCOPY

Tendoscopy is a newer and advanced, minimally invasive technique used to directly visualize the posterior tibial tendon and peroneal tendons. Reported indications are mainly to treat adhesive tenosynovitis and evaluate and/or debride degenerative tendinopathy, tendon subluxation or tendon rupture.[33,34] Initial outcomes appear to be promising but require further study.

For peroneal tendoscopy, the patient can be positioned supine or lateral decubitus. Oftentimes, this procedure is done in conjunction with ankle arthroscopy and the traction system on the ankle is released so that tendoscopy can be performed. The leg is supported by a sterile bump in these cases. A 2.7-mm 30° arthroscope is utilized. The landmarks of the distal tip of the fibula, longitudinal axis of the fibula, superior peroneal retinaculum and location of the peroneal tendons are determined as diagrammed in Figure 9. The distal portal is created first, approximately 2 cm distal to the fibular tip in line with the longitudinal axis of the fibula in order to prevent damage to the superior peroneal retinaculum. A small stab incision is made with a # 11-blade and a small curved hemostat bluntly creates the portal to enter into the peroneal tendon sheath. The calcaneofibular ligament is deep to the peroneal tendons and so, iatrogenic damage is rare. The arthroscope is then introduced into the peroneal tendon sheath. A superior portal is then localized with a spinal needle and is made approximately 3 cm proximal to the distal fibular tip and directly over the peroneal tendons. Now, the normal vincula that separates the proximal portion of the brevis from the longus can be seen proximally.

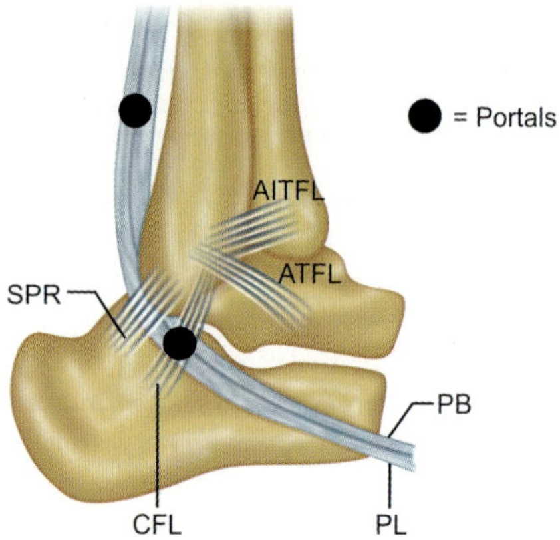

Fig. 9: Peroneal tendoscopy: Diagram of important structures and location of superior and inferior portal placement. Structures that are depicted include: superior peroneal retinaculum (SPR), calcaneofibular ligament (CFL), anterior talofibular ligament (ATFL), anterior-inferior tibiofibular ligament (AITFL), peroneus brevis (PB), and peroneus longus (PL)

A thorough examination of the brevis and longus tendons is done by using a probe to help rotate the tendons and assist in placing the scope superiorly and inferiorly to each tendon as shown in Figures 10A to D. The tendons are followed distally to the fibular groove via visualization from the superior portal as depicted in Figures 11A to C. If tenosynovitis or a small tear is found, then an oscillating shaver is used for debridement under direct visualization. More extensive tears or subluxations or ruptures may require the surgeon to perform an open approach in order to properly repair or reconstruct the damaged tendons or superior peroneal retinaculum. After irrigation, the portals are closed with 4-0 nylon and a dressing with posterior short leg splint is applied. Patients are initially non-weight bearing for 5–10 days after tendoscopy to allow resolution of initial inflammation. Then, after follow-up in the office, patients are generally started in a CAM walker boot weight bearing and physical therapy is started with the protocol depending on the amount of tendon damage.

For tendoscopy of the posterior tibial tendon, the use of the arthroscope is similar and portals are carefully placed via the knick and spread technique as described above. The inferior or distal portal is placed approximately 1.5–2 cm distal to the

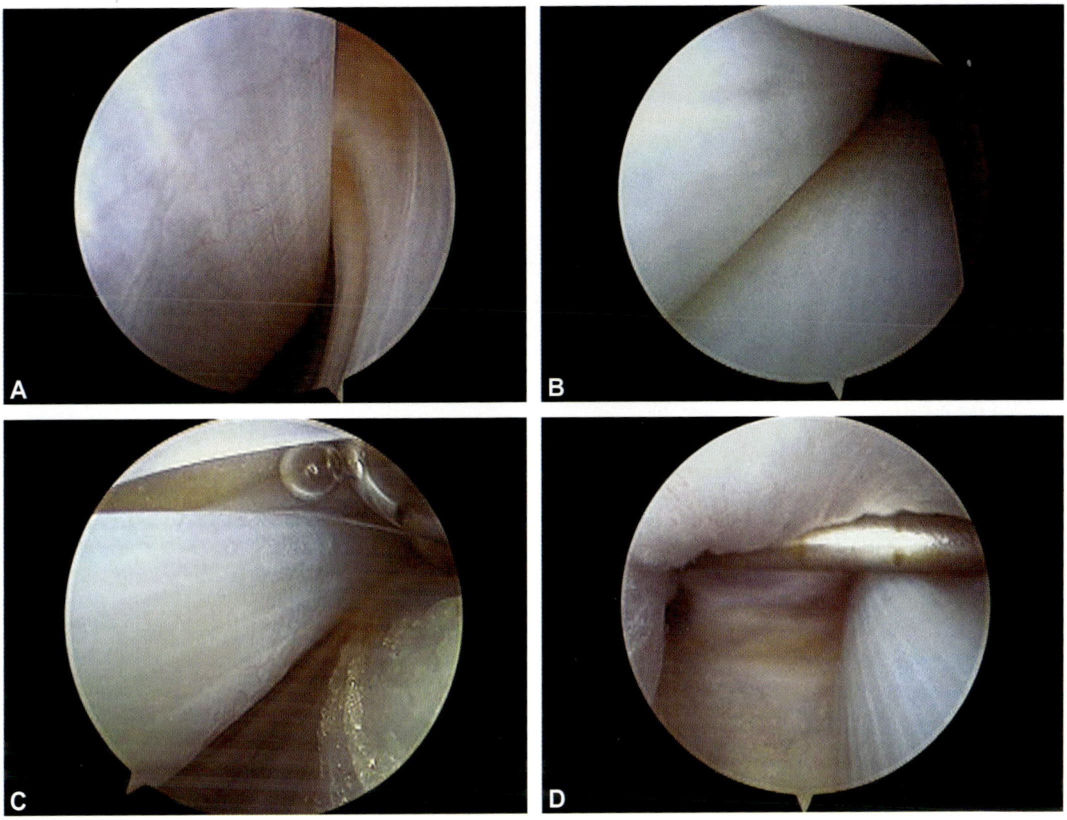

Figs 10A to D: Peroneal tendoscopy: Peroneal tendons are evaluated with a probe in the superior portal while visualizing with the arthroscope in the inferior portal. (A) Posterolateral surface of the longus tendon with intact peroneal tendon sheath demonstrated (right side of picture); (B) Brevis and longus are seen; (C) Probe placed in between the longus and brevis to rotate around and evaluate the tendons; (D) Anterior surface of the brevis is seen

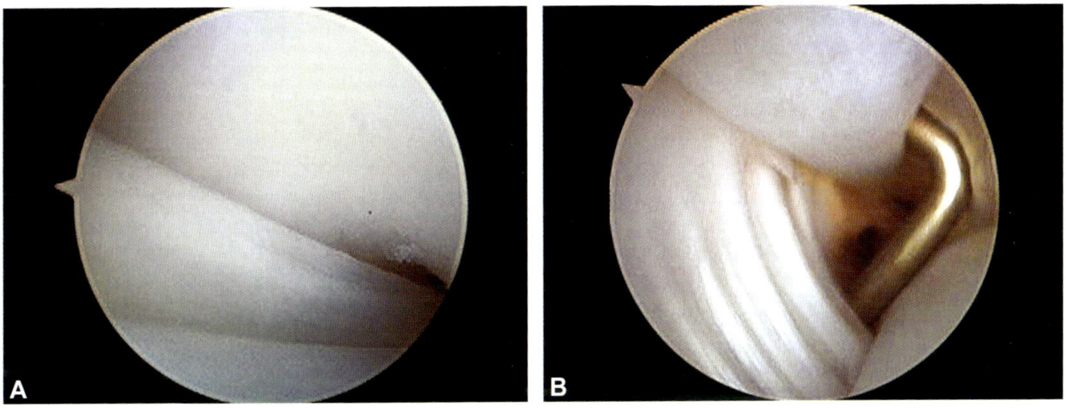

Figs 11A and B

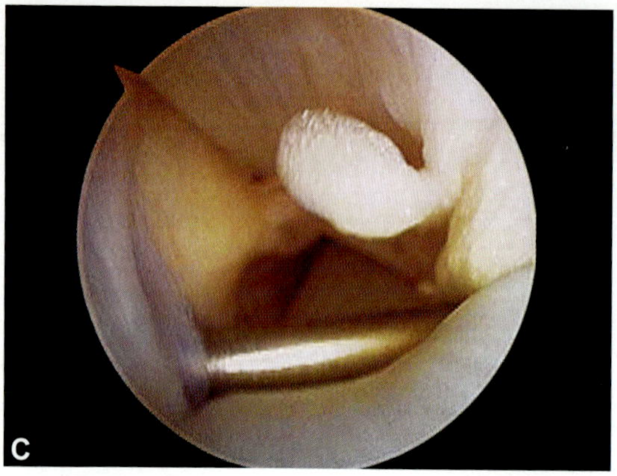

Figs 11A to C: Peroneal tendoscopy: Peroneal tendons are evaluated at the distal fibular groove area with the arthroscope placed in the superior portal and the probe placed through the inferior portal. (A) Initial look at the brevis and longus in the distal fibular groove (located superiorly in picture) and no subluxation is observed; (B) Tendons are probed to determine whether any pathology is present (brevis superior and longus inferior in picture, undersurface of superior peroneal retinaculum well visualized superior to probe); (C) Probe is placed around longus to retract the tendon and better visualize the brevis which has minimal tenosynovitis and a low-lying muscle belly but no tendon tearing is seen

medial malleolus right over the area where the tendon is located. The superior portal is localized with a spinal needle at a point over the posterior tendon sheath about 2 cm proximal to the medial malleolar tip. The posterior tibial tendon then can be evaluated down to its attachment on the navicular, via use of the inferior portal. Both portals can be used to determine the status of the posterior tibial tendon along its course. Tenosynovectomy can be performed with an arthroscopic shaver as indicated. Postoperative course and rehabilitation are similar to that described for peroneal tendoscopy.

CONCLUSION

Subtalar arthroscopy, hindfoot endoscopy and tendoscopy were presented in this chapter. These techniques are helpful in accessing and treating pathological conditions of the posterior ankle joint, subtalar joint, extra-articular hindfoot and ankle, flexor hallucis longus, retrocalcaneal bursa, Achilles tendon, peroneal tendon and posterior tibial tendon in a minimally invasive fashion. These cases can be challenging and knowledge of anatomy, careful portal placement and previous practice in a cadaver lab can improve surgeon confidence and prevent complications. Early outcomes demonstrate a faster return to activities, less wound difficulties and better cosmesis as compared to open surgical techniques. However, in more complicated cases, the surgeon should always be prepared to convert to an open approach, as sometimes a minimally invasive technique does not allow the surgeon proper access, exposure or the ability to repair or reconstruct the damaged structures.

REFERENCES

1. Guo QW, Hu YL, Jiao C, et al. Open versus endoscopic excision of a symptomatic os trigonum: a comparative study of 41 cases. Arthroscopy. 2010;26(3):384-90.
2. Leitze Z, Sella EJ, Aversa JM. Endoscopic decompression of the retrocalcaneal space. J Bone Joint Surg Am. 2003;85:1488-96.
3. Ortmann FW, McBryde AM. Endoscopic bony and soft-tissue decompression of the retrocalcaneal space for the treatment of Haglund deformity and retrocalcaneal bursitis. Foot Ankle Int. 2007; 28(2):149-53.
4. Sammarco G, Taylor A. Operative management of Haglund's deformity in the non-athlete: a retrospective study. Foot Ankle Int. 2000;19:724-9.
5. Willits K. Outcomes of posterior ankle arthroscopy for hindfoot impingement. Arthroscopy. 2008; 24(2): 196-202.
6. Ferkel RD, Scranton PE. Arthroscopy of the ankle and foot. J Bone Joint Surg. 1993;75A:1233-42.
7. Rammelt S, Amlang M, Barthel S, et al. Percutaneous treatment of less severe intraarticular calcaneal fractures. Clin Orthop Relat Res. 2010;468(4):983-90.
8. Scranton PE. Comparison of open isolated subtalar arthrodesis with autologenous bone graft versus outpatient arthroscopic subtalar arthrodesis using injectable bone morphogenic protein-enhanced graft. Foot Ankle Int. 1999;20(3):162-5.
9. Williams MM, Ferkel RD. Subtalar arthroscopy: indications, technique and results. Arthroscopy. 1998;14:373-81.
10. Frey C, Gasser S, Feder K. Arthroscopy of the subtalar joint. Foot Ankle Int. 1994;15:424-8.
11. Ferkel RD. Arthroscopic surgery: the foot and ankle. Philadelphia: Lippincott-Raven;1996.
12. Muraro GM. Arthroscopic arthrodesis of the subtalar joint. Foot Ankle Clin. 2011;16(1):83-90.
13. Beimers L, de Leeuw PA, van Dijk CN. A three portal approach for arthroscopic subtalar arthrodesis. Knee Surg Sports Traumatol Arthrosc. 2009;17:830-4.

14. Amendola A, Lee KB, Saltzman CL, et al. Technique and early experience with posterior arthroscopic subtalar arthrodesis. Foot Ankle Int. 2007;28: 298-302.
15. Lee KB, Saltzman CL, Suh JS, et al. A posterior 3-portal approach for isolated subtalar arthrodesis. Arthroscopy. 2008;24:1306-10.
16. Tasto JP. Arthroscopic subtalar arthrodesis. Tech Foot Ankle Surg. 2003;2:122-8.
17. Ferkel RD, Fischer SP. Progress in ankle arthroscopy. Clin Orthop Relat Res. 1989;240:210-20.
18. van Dijk CN. Hindfoot endoscopy. Foot Ankle Clin. 2006;11:391-414.
19. Frey C. Surgical advancements: arthroscopic alternatives to open procedures: great toe, subtalar joint, Haglund's deformity, and tendoscopy. Foot Ankle Clin. 2009;14(2):313-39.
20. Nickisch F, Barg A, Saltzman CL, et al. Post-operative complications of posterior ankle and hindfoot arthroscopy. J Bone Joint Surg Am. 2012;94(5):439-45.
21. Beals TC, Junko JT, Amendola A, et al. Minimally invasive distraction technique for prone posterior ankle and subtalar arthroscopy. Foot Ankle Int. 2010;31: 316-9.
22. Urguden M. Effect of joint motion on safety of portals in posterior ankle arthroscopy. Arthroscopy. 2009;25(12):1442-6.
23. Webb J, Moorjani N, Radford M. Anatomy of the sural nerve and its relation to the Achilles tendon. Foot Ankle Int. 2000;21:475-7.
24. Phisitkul P, Amendola A. False FHL: a normal variant posing risks in posterior hindfoot endoscopy. Arthroscopy. 2010;26:714-8.
25. Hampton CB, Shawen SB, Keeling JJ. Positioning technique for combined anterior, lateral, and posterior ankle and hindfoot procedures: technique tip. Foot Ankle Int. 2010;31(4):348-50.
26. Lawson JP. Clinically significant radiological anatomic variants of the skeleton. Am J Roentgenol. 1994;163:249-55.
27. Haglund P. Beitrag zur Klinik der Achillessehne. Zeitschr Orthop Chir. 1928;49:49-58.
28. Schneider W, Niehas W, Knahr K. Haglund's syndrome: disappointing results following surgery: a clinical and radiographic analysis. Foot Ankle Int. 2000; 21:26-30.
29. van Dijk CN, Scholten PE, Krips R. A 2-portal endoscopic approach for diagnosis and treatment of posterior ankle pathology. Arthroscopy. 2000;16:871-6.
30. Frey C, Rosenburg Z, Shereff MJ, et al. The retrocalcaneal bursa: anatomy and bursography. Foot Ankle Int. 1992;13:203-7.
31. Kolodziej P, Glisson RR, Nunley JA. Risk of avulsion of the Achilles tendon after partial excision for treatment of insertional tendonitis and Haglund's deformity: a biomechanical study. Foot Ankle Int. 1999;20(7):433-7.
32. van Dijk CN, van Dyk GE, Scholten PE, et al. Endoscopic calcaneoplasty. Am J Sports Med. 2001; 29:185-9.
33. Sammarco VJ. Peroneal tenoscopy: indications and techniques. Sports Med Arthrosc. 2009;17(2):94-9.
34. van Dijk CN, Kort N, Scholten P. Tendoscopy of the posterior tibial tendon. Arthroscopy. 1997;6: 692-8.

SECTION 5

Ankle Problems

Chapters Outline

28

Lateral Instability of the Ankle

John S Gould

EVALUATION OF THE CHRONIC PROBLEM

There is a history of "giving way" of the ankle, typically following a classic "sprain" or "turning" of the ankle acutely at some point in time prior to the onset of these symptoms. At times, the patient will report a feeling of insecurity, that the ankle "might" give way. Often, the patient will report recurrent swelling over the lateral ligament area.

When chronic ligament laxity does exist, there is point tenderness directly over the anterior talofibular ligament and/or calcaneofibular ligament (Fig. 1).[1] Unless there is bilateral laxity, an inversion stress with the ankle in some plantarflexion will demonstrate more inversion on the symptomatic side than the normal one. The patient may complain of pain with this maneuver as well. The "end feel" with the varus stress is "soft" suggesting that the ankle will move into further varus if you push a little harder, rather than a "hard end feel" which is an abrupt stop when the stress is applied. During this examination, it is always essential to observe the patient for a varus heel or varus moment on heel strike due to pathology more proximally in the tibia or knee. Failure to correct such an entity will lead to failure of any surgical reconstruction and a recurrence of ankle symptoms, even with a good conservative or postoperative regimen. In addition, the surgeon looks for evidence of systemic ligamentous laxity, which might be a confounding factor in the occasional patient.

The differential diagnosis includes loose bodies within the joint, joint surface erosions, osteochondral lesions of the talus, subtalar joint laxity, peroneal tendon pathology, and fracture nonunions of the lateral process of the talus, and anterior process of the calcaneus.[2] Palpation for tenderness may reveal a positive finding over these locations and possible crepitus.

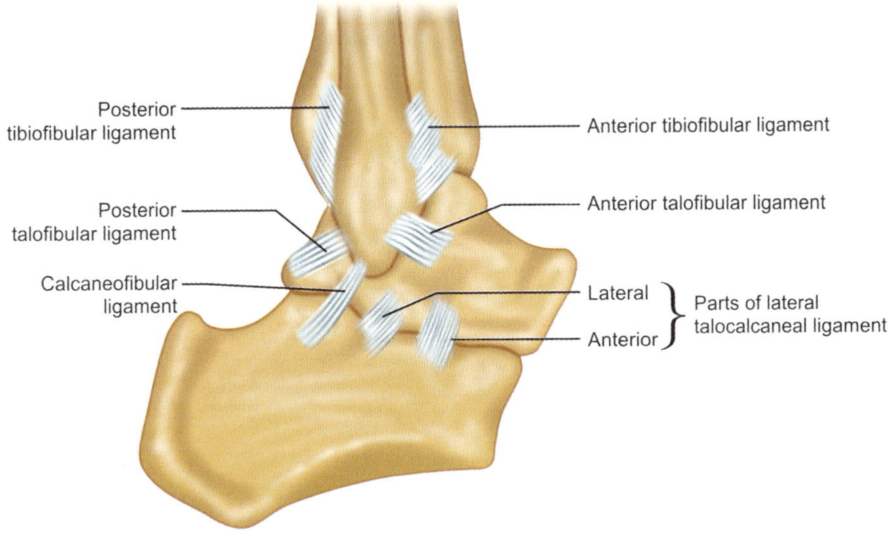

Fig. 1: Lateral ankle ligaments

Plain X-rays may confirm or rule out various entities in the differential list. A magnetic resonance imaging (MRI) may reveal the diagnosis and demonstrate the actual pathology in the ligament. An ultrasound examination is particularly useful in delineating the peroneal tendon diagnosis and would be advisable when other clues lead to this anatomy. This modality may reveal subluxation dynamically of the tendon. A computed tomography (CT) scan may also provide accurate information about an osteochondritis dissecans (OCD) of the talus.

In the author's experience, the history and physical examination are the keys to diagnosis with the ancillary examinations of a plain X-ray and the MRI.[3] This covers most of the possible diagnoses. An examination of the ankle under general anesthesia with stress testing of the stability is done, comparing the involved side against absolute values and to the other apparently normal asymptomatic contralateral side. We do a varus stress test (lateral tilt) under fluoroscopy (Fig. 2), as well a varus stress Broden's view (foot internally rotated, bimalleolar view with the X-ray tube pointed cephalad 30°, 45°, and 60°) to view opening of the posterior facet of the subtalar joint. At one of these degrees of upward tilt of the tube, a clear view of the facet is produced. Finally, we do an anterior drawer test of the talus with the tibia stabilized, with a sagittal view to demonstrate excessive motion of the talus forward under the tibia in the mortise. We then carry out an arthroscopic examination of the ankle with a 2.7 mm 30-degree-angled arthroscope. The joint surfaces are inspected and a "drive through" test is performed to demonstrate laxity on the lateral side. During the examination, one has the opportunity to remove loose bodies, debride chondral lesions or more thoroughly evaluate them, treat an OCD, and do a synovectomy.

As an immediate reconstruction for lateral ligament laxity is delayed to allow the joint to "dry out" and for motion to be restored, a decision is then made with an awake and recovered patient on the further plan of action.

CONSERVATIVE TREATMENT

Peroneal strengthening exercises may relieve the minimally lax ankle in some patients. A 6-week program is instituted with the help of physical therapists. If progress is being made, the program may be continued at home for another 6 weeks. If there is insufficient progress or the patient's ankle relapses, surgery is recommended.

SURGICAL REPAIR

The two current techniques available for repair of the lax lateral ligament in the chronic case are an extra-articular and an "anatomic repair".[4,5] The author opts for the "anatomic repair" in most instances, saving the non-anatomic approach for patients without sufficient tissue remaining for the more desired "anatomic" or in some recurrent cases. The "anatomic" technique consists of imbrication or reinsertion of the old torn ligament tissue (Fig. 3) and reinforcement with inferior extensor retinaculum (The "Brostrom-Gould" repair)[6] (Fig. 4). There are multiple variations of this technique including the use of drill holes through the fibula for reattachment (Hughston modification),

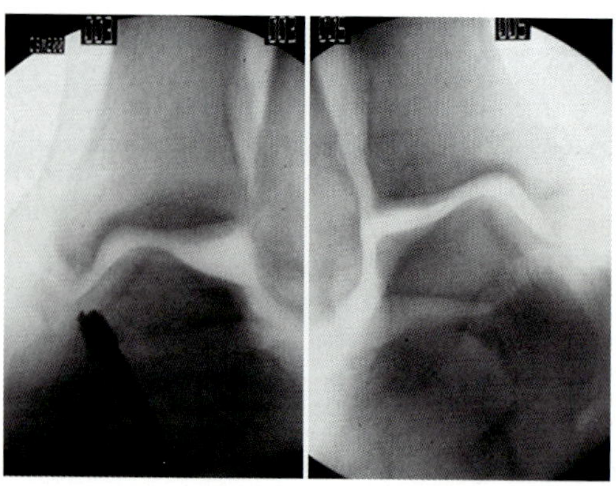

Fig. 2: Lateral tilt test
Note: With a fusion of the subtalar joint, the instability is very obvious and significant

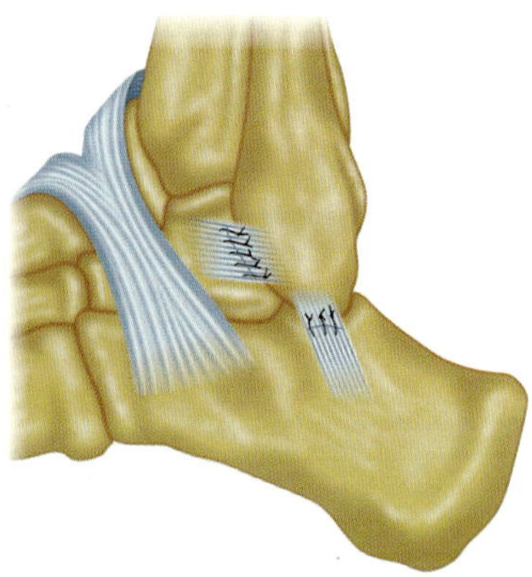

Fig. 3: The Brostrom component of the lateral ligament reconstruction: imbrication of the existing lateral ligaments

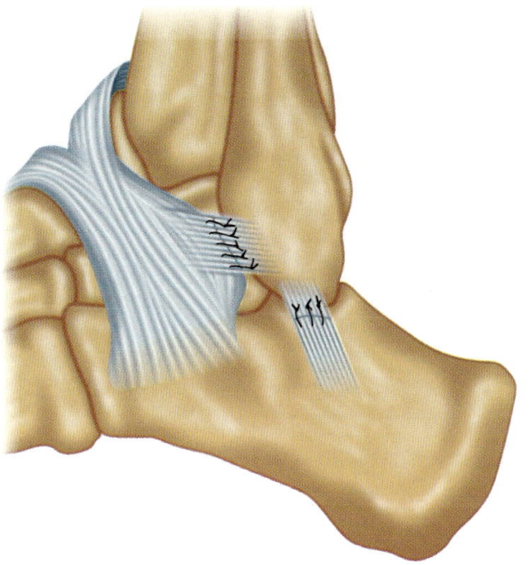

Fig. 4: The Gould component of the lateral ligament reconstruction: the reefing and advancement of the inferior retinaculum

and addition of a distal portion of the peroneus brevis (Evans addition),[7] or a free allograft supplement (Coughlin).[5] The non-anatomic method is multiple variations using the peroneus brevis tendon (Watson Jones)[8] or a portion of it, woven through bony structures including the fibula and calcaneus. The most frequently used of the techniques is the Chrisman-Snook repair.[9]

Brostrom-Gould Repair (Figs 5A to E)

The patient is placed in the supine position with a bump under the ipsilateral hip and the knee is flexed to provide easy access to the lateral ankle area. After tourniquet inflation, a curvilinear incision is made around the fibula, starting about a cm anterior to this structure at the level of the proximal end of the talofibular ligament and extending distally and posteriorly to the easily palpable peroneal sheath, staying about a cm from the fibula. A lateral branch of the intermediate cutaneous nerve of the foot (from the superficial peroneal) may be encountered in this incision and should be protected. Posteriorly, the sural nerve is close to the most posterior extent of the incision but is usually not seen. Careful dissection should reveal the edge of the inferior extensor retinaculum, which also attaches to the peroneal sheath, and this structure should be well delineated, anteriorly to posteriorly. The peroneal sheath should be opened to allow easy retraction of the peroneal tendons during the next step. A more extensive opening of the sheath may need to be done if there has been evidence of peroneal disease and this has to be managed during this procedure.

Palpating with a curved hemostat just anterior to the fibula, at the level of the distal tibiofibular syndesmosis, it should be easy, with a little pressure, to enter the interval between the fibula and the talus just above the anterior talofibular ligament. With the tip of the instrument pointing superficially and in the direction of the incision, the hemostat is advanced under the ligament toward the tip of the fibula. A knife with a #15 blade or a Beaver blade (#64), is used to cut down over the hemostat as it is advanced around the fibula toward the peroneals. If one cuts over the center of the underlying instrument, a cuff of tissue is left on both sides of the attenuated overlying ligament. As one approaches the peroneals, a curved right-angled retractor is used to move them more posteriorly, providing protection for them and allowing access to the calcaneofibular ligament. A synovectomy of the deep lateral recess of the ankle can be done, with removal of loose bodies or a fragment of bone in the ligament, if present.

The repair is now started, using size 0 braided permanent suture with a small stout tapercut needle. The reconstruction is begun posteriorly, advancing anteriorly, and all the sutures are inserted and clamped prior to tying. The concept is to imbricate this elongated tissue in a "vest over pants" manner, using horizontal mattress suture technique. The first stitch is begun on the fibular side, skiving the periosteum on the fibula, emerging at the center of the tip. The needle is then placed through the detached calcaneofibular ligament, through the top of the ligament, from superficial to deep and then back through it from deep to superficial. The needle is then brought back through the tip of the fibula, skiving as before, to emerge adjacent to the initial entry point. About half of the length of suture is used and the two ends are clamped with a hemostat. The next stitch is placed just anterior to the first. Hemostats of the same size are used and as they clamp the suture ends, the ring on the handle is assembled over an Army-Navy retractor in the order that the sutures are placed. Typically, six to eight sutures are used in this layer. The deep layer of sutures are all placed and then tied in succession, as the retractor holding the hemostats is reversed,

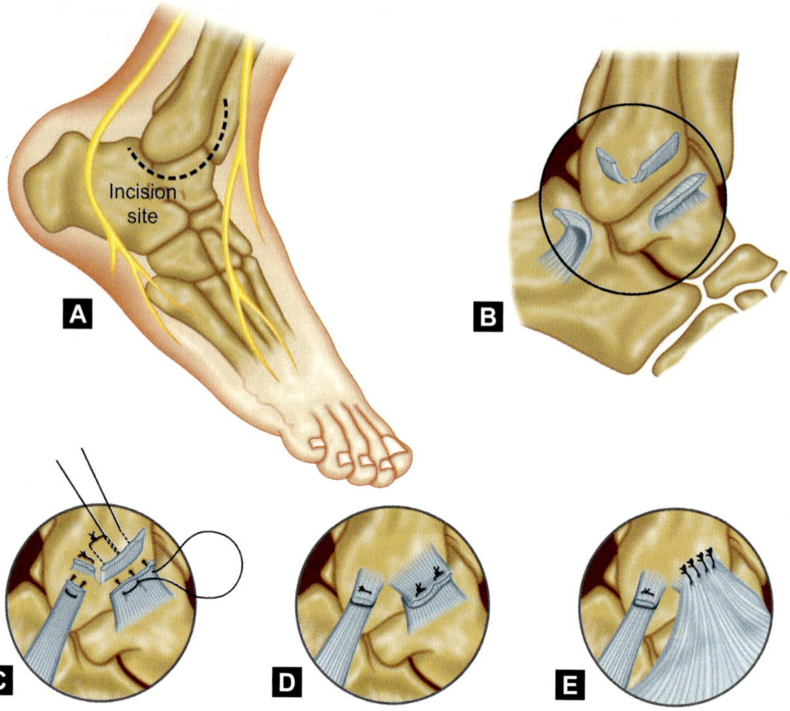

Figs 5A to E: The Brostrom-Gould anatomic lateral ankle reconstruction

allowing the assistant to take each instrument off in the original order of placement, and allowing the surgeon to tie the sutures without tangling with the other untied sutures. The second assistant holds the foot and ankle "everted and plantarflexed," thereby reducing the lax lateral ankle.

The next layer repairs the inferior extensor retinaculum to the fibula. While an assistant maintains the everted position, horizontal mattress sutures are taken between the edge of the retinaculum and the soft tissue overlying the fibula. The ring of sutures begins anteriorly and ends with a repair of the peroneal sheath and with sutures between the edges of the sheath distally and more proximally on the fibula. Care is taken not to incorporate the tendons. Permanent suture is again used and about four or five sutures are used in this layer.

The final step is to do the "gravity test," whereby the repaired foot is elevated to see if the ankle will sag out of the everted position. The foot will sag in the midfoot, but the ankle should stay everted. If it does not, the repair is too loose and will have to be redone. The subcutaneous tissue is closed with Monocryl™, and the skin with nylon. Care is taken to not catch a nerve branch with the suture. A bulky dressing with a fiberglass shell is applied in the operating room. Sutures are removed at 2 weeks, and cast immobilization is continued up to the 6-week interval. Physical therapy is started with range of motion and peroneal strengthening exercises. *Instructions are given to not use inversion exercises ever, and to delay balance board proprioceptive exercises only after 6 weeks of therapy.* Some surgeons have more aggressive postoperative regimens, and use earlier range of motion with protective splinting. We have not seen any earlier return to activity with this approach.

A few comments on variations in technique and on wound healing are in order. When the injured ligament has been avulsed from the bone, usually from the fibular side, reattachment can and should be done by suturing with drill holes through the fibula,[10] or with suture anchors. When the retinaculum is very flimsy or one is doing a revision from a prior failed procedure, various supplemental steps have been described, including use of half of the distal peroneus brevis tendon[7] or allograft tendon.[5] In some cases where there is simply no reasonable ligament and/or retinaculum remaining, there is an indication to use a non-anatomical tenodesis technique, such as the Chrisman-Snook.[9]

The concept of using previously injured attenuated ligament has validity and has been used for acromioclavicular ligament and ulnar collateral ligament repairs in the thumb, and very likely many other unreported areas. The repairs heal, remodel along lines of stress (Wolfe's law), and develop tensile strength. In addition, joint stability is re-established by the anatomical repair, and ankle range of motion, including "inversion," is re-established.[6,10] Tenodesis procedures with both autografts and allografts do not remodel or gain strength after repair and loss of range of motion and excessive ankle tightness leading to the development of osteoarthritis is a concern.[11] Consequently, the supplement of allograft or tenodesis as a supplement to the Brostrom-Gould carries the same risks, and while adding initial strength, may lead, at least theoretically, to a less desirable late outcome. These additions to the initial repair methods have been done too recently, with too short a follow-up, to validate this comment.

Ankles with a Varus Heel

When a varus heel, commonly with a cavus foot, coexists with the lateral ligament laxity, ligament reconstruction without attention to the varus is doomed to failure.[12] Reconstruction of the cavus foot, as described in an earlier chapter, may be indicated along with the lateral ligament procedure. When the cavus is fairly subtle, and the primary complaint is the ankle laxity, a concomitant valgus wedge, lateral displacement osteotomy of the calcaneus with the ligament procedure can be done. The author usually does both procedures with the patient in the lateral "beanbag" position. The postoperative course is unaltered.

Outcomes, Complications and Salvage

Outcome reports in the literature with the Brostrom-Gould have been almost universally very satisfactory, providing stability and flexibility.[13-15] The author's series has provided similar findings with two exceptions: neurogenic symptoms probably related to tethering of a branch of the intermediate cutaneous nerve, and a new appreciation by the patient of decreased inversion of the ankle compared to the chronic lax state. In a series of patients studied with a questionnaire concerning long-term outcome and subsequent examination and questioning, over 25% of patients described either transient or lingering numbness or vague pain in the distribution of the lateral nerve branch. Interestingly enough, this finding was rarely offered spontaneously, but brought out with specific questioning. The decreased inversion was not dysfunctional and essentially all patients achieved between 20° and 30° of inversion. One patient volunteered that she could no longer sit on her foot and ankle (with the ankle inverted), although it was not problematic and she had returned to full athletic activities after 4 years of instability complaints.

With the Brostrom-Gould repair, the main complication has been persistent or recurrent instability.[14] The reported success rates range from 82 to 87%;[4] although N Gould[6] and others including our own series, have had closer to 100% without recurrent laxity. An inadequate repair may occasionally be the cause of failure, as well as inadequate repair tissues; and systemic excessive ligament laxity is always a possibility. The far and away most common source of failure has been, however, untreated or unappreciated varus of the heel or a varus thrust on heel strike due to a more proximal anatomic problem.[16] It is essential, therefore, to examine patients adequately preoperatively to rule out the varus component, including the observation of the patient's gait from the posterior perspective.

Salvage has included correction of varus, reconstruction of the lateral ligaments, reusing the available tissues, or reverting to a tenodesis procedure.

Reconstruction of the Lateral Ligament in Association with Total Ankle Arthroplasty

In some instances, the Brostrom-Gould procedure may be satisfactory. The standard tenodesis procedures are technically more difficult and potentially risk fracture of the lateral malleolus if done concomitantly. Among the options for repair is the "O'Phalen technique" (Coetzee) in which the peroneus brevis tendon is used. At the completion of the total ankle arthroplasty procedure, one may note lateral ankle laxity or anteroposterior laxity of the talus. An incision is made proximal to the lateral malleolus into the sheath of the peroneals. The peroneus brevis tendon in its entirety is harvested at the musculotendinous junction. In fact, a portion of the aponeurosis proximal to the junction is taken with the distal tendon as well. The tibial cortex above the implant is burred or scarified. With lateral laxity alone present, the proximal tendon and aponeurosis (with the distal insertion of the structure intact) is brought anterior to the fibula and secured to the anterior tibia with suture anchors or staples. Traction is maintained on the tendon during the attachment and lateral laxity assessed to make sure the repair is secure. In the absence of the peroneus brevis, the peroneus longus has been used in a similar fashion, as well as an allograft tendon (with drill holes in the calcaneus and fibula, using suture anchors or interference screws for fixation). When anteroposterior instability exists, or lateral instability as well, the tendon is redirected posteriorly around the fibula and through the interosseous membrane to the anterior tibia proximal to the total ankle tibial component and attached as above. These procedures have been utilized for over 7 years to date but have not been reported. There have been no instances of recurrent lateral instability. The postoperative ankle with such a repair has been protected in a cast for 6 weeks; whereas, the ankle procedures alone are typically mobilized much earlier as reported in Chapter 40.

Chrisman-Snook Repair[9]

The Watson-Jones[8] repair, using the entire tendon of the peroneus brevis, is the forerunner of all the subsequent tenodesis non-anatomic repairs. The Elmslie,[17] Evans,[7] and others, using the distal half of the tendon, with the insertion remaining intact on the base of the 5th metatarsal, with various weaves through drill holes in the fibula followed.

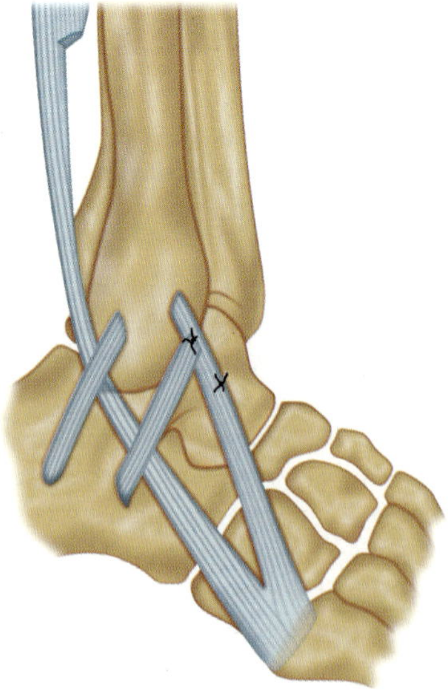

Fig. 6: The Chrisman-Snook extra-articular lateral ankle reconstruction

The Chrisman-Snook technique[9] (Fig. 6) provides a weave, as illustrated, which attempts to simulate, albeit more superficially than the actual ligaments, the direction of attachment of the calcaneofibular and anterior talofibular ligaments. Drill holes are made in the fibula, the calcaneus inferior to the tip of the lateral malleolus and the tendon drawn through these tunnels with a Hewson suture passer until it is finally secured over the talus in the inferior retinaculum. The ankle is held in the reduced position as the tendon is tensioned. The postoperative course is the same as that used with the Brostrom-Gould procedure. The primary problem with this repair is the significant potential for decreased dorsiflexion, lost subtalar motion, particularly inversion, loss of anterior talar rotation and rotary instability.[18] The additional complication is ankle tightness, loss of inversion, and later arthritis. Salvage for recurrent laxity includes concern for untreated or unappreciated heel varus, as noted above. Redo of the procedure has included free autograft using hamstring or allograft. Treatment of the arthritic ankle will be discussed in Chapters 38–41, but includes arthrodesis and arthroplasty.

REFERENCES

1. Burks R, Morgan J. Anatomy of the lateral ankle ligaments. Am J Sports Med. 1994;22:72-7.
2. Lee J, Hamilton G, Ford L. Associated intra-articular ankle pathologies in patients with chronic lateral ankle instability: arthroscopic findings at the time of lateral ankle reconstruction. Foot Ankle Spec. 2011; 4(5):284-9.
3. Stasko PM, McSpadden CK, Jung R, et al. Incidence of talar dome lesions with concomitant peroneal tendon pathologic features: a magnetic resonance imaging evaluation. J Foot Ankle Surg. 2012;51(5):579-82.
4. Karlsson J, Eriksson B, Bergsten T, et al. Comparison of two anatomic reconstructions for chronic lateral instability of the ankle. Am J Sports Med. 1997;25(1):48-53.
5. Coughlin MJ, Schenck RC, Grebing BR, et al. Comprehensive reconstruction of the lateral ankle for chronic instability using a free gracilis graft. Foot Ankle Int. 2004;25(4):231-41.
6. Gould N, Seligson D, Gassman J. Early and late repair of lateral ligament of the ankle. Foot Ankle. 1980;1(2):84-9.
7. Evans DL. Recurrent instability of the ankle; a method of surgical treatment. Proc R Soc Med. 1953;46(5):343-4.
8. Watson-Jones R. Recurrent forward dislocation of the ankle joint. J Bone Joint Surg Br. 1952;34(3):519.

9. Chrisman OD, Snook GA. Reconstruction of lateral ligament tears of the ankle. An experimental study and clinical evaluation of seven patients treated by a new modification of the Elmslie procedure. J Bone Joint Surg Am. 1969;51(5):904-12.
10. Hamilton W, Thompson F, Snow S. The modified Brostrom procedure for lateral ankle instability. Foot Ankle. 1993;14(1):1-7.
11. Ellis SJ, Williams BR, Pavlov H, et al. Results of anatomic lateral ankle ligament reconstruction with tendon allograft. HSS J. 2011;7(2):134-40.
12. Strauss JE, Forsberg JA, Lippert FG. Chronic lateral ankle instability and associated conditions: a rationale for treatment. Foot Ankle Int. 2007;28(10):1041-4.
13. Rosenbaum D, Becker HP, Sterk J, et al. Functional evaluation of the 10-year outcome after modified Evans repair for chronic ankle instability. Foot Ankle Int. 1997;18(12):765-71.
14. Brodsky AR, O'Malley MJ, Bohne WH, et al. An analysis of outcome measures following the Broström-Gould procedure for chronic lateral ankle instability. Foot Ankle Int. 2005;26(10):816-9.
15. Liu SH, Baker CL. Comparison of lateral ankle ligamentous reconstruction procedures. Am J Sports Med. 1994;22(3):313-7.
16. Sammarco VJ. Complications of lateral ankle ligament reconstruction. Clin Orthop Relat Res. 2001;(391): 123-32.
17. Elmslie RC. Recurrent Subluxation of the Ankle-Joint. Ann Surg. 1934;100(2):364-7.
18. ZD Ng, S Das De. Modified Brostrom-Evans-Gould technique for recurrent ankle lateral ligament laxity. J Orth Surg. 2007;15(3):306-10.

29

Medial Instability of the Ankle

Emilio Wagner, Cristian Ortiz, Pablo Wagner

INTRODUCTION

Medial ankle instability is a relatively new diagnosis known over the last 10 years in foot and ankle surgery. Previously ankle instability only considered lateral ligament instability, with its well known treatment strategy, including anatomic or non-anatomic ligament reconstruction. Concern was raised in some patients where although obtaining excellent anatomical surgical repair of the lateral ankle ligaments, average or poor results were seen. Literature shows up to 50% of long-term sequelae from ankle sprains, and this may be due to medial ankle instability not previously diagnosed.[1] Damage of the medial deltoid ligament in chronic lateral ankle instability can be demonstrated in imaging studies. Up to 72% of these patients with recurrent lateral ankle instability, without medial pain, have deltoid injuries considering the deep and superficial components (Fig. 1).[2] Articles dealing with these issues have appeared over the last two years, where medial and lateral ankle ligament reconstruction has been performed, trying to decrease rotational instability of the ankle joint.[3]

Besides the classic clinical scenario of recurrent ankle sprains, there are other situations where medial ankle instability can be seen, which are the final stages of posterior tibial tendon insufficiency, which has been named as stage IV of the modified Johnson and Strom classification by Myerson, and medial instability seen after varied hindfoot reconstructions such as triple arthrodesis or procedures associated with a total ankle arthroplasty (Fig. 2).[4] These conditions are more difficult to analyze, as they have evolved over long time, and the severity of tissue damage is varied.[5] In acquired flatfeet, not only the medial ankle ligaments can fail but also the complete medial column of the foot can result with damage and become attenuated over time. The medial column includes the spring ligament, plantar ligaments, talonavicular, naviculocuneiform and tarsometatarsal joints. In hindfoot pathology, not only a diffuse damage of ligaments can be found as stated in the previous sentence, but also different biomechanical conditions can influence and increase medial ankle instability. Long standing calcaneovalgus, subtalar arthrodesis in valgus

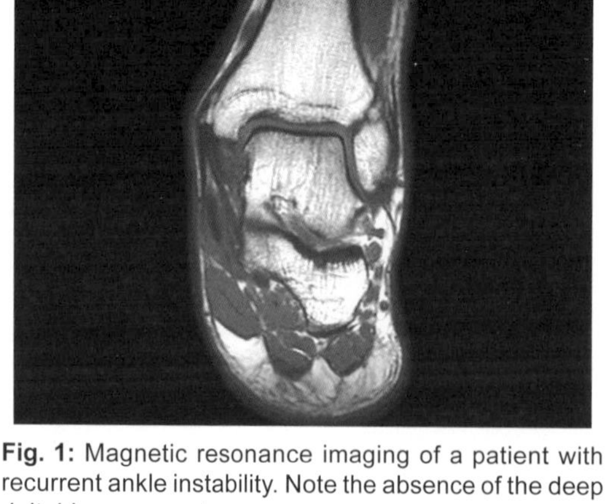

Fig. 1: Magnetic resonance imaging of a patient with recurrent ankle instability. Note the absence of the deep deltoid component

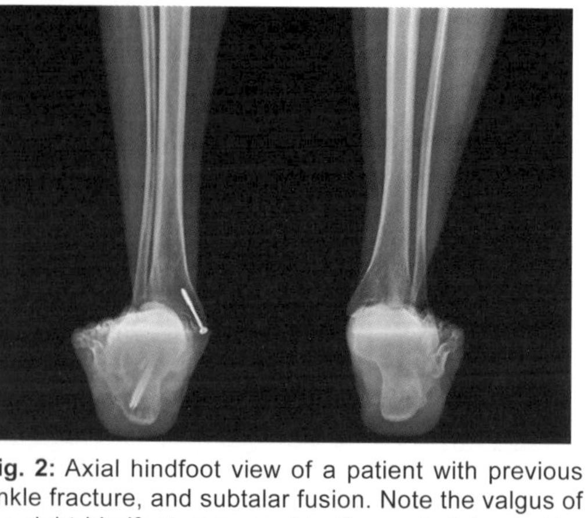

Fig. 2: Axial hindfoot view of a patient with previous ankle fracture, and subtalar fusion. Note the valgus of the right hindfoot compared to the contralateral side, mainly through the ankle joint

malposition, malunited fractures and medial column insufficiency all can lead to a skeletal misalignment which will influence negatively the outcome of any proposed medial ligament reconstruction.

ETIOLOGY AND PATHOPHYSIOLOGY

The anatomy of the deltoid ligament has to be well known in order to correctly understand the pathology, and propose a reconstruction. Different components of the medial deltoid can be identified although different authors find different ligaments more constantly than others. Two main components are identified, the superficial and the deep component. The superficial crosses two joints, the tibiotalar and the subtalar joint. The deep layer just spans the ankle joint. Apparently the most constant ligaments of the superficial component are the tibiospring and the tibiocalcaneal ligaments. Although a tibionavicular ligament has also been described, it may be just a reinforced area of the capsule of the ankle joint.[6] The tibiospring ligament is the strongest superficial component of the medial ankle ligaments.[1] Regarding the deep component of the deltoid, anterior and posterior deep ligaments can be found, besides a slightly more superficial component called the superficial tibiotalar ligament. The proximal insertion of the deltoid ligament corresponds to an area approximately 5–8 mm cranial to the apex of the medial malleolus. Distally the different components insert depending on their name, on different bony prominences or ligaments, as for example the tibiocalcaneal ligament inserts distally on the medial border of the sustentaculum tali. The insertion on the talus corresponds to an area just distal and under the cartilage limit on the medial side of the talus.

Regarding function, the deltoid ligament is the strongest restraint that limits talar abduction. The tibiocalcaneal ligament resists talar pronation, and the deep component of the deltoid resists external rotation. This medial complex unites the tibia and talus for the coupling mechanism at the ankle joint, which is essential in transferring motion, shock absorption and function between the foot and the leg.[1] Commonly the subtalar joint compensates tibial rotation under the talus, thus leading to an inverted or everted position. With ankle instability, Hintermann has postulated that inversion or eversion may originate at the ankle joint, thus creating a rotational instability, an idea which is also shared by the authors. The importance of determining exactly the origin of ankle instability is to be able to determine the origin of the pathology in order to treat it correctly. It has been shown that when comparing an articular step-off versus ankle instability in terms of potential damage to the ankle cartilage, isolated ankle instability is more important than ankle incongruity.[7] Indeed it has been shown that in vivo cartilage strains shift significantly in an anterior and medial direction within the ankle joint in patients with lateral ankle instability, changes that correspond to the area of clinically observed arthrosis.[8] These articles deal only with lateral ankle instability and it can be argued that combined medial and lateral ankle instability should have increased deleterious effects over the joint cartilage.

DIAGNOSIS

Medial ankle instability has to be suspected when medial ankle pain appears in patients with history of recurrent ankle sprains, previously asymptomatic flatfeet or acquired flatfeet deformities with a break in their natural history, previous hindfoot reconstructions, and ankle replacements.

After ankle sprains, if medial ankle pain develops or a change in the static alignment of the foot occurs, our suspicion of subjacent medial ankle instability should be high. Generally these patients have been treated for lateral ankle instability for long time, with physical therapy and orthosis. Medial lesions should occur more frequently after external rotation injuries, although the authors have seen patients where only inversion injuries have progressed to combined medial and lateral ankle instability. Pain in the medial gutter of the ankle can be found in almost all patients. In physical examination, in the standing position no alteration can be observed or a slight valgus of the hindfoot in stance position can be observed. This valgus position has to correct itself when standing on the tip of the toes, as the posterior tibial tendon is absolutely normal and no medial column insufficiency has yet developed.[1] Clinically, differences can be found when testing anterior stability with the anterior drawer test, although this difference is very subjective and difficult to quantify.

When dealing with patients with acquired flatfeet or with hindfoot reconstructions, where medial instability is suspected, the most important characteristic is that they present peritalar instability. This is a new concept that has received almost no attention except in cases where traumatic peritalar dislocations are present. No studies are out there that deal with chronic peritalar instability, until recently.[9] Hintermann described patients with peritalar instability where the dysfunction occurs on all the structures surrounding the talus, namely the subtalar, and talonavicular joints. Depending on the patient, the subtalar joint can compensate or not in valgus or varus orientation, thus differentiating peritalar instability in varus or valgus types. The importance of this diagnosis is that peritalar instability can never be corrected only through the ankle joint. Surgical procedures to realign completely the foot have to be undertaken. Osseous balancing through supramalleolar osteotomies, calcaneal osteotomies, lateral column lengthening procedures, and subtalar arthrodesis have to be considered as they supposedly will be more reliable for a long-lasting rebalancing procedure. The authors fully agree on this concept and thus postulate a complete osseous realignment before a medial ankle ligament reconstruction is planned when treating these types of patients. Regarding symptoms, medial ankle pain is the most frequent complaint. Pain can also be reported laterally, besides tarsal tunnel symptoms. There is also a history of progressive deformity and shoeware modifications. As these are cases of a chronic nature, there are other signs of deformity such as calluses under the talar head, triceps surae contracture and decreased muscular strength.[5]

Imaging

Radiographic imaging is very important, especially when dealing with post-traumatic cases, hindfoot reconstruction or ankle arthroplasty. In these cases, besides the standard weight-bearing X-rays of the leg, ankle and foot to determine possible sites of deformity, hindfoot alignment views should be obtained to evaluate which joint primarily contributes to the deformity. Joint arthritis should be evaluated with computed tomography (CT) scans. In patients with only ankle sprains and probable medial ankle instability, magnetic resonance imaging (MRI) may have a role, as it may rule out other diagnoses and show where the lesion is in the deltoid ligament.

TREATMENT

Medial Ankle Instability

Conservative Treatment

Conservative treatment may be attempted with total contact insoles with medial support, physical therapy with strengthening of the posterior tibialis tendon and modifications of daily life activities. If the patients does not experience relief a surgical treatment should be recommended. No results are published relative to success of conservative treatment, but apparently patients with open physes have a healing potential, and medial deltoid and even spring ligament injury could be treated conservatively with some chance of success.

Surgical Treatment

A difference has to be made between medial ankle instability and peritalar instability. For medial ankle instability alone, we consider young patients which have sustained recurrent ankle sprains, and have no associated damage of other ligaments of the foot. In these cases, a certification of the diagnosis can be made arthroscopically. It has been suggested that medial ankle instability is present if with a normal 4.0 mm knee scope, the cannula can be inserted through the medial tibiotalar space (Fig. 3). If this is possible, it is more probable that we are facing true medial ankle instability. In these cases, an open reconstruction is performed as suggested by Hintermann.[1]

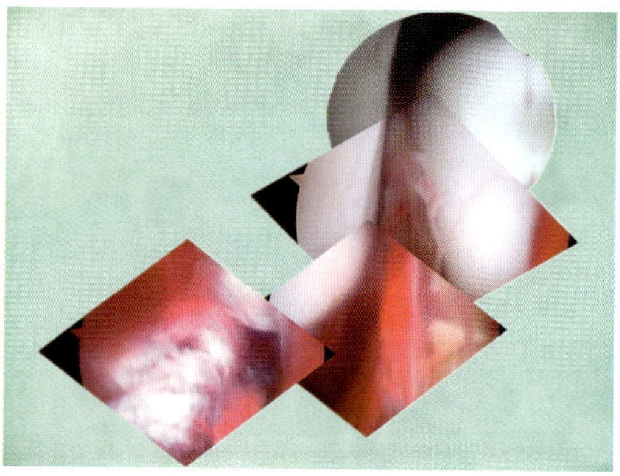

Fig. 3: Arthroscopic view of deltoid injury. Notice the detachment from the talar insertion site, with remnant tissue adjacent to the tip of the medial malleolus

Surgical Technique

On the medial side of the ankle joint, a curved incision is performed measuring approximately 6 cm in length, from the tip of the medial malleolus towards the navicular bone. The superficial component of the deltoid is inspected and also the sheath of the tibialis posterior tendon is divided to get access to its floor where the spring ligament is situated. A macroscopic evaluation of these structures is performed as well. Depending on the arthroscopic examination and the MRI, a deep ligament reconstruction can be performed, where anchors are placed in the tip of the medial malleolus, 6 mm cephalic to the tip of the malleolus, and a reefing of the remaining ligaments is done. The same can be done inserting an anchor on the talus, trying to leave it on the original insertion of the deep tibiotalar ligaments (Fig. 4). Generally a 5 mm metallic anchor is used, with FiberWire attached to it which is used after closing the deep interval, to close the superficial deltoid ligaments. If only the superficial deltoid is compromised, it is repaired with direct suturing or also using an anchor on the medial malleolus. The most commonly damaged superficial ligament is the tibionavicular ligament and the tibiospring ligament.[1]

Additional procedures should be considered as many of these patients can have also lateral ankle instability. A classic Brostrom-Gould lateral ligament reconstruction is preferred by the authors. Relative to osseous alignment, although stated previously that these are relatively acute damages to the deltoid with no associated damage, the presence of a flatfeet can deteriorate a medial ankle reconstruction. A calcaneal lengthening osteotomy should be considered if significant abduction and pronation of the foot is present.

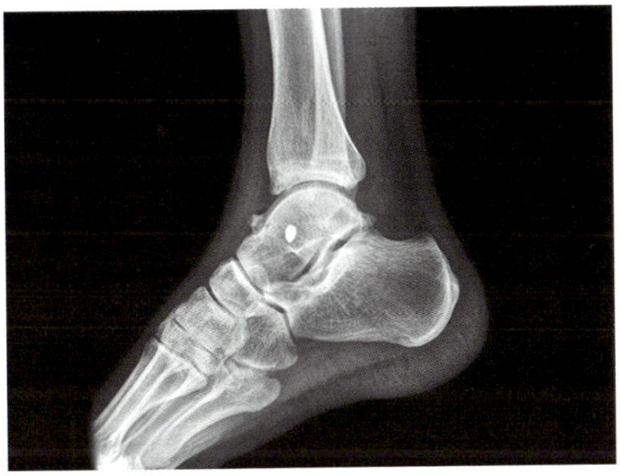

Fig. 4: Lateral X-ray view of deltoid reconstruction using an anchor placed in the talus. Superficial reconstruction also was performed reefing the tibionavicular and tibiospring ligaments

Postoperatively patients are kept non-weight bearing for 2 or 3 weeks in a cam walker, and then are allowed full weight bearing as tolerated. Physiotherapy is started at this point.

Results

The few results in the literature are primarily from Hintermann and associates. He showed results in 54 patients with medial ankle instability, where the most frequent area of damage was at the proximal insertion of the deltoid. He reported good to excellent results in 89% of the cases treated, with additional procedures performed in the majority of the cases, as repair of the spring ligament (20%), repair of lateral ligaments of the ankle (70%), and calcaneal lengthening osteotomy in 27%.[1]

Peritalar Instability

We consider a diagnosis of peritalar instability in patients who developed medial ankle instability in a chronic situation, and which have other conditions on the hindfoot, like a previous reconstruction, fusion or ankle arthroplasty. As said before, these cases are extremely difficult to manage as there is an osseous imbalance and a ligament abnormality. If these patients are treated just with medial deltoid reconstruction, the chance of failure is high as there are many other structures involved and weakened. The main goal in surgery should be to realign first the bony anatomy, trying to push slightly the limit of normal skeletal alignment. This means that patients with valgus ankle alignment should be treated with osteotomies or arthrodesis which achieves a slight varus tendency, so as to have a protective mechanical effect over the medial ligaments of the ankle and the foot. Only after a complete supramalleolar, ankle, hindfoot and midfoot realignment has been obtained, where mild varus is obtained can a medial ligament reconstruction be attempted.

These cases present with a medial tilt of the talus which can be observed in the radiological examination. Sometimes subtalar valgus malalignment is present and also has to be addressed. A complete examination of the leg, hindfoot and foot alignment has to be done, with complete X-rays and CT scans. Surgery can be divided into skeletal and ligamentous procedures.

Skeletal Procedures

The surgical decision-making process goes proximal to distal. If a valgus tilt at the supramalleolar level is found, realignment surgery should be performed at that level. If subtalar valgus malalignment without arthrosis is present, a medializing calcaneal osteotomy can be attempted. If subtalar arthrosis is present, a corrective subtalar fusion should be performed leaving it in slight varus. Then the medial column has to be examined. Joint collapse at the talonavicular, naviculocuneiform and/or tarsometatarsal joint should be addressed with localized fusions, using the same concepts as for flatfoot treatment. Abduction of the forefoot associated to a valgus hindfoot should be treated with a calcaneal lengthening osteotomy.[10]

Surgical Techniques

- *Supramalleolar osteotomies*: A medial incision is performed 3 cm proximal to the ankle joint. A wedge is resected from the medial side of the tibia, calculated to obtain a mild overcorrection of the valgus inside the ankle joint (within 5° of normal). The osteotomy is closed and fixed with an angular stable small fragment plate (Fig. 5).
- *Calcaneal osteotomies*: Realignment osteotomies are performed from the lateral aspect, displacing medially 1 cm the posterior tuberosity of the calcaneus. We fix it with two cancellous large fragment screws, generally 45 mm in length (Fig. 6).
- Calcaneal lengthening osteotomies are performed through a small lateral approach just plantar to the sinus tarsi approach. The osteotomy is performed in a vertical direction just distal to the posterior facet of the subtalar joint. We prefer to use the Hintermann distractors, and we elongate 1 cm the calcaneus trying to keep the medial cortex intact. The gap produced can be filled with cancellous or synthetic material. Fixation is accomplished by one small fragment screw from distal dorsal to proximal plantar.
- *Subtalar-talonavicular-naviculocuneiform-tarsometatarsal arthrodesis*: These are performed as generally described in the literature, always achieving good bone contact, very seldom needing bone graft. The subtalar joint is fixed preferably with two screws, one for compression and one to control rotation. The talonavicular arthrodesis is fixed with three screws from distal to proximal, generally small fragment screws. The naviculocuneiform and tarsometatarsal joints are fixed with two crossed screws.

Pantalar fusion is avoided, as although they are successful in achieving a plantigrade foot, there is more energy consumption and less functionality.[11]

Deltoid Reconstruction

Previous attempts to reconstruct the dysfunctional deltoid describe reefing of native tissue to retighten the medial collateral complex, medial malleolus vertical osteotomies with proximal displacement with the same idea of achieving greater tension

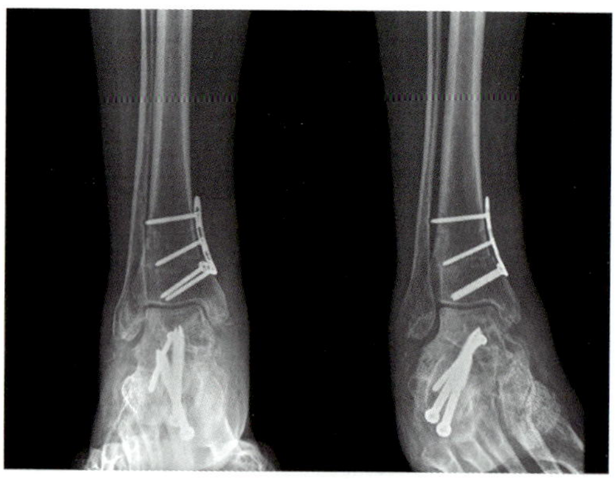

Fig. 5: Anteroposterior and oblique X-ray view of same patient indicated in Figure 2. A supramalleolar osteotomy was performed, 3 cm above the ankle joint, correcting the mechanical axis into a slight varus. A combination with a calcaneal medializing osteotomy was done in order to correct completely the weight-bearing axis

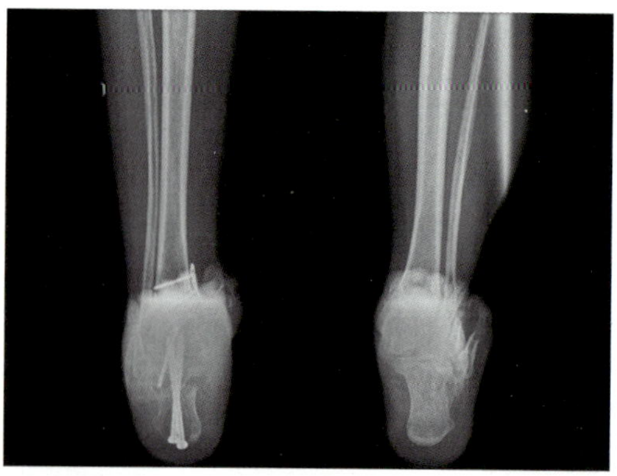

Fig. 6: Same patient as indicated in Figures 2 and 5. Hindfoot axial view showing the correction obtained after a supramalleolar and calcaneal osteotomy. Compare to Figure 2

of the damaged ligament, and imbrication of the ligament fascicles.[5] Although the idea of retightening the ligament may work, no published results are available. Newer attempts to reconstruct the deltoid have been published. In 2010, a medium term follow-up result was published by Ellis where five patients were followed for 8 years.[12] The reconstruction tried to replace the deep component of the deltoid, with an autograft which spans the tibiotalar joint. They show satisfactory results, and comment that they recommend using Achilles allograft to avoid donor morbidity. Another reconstruction was presented in 2010 using the anterior tibialis tendon which was divided into two limbs, one to reconstruct the superficial portion of the deltoid and the other to reconstruct the deep component. The proximal band was fixed to the medial malleolus. This was a cadaveric study where the strength of the reconstruction was tested to be similar to the intact specimens. No clinical studies are available.[13] A minimally invasive deltoid reconstruction study was published in 2011, where the authors used allograft hamstring tendon which was divided in two limbs, one to reconstruct the superficial portion of the deltoid and the other to reconstruct the deep portion. Five of eight patients were considered to have a successful outcome and a limit of 10° of valgus tibiotalar tilt was suggested as the upper limit to perform this procedure.[14]

None of these proposed techniques have shown consistent clinical results, and thus they still cannot be used in a widespread way. The authors think that the most reliable way to correct these complex situations is to address all skeletal malalignment issues, slightly overcorrecting the mechanical axis to a varus situation, and just reefing the remnant ligament fascicles, until a reliable deltoid ligament reconstruction is available.

SUMMARY

Medial ankle instability has different clinical presentations, being the most common scenario after multiple ankle sprains. It is also seen in posterior tibial tendon dysfunction stage IV or after reconstructive procedures including ankle replacement or hindfoot reconstruction. A thorough clinical analysis has to be considered before attempting surgical treatment, and there is no general consensus relative to the correct surgical procedure.

REFERENCES

1. Hintermann B. Medial ankle instability. Foot Ankle Clin. 2003;8(4):723-38.
2. Crim JR, Beals TC, Nickisch F, et al. Deltoid ligament abnormalities in chronic lateral ankle instability. Foot Ankle Int. 2011;32(9):873-8.
3. Buchhorn T, Sabeti-Aschraf M, Dlaska C, et al. Combined medial and lateral anatomic ligament reconstruction for chronic rotational instability of the ankle. Foot Ankle Int. 2011;32(12):1122-6.
4. Hintermann B, Knupp M, Pagenstert GI. Deltoid ligament injuries: diagnosis and management. Foot Ankle Clin. 2006;11(3):625-37.
5. Bluman EM, Myerson MS. Stage IV posterior tibial tendon rupture. Foot Ankle Clin. 2007;12(2):341-62.
6. Boss AP, Hintermann B. Anatomical study of the medial ankle ligament complex. Foot Ankle Int. 2002;23(6):547-53.
7. Tochigi Y, Rudert MJ, McKinley TO, et al. Correlation of dynamic cartilage contact stress aberrations with severity of instability in ankle incongruity. J Orthop Res. 2008;26(9):1186-93.
8. Bischof JE, Spritzer CE, Caputo AM, et al. In vivo cartilage contact strains in patients with lateral ankle instability. J Biomech. 2010;43(13):2561-6.
9. Hintermann B, Knupp M, Barg A. Peritalar instability. Foot Ankle Int. 2012;33(5):450-4.
10. Pagenstert G, Hintermann B, Barg A, et al. Realignment surgery as alternative treatment of varus and valgus ankle osteoarthritis. Clin Orthop Relat Res. 2007;462:156-68.
11. Smith J, Bluman E. Update on stage IV acquired adult flatfoot disorder: when the deltoid ligament becomes dysfunctional. Foot Ankle Clin. 2012;17(2):351-60.
12. Ellis SJ, Williams BR, Wagshul AD, et al. Deltoid ligament reconstruction with peroneus longus autograft in flatfoot deformity. Foot Ankle Int. 2010;31(9):781-9.
13. Haddad SL, Dedhia S, Ren Y, et al. Deltoid ligament Reconstruction: a novel technique with biomechanical analysis. Foot Ankle Int. 2010; 31(7):639-51.
14. Jeng CL, Bluman EM, Myerson MS. Minimally invasive deltoid ligament reconstruction for stage IV flatfoot deformity. Foot Ankle Int. 2011;32(1):21-30.

30

Ankle Arthroscopy

Shana N Miskovsky

INTRODUCTION

This chapter will serve as an overview of arthroscopic techniques successfully utilized in the minimally invasive treatment of a multitude of ankle disorders. It is important for the surgeon to be familiar with the indications, portal anatomy, complications, and outcomes of these arthroscopic techniques as they are associated with improved joint visualization, lower postoperative morbidity, less postsurgical pain, and earlier functional recovery than more traditional, open surgical techniques.[1-3] Posterior ankle arthroscopy and hindfoot endoscopy will be discussed in a later chapter.

ANKLE

Ankle Arthroscopy

In this section, ankle arthroscopy will be discussed in detail including indications, complications, anatomy, and step-by-step surgical technique. Also an overview of the conditions treated via ankle arthroscopy will be reviewed along with surgical technique pearls, outcomes and postoperative rehabilitation pointers where appropriate.

Indications

Ankle arthroscopy is indicated in the treatment of ankle impingement, osteochondral defects of the talus or tibia, and ankle arthritis requiring arthrodesis.[4] Other indications reported in the literature for ankle arthroscopy require further evidence-based investigation and include treatment for loose bodies, ankle instability, septic arthritis, synovitis, tumors, ankle fractures, and arthrofibrosis.

Ankle arthroscopy can be performed with or without non-invasive distraction, depending on the pathologies anticipated and being treated. The distraction aids in visualization of the cartilage for osteochondral lesions but may be less helpful in the situation of loose bodies in the anterior compartment of the ankle which may dislodge and travel into the more difficult to access posterior portion of the joint. The visualization and examination of the central and posterior ankle has been shown to be better utilizing traction, and the anterior compartment was appropriately evaluated in 90% of cases.[5] If the surgeon would like to use dorsiflexion instead of distraction, one can stand at the foot of the bed and place the ankle in dorsiflexion by leaning forward on the foot. The advantage would be that the anterior capsule is looser in this position creating more working space in the anterior compartment of the ankle and better access to the lateral gutter as noted in one study.[5] Distraction tightens the capsule theoretically making it more difficult to remove impingement spurs of the distal tibia and talus.[6] Most authors recommend use of a 2.7 mm 30° arthroscope to allow for easier transit through the joint. However, the 4.0 mm 30° arthroscope can be used and is often utilized for posterior hindfoot or ankle arthroscopy in order to move soft tissues and make more working space for the surgeon.

With respect to patient positioning for ankle arthroscopy, there are several options including supine, lateral decubitus, or prone positions. The supine technique is used most often due to ease of setup and surgeon orientation with respect to anatomy and will be discussed in detail later in this chapter. There are reported drawbacks with respect to accessing the posterior ankle and hindfoot compartments. However, adequate access using the supine position without repositioning the patient have been reported with the use of double posteromedial portals with no significant adverse effects.[7] The main advantage of lateral decubitus technique includes no need to reposition the patient to do additional procedures such as a lateral ligament reconstruction or hindfoot endoscopy.[8]

Portal Options and Anatomy

The anteromedial portal location is identified by following the medial malleolar tip and heading up towards the joint line where there is a soft spot just medial to the tibialis anterior tendon. The structure at risk is the saphenous nerve. The accessory anteromedial portal location lies just anterior and lateral to the tip of the medial malleolus.

The anterolateral portal is placed lateral to the peroneus tertius. The structure at risk is the superficial peroneal nerve and its branches (intermediate dorsal cutaneous, medial dorsal cutaneous). From the start point of a 10° plantarflexed ankle and inverted hindfoot, it has been shown that the superficial peroneal nerve moves laterally 3.6 mm with movement from the starting position into 5° of dorsiflexion, and the nerve moves laterally 2.4 mm from the starting position into neutral dorsiflexion.[9] Thus, it may be helpful to place the anterolateral portal slightly medial to the preoperative marking on the skin where the superficial peroneal nerve is identified (easy to see and palpate the nerve branches with the foot plantarflexed and inverted). The accessory anterolateral is located just in front of and medial to the distal fibular tip.

The posterolateral portal is placed approximately 1 cm proximal to the level of the distal fibular tip, directly alongside the lateral border of the Achilles. Structures at risk with this portal are the sural nerve and small saphenous vein. The mean distance of this portal to the sural nerve was 9.7 mm in one study.[10]

The anterocentral portal located in between the tendons of the extensor digitorum communis is not generally recommended as the deep peroneal nerve and dorsalis pedis are at risk.

The posteromedial portal is not used often and usually sufficient access to the posterior joint is afforded by a good posterolateral portal. It is placed just medial to the Achilles border and lateral to the flexor hallucis longus tendon and approximately at a level 1 cm proximal to the distal fibular tip. Structures at risk include the calcaneal nerve branches and posteromedial neurovascular bundle. The mean distance of this portal to the posterior tibial nerve was 13.3 mm in one study.[10]

Complications

Overall, the rate of complications related to ankle arthroscopy ranges in the literature from 3.4% to 17%, the majority of which are neurological.[11-15] Damage to the superficial peroneal nerve is the most commonly encountered and is associated with the use of the anterolateral portal. With respect to the commonality of the remaining neurological complications, sural nerve injuries follow with posterolateral portal placement, then saphenous nerve injuries with anteromedial portal placement, and finally deep peroneal nerve injuries with anterocentral portal placement.[14] Careful technique of portal creation and closure is important to prevent inadvertent laceration or suture entrapment of the nerves, respectively. Other complications reported include iatrogenic articular surface damage, instrument breakage, chronic regional pain syndrome, infection, and other neurovascular injuries. In one study,[15] workman's compensation patients had a complication rate of 21% with particularly nerve-related symptoms compared to a 4.7% complication rate in other patients. Out of 294 consecutive arthroscopies, the authors reported one deep venous thrombosis (DVT), one prolonged drainage from a portal site, and two superficial infections. Fortunately, most complications related to foot and ankle arthroscopy tend to resolve over a 6-month period of time.[16]

Ankle Arthroscopy: Step-by-Step Technique

Anesthesia

The patient undergoes general anesthesia with muscle relaxation to aid in non-invasive distraction of the ankle joint. To aid with postoperative pain control, a popliteal block is placed by anesthesia usually immediately prior to the procedure.

Equipments

- 2.7 mm 30° arthroscope, double cannula (one for inflow, one for suction) to aid in visualization and negates need for additional fluid inflow portal
- 4.0 mm scope can be used but more difficult and iatrogenic cartilage damage more likely
- Small joint arthroscopy set with curved and straight punches, graspers, ring and closed curettes, probe (with 1 mm hatch marks to aid in measurements), osteotome probe, tissue elevators
- Sterile non-invasive distractor system with disposable sterile ankle stirrup sling

- Small joint oscillating shaver (short handle) 3.5 mm or 2.5 mm full radius shaver (less aggressive)
- Small joint burr (short handle) 3.0 mm hooded burr
- Micro vector guide (Smith and Nephew, Andover MA) with K-wire guides for 0.045" (1.1 mm), 0.062" (1.6 mm), 0.125" (3.2 mm) or use an anterior cruciate ligament (ACL) targeting guide to assist for aiming for retrograde drilling of osteochondritis dissecans (OCD) or for placing guidewires for arthroscopic fusion procedures
- Subchondral picks (45° or more acute angles are most useful)
- 18 gauge spinal needle for help with portal localization
- 10 cc syringe and connector tubing to attach to spinal needle for joint insufflation
- No. 11-blade, small mosquito hemostats
- Arthroscopy pump with pressure set at 30 mmHg
- Basic foot instrument tray with small retractors, osteotomes, curettes, etc.

Patient Positioning

The patient is positioned supine on the operating table with the patient's knees at the same level as the break in the table to allow for lower leg and foot elevation or depression. In cases using a non-invasive ankle distraction system, this positioning enables the surgeon to increase ankle distraction by lowering the foot of the bed. Then, a bump, consisting of a 3L bag of saline with towel secured around it, is placed underneath the ipsilateral hip so that the lower leg is rotated properly and the ankle is oriented straight up and down, eliminating external rotation of the leg during the procedure. While the hip is flexed at least 45° and held by an assistant, a foam-padded leg holder is placed approximately four fingerbreadths proximal to the popliteal crease to protect the neurovascular bundle, support the thigh, and provide a stable base on which to apply traction to the ankle. For ease of positioning, the longer metal arm of the leg holder should be kept vertical. Holder position is then secured by use of a clamp which attaches to the bed and is tightened with an interlocking teeth mechanism. The medial to lateral location of the foam pad support of the thigh can be adjusted by sliding the apparatus on the shorter metallic arm of the leg holder. An example of patient positioning and placement of video monitor is shown in Figures 1A and B. As a reference, after the leg holder is positioned, the leg naturally rests with the knee flexed and the foot lies just above the table's surface. If posterior portals are planned or anticipated, the surgeon has to take into account the length of the instruments to be used posteriorly; otherwise, there may not be sufficient room to manipulate or move the instruments due to interference with the OR table. A few inches of additional working room for instrumentation placed through the posterolateral portal can be obtained by removing the padded base of the foot of the bed. In this situation, to prevent pressure sores, the straight contralateral limb is supported with blankets or padding, keeping the heel elevated of the table.

Tourniquet

A well-padded tourniquet is placed on the upper thigh of the operative extremity after adequate padding has been placed. Tourniquet is elevated to 280 mm Hg for a maximum of 2 hours.

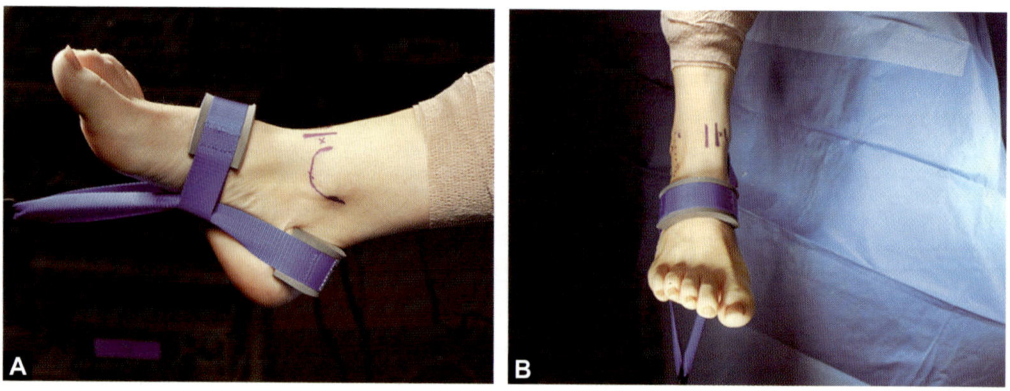

Figs 1A and B: Example of proper patient positioning for ankle arthroscopy and equipment location

Step-by-Step Surgical Technique

After sterile prepping and draping, the non-invasive, sterile ankle distractor clamp is attached over the last sterile extremity sheet to the operating table and slid until the end of the table's rail. While draping, it is important not to have multiple layers of sheets over the rail where the clamp is applied. The drapes may bunch up and prevent the surgeon from advancing the table clamp to the end of the table rail and could limit the amount of traction that can be applied. The hinged distal portion of the clamp is oriented superiorly so that the clamp can be easily tightened and secured to the table. The L-shaped support bar is temporarily secured to the table clamp. The distractor's excursion ring is twisted and set to allow for maximum flexibility in the amount of traction applied, and the distractor is attached to the support bar.

A sterile ankle stirrup sling is placed on the operative ankle with the posterior heel pad placed just above the posterior tuberosity of the calcaneus, and the dorsal footpad is placed over the midfoot between footpad and to protect the dorsalis pedis neurovascular bundle. The portion of the ankle stirrup with a clip to attach to the distractor comes out plantar to the foot, making sure that the straps that run alongside the foot are not twisted. It is important not to get the foot and ankle or the ankle stirrup wet as either will otherwise slip (but can use coban to help secure in those cases). A picture of the setup is shown in Figure 2. The support bar is secured in the table clamp in a position that has the maximum height from the OR table to allow for enough room for use of instruments in posterior portals.

Once the ankle is positioned and traction is set to the desired amount, anatomical landmarks about the ankle are drawn with a skin marker or identified: medial malleolar tip, saphenous neurovascular bundle, tibialis anterior tendon, peroneus tertius tendon, superficial peroneal nerve branches, lateral malleolar tip, lateral border of the Achilles tendon (Figs 3A to D).

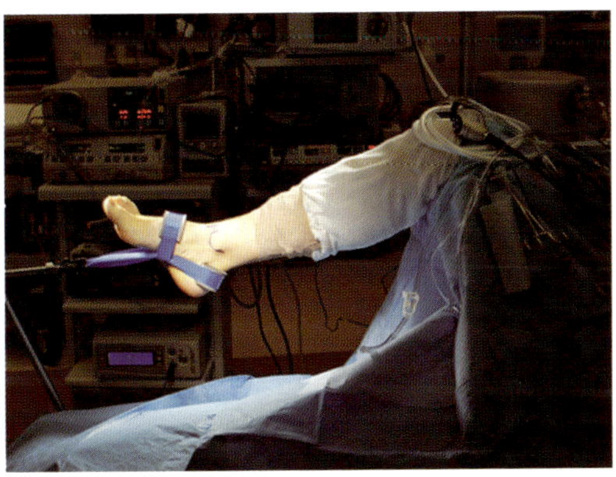

Fig. 2: Intraoperative setup for non-invasive distraction is pictured

With the surgeon's thumb, a soft spot is felt in between the medial border of the tibialis anterior tendon and the shoulder area of the medial malleolus and this anteromedial portal location is temporarily marked with an "x" in the middle of the surgeon's thumbnail print. An 18 gauge spinal needle directed 90° with respect to the tibial longitudinal axis and 45° with respect to the axial plane in placed in the proposed anteromedial portal site (Fig. 4A). By gently moving the needle up and down, the surgeon can feel the tibia and talus respectively and confirm position within the joint. Sterile saline is injected into the ankle for insufflation (Fig. 4B) and no significant resistance should be felt initially until 5 or so milliliters of fluid is injected. The inner trocar of the spinal needle is removed (Fig. 4C) and drops of synovial fluid are seen coming out of the spinal needle confirming intra-articular position. No more than 5–10 cc of fluid needs to be injected to get adequate backflow.

The surgeon carefully takes a no. 11-blade (with the blade facing superiorly) and creates a longitudinal small skin incision using only the tip of the blade under direct visualization, careful not to plunge deeper into the soft tissues to avoid iatrogenic injury to the saphenous nerve. The surgeon stabilizes his or her hand by putting the small and ring finger against the skin while the incision is made. The portal then is created with a blunt, small curved mosquito hemostat. To aid in instrument control and avoid inadvertent cartilage damage with joint entry, the surgeon places his or her index finger along the shaft of the hemostat (Fig. 5A) and the surgeon feels a "pop" as the joint is entered. Hemostat is removed.

The blunt trocar and cannula for the 2.7 mm 30° arthroscope is placed into the ankle keeping the same trajectory (Figs 5B and C). The arthroscope is introduced. The fluid is turned on and the scope light cord is rotated to look at the anterolateral aspect of the ankle joint. The anterolateral portal is localized with a spinal needle so that the needle enters the joint under direct visualization. The arthroscopist then checks to ensure that the portal enters at the level of the tibiotalar joint and will allow access to the posterior aspects of the ankle. The spinal needle

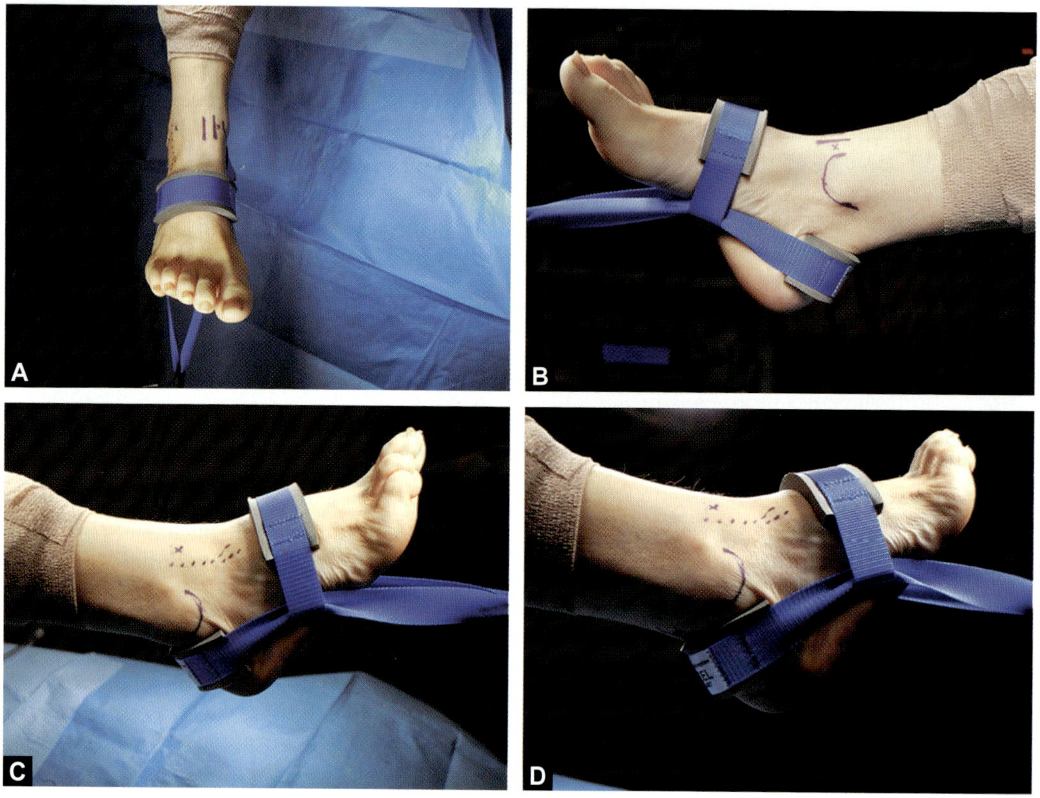

Figs 3A to D: (A) Superior view of the ankle with anterior landmarks of the anteromedial joint line (x), tibialis anterior (most medial tendon), anterolateral portal site, superficial peroneal nerve (dotted line) branches; (B) Medial view showing landmarks; (C) Lateral view with landmarks depicted; (D) Posterolateral view showing an x where the posterolateral portal can be placed

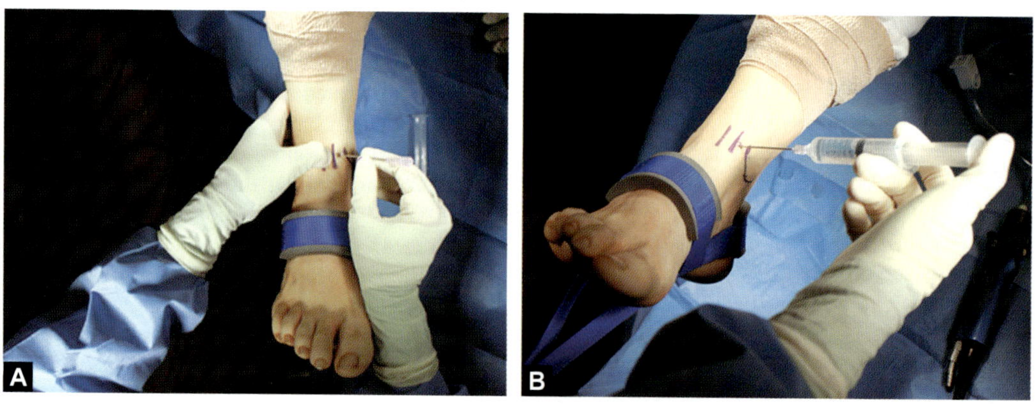

Figs 4A and B

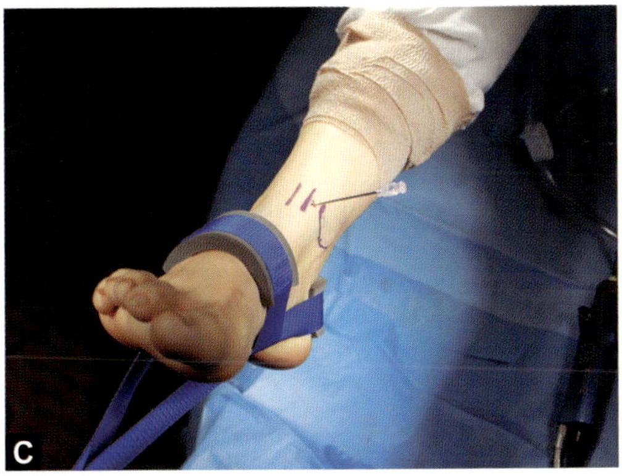

Figs 4A to C: Steps in the establishment of the anteromedial portal (see text)

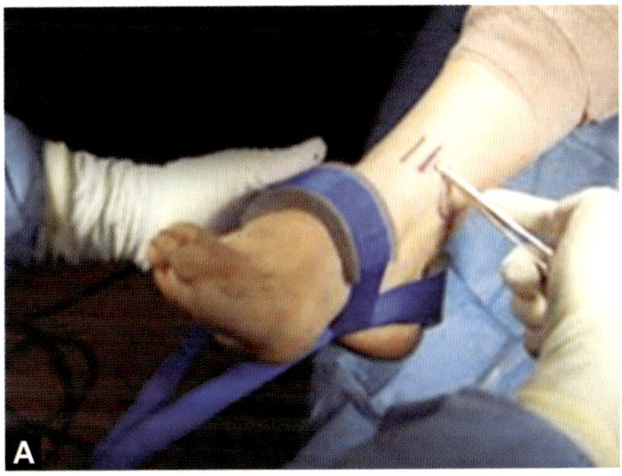

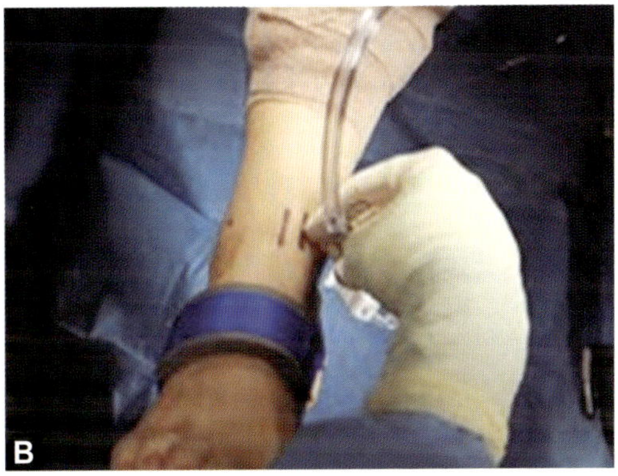

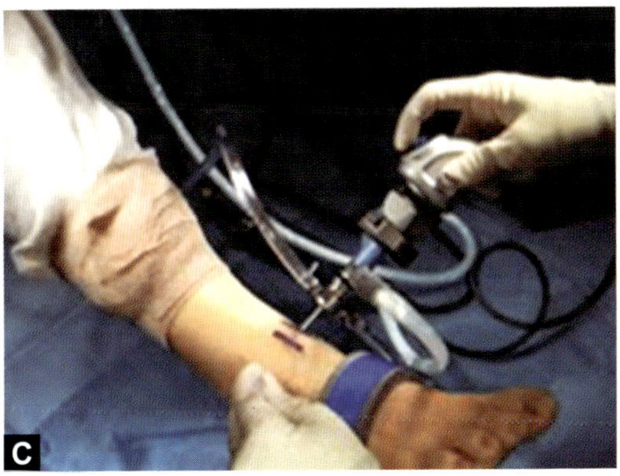

Figs 5A to C: Ankle joint entry and creation of an anterolateral portal

is removed and no. 11-blade is used to create a nick in the skin only. A blunt curved hemostat is then placed through the anterolateral portal and the tissue is spread slightly to enlarge the portal.

Once two working portals are created, the thorough examination of the ankle joint can commence. If extensive synovitis in the medial and lateral gutters is obstructing the view, an oscillating shaver is used to clear the red, inflamed tissue. Anteriorly, there may also be synovitis. The tissue is carefully removed under direct visualization as once fatty tissue is encountered debridement stops in order to prevent injury to the dorsalis pedis neurovascular bundle. Plicas also do exist in the ankle and can sometimes abrade the cartilage in the area and obstruct the arthroscopic view.

The ankle joint is examined in a reproducible way every time in order not to miss any pathology.

The scope begins in the anteromedial portal and the following structures or areas are evaluated:

- Anteromedial talus and tibia (Fig. 6A)
- Medial gutter (all the way down approaching the subtalar joint (Fig. 6B)
- Medial malleolar tip, posteromedial and posterior-central talus and tibia and posteromedial talus with flexor hallucis longus (FHL) reflection (Fig. 6C)
- Posterior-central tibia and talus (Fig. 7A)
- Posterior-lateral tibia and talus (Fig. 7B)
- Lateral ankle and distal fibula and syndesmosis (Fig. 7C)
- Anterior-central tibia and talus, anterior-lateral tibia and talus and anterior inferior tibiotalalar ligament (Figs 8A to C)
- Distal edge of lateral tibial plafond, distal and anterior portion of talar dome (Fig. 9A)
- Dorsolateral aspect of talar neck area (Fig. 9B) anterior talar dome.

A probe placed through the anterior-lateral portal is used to assess cartilage integrity in the above areas.

In order to see the cartilage surfaces well and to minimize iatrogenic cartilage injury, the surgeon's hand should minimally move the scope side to side or up and down as rotation of the light cord can yield actually quite an extensive view of the ankle joint. This is particularly important when attempting to view the posterior aspects of the joint through the anterior portals. The notch of the distal tibial plafond as it comes down to the malleolus or the shoulder of the distal tibia is identified and the scope is pushed gently posteriorly into the joint in that interval and the light cord is rotated to evaluate the posterior joint (Fig. 7A). The scope is carefully backed out of the notch area.

The arthroscope then is switched to the anterior-lateral portal to assess the following areas of the ankle:

- Anterolateral talus and tibia
- Lateral malleolar tip
- Lateral gutter (all the way down approaching the subtalar joint)
- Lateral-central tibia and talus
- Lateral-posterior tibia and talus
- Tibial slip, central tibia and talus
- Inner surface of medial malleolus
- Medial talus and tibia, anterior border of distal tibia

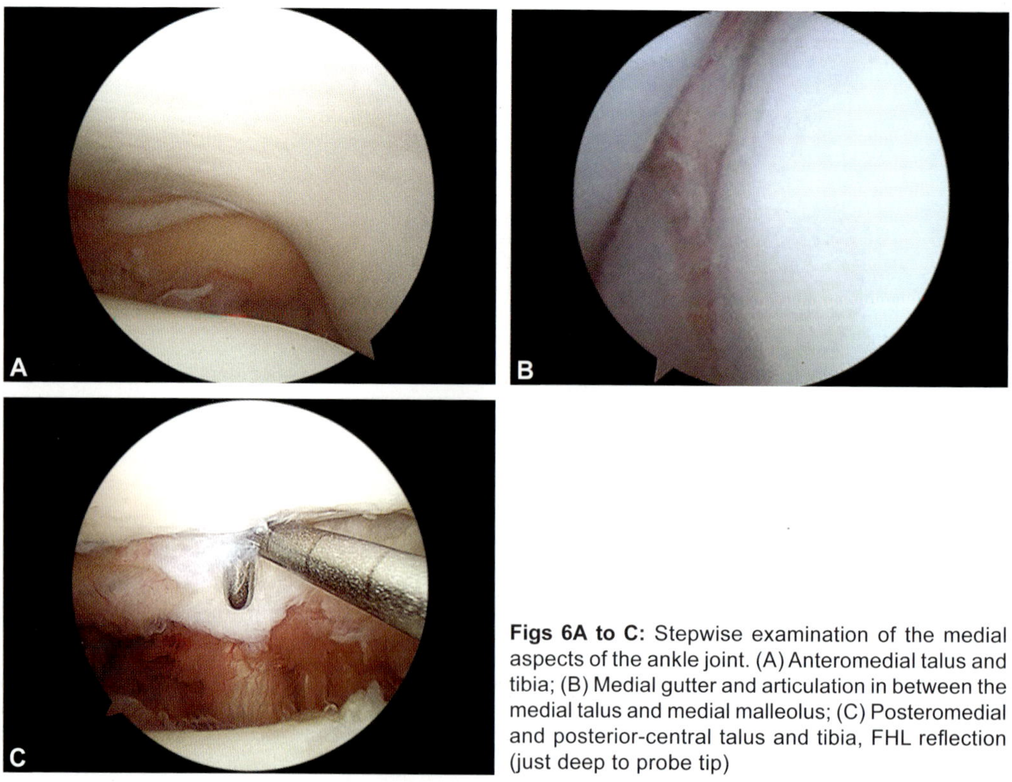

Figs 6A to C: Stepwise examination of the medial aspects of the ankle joint. (A) Anteromedial talus and tibia; (B) Medial gutter and articulation in between the medial talus and medial malleolus; (C) Posteromedial and posterior-central talus and tibia, FHL reflection (just deep to probe tip)

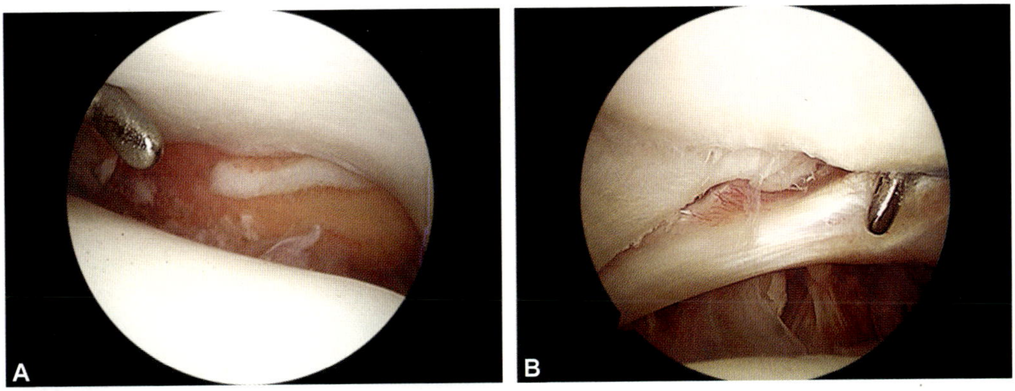

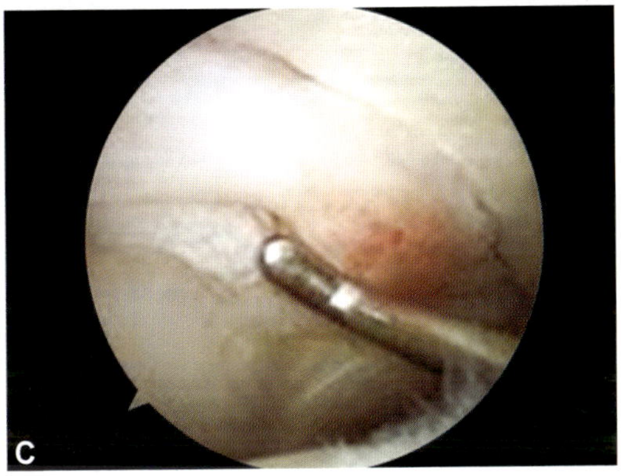

Figs 7A to C: Stepwise examination of the central and lateral aspects of the ankle joint. (A) Central and central-posterior tibia and talus; (B) Posterolateral talus and tibia, probe on tibial slip (transverse tibial ligament runs superiorly to the tibial slip); (C) Lateral aspect of the ankle with probe tip in between the distal fibular articular cartilage noted below and the proliferative tissue of the syndesmosis (formerly known as a meniscoid lesion) is above

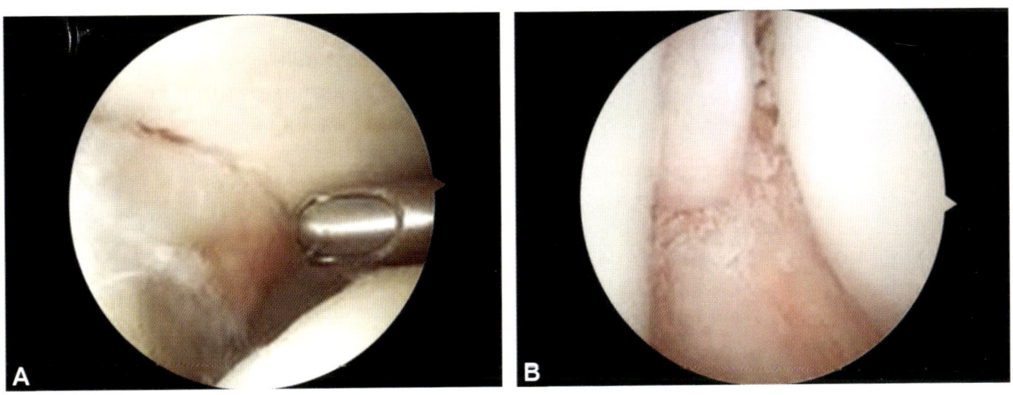

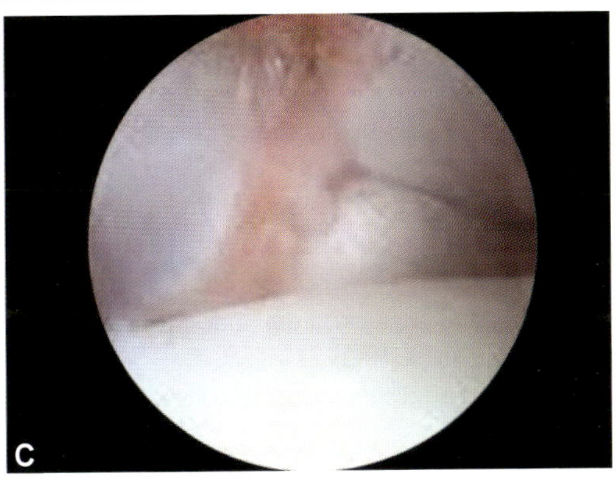

Figs 8A to C: Examination of the anterolateral structures of the ankle. (A) Anterolateral talus and tibia as viewed from the anterolateral portal; (B) Lateral gutter and the articulation between the lateral talus and the fibula noted; (C) Anterolateral talus and tibia, along with the distal fibula and the anterior tibiofibular ligament (AITFL) which is the vertical structure that runs just anteriorly to the borders of the tibia and the fibula

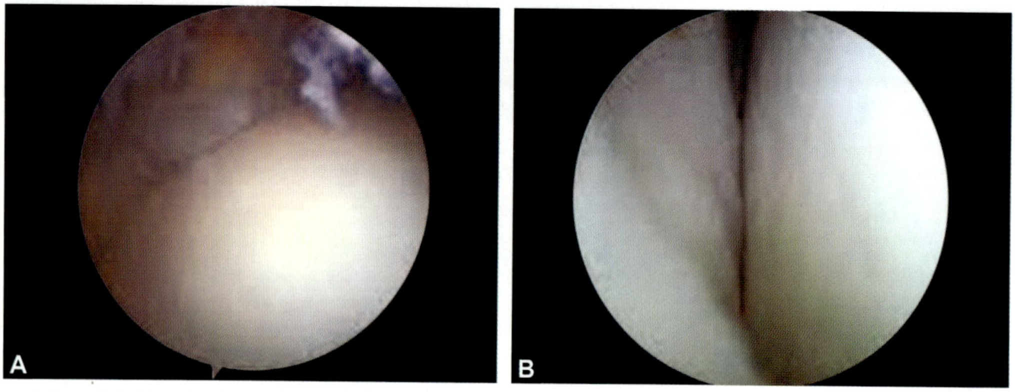

Figs 9A and B: Examination of essentially the anterior gutter or compartment of the ankle. (A) Distal anterior and central talar dome; (B) Dorsolateral and central talar neck area

- Anterior border of medial malleolus and
- Dorsomedial neck of the talus.

In cases where there are OCD defects, loose bodies, or further visualization of the posterior compartment is necessary, a posterolateral portal is localized 1 cm proximal to the fibular tip with a spinal needle (Fig. 10) while the scope is in the anteromedial portal to aid the surgeon in triangulation. Entry of the spinal needle should be inferior to the tibial lip to allow for unimpeded movement posteriorly. The joint then is inspected with the scope in the posterolateral portal and the following structures are identified and evaluated (Fig. 11): posteromedial talus and tibia, posterior-central talus and tibia, and posterolateral talus and tibia. The probe can be placed through either anterior portals to assess cartilage integrity.

After completion of the procedure, the portals are closed with 4-0 nylon simple sutures in order to prevent synovial fistula or sinus formation. As needed to supplement the block and provide postoperative pain relief, a ropivacaine and morphine mixture is injected into the joint (5 cc total) and 0.5% marcaine without epinephrine is injected only into the skin incisions. A drain is not routinely placed but if needed a 7 French round drain with Jackson-Pratt attachment can be placed into the joint under arthroscopic visualization by use of a small mosquito clamp. Dressings are placed over the incisions and the foot and ankle is placed into a well-padded posterior and sugar tong plaster splint. Patients are kept non-weight bearing a few days to 4–6 weeks depending on the procedure(s) performed.

Overview of Ankle Conditions Treated Arthroscopically

This section will serve as a short review of clinical conditions affecting the ankle for which arthroscopic treatment has been successful. The discussion will also include surgical technique pearls, presentation of assorted pathological picture, and rehabilitation guidelines where appropriate.

Loose Bodies

Loose bodies such as those due to trauma or synovial chondromatosis (Figs 12A and B) can be difficult to remove arthroscopically and can potentially cause the surgeon much angst during a case. There are technique tips for removing loose bodies from the ankle joint that may be helpful and include the following:

- Turn-off the pump inflow as you enter the joint with a grasper
- Delay applying full traction on the ankle to trap the fragments in the anterior compartment of the joint so that you can reach them and remove them
- Always push the grasper in a little past the loose body so that when the jaws close the loose body is not pinched out of the grasper
- If a loose body disappears it most likely is in the posterior recesses, use your hand to palpate and push in and out over (cycle) the posterolateral ankle and posteromedial ankle joint line to flush out the loose body
- Have available suction graspers

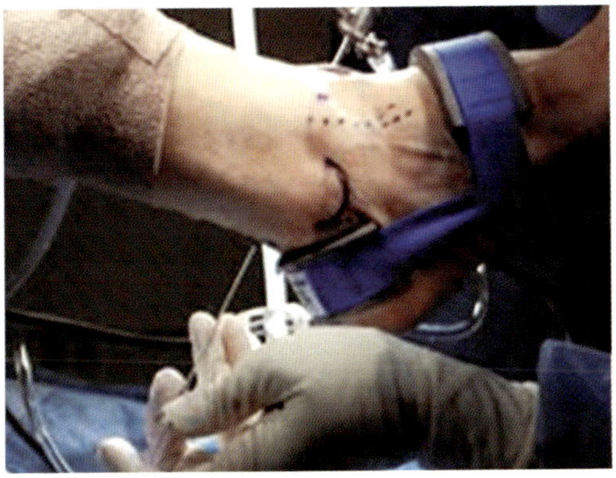

Fig. 10: Landmarks and method for creation of a posterolateral portal

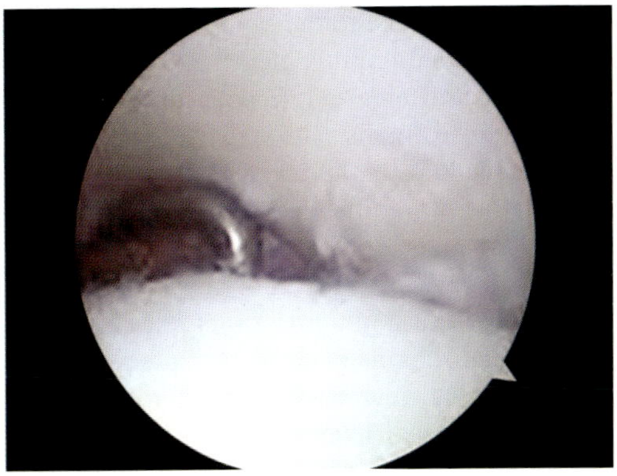

Fig. 11: Visualization of probe brought into the ankle joint from the posterolateral portal (see text)

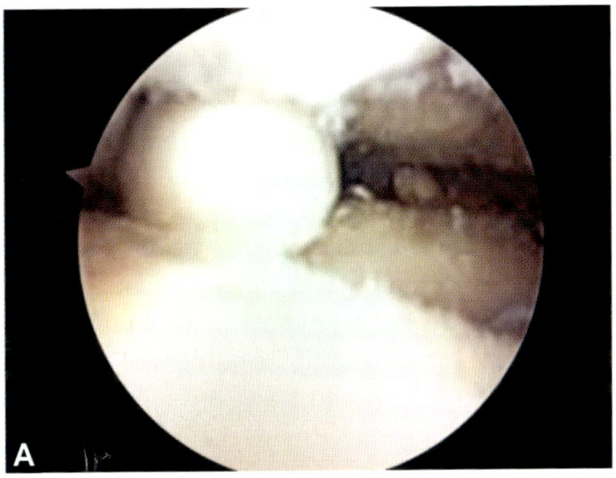

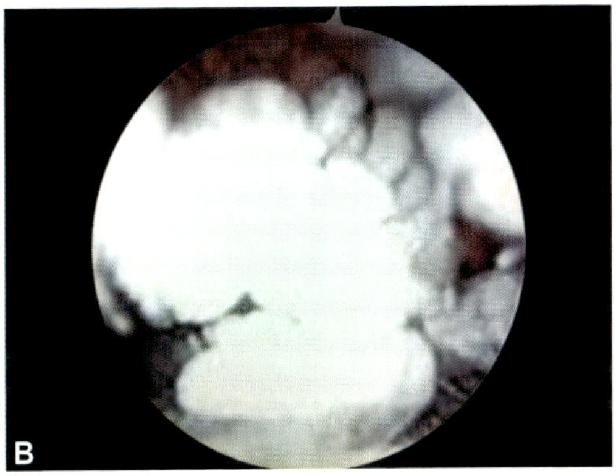

Figs 12A and B: Loose bodies are identified. (A) Loose body caught in between the articular cartilage surfaces and causing damage; (B) Synovial chondromatosis is pictured

- Use a spinal needle and spear the loose body to keep it stationary until you can get a grasper around it
- Gently twist the grasper as you work the loose body through the soft tissues, the portal incision and then out of the joint (don't be afraid to extend the portal incision so that it is easier to remove a larger sized loose body)
- If the loose body is large, trap it in the anterior compartment of the ankle and use a small osteotome placed through one of the anterior portals and under direct visualization cut the loose body in half using the anterior surface of the tibia as a cutting block or use an aggressive oscillating shaver and try to separate the loose body into smaller pieces that can be more easily removed
- If all else fails, it is ok to make an open arthrotomy incision.

ANKLE IMPINGEMENT

Anterior ankle impingement was first described as "footballer's ankle" due to its predominance in soccer athletes. This nomenclature refers to spur formation over the anterior and distal tibia and the dorsal surface of the talus that limits ankle dorsiflexion. Etiology appears to be from repetitive forced dorsiflexion injury, acute ankle sprains, supination stresses, or chronic ankle instability. Spurs form as part of the reparative process. Patients will have pain with squatting, jump landing, stair-climbing, or activities that require a larger amount of dorsiflexion. On exam, anterior joint line tenderness may be elicited with passive hyperdorsiflexion of the ankle. Also, the location of soreness to palpation differentiates between the subtypes of anterior ankle impingement:

- Over area lateral to the peroneus tertius (anterolateral impingement)

- Over area medial to the tibialis anterior tendon (anteromedial impingement), and
- Over central area of the anterior joint line in between the tibialis anterior and peroneus tertius (anterocentral impingement).

The clinical significance of each subtype is still being elucidated. Standard anteroposterior (AP), lateral, and oblique X-ray views of the ankle often do not show the impinging spurs and an oblique anteromedial impingement view can be ordered.[17] To perform this view, the foot is externally rotated 30° from the usual lateral X-ray position and the ankle is plantarflexed slightly. The beam then is oriented 45° in a craniocaudal direction. Surgical treatment is initiated if conservative treatment modalities fail (i.e. heel lift, anti-inflammatory medication, activity modification, physical therapy, and rare cortisone injection).

Anterior Ankle Impingement Excision: Surgical Steps

When using an ankle distractor, the surgical steps after portal placement include the need to clean off the distal tibia soft tissue by keeping the blade of the 3.5 mm oscillating shaver turned away from the anterior capsule and staying on the anterior and distal surface of the tibia as the spur is excavated and exposed (Fig. 13A).

The arthroscope is switched to the anterolateral portal and the shaver is used to clear off the soft tissues of the central and medial distal tibia and medial malleolar area to expose all of the osteophytes. With the light cord for the arthroscope looking superiorly, a demarcation is observed in between the normal vertical contour of the distal tibia and the osteophytes (Fig. 13B).

In a systematic fashion, a burr is introduced through the anteromedial portal and the spur is taken down in smooth, long strokes of the burr from above the superior aspect of the spur going inferiorly with controlled motions to avoid plunging into the talus. Spur excision starts medially at the rim of the medial malleolus and shoulder area of the tibia (as there is less spur formation in those locations generally and the normal contour/orientation of the distal anterior tibial surface can be appreciated) and moves laterally as far as visualization allows (usually at least half the way across the distal tibia). Usually, the spur comes off easily as the bone is soft. Once the surgeon debrides down to healthy bone, the bone is harder and more difficult to remove with the burr. Generally, the amount of bone removed related to a spur is at least the width of the burr or 5 mm. A shaver then is used to remove any loose flaps of cartilage or bone debris.

The scope is switched to the anteromedial portal and the burr brought through the lateral portal. The normal demarcation of the distal tibia is now seen well and excision starts laterally and moves medially towards the area already completed. The final appearance of tibia is shown in Figure 13C.

The talus also should be evaluated early in the case for any spur formation (usually anteromedially) before there is soft tissue swelling related to the arthroscopic fluid that will decrease working space dorsally. To aid in visualization, any synovitis of the medial gutter, anterior compartment or lateral gutter is removed with an oscillating shaver. The plica generally has to be elevated and released. The scope placed in the anterolateral portal looking down the dorsal surface of the talar dome and neck of the talus as you follow the instrument (oscillating shaver) from the anteromedial portal entrance to the talar neck region. Keeping the blade away from the dorsal soft tissue, exposure of the talar spur is accomplished safely and the borders of the spur are outlined (Figs 14A and B). A 3.0 mm rounded-tip burr is then introduced with the hood towards the dorsal soft tissues and long strokes with the burr are done in a lateral to medial direction starting at the superior-most extent of the spur so that the spur does not affect positioning of the burr.

The arthroscope is switched to the anteromedial portal and the shaver is placed in anterolateral portal. The plica is released to have room to travel to the dorsal aspect of lateral talar dome and neck region to make sure that the entirety of the impingement spur has been removed.

Traction is then released partially and the ankle is dorsiflexed with the scope in the joint to see whether bony or soft tissue impingement occurs in dorsiflexion. Fluoroscopic evaluation of spur excision can also be used, but the arthroscopic exam is the most helpful to confirm that there is no impingement within the normal limits of ankle motion. Depending on concomitant procedures, a drain can be placed intra-articularly to prevent hematoma formation if that is a concern.

Portals are closed with 4-0 nylon, dressings are placed, and a well-padded non-weight-bearing short leg splint is applied. Patients are seen in the office a few days after surgery when their splint is

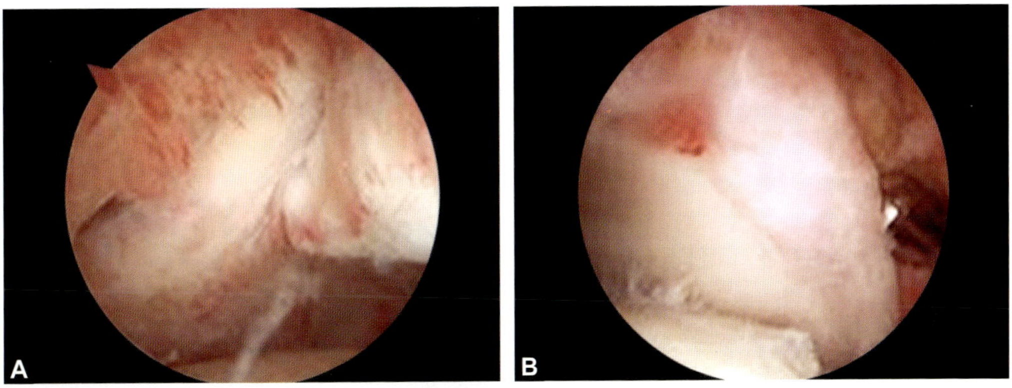

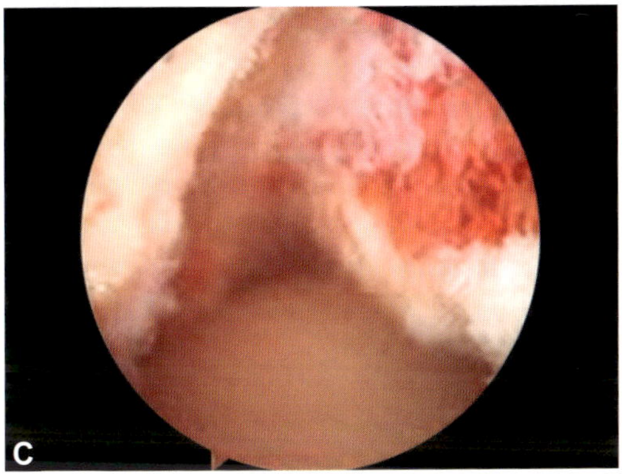

Figs 13A to C: Tibial-sided anterior ankle impingement (usually anterolateral). (A) Distal anterolateral tibial spur formation in a patient with some AITFL hypertrophy due to injury to the syndesmosis; (B) Anterior and anteromedial border of the medial malleolar area with large osteophyte formed; (C) Final appearance of tibia after spur excision

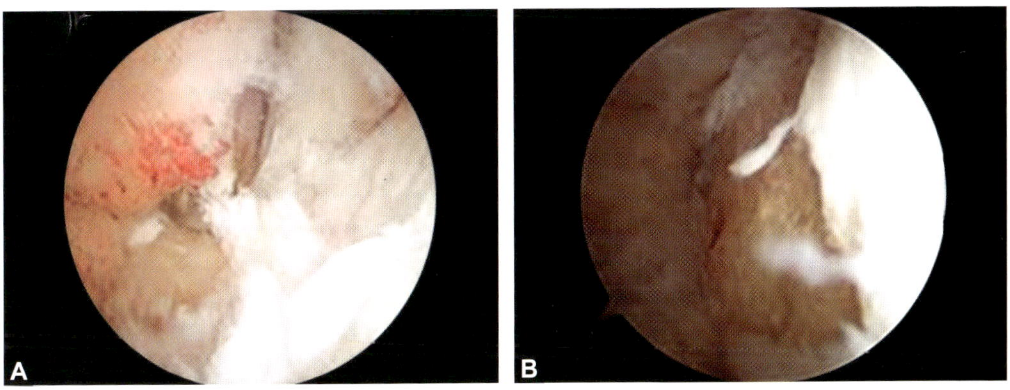

Figs 14A and B: Talar-sided anterior ankle impingement (usually dorsomedial). (A) Exposure of spur is performed and burr is on the superior most surface outlining the extent of spur formation; (B) Completed excision of talar spur

removed, dressing is changed, and they are placed in a tall cam walker boot. Patients start weight-bearing in the boot, early range of motion exercises, and physical therapy. Early recovery is 6–8 weeks with return to more rigorous activities such as running usually after 10–12 weeks.

Successful outcomes from arthroscopic excision of anterior ankle impingement spurs range from 73–96%, with poorer results noted in patients with joint space narrowing already present.[6,18] Patients should be counseled preoperatively that it is likely that the osteophytes could recur.

Lastly, there are other types of ankle impingement. Subfibular or submalleolar impingement can result from ossicle formation related to old ankle sprain injury. Accessory anterolateral or anteromedial portals respectively can aid the surgeon in visualizing with the arthroscope in the traditional portal and using instrumentation through the appropriate accessory portal to access and remove the ossicle. Posterior ankle impingement will be discussed in more detail later in the chapter covering subtalar arthroscopy and hindfoot endoscopy.

OSTEOCHONDRAL DEFECTS

Osteochondral defects of the talus occur mainly due to trauma (micro or macro) and represent sequelae of acute lateral ankle ligament sprains in 4–7% of cases. Medial defects tend to be more common, involve the middle or posterior third of the talar dome, and characteristically are deep and cup-shaped. Lateral defects are often more symptomatic and displaced, involve the middle or anterior portions of the lateral talar dome, and are wafer-shaped. Patients complain of persistent ankle pain after a sprain, recurrent swelling, and a deep catching or locking sensation within the joint. Examination shows an effusion and localized tenderness over the joint line and occasionally palpable crepitus over the talar dome with motion. X-rays are generally done and unless the process is chronic or there is an osteochondral fracture, findings are limited. Due to clinical suspicion, further imaging with a magnetic resonance imaging (MRI) or CT scan is performed. MRI staging systems of the OCD lesion are based off of the original Berndt and Harty classification:[19]

Stage I: Subchondral trabecular compression
Stage II: Incomplete separation of fragment
Stage IIA: Formation of subchondral cyst
Stage III: Presence of unattached and undisplaced fragment with synovial fluid undermining the lesion, and
Stage IV: Displaced osteochondral fragment.

It appears that compared with arthroscopy, MRI predicted the presence and stability of OCD lesions of the talus relatively well.[20] However, the clinician cannot depend on one grading system to determine optimal treatment and essentially the decision depends on a multitude of factors:

- Stable or unstable lesion
- Symptomatic or asymptomatic incidental lesion
- Size of the lesion
- Character of the lesion
- Location of lesion
- Age of the patient, and
- Patient activity level.

For the most part, unstable lesions associated with mechanical symptoms and acute or chronic Stage III or IV lesions require surgical intervention.

The arthroscopy-based treatment options for OCD of the talus include subchondral drilling, or microfracture, retrograde drilling, or fragment fixation in cases of osteochondral fracture. Bone marrow stimulation techniques such as microfracture tend to have better outcomes in patients less than 50 years of age, lesions less than 10 mm in size, noncystic lesions, and lateral lesions.[2,21,22] Outcomes seem to be negatively affected by a higher body mass index, presence of osteophytes, and increasing age. Intralesional debridement and microfracture was associated with 86% good to excellent results in a large systematic review.[23] More recently, equivalent results at 2 years were reported for microfracture, osteochondral autograft transplantation surgery (OATS), and chondroplasty.[24] Despite these clinical outcomes after microfracture, MRI appearance does not improve much after surgery.[25]

Microfracture Surgical Technique: Step-by-Step

The setup and equipment are the same as described earlier for supine ankle arthroscopy.

The surgeon has to keep in mind the size and location of the OCD. Most lesions can be accessed arthroscopically. If reasonable plantarflexion of the ankle can be done during the operation, anterior portals can give the surgeon access to the anterior half of talus and to the anterior 50% of the posterior half of talus.[26] The posterolateral portal can be used to access posterior lesions. With respect to using the microfracture awls and equipment management, if the OCD is located anterolaterally, the arthroscope is placed in the anteromedial portal. Instrumentation then is shuttled through the anterolateral portal in order to directly view the extent of the OCD and get a measurement utilizing a calibrated probe. If the OCD is a central or anteromedial lesion, the arthroscope is positioned in the anterolateral portal and the instrumentation is introduced via the anteromedial portal.

When preparing a stable rim around the defect, the surgeon can switch portals to access different portions of the lesion with curettes, prepare a perpendicular edge around the defect, and prevent injury to the healthy surrounding cartilage surface. A prepared OCD defect is shown in Figures 15A to C.

The most angled of the subchondral picks available is chosen and carefully placed through the portal following the curve of the instrument for easy joint entry. The pick is positioned as perpendicular as possible with respect to the surface of the lesion (Fig. 15D). Different portals are used to access different portions of the lesion with the subchondral picks. Gentle tapping with a mallet under direct visualization is performed to ensure that the pick does not skid or lose position. Each drill hole should be spaced apart by a few millimeters.

Once finished with the microfracture, the fluid to the scope is temporarily stopped to determine whether adequate bleeding occurs at the OCD site (Fig. 15E).

The joint is copiously irrigated. The arthroscopic equipment is removed. Portals are closed with 4-0 Nylon and a dressing is placed. The operative leg is placed in a well-padded posterior splint.

Postoperatively, patients are non-weight bearing and released to home the same day if they fulfill discharge criteria. Patients are seen in the office within a week and changed to tall cam walker boot. A continuous passive motion machine protocol is then started for 4–6 hours a day for 4–6 weeks. Physical therapy is started. Patients then progress

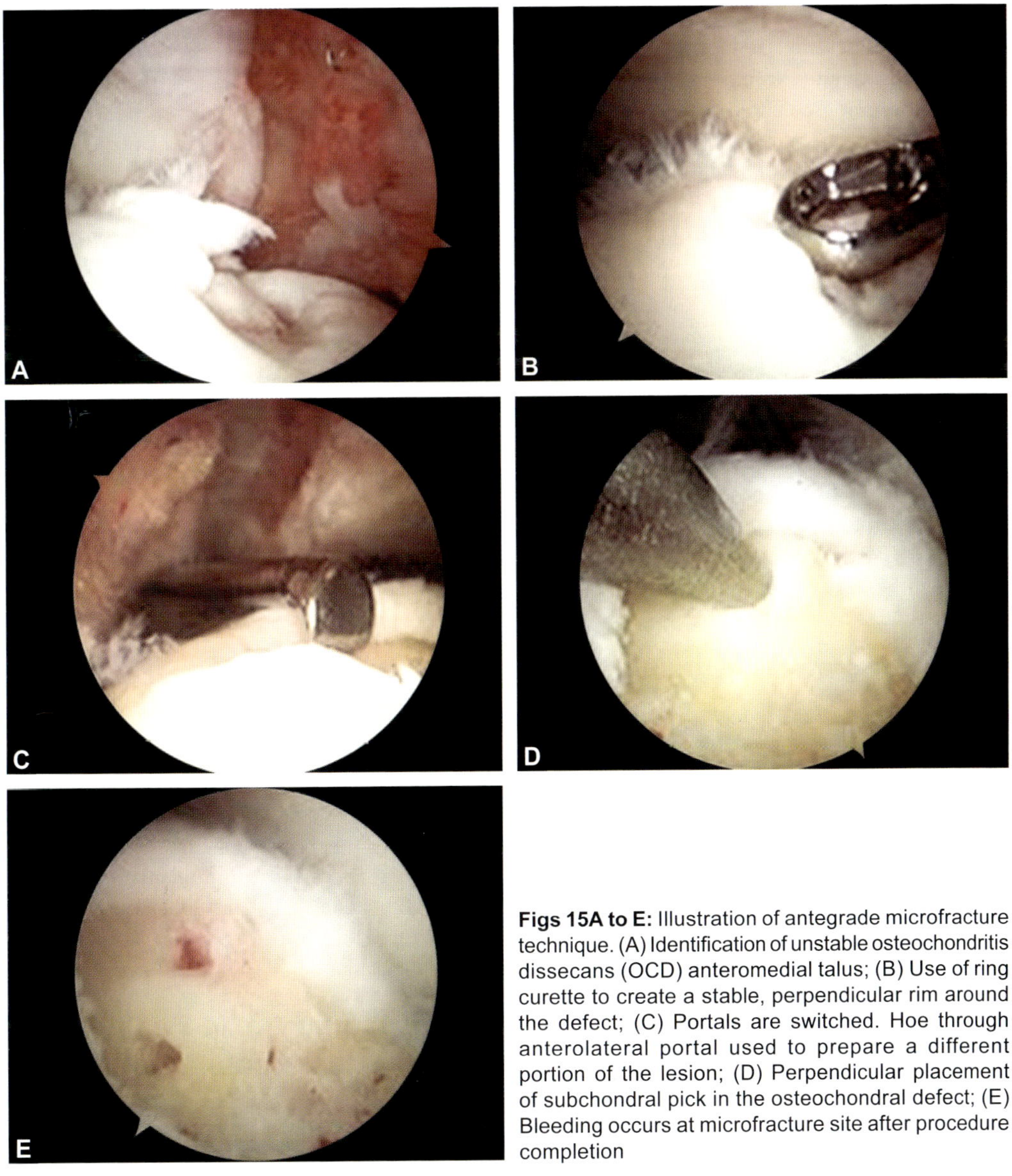

Figs 15A to E: Illustration of antegrade microfracture technique. (A) Identification of unstable osteochondritis dissecans (OCD) anteromedial talus; (B) Use of ring curette to create a stable, perpendicular rim around the defect; (C) Portals are switched. Hoe through anterolateral portal used to prepare a different portion of the lesion; (D) Perpendicular placement of subchondral pick in the osteochondral defect; (E) Bleeding occurs at microfracture site after procedure completion to weight-bearing as tolerated in cam boot brace usually at 6th week, postoperatively. Impact activities and running are initiated after 12 weeks. Sports return takes at least 4–6 months.

There are other options with respect to subchondral drilling of OCD lesions. Transtalar retrograde drilling of an OCD lesion may be selected as the treatment of choice in situations where there is an intact cartilaginous cap and an associated subchondral cyst.[27] A guide or cruciate guide is used to localize the lesion. A K-wire is drilled through the sinus tarsi (Fig. 16) to treat a medial defect. Several passes with the K-wire through the guide can be done to make holes in the sclerotic bone and encourage bone healing. If there is a significant cyst, then a cannulated trephine or small reamer used with the guide can remove a core of bone or cyst material. The surgeon then can back fill the previous cyst area with cancellous bone graft (obtained from the calcaneus or proximal tibia). Sometimes it is technically difficult to localize the lesion. If one can see the lesion on X-ray, then fluoroscopy may be helpful intraoperatively. A picture of the posteromedial lesion after retrograde drilling through the posterolateral portal is shown in Figures 17A and B. The surgeon can monitor the lesion arthroscopically while packing the bone graft and observe that the contour and firmness of the talus subtly improves. Rarely, transmalleolar anterograde drilling can be performed. This technique has the disadvantage of the surgeon having to drill through healthy cartilage of the tibia in order to reach the OCD of the talus.

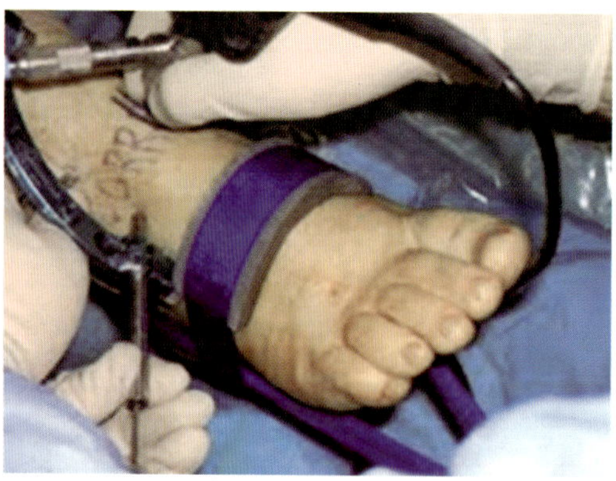

Fig. 16: Example of transtalar retrograde drilling for a medial osteochondral lesion of the talus. Guide is seen in place and K-wire is introduced into the talus via the sinus tarsi

Osteochondral Defects of the Tibia

Osteochondral defects of the tibia also do occur, albeit less commonly. There is a sparsity of information regarding the treatment, location, and prognosis of these lesions. An example of a posteromedial tibial OCD lesion is shown in Figures 18A and B. Microfracture was performed utilizing the same principles as outlined above.

Osteochondral Fractures of the Talus

Finally, osteochondral fractures of the talus can be managed arthroscopically. However, proper access to the lesion and the selection of fixation implant make treatment of these fractures challenging. Ankle arthroscopy is performed as usual. If there is enough subchondral bone attached to healthy cartilage cap, then the fracture bed is debrided and prepared. If it is a central or posterior lesion, access for perpendicular placement of implants is restricted or difficult. The posterolateral portal can be employed in addition to dorsiflexion to provide some access for posterior lesions. Traction can be released somewhat to allow for more plantarflexion of the ankle which can give the surgeon room to work for anterior and central lesions. A K-wire is temporarily placed in the central part of the fracture fragment via a more proximal incision above the ankle joint to enable correct trajectory. Newer fixation options include bioabsorbable implants which can provide compression of the fracture fragment. An example of an osteochondral fracture of the lateral talar dome that was fixed is shown in Figures 19A to C.

ARTHRITIS

Arthroscopic ankle fusion is indicated in patients who have failed a full course of conservative treatment for their ankle arthritis and have normal weight-bearing alignment or very mild malalignment.[28] This procedure is contraindicated in situations where there is bone loss, a large area of avascular necrosis, or significant deformity. With arthroscopic techniques, it is technically difficult to correct more than 5° of varus or significant anterior-to-posterior plane malalignment.

Arthroscopic Ankle Fusion: Step-by-Step Technique

Patient setup is the same as described for supine ankle arthroscopy with one modification to facilitate

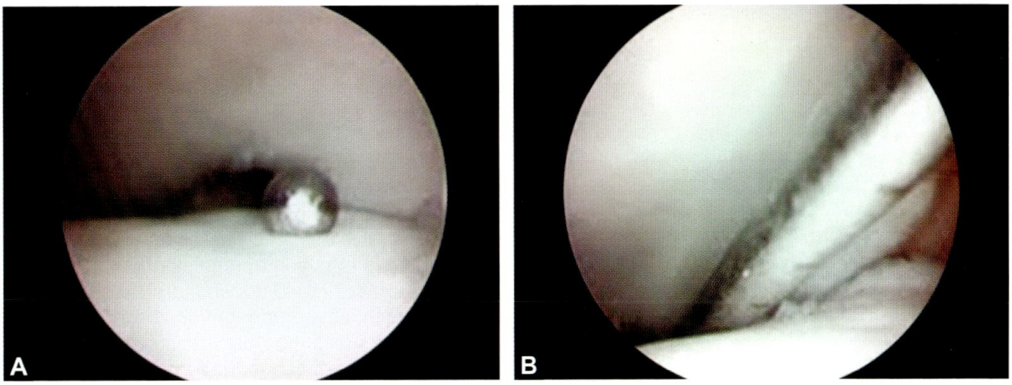

Figs 17A and B: Example of retrograde drilling of a posteromedial osteochondral defect of the talus. (A) View from the posterolateral portal with aiming guide placed through medial portal (tip of guide seen in resting gently in the central area of the lesion); (B) Calibrated probe assists in measurement of the size of the lesion for comparison purposes to magnetic resonance imaging (MRI) images

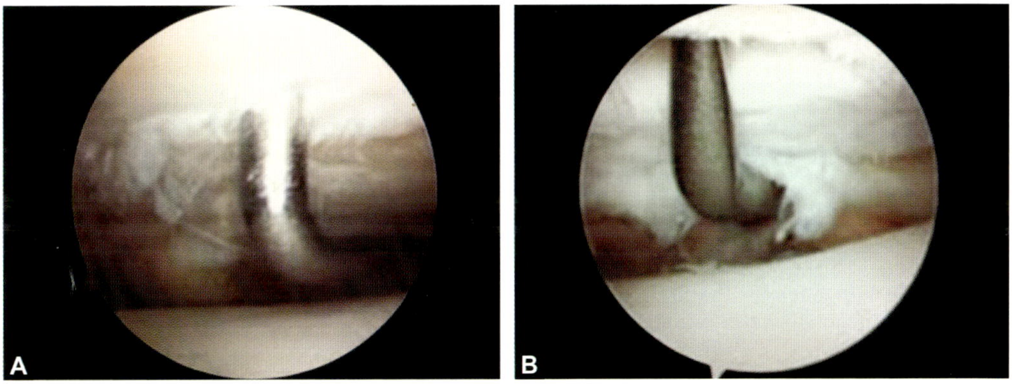

Figs 18A and B: Example of OCD lesion of the posteromedial tibia. (A) Defect identified after thorough evaluation of the joint; (B) Rim of lesion prepared and subchondral pick brought into joint through posterolateral portal in order to access lesion for microfracture

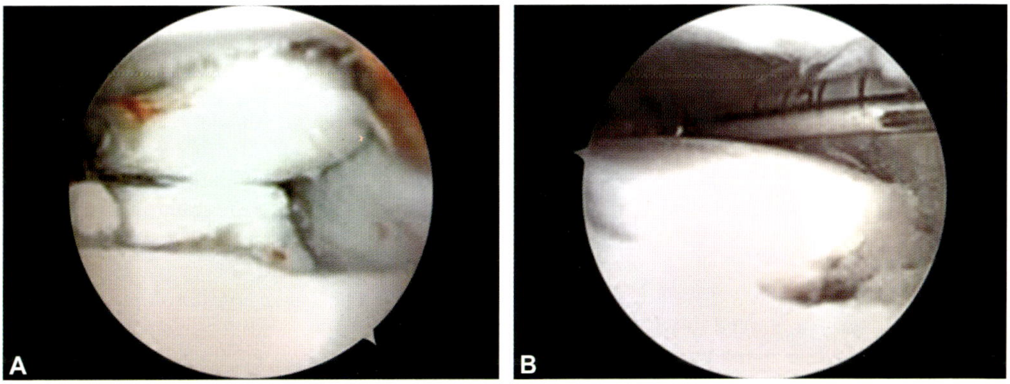

Figs 19A and B

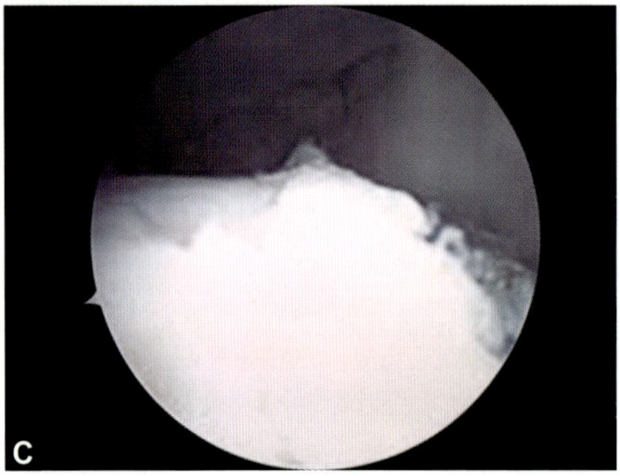

Figs 19A to C: Example of an anterolateral osteochondral fracture stabilized by use of bioabsorbable fixation. (A) Traumatic osteochondral fragment from the anterolateral talus is flipped 180° so that the cancellous bone portion is brushing up against the tibial plafond cartilage surface; (B) Osteochondral fragment after being flipped into the proper orientation in the anterior gutter and then reduced back to its prepared bed; (C) Final view of osteochondral fragment after fixation

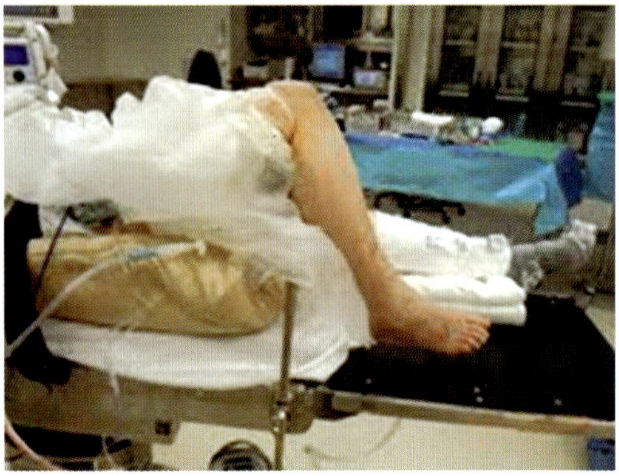

Fig. 20: Patient positioning performed with modification to improve working space for the arthroscope and instrumentation through the posterolateral portal

the use of the posterolateral portal and increase working space. The pad at the foot of the bed is removed and the contralateral leg is protected (Fig. 20). The anteromedial portal is established first followed by the anterolateral portal. A posterolateral portal also is created in order to prepare the posterior joint surfaces.

Typically, the large anterior osteophytes on the tibia have to be removed with a burr in order to gain better joint access. If a large osteophyte is on the dorsal aspect of the talus which will prevent proper positioning of the talus under the tibia when fusing, then the talar spur also will be excised.

The surgeon then starts preparing the joint for fusion in a systematic fashion with a curette (open or closed), oscillating shaver, burr (Fig. 21A). Unhealthy cartilage is removed down to bleeding subchondral bone while maintaining the contour of the talus and tibia. With the scope in the lateral portal and instruments in medial portal, the surgeon can start anterior-medially and work posteriorly including preparations of the articulation between the medial talus and medial malleolus. Then, the surgeon works centrally as far as able. After portals are switched with instrumentation in the anterolateral portal, joint preparation start laterally from anterior to posterior, including the articulation between the lateral talus and distal fibula. Intermittent suction with oscillating shaver or through a port on scope is performed regularly to clear out debris and improve visualization.

Instrumentation is placed through the posterolateral portal with the scope in the anteromedial portal. Posterior joint surfaces are prepared.

Once initial preparations are done and contours are maintained, the surgeon can make minor adjustments with respect to alignment of the fusion (i.e. if ankle in varus slightly then take more bone laterally). Vascular channels to enhance fusion are created in the tibia and talus with a burr every several millimeters maintaining the overall bony contour.

If bone graft is needed, a trephine system is used to harvest autologous graft from the proximal tibia through a small incision centered on the anteromedial face of the proximal tibia. Dissection proceeds down to the periosteum and periosteal flaps are elevated. A sharp entry trocar is placed, centered in between the anterior and posterior cortices, and malleted to form an entry hole or start point for the trephine. The drill with an appropriately sized trephine is advanced through the first cortex until it reaches second cortex. The drill is stopped and carefully removed with a core of cancellous bone which is then put into a sterile container and placed carefully on the back table. Several passes with the drill can be made depending on the amount of bone graft needed. Gelfoam with thrombin is placed in area of bone graft harvest and then the periosteum and deep tissues are closed with absorbable sutures. Finally, the skin is closed with 4-0 nylon or staples.

A Micro Vector (Smith and Nephew, Andover MA) type guide is used for placement of guidewires for cannulated screws, usually two (6.5 or 7.3 mm) cannulated screws are placed. The medial screw is directed from posterior to anterior and the lateral screw is aimed from anterior to posterior (due to fibula). The guide is placed into the ankle under direct visualization with the scope. Small stab incisions are made with a no. 15-blade, blunt dissection down to bone is performed, and retractors are used as needed to protect the skin and deep tissues. Threaded guide pins for the cannulated screws are then advanced into tibia with only the tips visualized in the tibia as seen with arthroscopy (Figs 21B to D) and the surgeon checks positioning and spacing of the pins. Fluoroscopy also is used to confirm pin position.

If pin position is adequate, the scope is removed and if needed, the bone graft is placed into the ankle with use of cannulas. Traction is released and the ankle is positioned appropriately for fusion (i.e. neutral dorsiflexion, correct rotation as compared to normal side and 5° of valgus). Guide pins are advanced into the talus and fluoroscopy evaluation ensures that the pins are placed appropriately. An additional third screw could be placed, if needed.

Clinical and radiographic alignment is closely inspected and evaluated. Measurement of screw lengths is done. Then, the guide pins are over-drilled with the proper reamer. The cannulated screws are placed one by one in sequence and tightened into place compressing the fusion site. Final fluoroscopy pictures are done and the guide pins are removed.

Copious irrigation of the small incisions is performed followed by wound closure. The surgeon can augment the popliteal block as needed with local anesthetic. Dressings are placed and a well-padded short leg splint is applied.

Postoperatively, patients are discharged home the same day if discharge criteria are fulfilled. DVT prophylaxis is instituted. The splint is changed to a

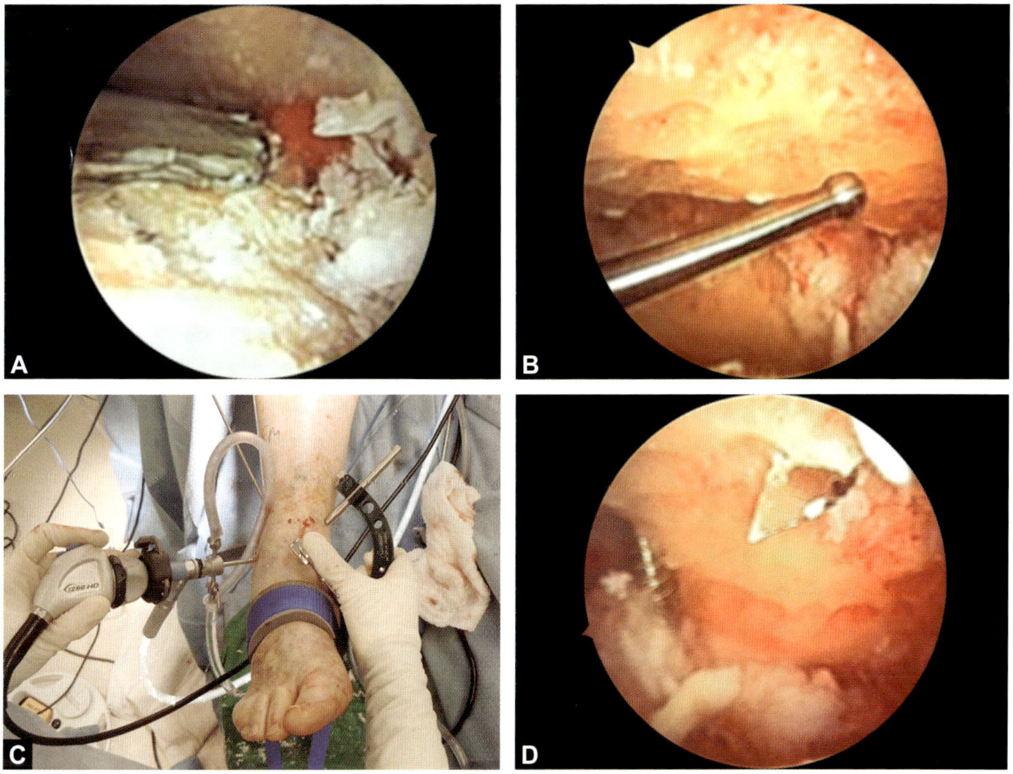

Figs 21A to D: Technique of arthroscopic ankle arthrodesis. (A) Joint preparation begins utilizing a curette and joint contour is preserved; (B) Vascular channels created to enhance fusion and tip of aiming guide brought into ankle joint to aid placement of guidewires for cannulated screws; (C) View of aiming guide and placement of second guidewire; (D) Arthroscopic view of guidewire positions in tibia prior to releasing traction, placing bone graft, positioning the ankle in properly for fusion and advancing the guidewires into the talus short leg cast after 10–14 days. They are non-weight bearing for 4–6 weeks. Then, if early healing on X-ray (Figs 22A to C), weight-bearing as tolerated in a tall cam walker boot for 2–4 weeks and then progression into shoe with a mild rocker bottom to start. Physical therapy is used as needed to aid the patient in gait training and leg strengthening.

Outcomes for arthroscopic ankle arthrodesis were reported in a large study of 35 patients with at least an average of 72 months follow-up. Results showed fusion rate of 97% with a time to fusion averaging 11.8 weeks (range was 8–18 weeks) and good to excellent results on outcomes assessments were 74–83%.[28]

Conditions Combined with Arthroscopic-Assisted Procedures

With the advent of arthroscopic techniques, knowledge concerning intra-articular injuries that are associated with ankle instability, ankle fractures, peroneal tendon disorders, and other conditions has lead to increased and combined use of ankle arthroscopy with open procedures to address extra-articular pathology.

Lateral ankle instability is commonly treated in one surgical setting. However, surgical treatment may be performed in a two-staged fashion depending on the amount of intra-articular work that has to be done. Arthroscopy of the ankle is performed efficiently and with the lowest pressure fluid flow as possible (or basically dry) to allow visualization and to prevent excessive fluid extravasation. Issues such as meniscoid lesions, anterior ankle impingement, soft tissue impingement, chondral injuries, loose bodies, osteochondral defects, and synovitis are addressed. Then, usually an open incision is performed to repair, reef, or reconstruct the lateral ankle ligaments. In one ankle arthroscopy study utilizing a modified Brostum-Gould technique,[3] intra-articular lesions were noted in 91% of cases.

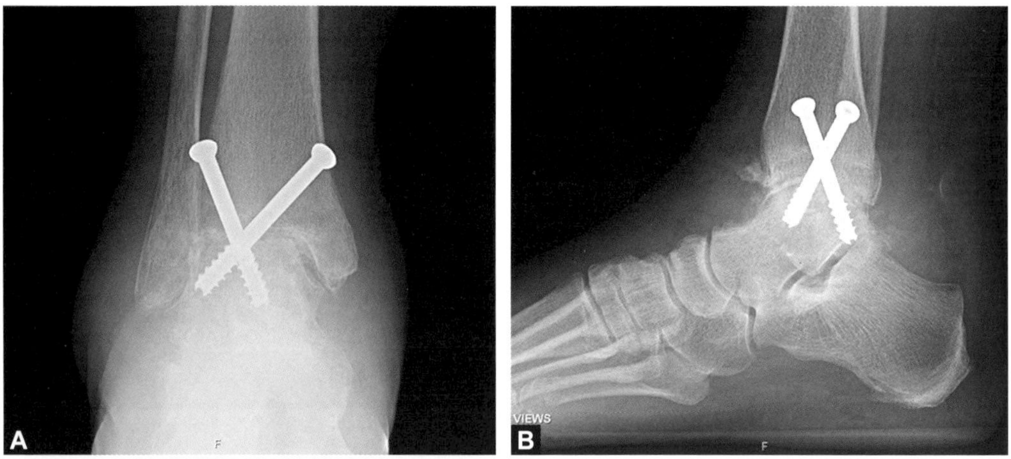

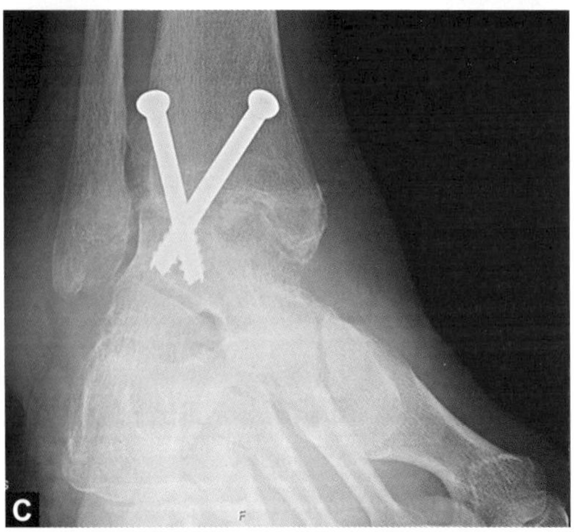

Figs 22A to C: Example of X-rays performed approximately 5 weeks after arthroscopic ankle fusion. (A) Anteroposterior view; (B) Lateral view; (C) Oblique view

The authors found that postoperative American Orthopaedic Foot and Ankle Society (AOFAS) outcome scores were significantly higher after surgery in relation to preoperative scores and significantly higher in patients without chondral lesions as compared to those with chondral lesions. Other authors have described their promising results utilizing a three-portal all arthroscopic approach for lateral ligament reconstruction, with further comparative studies needed.[29]

Ankle fractures also can be treated with an arthroscopic-assisted approach. In one investigation of 84 patients who underwent open reduction internal fixation of their ankle fracture combined with ankle arthroscopy,[30] 73% were found to have chondral lesions that were treated. The number of associated intra-articular chondral lesions was significantly higher in more severe injury patterns, particularly pronation-external rotation and supination-external rotation type IV fractures. An example of a distal fibular fracture combined with an avulsion fracture of the distal anteromedial tibia not appreciated on plain X-rays is pictured (Figs 23A and B). The role of arthroscopy in the treatment of ankle fractures is currently in evolution.

Other Conditions (Synovial Disorders, Arthrofibrosis)

Ankle arthroscopy has been reported as a less invasive option than open procedures for challenging conditions such as synovial disorders [i.e. hemophilia, synovial chondromatosis, pigmented villonodular synovitis (PVNS), rheumatoid arthritis] and arthrofibrosis of the ankle. Studies are few and the patient numbers are small. But, ankle arthroscopy can be a viable treatment option in these difficult to manage patients. Hemophiliacs develop recurrent hemarthroses which lead to synovial proliferation. Imbibement of the synovial membrane with hemosiderin and iron is thought to cause catabolic effects on the cartilage matrix. If initial radiosynovectomy interventions do not work, arthroscopic synovectomy can be reliably performed with a thorough evaluation of the joint[31] (Figs 24A and B). Though rare in the ankle, synovial chondromatosis also can be reliably treated with arthroscopy (Fig. 12B).[32] Synovial tumors such as PVNS are challenging due to recurrence issues and tumor bulk (Fig. 25).

Finally, ankle arthrofibrosis after trauma, ankle fracture, or surgery can cause significant functional disability in patients. Most may also have a neuritic type of pain component in addition to the ankle stiffness. In these patients, arthroscopic management proceeds in an organized fashion. The ankle is tight upon entry of the scope (Fig. 26A). Once the lateral gutter is developed, the arthroscope is placed in the anterolateral portal and the anterior compartment and medial gutter are debrided. The gutters are cleared of thick, synovial tissue and scar tissue (Figs 26A to C) with either a shaver or sometimes an arthroscopic punch. Any bony impingement is also addressed. At procedure completion, the surgeon can now move throughout the joint and evaluate the degree of secondary damage to the articular cartilage surface due to abrasion (Fig. 26D). Postoperative rehabilitation generally involves the use of controlled passive motion machine, intense physical therapy, pain control and bracing techniques.

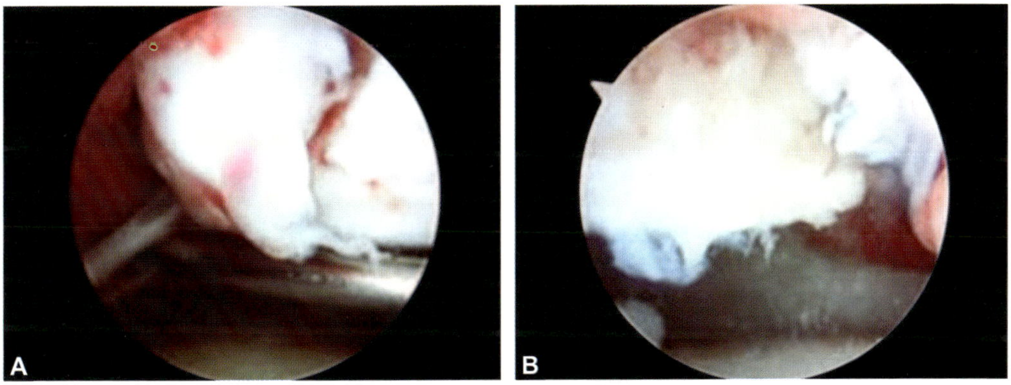

Figs 23A and B: Arthroscopic view of distal fibular fracture. (A) Loose avulsion fragment anteromedial tibia not noted on preoperative imaging; (B) Fracture line seen in distal fibula prior to open reduction internal fixation

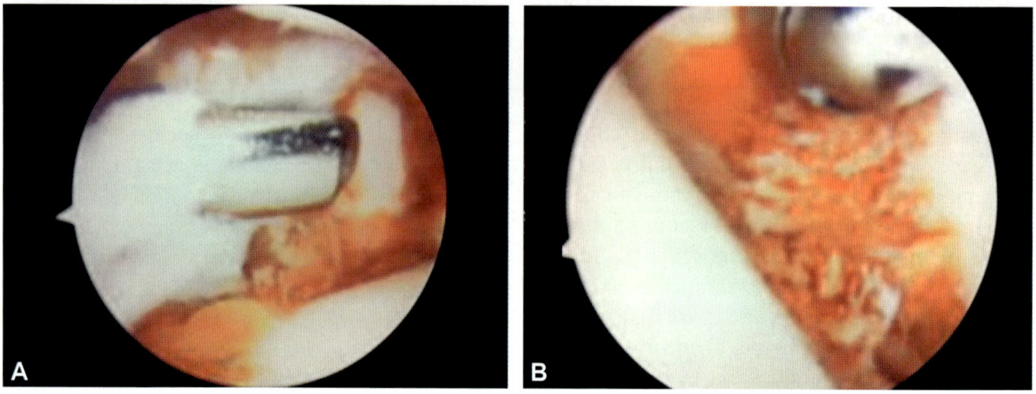

Figs 24A and B: Example of arthroscopic synovectomy for hemophilia. (A) Extensive hemosiderin deposition and synovitis in the lateral gutter; (B) Distal aspect of medial gutter

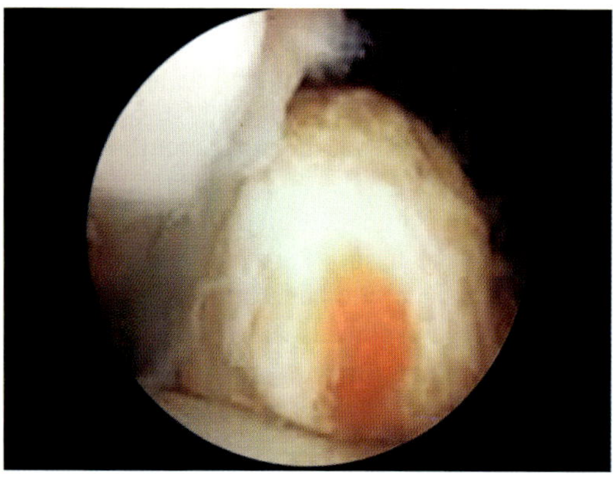

Fig. 25: Example of large nodule formation associated with pigmented villonodular synovitis involving the anterior compartment of the ankle (tibia in upper left side of picture, talus on bottom)

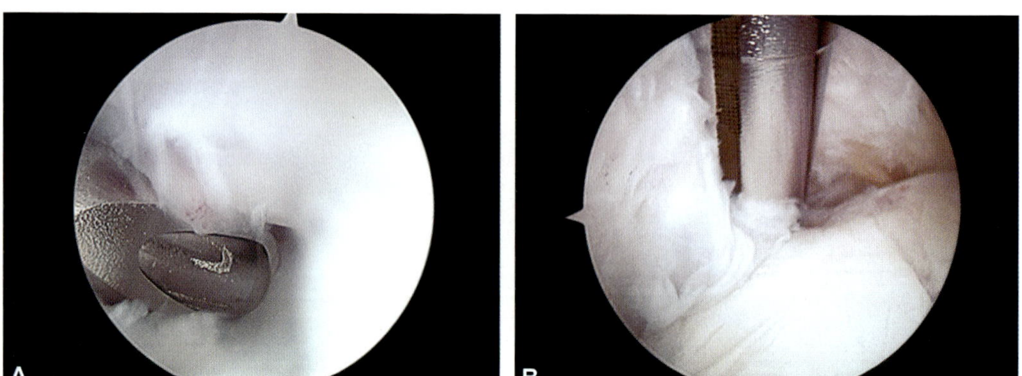

Figs 26A and B

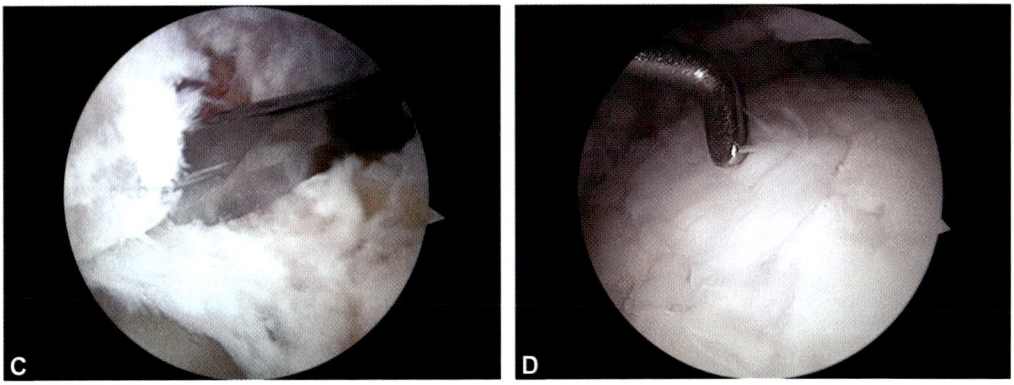

Figs 26A to D: Example of arthrofibrosis of the right ankle developing after trauma. (A) View from the anteromedial portal with oscillating shaver placed through anterolateral portal. Extensive, thick scar tissue is encountered as attempts are made to excavate the anterior compartment; (B) Gutters are cleared of scar tissue; (C) Thick band of tissue is released with a punch in order to access the anteromedial portion of the joint; (D) Chondral damage over anterior talus noted as a consequence of arthrofibrosis (probe tip)

CONCLUSION

A careful study of the applied anatomy and practice of arthroscopic techniques is essential as the joints of the foot and ankle are smaller, more constrained, and more technically demanding, even for the experienced arthroscopist. In general, a broad range of conditions can be addressed arthroscopically ranging from soft tissue impingement to osteochondral defects to fractures to fusions. Anterior ankle pathology is more easily accessible as compared to that in the posterior ankle compartment which will be discussed in a forthcoming chapter. The development of newer equipment and hindfoot endoscopy techniques has aided access to and treatment for these challenging posterior lesions. For these minimally invasive arthroscopic techniques, the future is promising with respect to further investigations evaluating the efficacy and further applications of the techniques as the technology and equipment improve.

REFERENCES

1. Scranton PE, McDermott JE. Anterior tibiotalar spurs: a comparison of open versus arthroscopic debridement. Foot Ankle. 1992;13:125-9.
2. Guo QW, Hu YL, Jiao C, et al. Open versus endoscopic excision of a symptomatic os trigonum: a comparative study of 41 cases. Arthroscopy. 2010;26(3):384-90.
3. Hua Y, Chen S, Li Y, et al. Combination of modified Broström procedure with ankle arthroscopy for chronic ankle instability accompanied by intra-articular symptoms. Arthroscopy. 2010;26(4):524-8.
4. Glazebrook MA, Ganapathy V, Bridge MA, et al. Evidence-based indications for ankle arthroscopy. Arthroscopy. 2009;25(12):1478-90.
5. Lozano-Calderón SA, Samocha Y, et al. Comparative performance of ankle arthroscopy with and without traction. Foot Ankle Int. 2012:33(9):740-5.
6. van Dijk CN, Tol JL, Verheyen CC. A prospective study of prognostic factors concerning the outcome of arthroscopic surgey for anterior ankle impingement. Am J Sports Med. 1997;25:737-45.
7. Allegra F, Mafulli N. Double posteromedial portals for posterior ankle arthroscopy in supine position. Clin Orthop Relat Res. 2010;468(4):996-1001.
8. Harbach GP, Stewart JD, Lambert EW, et al. Ankle arthroscopy in the lateral decubitus position. Foot Ankle Int. 2003;24(8):597-9.
9. de Leeuw PA, Golanó P, Sierevelt IN, et al. The course of the superficial peroneal nerve in relation to the ankle position: anatomical study with ankle arthroscopic implications. Knee Surg Sports Traumatol Arthrosc. 2010;18(5):612-7.
10. Urgüden M, Cevikol C, Dabak T, et al. Effect of joint motion on safety of portals in posterior ankle arthroscopy. Arthroscopy. 2009;25(12):1442-6.
11. Ferkel RD, Heath DD, Guhl JF. Neurological complications of ankle arthroscopy. Arthroscopy. 1996;12:200-8.
12. Barber FA, Click J, Britt BT. Complications of ankle arthroscopy. Foot Ankle. 1990;10:263-6.
13. van Dijk CN. Hindfoot endoscopy. Foot Ankle Clin. 2006;11:391-414.
14. Ferkel RD. Arthroscopic surgery: the foot and ankle. Philadelphia: Lippincott-Raven;1996.

15. Young BH, Flanigan RM, DiGiovanni BF. Complications of ankle arthroscopy utilizing a contemporary noninvasive distraction technique. J Bone Joint Surg Am. 2011;93:963-8.
16. Ferkel RD, Small HN, Gittins JE. Complications in foot and ankle arthroscopy. Clin Orthop Rel Res. 2001; 391:89-104.
17. Tol JL, Verhagen RA, Krips R, et al. The anterior ankle impingement syndrome: diagnostic value of oblique radiographs. Foot Ankle Int. 2004;25:63-8.
18. Baums MH, Kahl E, Schultz W, et al. Clinical outcome of the arthroscopic management of sports-related "anterior ankle pain": a prospective study. Knee Surg Sports Traumatol Arthrosc. 2006;14:482-6.
19. Berndt AL, Harty M. Transchondral fractures (osteochondritis dissecans) of the talus. J Bone Joint Surg Am. 1959;41:988-1020.
20. Tuite MJ, DeSmet AA. MRI of selected sports injuries: muscle tears, groin pain and osteochondritis dissecans. Semin Ultrasound CT MR. 1994;15(5): 318-40.
21. Chuckpaiwong B, Berkson EM, Theodore GH, et al. Microfracture for osteochondral lesions of the ankle: outcome analysis and outcome predictors of 105 cases. Arthroscopy. 2008;24(1):106-12.
22. Kumai T, Takakura Y, Higashiyama I, et al. Arthroscopic drilling for the treatment of osteochondral lesions of the talus. J Bone Joint Surg Am. 1999;81(9) 1229-35.
23. Verhagen RA, Struijs PA, Bossuyt PM, et al. Systematic review of treatment strategies for osteochondral defects of the talar dome. Foot Ankle Clin. 2003;8: 233-42.
24. Gobbi A, Francisco RA, Lubowitz JH, et al. Osteochondral lesions of the talus: Randomized controlled trial comparing chondroplasty, microfracture, and osteochondral autograft implantation. Arthroscopy. 2006;22:1085-92.
25. Takao M, Ochi M, Naito K, et al. Arthroscopic drilling for chondral, subchondral, and combined chondral-subchondral lesions of the talar dome. Arthroscopy. 2003;19(5):524-30.
26. Schuman L, Struijs PAA, van Dijk CN. Arthroscopic treatment for osteochondral defects of the talus: Results at follow-up at 2 to 11 years. J Bone Joint Surg Br. 2002;84:364-8.
27. Taranow WS, Bisignani GA, Towers JD, et al. Retrograde drilling of osteochondral lesions of the medial talar dome. Foot Ankle Int. 1999;20:474-80.
28. Ferkel RD, Hewitt M. Long-term results of arthroscopic ankle arthrodesis. Foot Ankle Int. 2006;26(4):275-80.
29. Nery C, Raduan F, Del Buono A, et al. Arthroscopic-assisted Brostöm-Gould for chronic ankle instability: a long-term follow-up. Am J Sports Med. 2011; 39:2381-8.
30. Leontaritis N, Hinojosa L, Panchbhavi VK. Arthroscopically detected intra-articular lesions associated with acute ankle fractures. J Bone Joint Surg Am. 2009;91(2):333-9.
31. Vanderhave KL, Caird MS, Hake M, et al. Musculoskeletal care of the hemophiliac patient. J Am Acad Orthop Surg. 2012;20:553-63.
32. Galat DD, Ackerman DB, Spoon D, et al. Synovial chondromatosis of the foot and ankle. Foot Ankle Int. 2008;29(3):312-7.

31

Osteochondritis Dissecans of the Talus

John S Kirchner, Beatriz Garcia-Cardona

INTRODUCTION

Etiology

The etiology of osteochondritis dissecans of the talus still remains unknown. Many theories including metabolic abnormalities, systemic vasculopathies, genetics, joint degeneration, and malalignment have been proposed but trauma remains the most commonly associated event. Nevertheless, osteochondritis dissecans can occur outside the setting of trauma. It was first described in the ankle by Kappis[1] who commented on the cases mentioned by Paget in 1870 and Konig in 1888, both of whom had observed loose bodies in the knee joint. The most popularized description of the lesions is based on images made by Berndt and Harty in 1959.[2] They proposed the concept of transchondral fracture as the etiology of osteochondritis dissecans of the talus. Cartilage is avascular and aneural; therefore, a chondral fracture could very well be the cause of avascular necrosis.

Pathophysiology

The histologic basis behind osteochondral lesions of the talus (OLTs) is a loss of glycosaminoglycans from extracellular matrix and a decreased number of chondrocytes. Chondroitin sulfate and keratan sulfate are increased in deep cartilage layers. After the reparative phase, hyaline cartilage is replaced by fibrocartilage. Subchondral bone remodeling with areas of bone resorption is observed around the lesions. Osteoclasts in the lacunae within cancellous bone trabeculae digest bone and osteoblasts replace bone. Fibrous tissue connects osteochondrotic cartilage to subchondral bone. As a result of an OLT, the surface contact area of the talus is reduced, thereby increasing the load to a smaller area of remaining cartilage. Two factors determine cartilage deformability, thickness and elasticity. The cartilage over the talus is relatively thin and therefore less elastic. It also has a high compressive modulus. There is an inverse relationship between cartilage thickness and the compressive modulus. An OLT is in essence a traumatic microfracture of the subchondral plate that creates a path for synovial fluid to flow into cartilage and the subchondral bone. Increased fluid pressure over time decreases normal bone perfusion. This in turn can cause osteonecrosis, bone resorption, and osteolytic resorption (Flow chart 1).

Malalignment can increase contact pressures to the cartilage within the mortise due to the position of the talus. Varus and supination cause increased contact pressure on the medial talus. On the other hand, valgus and pronation cause

Flow chart 1: Progression leading to formation of osteochondral lesion of the talus (OLT)

Damaged subchondral plate is not able to support overlying cartilage

↓

Loss of negatively loaded glycosaminoglycans and hydrophilic proteoglycans

↓

Decreased water containment
Every step (loading moment) causes fluid to flow into microfractured areas

increased contact pressure on the lateral talus. Most OLTs of the talus have been subdivided into lateral and medial talar dome lesions. Berndt and Harty[2] described the exact mechanism by which each of these lesions occurs. When the foot is inverted and plantarflexed, the posteromedial edge of the talar dome is occupying the mortise and subject to injury. This mechanism usually causes deeper and smaller lesions (Fig. 1A). On the other hand, if the ankle is dorsiflexed and inverted, the anterior two-thirds of the lateral talar dome can impact upon the fibula. This would produce a shallow and larger lesion (Fig. 1B). Central lesions of the talar dome are very rare. They usually occur as a result of axial trauma and may be associated with a tibial plafond cartilage lesion. Due to the fact that this is an area of high compressive loads, early treatment is paramount.

MAKING THE DIAGNOSIS

History and Physical Examination

Patients rarely present acutely, especially if the lesion is undisplaced. Swelling and pain after the initial trauma might disguise the symptoms. Patients might present with finding as subtle as decreased range of motion. X-rays may be negative. Symptoms for more than 4–6 weeks after an ankle sprain should alert the surgeon of further pathology, such as an osteochondral lesion (OLT). Locking and catching are frequent symptoms which can be caused by a displaced fragment. Therefore, a chronic presentation is much more common. Patients complain of persistent intermittent deep ankle pain during or after activity. They may have normal ankle motion and absence of swelling, locking, or catching but this does not rule out an osteochondral defect. The physical examination consists of palpation of discrete points of tenderness. A proper neurovascular assessment should be obtained. Range of motion of the injured and uninjured ankle and hindfoot should be compared. The ankle should be tested for ligamentous instability with an anterior drawer test and talar tilt test with the ankle in both plantarflexion and dorsiflexion. Inversion and eversion stress testing are appropriate. A diagnostic anesthetic ankle injection is in order if intra-articular pathology is in question. Residual pain after such injection could point towards a different pathology other than an OLT. Bone marrow has abundant innervation and patients may experience pain sooner than periosteal involvement appears in X-ray. Pain develops as a rise of fluid pressure and decrease in pH. This activates ion channels in nerve endings of subchondral bone to send nociceptive signals.

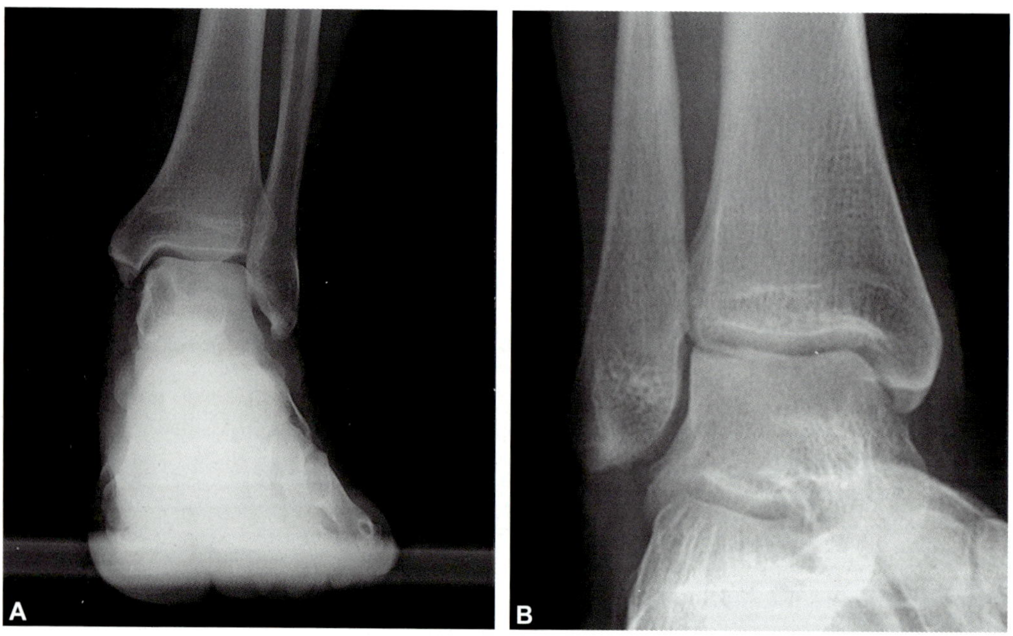

Figs 1A and B: Osteochondral lesions of the talus. (A) Medial; (B) Lateral

X-Rays

Routine anteroposterior (AP), lateral, mortise views, as well as stress views are indicated. They are the basis for the Berndt and Harty classification which refer to four stages:

Stage I: Minimal subchondral compression
Stage II: A partially detached fragment
Stage III: Non-displaced detached fragment
Stage IV: Completely detached and displaced fragment.[2]

The changes observed may be as subtle as a loss in the cortical margin of the talar dome, or as obvious as subchondral lucency with surrounding sclerosis. In the early stages of the disease or in the case of small lesions, X-rays might even be negative. Further imaging is usually necessary to attain the full extent of the cartilage damage.

Computed Tomography Scan

It is considered as a reliable tool to assess the subchondral damage. It cannot, however, detect early changes in the overlying cartilage. It does help to estimate the size of the subchondral cyst if it was present which could be of great importance for preoperative planning. Cyst formation is caused by damaged cartilage valve mechanism which allows hydrostatic influx of synovial fluid from joint space into subchondral bone and not vice versa. There is a classification based on computed tomography (CT) scan findings described by Ferkel.[3]

Stage I: Cystic lesion within the talar dome with intact roof
Stage IIA: Cystic lesion with communication to the talar dome surface
Stage IIB: Open articular surface lesion with overlying non-displaced fragment
Stage III: Non-displaced lesion with lucency
Stage IV: Displaced fragment.

Magnetic Resonance Imaging

Magnetic resonance imaging (MRI) is by far the most sensitive test to diagnose cartilage injury (Figs 2A and B). Studies have shown sensitivity of 95%, specificity of 100%, negative predictive value of 88%, and positive predictive value of 100%.[4] It can detect the most subtle bone bruise, cartilage damage, or any other soft tissue pathology. Nevertheless, many believe it can overestimate the severity of the true lesion. Early changes include edema and subchondral contusion. In chronic OLTs, a subchondral cyst may be evident (Fig. 3). Hepple[20] described an MRI classification of OCLs of the talus.

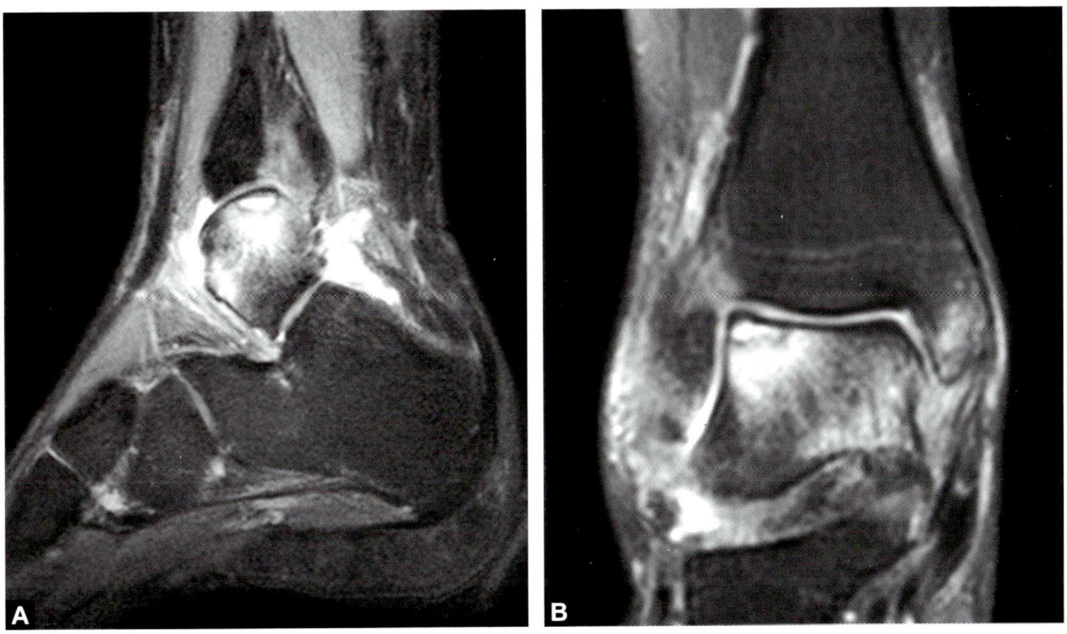

Figs 2A and B: Magnetic resonance imaging of a lateral osteochondral lesion of the talus. (A) Lateral; (B) Anteroposterior

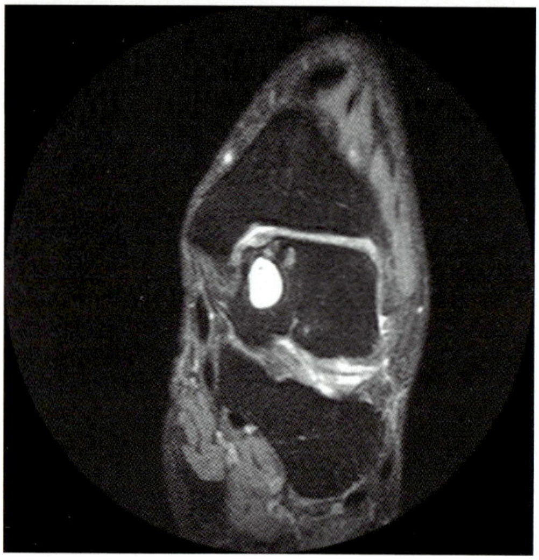

Fig. 3: Osteochondral lesion with unstable brim and associated large subchondral cyst

Stage I: Articular cartilage edema
Stage IIA: Cartilage injury with underlying fracture and surrounding bony edema
Stage IIB: A stage IIA without bony edema
Stage III: Detached but non-displaced fragment
Stage IV: Detached and displaced fragment
Stage V: Subchondral cyst formation.

MANAGEMENT (FLOW CHART 2)

Nonoperative treatment should always be attempted first, unless the lesion is grossly unstable. Some patients might undergo complete resolution of the symptoms even though the imaging studies show that the OLT has not completely healed. Chances of success with nonoperative treatment have been estimated between 45–53%.[5-7] Acute lesions have a slightly higher likelihood of healing with nonoperative treatment as compared to chronic lesions. Acute lesions should be initially casted for immobilization for 3 weeks to 4 months. The rationale for this treatment is unloading the cartilage to reduce edema and prevent avascular necrosis and possibly heal an undetached fragment of cartilage to underlying bone. Rest or cessation of sports often is used in collaboration with or without nonsteroidal anti-inflammatories. The goal is similar to that of placement of a cast. Physical therapy after a period of immobilization is essential to regain range of motion and overall strengthening of the muscles that control ankle motion. It is also key to work on proprioception exercises to help prevent future lesions or injuries about the ankle.

Surgery is considered an option for patients that have symptomatic focal lesions who have been through a 6 weeks course of non-surgical management and have failed. Also surgery should be utilized in patients with acute, unstable, displaced cartilage fragment. Many factors have been identified as prognostic in the surgical treatment of OLTs of the talus. Cuttica et al.[8] determined that the most important of these factors were age, size of the lesion, and lesion containment.

Size of the lesion has always been associated with a poor outcome. Hunt et al.[10] did a study on cadaveric ankles to prove the effect of size of OLTs. In this study, a threshold of 1 cm was found to be significant. In other studies, 1.5 cm is the cut-off to consider the lesion as a large or small defect. It has been proven that after these benchmarks the contact area decreases and the peak stresses in the ankle joint increase, further destabilizing the OLT.

Lesion containment is very important as it creates a stable brim around the cartilage defect which reduces the stress around the lesion and improves the likelihood that it may heal with fibrocartilage after surgical intervention. For this reason, unstable lesions are associated with less favorable outcomes.

Lastly, age is also considered a predictor of outcome. Multiple authors have hypothesized that open physes are a good indication of abundant subchondral microvasculature which suggest a higher chance of healing an OLT. In the study by Cuttica et al.[8] age was significant until 33 years of age, after which no significance was found.

Operative Procedures

The decision to proceed with operative treatment depends on the chronicity as well as the nature of the symptoms the patient is experiencing. The size of the lesion also has to be factored when choosing one surgical option over another. Lesions that do not reach the subchondral plate have a low likelihood of healing. The location of the lesion is also taken into consideration. Whether the lesion is central, lateral, medial or posteromedial is of great importance when considering the approach to be used. The utmost goal of surgery is to create a

Flow chart 2: Algorithm for treatment of osteochondral lesion of the talus OLT

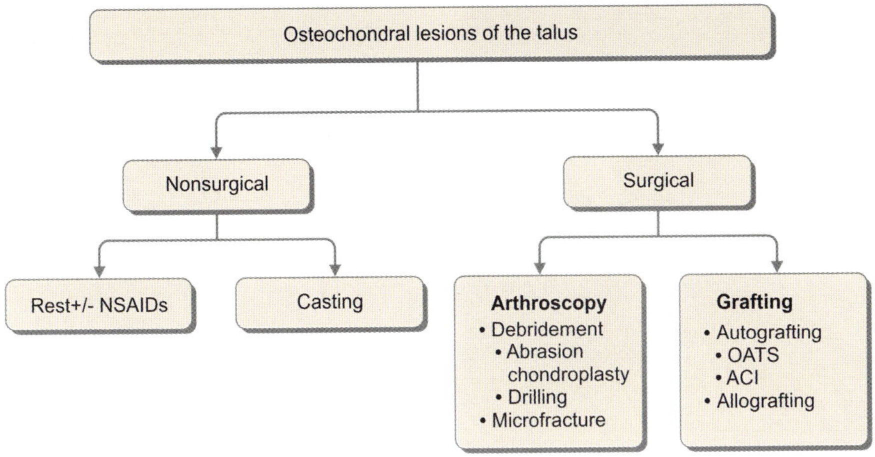

stimulus to the marrow cells in the subchondral bone to produce cells that can regenerate the defect. The options that are available vary from arthroscopic debridement, retrograde or antegrade drilling, microfracture, abrasion chondroplasty, fragment excision or internal fixation, osteochondral autograft or allograft, and autologous chondrocyte transplantation.

Arthroscopic debridement with or without bone marrow stimulation techniques is considered the initial procedure of choice by most authors. After arthroscopic debridement of the OLT and a bone marrow stimulating procedure, the patient can expect to be non-weight bearing anywhere from 2–4 weeks depending on the size of the lesion. Therapy focused on the range of motion should start right after the portals have healed, which is usually about a week after surgery. Longevity of the procedure can be estimated on the basis of the outcomes and the time of follow-up. In most series the follow-up averages from 1 year to 4 years. Most patients have good to excellent outcomes in terms of durability in this time range. Rates of success have been estimated between 84% open procedures and 86% arthroscopic procedures.[12-15]

Technique

Patient positioning is usually surgeon's preference, but for most techniques a supine positioning is favored. A well-padded leg holder is used with a thigh tourniquet and noninvasive ankle distraction. Instruments needed are primarily the small joint arthroscopy equipment including a 2.7 mm with 30-degree-angle arthroscope, Kirschner (K) wires or arthroscopic picks/awls with varied angles, a shaver and a burr. A gravity-assisted pump usually suffices for adequate low pressure flow.

Standard anteromedial and anterolateral portals are utilized. Using a non-invasive distractor, distraction with slight plantar flexion will expose most of the talar dome. The lesion should be probed to determine if the cartilage is stable or unstable. Synovectomy, removal of loose bodies, and debridement can be achieved with the shaver. If the lesion is unstable it should be debrided until a stable rim of cartilage is accomplished. This can be accomplished with a ring curette or an arthroscopic knife. If drilling of the defect is the preferred technique, the surgeon must take into account whether the cartilage cap is unstable. If the cap is stable, retrograde drilling should be considered. This is done by inserting a K-wire through the sinus tarsi under fluoroscopic guidance, using a guidewire, and arthroscopically assisted visualization is used to confirm the cartilage is not penetrated. On the other hand, if the cap is unstable the cartilage should be removed and antegrade drilling into the subchondral bone or pick chondroplasty is preferred.

Microfracture is an acceptable technique when the lesion is unstable and the cartilage has been removed. For this technique to be employed, an awl (or pick) can be tapped into the subchondral bone until bleeding is seen (Fig. 4). Ideally, microfracture holes should be spaced approximately 3–4 mm apart so that they do not break into each other and destabilize the subchondral plate.[21] The order in which the technique should proceed would be starting in the periphery and working towards the

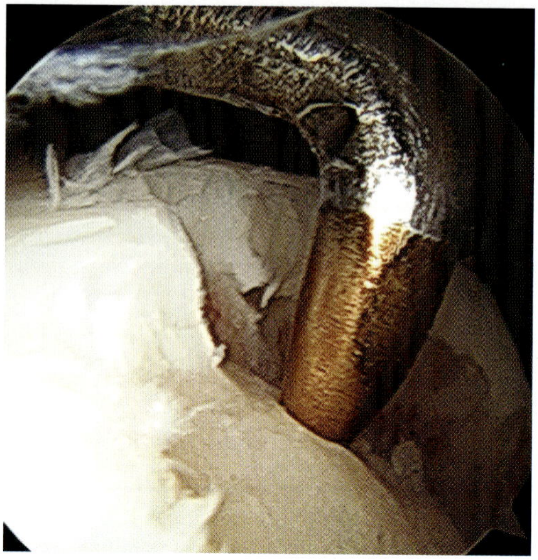

Fig. 4: Microfracture technique using an awl or pick

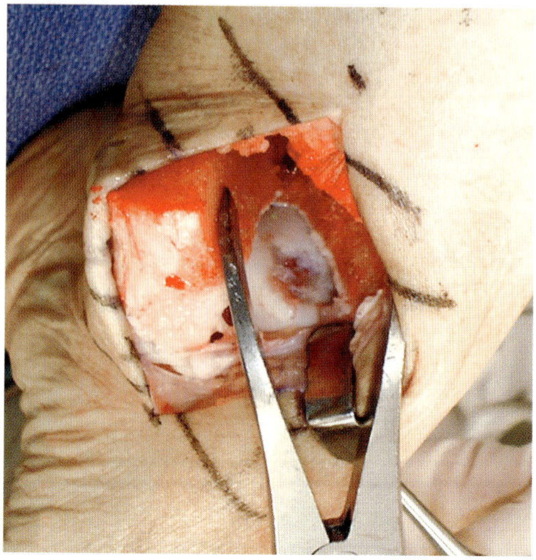

Fig. 5: Medial malleolar osteotomy

center of the lesion and leaving space between the fracture points.

Other Surgical Alternatives

Open treatment of an OLT of the talus is usually considered if arthroscopic management fails to provide relief or for those lesions that are too large and associated with a substantial subchondral cyst which would most likely require an autograft or allograft reconstructive procedure.

APPROACHES

When dealing with posterior or posteromedial talar dome lesions most authors consider a medial malleolar osteotomy as the best approach (Fig. 5). The actual line of the osteotomy is of some significance. It should be planned preoperatively such that the osteotomy line exits away from the lesion. The surgeon must be sure that a perpendicular access to the lesion will be achieved with the osteotomy. An anterior medial arthrotomy is done to visualize the joint line. Before performing the osteotomy the soft tissue structures must be protected. Two parallel screw holes should be predrilled for later fixation. The osteotomy is started with a saw and completed with an osteotome to decrease the risk of removing excess bone. For anterior or lateral talar dome lesions, a lateral malleolar osteotomy, pyramidal osteotomy, or anterolateral arthrotomy is needed. The incision is carried out along the distal fibula. The anterior talofibular ligament (ATFL) and calcaneofibular ligament (CFL) are incised leaving a cuff for later repair. If a fibular osteotomy is required, an oblique orientation is preferred. Also predrilling for plate fixation is recommended. Pyramidal osteotomy of the tibia (Figs 6A and B) allows easier access to the central talar dome. Two parallel cuts are done and a proximal oblique cut is then done.

TECHNIQUES

Osteochondral Autograft/Allograft Transfer System or Mosaicplasty

The donor site most commonly used is the non-weight bearing portion of the ipsilateral knee, ipsilateral non-weight bearing portion of the talus, or from an allograft talus. To attain a press fit in the recipient site, the graft should be 1 mm larger than the defect in respect to the diameter. In terms of depth, the graft should be 10 mm. This will decrease the energy that must be driven to place the graft flush to the level of the recipient site as well as decrease the shear forces. Perpendicular alignment of the graft and recipient site is paramount. The graft is transferred from the donor to the recipient talus within the chisel and when positioned in the recipient site it is advanced with a bone tamp. Care should be taken not to countersink the graft. It should lay flush with the talar cartilage surface. Multiple grafts could be required for large lesions.

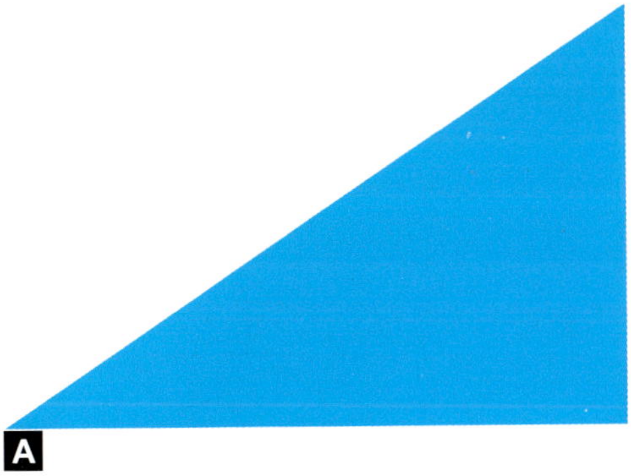

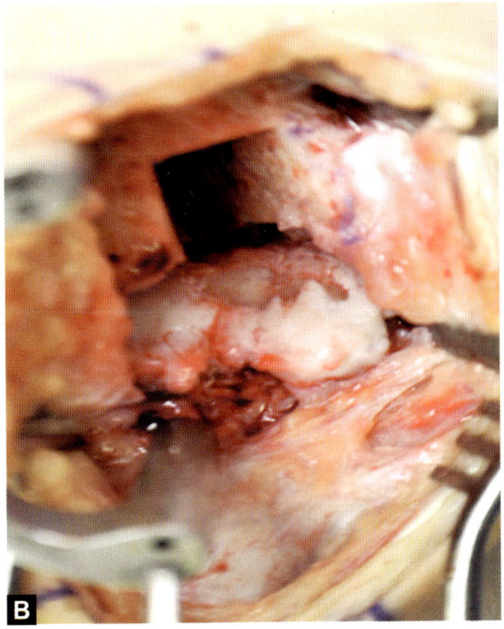

Figs 6A and B: Pyramidal osteotomy of the distal tibia and underlying osteochondral lesion of the talus. (A) Lateral outline of the osteotomy; (B) Clinical photograph

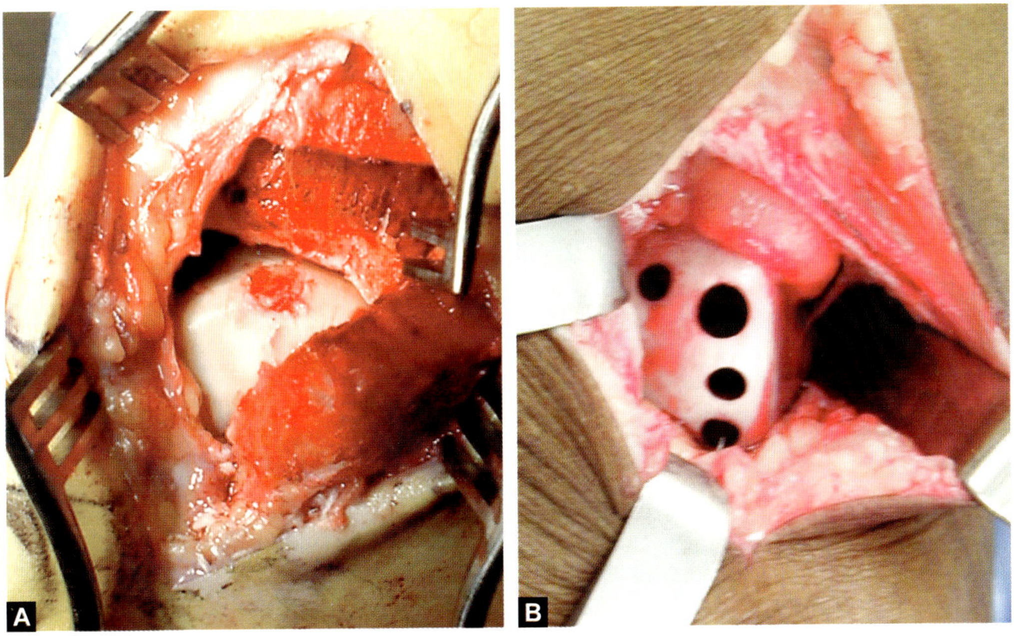

Figs 7A and B: (A) Mosaicplasty osteocartilaginous graft; (B) Donor site for grafts from lateral supratrochlear ridge of the femur at the knee

If mosaicplasty is necessary (Figs 7A and B), then small bone bridges between the grafts are needed. The peripheral grafts should not be closer than 1.5 mm from the shoulder to decrease break out from the talus.

Autologous Chondrocyte Implantation

Carticel® (Genzyme Corporation) is the only food and drug administration (FDA) approved product

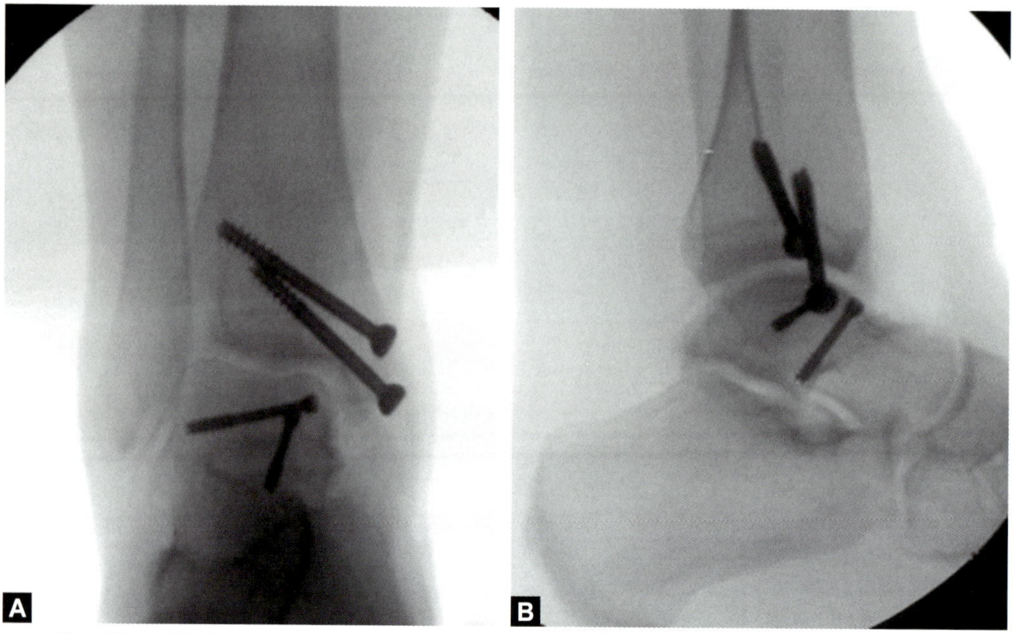

Figs 8A and B: (A) Anteroposterior X-ray of a patient who underwent osteochondral structural allografting of the talus through a medial malleolar osteotomy; (B) Lateral X-ray

for autologous chondrocyte implantation (ACI). The first stage involves taking a small biopsy arthroscopically from the knee. The preferred sites for biopsy are either the margins of the femoral condyles or the intercondylar notch. The sample is harvested and cultured until it reaches 10–12 million chondrocytes, which takes around 2 weeks. The second stage entails debriding the OLT, harvesting a periosteal flap to cover the OLT and injecting the suspension with the chondrocytes under the periosteal flap. The periosteal flap may very well be taken from the distal tibia, and should be 1–2 mm larger than the size of the actual lesion. It is sutured to the outlining cartilage with interrupted sutures. The repair should be water tight and this can be confirmed by injecting saline. The chondrocyte suspension is injected and the periosteum is sealed with fibrin glue. Due to the confines of the ankle this is a very technically demanding procedure.

Structural Allograft Transplantation

This procedure may be indicated when osteochondral autograft transfer system (OATS) or ACI have failed, the lesion occupies a wide area on the talus, if the lesion is uncontained, or it occupies the shoulder of the talus. A CT scan is essential to measure the defect and find a sized matched graft. The talus allograft should be used in a window of 14 days to ensure the viability of the chondrocytes. The lesion on the talus as well as the graft from the allograft talus is removed with a microsagittal saw. The graft should be cut 2 mm larger than the host to compensate for the 2 mm kerf of the saw blade. To lessen the immunogenicity of the allograft, it is recommended to meticulously irrigate before implantation. Press fit of graft and recipient site is desired. Stable fixation of the graft with screws decreases the chances of graft migration during healing (Figs 8A and B).[11,18-20]

COMPLICATIONS

Graft resorption or failure is the most feared complication. Patients with persistent pain or imaging studies consistent with this complication are candidates for an arthroscopic second evaluation. Failure to debride the OLT appropriately can cause progression of the lesion or delamination. If the graft failed to integrate or there is articular delamination, repeat debridements or salvage procedures are possible. If scar tissue is identified as the cause of the symptoms, it can be arthroscopically debrided. Medial or lateral malleolus osteotomy non unions can occur. As long as the X-rays evidence steady progression of the healing process, no further treatment is necessary. If no improvement is seen in serial examinations, consider revision open reduction internal fixation with bone graft. Knee graft harvesting can cause patellofemoral symptoms. These usually subside with time, but in a very low subset of the patients may persist.

SALVAGE PROCEDURES

Total ankle replacement, arthrodesis, and joint realignment procedures serve as salvage for continued symptoms, progression of disease, or contraindications to the previous mentioned options. Candidates for ankle replacement should be evaluated for adequate bone stock and possible subtalar arthritis. A CT scan can further assess the joint and rule out arthritis in the adjacent joints. Ankle arthrodesis is an option when the extent of the arthrosis is not amenable for other reconstructive procedures or patient demographics preclude it. It is crucial to rule out arthritis in the surrounding joints, including talonavicular and subtalar joints. An ankle with very limited and painful range of motion is traded for a plantigrade, stiff, non-painful ankle. Joint realignment osteotomies can be considered an acceptable option if the ankle is clearly in varus or valgus malalignment or as a temporary procedure. Either an opening or closing wedge osteotomy of the tibia is suitable to prevent overload on a specific area within the ankle joint.

REFERENCES

1. Kappis M. Weitere beitrage zur traumatisch-mechanischen entstehung der "spontanen" knorpela biosungen". Deutsche Zeitschrift für Chirurgie. 1922;171:13-29.
2. Berndt AL, Harty M. Transchondral fractures of the talus. J Bone Joint Surg Am. 1959;41-A:988-1020.
3. Ferkel RD, Sgaglione NA, Del Pizzo W. Arthroscopic treatment of osteochondral lesions of the talus: Technique and Results. Orthopaedic Transactions. 1990;14.
4. Mintz DN, Tashjian GS, Connell DA, et al. Osteochondral lesions of the talus: a new magnetic resonance grading system with arthroscopic correlation. Arthroscopy. 2003;19(4):353-9.
5. Shearer C, Loomer R, Clement D. Nonoperatively managed stage 5 osteochondral talar lesions. Foot Ankle Int. 2002;23(7):651-4.
6. Pettine KA, Morrey BF. Osteochondral fractures of the talus. A long-term follow-up. J Bone Joint Surg Br. 1987;69(1):89-92.
7. Huylebroek JF, Martens M, Simon JP. Transchondral talar dome fracture. Arch Orthop Trauma Surg. 1985;104(4):238-41.
8. Cuttica DJ, Smith WB, Hyer CF, et al. Osteochondral lesions of the talus: predictors of clinical outcome. Foot Ankle Int. 2011;32(11):1045-51.
9. Ferkel RD, Zanotti RM, Komenda GA, et al. Arthroscopic treatment of chronic osteochondral lesions of the talus: long-term results. Am J Sports Med. 2008;36(9):1750-62.
10. Hunt KJ, Lee AT, Lindsey DP, et al. Osteochondral lesions of the talus: effect of defect size and plantar flexion angle on ankle joint stresses. Am J Sports Med. 2012;40(4):895-901.
11. Emre TY, Ege T, Cift HT, et al. Open mosaicplasty in osteochondral lesions of the talus: a prospective study. J Foot Ankle Surg. 2012;51(5):556-60.
12. Easley ME, Latt DL, Santangelo JR, et al. Osteochondral lesions of the talus. J Am Acad Orthop Surg. 2010;18(10):616-30.
13. O'Loughlin PF, Heyworth BE, Kennedy JG. Current concepts in the diagnosis and treatment of osteochondral lesions of the ankle. Am J Sports Med. 2010;38(2):392-403.
14. Gobbi A, Francisco RA, Lubowitz JH, et al. Osteochondral lesions of the talus: randomized controlled trial comparing chondroplasty, microfracture and osteochondral autograft transplantation. Arthroscopy. 2006;22(10):1085-92.
15. Qin-wei G, Yue-lin H, Chen J, et al. Arthroscopic treatment for osteochondral lesions of the talus: analysis of outcome predictors. Chin Med Journal. 2010;123(3):296-300.
16. Stufkens SA, Knupp M, Horisberger M, et al. Cartilage lesions and the development of osteoarthritis after internal fixation of ankle fractures: a prospective study. J Bone Joint Surg Am. 2010;92(2):279-86.
17. Zengerink M, Struijs PA, Tol JL, et al. Treatment of osteochondral lesions of the talus: a systematic review. Knee Surg Sports Traumatol Arthrosc. 2010;18(2):238-46.
18. El-Rashidy H, Villacis D, Omar I, et al. Fresh osteochondral allograft for the treatment of cartilage defects of the talus: a retrospective review. J Bone Joint Surg. 2011;93:1634-40.
19. Haene R, Qamirani E, Story RA, et al. Intermediate outcomes of fresh talar osteochondral allografts for treatment of large osteochondral lesions of the talus. J Bone Joint Surg Am. 2012;94(12):1105-10.
20. Hepple S, Winson IG, Glew D. Osteochondral lesions of talus: a revised classification. Foot Ankle Int. 1999;20(12):789-93.
21. Gomoll AH, Farr J, Gillogly SD, et al. Surgical management of articular cartilage defects of the knee. J Bone Joint Surg Am. 2010;92(14):2470-90.

32

Ruptures of the Tendo-Achilles

Shana N Miskovsky, Christopher Orr

INTRODUCTION

Achilles tendon ruptures most commonly result from sports-related activities. The true incidence of ruptures is not entirely known but estimated to be 18 per 100,000 people.[1] The majority occur in the 3–5 decades of life with males outnumbering females by a 5:1 ratio. The mechanisms of injury are noncontact for the most part, with direct contact, laceration, and crush injuries being less frequent. Rupture can occur about the length of the Achilles but the majority occur at the intratendinous region (4–6 cm proximal to insertion site) (73%), followed by the musculotendinous junction (24%), and then the insertion (4%).[2]

There are identifiable risk factors associated with acute Achilles rupture. Ruptures are common in both competitive and recreational athletes and in manual laborers. In North America, ruptures frequently occur in sports such as football, basketball, baseball, tennis, and downhill skiing. A substantial change in training regimen, intensity, or activity is usually noted. Also, medical conditions can predispose to rupture: inflammatory arthritides (rheumatoid arthritis, lupus, gout), endocrinopathies (renal failure, hypothyroidism, diabetes), hypercholesterolemia, renal transplantation, tumors, and infections. Additionally, fluoroquinolone use has been implicated with reports of Achilles ruptures a few weeks after therapy was begun.[3,4] Fluoroquinolone-related tendon disorders are estimated at a rate of 15–20 per 100,000 patients, with Achilles tendinitis the most common. Patients with higher risk for rupture while on a fluoroquinolones include the elderly, transplant patients, those with renal failure, and chronic corticosteroid users. The estimated risk for ciprofloxacin alone is one case generated per 779,600 treatment days.[3]

Anatomical factors appear to play a role in the acute rupture of the Achilles tendon. The Achilles tendon is one of the strongest tendons in the body, handling forces up to ten times of body weight during high impact activities such as running.[5] Its dimensions at the ankle level range from 1.2 cm to 2.5 cm wide and 5–6 mm thick.[6] Proximally, the separate aponeuroses of the gastrocnemius and soleus form tendons and the fibers from each tendon eventually coalesce to form the Achilles tendon at a point 5–6 cm proximal to the calcaneus.[7] Rotation of the Achilles tendon starts at about 15 cm proximal to its calcaneal insertion when the soleus contributes fibers to the tendon. Proceeding distally, maximum twisting of the Achilles then develops at 5–6 cm from its insertion, creating an area of high stress in the tendon which happens to coincide with an area of hypovascularity.[8] Both factors are thought to contribute to the more commonly seen noninsertional (or proximal) Achilles tendon rupture.

Vascularity of the Achilles tendon has additionally been mentioned as a possible etiological factor. The tendon is surrounded by a vascularized and innervated paratenon, a two-layered membrane without a synovial lining. Mesotenon connects the inner visceral layer to the outer parietal layer of the paratenon. The paratenon is confluent proximally with the investing fascia of muscle and distally with the periosteum of the calcaneus. Transverse vincula are conduits through which blood vessels travel to supply the mid-portion of the tendon. Proximally, the tendon's blood supply is via the recurrent branch of the posterior tibial artery and distally by the rete arteriosum calcane, formed from the fibular and posterior tibial arteries.[9] Mesotenal vessels are distributed evenly along the entire length of the paratenon anteriorly and posteriorly.[10] However, there is a decrease in the number and mean percentage area of blood vessels in the tendon from 2 cm to 6 cm proximal to its insertion, consistent with a low metabolic rate, decreased healing potential, and increased susceptibility to ischemia.[11] The other two main sources of blood supply to the Achilles tendon at its ends arise from the musculotendinous junction and osseous insertion.[7]

Finally, the method by which the muscle-tendon unit is loaded has been considered to be a factor in Achilles ruptures. The most forceful mode of muscular contraction is eccentric, utilized in acceleration and deceleration activities. Rapid loading of the viscoelastic muscle-tendon unit increases stiffness and increases susceptibility to rupture. Achilles ruptures commonly occur with no preceding symptoms or signs, particularly in sports requiring quick changes of direction, jumping, or running. Only a small fraction of patients describe prodromal symptoms (10% or less) and even fewer have a history of steroid injections into the Achilles. It is thought that the rupture either occurs (1) due to the extremely high loads generated during performance of sports activities combined with fatigue and/or failure of neuromuscular control or coordination or (2) due to subclinical tendon degeneration.

MAKING THE DIAGNOSIS OF ACUTE ACHILLES TENDON RUPTURE

The evaluation of Achilles tendon rupture is guided by clinician suspicion incited by a thorough patient interview. This can be challenging with the commonality of ankle presentations in primary and specialty practices and as many as 25% of acute ruptures are missed initially.[12] In the history, the physician can elicit the mechanisms leading to rupture: (1) significant dorsiflexion force applied to a plantarflexed ankle, (2) forceful, sudden ankle dorsiflexion, and (3) forceful push-off from a planted foot while the knee is straight. In a nonacute presentation, one must consider the cumulative impact loading and microtrauma that can be seen in runners and in those with degenerative tendinopathy.

The classic presentation with an acute rupture is reported as a sudden severe pain in the calf, sometimes accompanied by an audible snap or "pop", and inability to bear weight.[12] The patient may also describe the inability to plantarflex the foot. There may be swelling and a submalleolar bruising pattern which extends plantarly, medially, and/or laterally. Chronic ruptures and missed ruptures may present with persistent pain along the Achilles, swelling, and plantarflexion weakness with push-off activities.

Several physical examination maneuvers have been found to be helpful in diagnosing ruptures, but each has limitations.[13] First, the palpation test is an evaluation of the course of the tendon by the examiner's finger to determine if there is a palpable defect in the tendon. This test can be useful initially but is less reliable once edema and organized hematoma have formed. Second, the calf squeeze test[14] (Fig. 1) involves evaluating a patient in the prone position while gentle compression is applied to the calf. Thompson found that plantarflexion depends on an intact soleus to the Achilles. Albeit the most commonly employed test in practice, this test can be limited by compensation of an intact tibialis posterior, peroneal group, and flexor hallucis longus (FHL). Contralateral comparison in this case is essential. The seated position with the knee bent to 90° also can be used but does not lend to an easy visual comparison of the injured vs noninjured side. Third, the Matles test[13] can be peformed in an awake patient and the patient is asked to flex the knees to 90°. An Achilles defect will be suspected if the foot on the affected side falls into neutral or slight dorsiflexion. The unaffected side should expectedly remain in slight plantarflexion. Other examination maneuvers such as the Copeland test and O'Brien tests are limited by patient compliance and, due to significant patient discomfort, will commonly be assessed under anesthesia.[12,15]

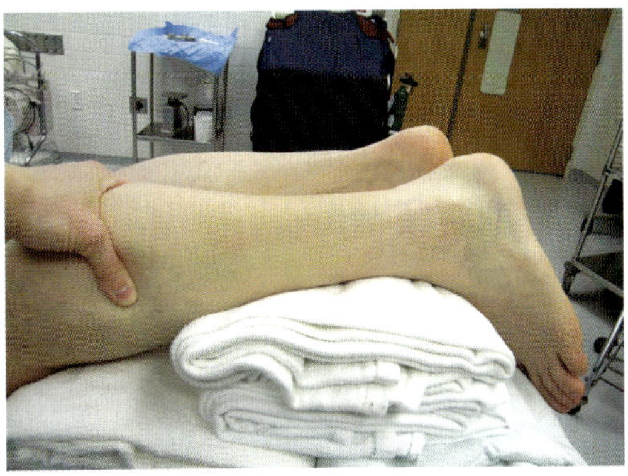

Fig. 1: Thompson test is positive on the left with no plantarflexion created after squeezing the calf

Each of the aforementioned tests offers their own benefit in the proper setting and correlation with patient presentation and mechanism of injury. A thorough interview and physical exam will identify ruptures in most cases and in a cost efficient manner. Imaging plays little role in identifying a rupture aside from examining for secondary contributors to rupture including tendinopathy with ossifications (proximal or distal) or posterior calcaneal bony avulsions. X-rays can be closely examined for signs of rupture including proximal migration and/or separation of tendinous ossifications (Fig. 2) and soft tissue swelling in Kagel's fat pad. When necessary to confirm the presence of rupture in less obvious cases and to determine the quality of the remaining tissue, imaging modalities of choice are usually limited to sonography and magnetic resonance imaging (MRI).

The use of ultrasonography was evaluated in 26 cases of Achilles tendon tears with clinical correlation.[16] The study showed high sensitivity, specificity, and accuracy. Concluding that sonography can be useful to distinguish between partial and full thickness tears, the cost-effective option over MRI in evaluating surgical candidacy is favorable. MRI is superior in distinguishing partial vs full thickness tears or tendinosis. In cases of partial tears and tendinosis, most can be treated nonsurgically and MRI scanning should be reserved for only those recalcitrant cases with persistent symptoms and functional limitations.

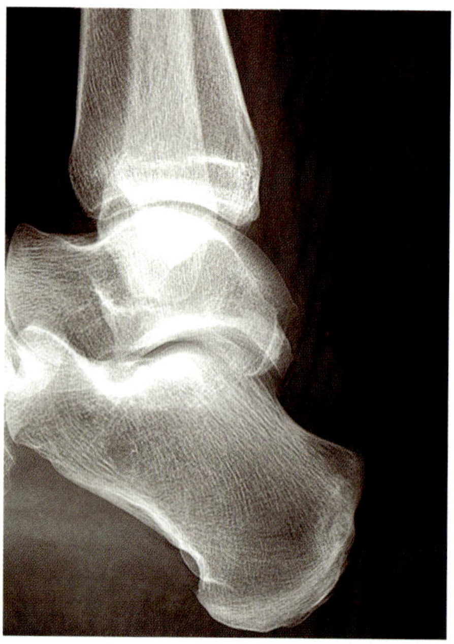

Fig. 2: Lateral X-ray of the ankle shows proximal migration of ossifications consistent with acute insertional Achilles tendon rupture in the setting of chronic tendinopathy

The diagnosis of Achilles rupture can be challenging, but adhering to the basics of a thorough patient interview and physical exam will identify the rupture in most cases. Special tests have been devised in this diagnostic effort, each with their own limitations requiring correlation with the exam and history for the diagnosis to be made and proper treatment rendered. In cases where tendon integrity is questionable or patient response to conservative measures is poor, advanced imaging with ultrasonography or MRI scanning will identify the rupture.

Options of Management

There is still controversy as to the optimal treatment of Achilles tendon ruptures, with some authors reporting similar patient functional outcomes from nonoperative treatment or surgical repair.[17] Pooling data from 12 trials with 844 participants, the latest Cochrane review[18] revealed a statistically significant lower risk of re-rupture with open surgical treatment as compared to conservative treatment. However, there was a significantly higher risk of infection, adhesions, and dysesthesias with surgery. No comment could be made with respect to functional outcomes or sporting activities due to incomplete or inconsistent reporting across the studies. When comparing open with percutaneous repairs, there was higher risk of infection with open repair but the patient numbers were small. Also, patients managed with a functional brace and early mobilization had a lower complication rate after surgery than those who were casted. The authors noted that the scientific methodology of many of these pooled studies was less than ideal, so further investigations are warranted to elucidate the best treatment regimen.

Numerous studies[17-22] have reported the rates of complications after treatment of Achilles tendon ruptures and the data vary somewhat but are listed: (1) re-rupture (2–15% nonoperative, 1–5% operative); (2) complications other than re-rupture such as wound infection, adhesions, sensory dysthesia (3% nonoperative, 34% operative); (3) postsurgical complications such as adhesions, infection, and keloid formation (36% cast group, 20% functional brace group); and (4) skin-healing complications (0.5% nonoperative, 2–15% operative). A study further evaluated the wound complications reported after open repairs and reported a rate of 12% for minor wound complications (superficial infection, wound hematoma, delayed wound healing, scar adhesion, suture granuloma, and skin necrosis) and a rate of 2% for major wound complications (deep infection and chronic fistula formation).[19]

It is extremely important that the surgeon have a long and detailed discussion with each patient sustaining an Achilles rupture regarding their expectations, desired activity level, modifiable health conditions (such as smoking cessation or improved diabetes control), and their ability to be compliant with the conservative or postoperative treatment protocol and extensive physical therapy. The risks and benefits should be clearly explained and the treatment selected should be based on a joint decision made by the well-informed patient and his or her surgeon. Treatment should be individualized.

Conservative Treatment

Nonoperative management can be successfully implemented in particular patient populations and types of Achilles tendon ruptures. Generally, nonoperative management is the preferred approach in patients with significant medical conditions that substantially increase risks of general anesthetic (i.e. severe cardiovascular and pulmonary disorders), that preclude the patient being positioned prone on the operating table safely, or that have a detrimental impact on soft tissue and wound healing (i.e. cigarette smoking, peripheral vascular disease, diabetes mellitus, skin disorders, autoimmune disorders). Conservative treatment should also be considered in cases where patients have limited ambulatory capacity and/or functional demands.

Conservative treatment success is defined by the apposition of tendon ends and healing of the ruptured tendon with good quality tissue resilient to re-rupture and by the return of the patient to their previous level of function. Traditionally, conservative treatment varied from immobilization of the injured extremity in a long leg splint or cast in equinus for the first 1–2 weeks and then transition into a short leg cast in equinus for 4 weeks or patients were just immobilized in a short leg cast for 6–8 weeks. Longer term immobilization however is associated with muscular atrophy, joint stiffness, and poorer quality healing tissue. As the basic science knowledge of tendon healing expanded, contemporary treatment protocols shorten the period of non-weight-bearing immobilization and utilize functional bracing to allow for earlier joint motion and rehabilitation without undue stress on the healing tissue. The success of a functional rehabilitation protocol is based on patient compliance and initial positioning of the ankle in 20° of plantarflexion. This position of 20° of plantarflexion has been shown to improve blood flow to the skin overlying the Achilles tendon[23] and to decrease plantarflexor muscular activity during gait.[24]

Studies have shown that patient satisfaction is increased and tendon healing is facilitated with contemporary protocols.[25,26] In one study, patients were immobilized in a short leg cast in equinus for 4 weeks and then were progressed to weight-bearing in an orthosis in 15° of ankle plantarflexion and physical therapy with respect to range of motion was started. The brace was discontinued at 4 weeks and physical therapy continued as the patient worked on strength and functional activities. The authors found a low 6% re-rupture rate, 98% patient satisfaction rate, and, of 72% of patients involved in athletics, 37% returned to the same or higher level of sport.[27]

Another study was a randomized trial of nonoperative vs operative intervention for acute Achilles tendon ruptures in 42 patients who underwent the same postoperative functional rehabilitation protocol.[28] Patients were made non-weight bearing with crutches for a total of 6 weeks. For the first ten days, patients were placed in a short leg cast in equinus. Then, they were put in a below-knee orthosis with 20° of built-in plantarflexion. Patients were instructed to sit and remove the brace and perform passive ankle plantarflexion and active dorsiflexion up to neutral position for 5 minutes every waking hour. At 4 weeks, the orthosis was set at zero degrees and the same range of motion protocol was continued. Patients were able to weight bear at 6 weeks in the orthosis. The orthosis was discontinued at 8 weeks and strengthening exercises, including toe raises, were started. These exercises were continued until the patient was able to easily perform a single leg-toe raise on the injured side. After analyzing the outcomes, the authors found no difference between the treatment groups with respect to ankle motion, complications, patient satisfaction, injured vs noninjured calf circumference. Re-rupture rates were low in both groups with no statistically significant difference. The authors felt that controlled active motion, started early, as part of their functional rehabilitation program was the key to a more successful outcome in patients treated nonoperatively.[28]

Additionally, there are specific tear characteristics that may aid the clinician in determining whether conservative treatment is appropriate for a patient's rupture. Dynamic ultrasound technique has delineated several favorable tear characteristics:

- Less than a 5 mm gap measured between the ruptured ends with the ankle positioned in maximum plantarflexion
- Less than a 10 mm gap with the ankle in neutral dorsiflexion, and
- Tendon end-to-end contact greater than or equal to 75% with the ankle in 20° of plantarflexion.[22,23,29]

Using ultrasound criterion of less than 5 mm of gapping, authors compared patient outcomes from conservative vs surgical intervention using the same functional rehabilitation protocol for both groups.[22] An overall complication rate of 7.4% was reported in the surgical group, as compared to 3.4% in the nonsurgical group. With respect to re-rupture rates, 1.5% was noted for the nonoperative group and 3.4% for the surgical group.

Other authors utilized the 75% tendon apposition and less than 10 mm gap criteria.[29] Patients were placed in a cast in equinus for 1–3 days and then were placed in a special boot that allows for 3 cm heel elevation and weight-bearing (Vario-Stabil, Orthotech GmBH, Gauting, Germany). Patients remained in the high-shaft boot for 8 weeks. Physical therapy protocol allowed isometric and gait training at 3 weeks, exercises done without the boot at 4 weeks and exercises to gain strength at 6 weeks. Ultrasound evaluations were done throughout the rehabilitation period, and if healing of the tendon was evident at 8 weeks, patients were allowed to wear a shoe with a 1 cm heel lift for 3 months. If the tendon was not healed, patients used the boot for another 2 weeks. If the tendon re-ruptured or did not heal, then the morphological appearance of the tendon on ultrasound was taken into account and either prolonged nonoperative treatment or surgical repair was chosen. Outcomes were reported: 6.4% re-rupture rate, return to work at a mean of 4.5 weeks, 75% return to athletic activities at the same level as prior to injury; 96% of patients reported no pain, and injured leg calf circumference with a mean 2.1 cm difference as compared to normal side.

Conservative treatment can be used successfully in selected patients with good functional outcomes and low re-rupture and complication rates. Throughout the recovery process, patients' ruptures can be monitored clinically and noninvasively with ultrasound (or MRI) to determine whether the tear is healing well. Patient satisfaction is higher with a functional rehabilitation protocol which allows for earlier weight-bearing and range of motion. However, if patients discontinue their immobilization or functional brace prematurely, then their outcomes will be poor, with lower function and higher re-rupture rates.

Some patients will not respond well to conservative treatment. To try to jumpstart the healing process, newer technologies are considered, including platelet-rich plasma (PRP) therapy, with injection into the rupture site. Platelets are storehouses of growth factors that aid in the healing process and create a temporary fill at defect sites with a matrix that allows for effective cell migration and tissue remodeling. Early results are promising in other clinical applications and in vivo animal models of Achilles ruptures with respect to the biomechanical and structural quality of the healing tissue. But, clinical validation of PRP's safety, proper dosing regimen, and efficacy is currently lacking.[30] Therapeutic ultrasound and laser treatments along with electrical stimulation and hyperbaric oxygen therapy are other modalities currently being studied in animal models. As investigations continue, the future may hold additional treatment strategies.

After institution of nonoperative treatment, surgery is then recommended in certain clinical situations. Surgical treatment is indicated when patients have persistent pain and swelling or significant functional limitations with loss of plantarflexion strength with push-off activities. Also, if patients sustain a re-rupture, have poor tissue fill of the tendon defect, or demonstrate changes on advanced imaging findings suggesting tendon discontinuity, then surgical repair is offered.

Operative Management and Procedures

As compared to conservative treatment, operative management of Achilles tendon ruptures has been shown in most studies to have a lower re-rupture rate, but a higher complication rate, particularly wound complications.[21] Functional outcomes with respect to plantarflexion strength and return to sport or previous activities also favor operative management, as the tendon ends are approximated and proper length of the muscle-tendon unit is restored. Surgical repair is favored and recommended in high-level athletes, young patients, and active patients with no significant risk factors.[31] In the literature, factors shown to increase wound complications after surgical repair include tobacco use, steroid use, and female gender. In patients who had one or more of the these risk factors (diabetic, smoker and/or steroid user), 42% had developed a wound complication in one study.[32] Careful consideration of these factors is important in determining whether a patient is a suitable candidate for operative repair.

The goals of surgical repair of Achilles tendon ruptures include:

- Establishment of proper muscle-tendon length, tension, and stiffness to allow for efficient and effective push-off and forward propulsion.
- Creation of a repair that is strong enough to allow for early rehabilitation and patient mobilization without the fear of resultant tendon elongation or gapping.
- Most importantly restoration of the patients' ability to function at their preinjury level.

The perfect repair is still elusive, as most patients are not functioning at a level equivalent to their preinjury state even at 2 years postsurgery[33] and may have chronic calf atrophy and loss of heel-rise height. The majority do not have any activity limitations and are able to return to athletic activities, but reportedly only 57% return to the same level of sport and the mean plantarflexion strength is generally 87% of normal.[20] After repair, re-rupture rates utilizing a functional rehabilitation protocol are reportedly 3–5%.[33,34] This may be due to the quality and organization of the resultant healing tissue.

In the literature, methods have been introduced to maximize the biomechanical strength of the repair and prevent tendon elongation during the healing process. Suture material choice tends to favor nonabsorbable braided sutures of caliber greater than or equal to # 2. Additionally, the quality of the tissue influences the friction or how well the tendon resists suture pullout. Locking-loop stitches, such as the Krackow, are excellent for holding and grasping tendon tissue. The location of where the knot is tied also can make a difference. The one disadvantage of Krackow stitches is that failure can occur through the knot at the site of rupture, as it creates a stress riser. A modified technique called the "gift box" technique[35] utilizes the Krackow stitch but ties the counterlimbs of the sutures away from the rupture site. Augmentation with epitenon repair also is recommended, due to increased gapping resistance and repair strength. Finally, tissue engineering has lead to the development of extracellular matrix xenograft which has been shown to decrease gapping at the repair site and improve strength and/or stiffness characteristics of the repaired tendon.[36] In the future, mesenchymal stem cells and growth factors may be helpful in improving repair tissue quality and early studies are promising. However, further study is needed as no conclusive information is available at this time to support common clinical use.

With respect to rehabilitation protocols, there is no standard, globally accepted protocol in the literature with proven results and controversy still exists as further studies are warranted. As these protocols are evaluated, it is important to consider the forces that the Achilles tendon experiences with common activities: ankle immobilized in neutral [370 newtons (N)], passive ankle range of motion (400N), walking with cam boot with ankle in neutral (590N), bicycling (1,000N), walking (1,500–2,000N), hopping (3,790N) and running (9,000N).[24,37] The Achilles tendon handles the most force of any tendon during ambulation. Interestingly, with current repair techniques, failure may occur with forces as little as 45–250N. Stronger repairs such as the four-strand augmented Krackow repair may fail at 323N.[38] It is postulated that suture techniques that resist tendon gapping may be more clinically important, rather than considering only strength and stiffness. Clinical failure of tendon repair is defined by gapping of 5 or more millimeters, resulting in poorer repair tissue characterized by increased granulation tissue, adhesion formation, and delayed collagen maturation. Finally, protocols implementing early, protected range of motion and weight-bearing have been shown to improve the patients' quality of life, lessen the potential for tendon elongation, and show a trend toward earlier return to work or sport.[39,40] The augmented Krackow repair is the only repair method shown to be able to handle early range of motion and weight-bearing with a 1 inch heel lift.[38]

Biomechanical knowledge and tendon healing physiology should be kept in mind as a protocol is implemented and modified according to the patient's injury, co-morbid conditions, tissue quality, and repair technique.

Minimal Incision Techniques

Percutaneous repairs are utilized for noninsertional (or proximal) ruptures and have the reported advantages of minimizing wound complications, lower overall complication rates, and equivalent functional outcomes as compared to open repairs.[21,41] Minimal incision techniques were first introduced in late 1970's with later concerns reported due to the high rate of sural nerve damage (13% incidence in one study) utilizing the Ma and Griffith technique.[42] Contemporary percutaneous repair techniques utilizing devices similar to the Achillon (Integra Life Sciences Corporation, Plainsboro, NJ, USA) where sutures are placed within or underneath the paratenon have led to a significant decrease in sural nerve stitch entrapment; with no sural nerve injuries reported in a large, multicenter study.[43] Other concerns with the percutaneous approach include the ability to coaptate tendon stump ends together and the strength of the resultant repair. This has been addressed with proper placement of a transverse incision at the rupture site for sub-paratenon placement of the guide and for direct visualization of the tendon ends after repair. This transverse incision can be extended proximally or distally as needed if further exposure is warranted to confirm coaptation or to repair the epitenon. Tensile strength of the percutaneous repair has been shown to be equivalent to a two-strand Kessler technique in a model utilizing sheep Achilles tendons.[44] Other devices (i.e. Arthrex, PARS System, Naples, FL) allow for placement of locking, nonabsorbable sutures which increase the strength of the repair. Another study estimated the repair strength of the percutaneous method was approximately 50% weaker than an open repair.[45] Thus, the authors recommended that early range of motion and weight-bearing is delayed in these repairs.[38]

The anatomy and course of the sural nerve deserves mentioning as it is variable, leaving the nerve at risk during percutaneous needle placement. However, as a guide, proximally, the sural nerve travels across the lateral border of the Achilles tendon about 9.8 cm from the calcaneus. Distally, the sural nerve tends to be a mean of 18.8 mm anterior and lateral from the lateral border of the Achilles as it inserts onto the posterior calcaneus.[46] Methods to prevent iatrogenic injury have included placement of an additional small incision or localization with ultrasound to determine the location of the sural nerve prior to suture placement.[47]

Indications for use of percutaneous repair technique are evolving. In a meta-analysis of six randomized controlled trials with 277 repairs comparing open repair to percutaneous repair or minimally invasive surgery (MIS), there was no statistically significant difference with respect to rates of re-rupture, tissue adhesion, sural nerve damage, deep infection, and deep venous thrombosis (DVT). The authors noted the MIS had a statistically significant lower risk of wound infection and patient satisfaction (rated as good to excellent results) was three times greater than conventional open repair.[48] Percutaneous repair also is associated with less adhesion formation, less soft tissue stripping, less devascularization, and a shorter operative time. Use of this technique can be considered in particular patient populations:

- Patients who are active but smoke or have medical conditions that predispose to wound healing problems.
- Middle-aged patients with reasonable tissue quality that need to get back to work as soon as possible with less pain and morbidity.
- Active elderly patients with poorer skin quality
- With respect to use in athletes, there are advantages but concerns exist regarding proper tendon end coaptation and repair strength and so such a decision is made on a case by case basis.

Percutaneous Repair Surgical Technique

Anesthesia

General anesthetic is utilized with popliteal block placed for postoperative pain control.

Tourniquet

After adequate padding has been placed, an upper thigh tourniquet is applied with the tubing directed towards the head of the table and tubing positioned on the posterior aspect of the leg (so that the patient is not lying on the tourniquet tubing while in the prone position). Tourniquet is set to 280 mm Hg for an hour.

Position

The patient is positioned prone on thoracic chest rolls (Fig. 3). A facial pillow with mirror combination is used so that the anesthesiologist can visualize and assure that eyes are not getting pressure. A pillow is placed to cushion the knees and blankets are used to support the lower legs. The operative leg is elevated above the nonoperative one with use of an extra blanket. The patient's arms are abducted and externally rotated on arm boards with padding to keep pressure off of the ulnar nerves.

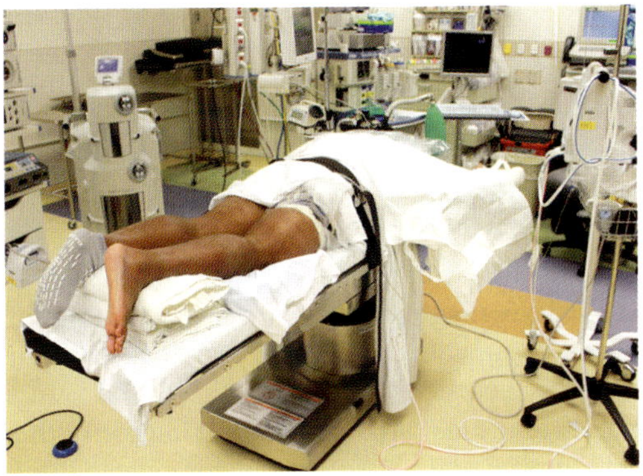

Fig. 3: Example of prone positioning used for Achilles tendon repairs. To obtain more exposure to the medial foot for flexor hallucis longus (FHL) tendon transfer, the operative leg is elevated on more blankets above the noninjured leg

Surgical Technique Steps and Details

After sterile prepping and draping, the tourniquet is elevated to 280 mm Hg.

A transverse incision (2–3 cm) (Fig. 4) is made at the location of rupture that approximates the width of the tendon and is large enough to accommodate proper positioning of the percutaneous repair jig. In cases where increased exposure is required for improved visualization of tendon ends, the incision can be extended proximally and distally.

The paratenon is identified and carefully split longitudinally. Tag sutures may be placed to ease identification of paratenon during wound closure.

Adhesions around the tendon stumps are released with blunt dissection and a Kocher clamp is gently placed at the distal end of the proximal tendon stump.

Distal traction is applied on the Kocher clamp, the percutaneous repair jig is slid underneath the paratenon, and the width of the jig arms is adjusted manually to fit the tendon width. The jig is then advanced to its base with its two arms snugly fit and centered along the sides of the medial and lateral aspects of the proximal Achilles stump (Fig. 5).

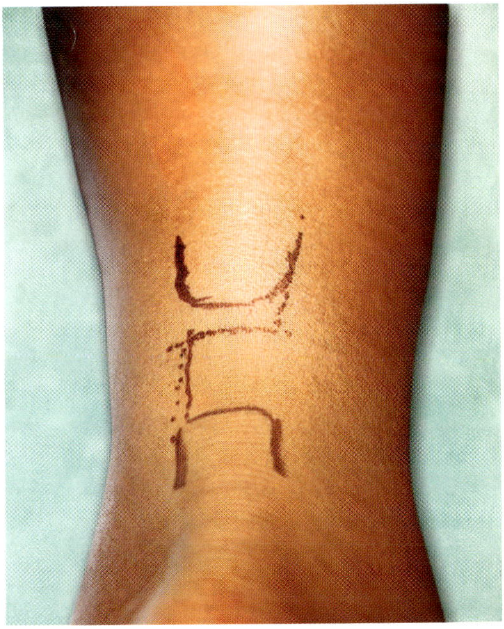

Fig. 4: The transverse percutaneous repair incision is marked with a skin marker. If the incision needs to be extended proximally or distally, the proposed incisions are also drawn out

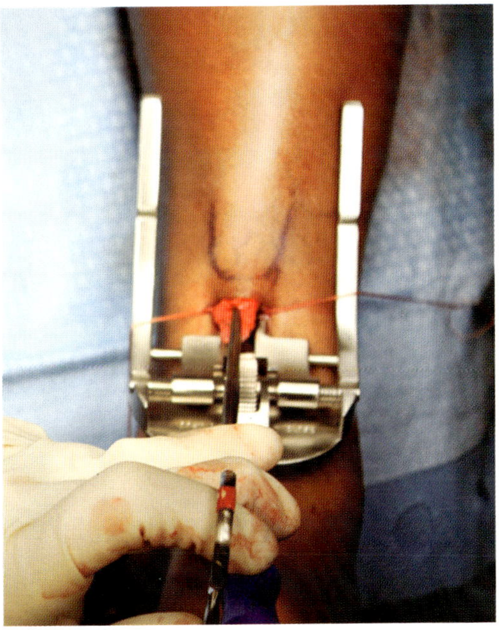

Fig. 5: The percutaneous repair jig is slid underneath the paratenon and the inner arms of the jig fit snugly around the proximal Achilles stump

While holding the position of the jig with one hand and placing mild digital pressure on the skin overlying the proximal Achilles stump with the other hand, the Keith needles with nonabsorbable sutures are passed one by one through the jig from lateral to medial (i.e. in a right Achilles tendon rupture). The surgeon can feel resistance with passage of the needles through the tendon. The needles are carefully retrieved from the medial side and the differently colored sutures are spread out and tagged.

The jig is then carefully pulled distally and the sutures follow (Fig. 6). Once the inner arms of the guide are out of the wound, the percutaneous sutures are then shuttled out of the outer arms of the jig so that they do not become entrapped in the targeting holes in the jig. Differently colored sutures now are out of the wound and the medial and lateral suture ends are carefully kept separated. Sutures are then organized as they were in the jig and spread out on the drapes and secured with clamps.

For locking suture loop capability, the looped end of the nonabsorbable passing suture is identified on the medial side. The adjacent suture located superiorly is brought underneath and up and through the loop. The lateral sided looped suture end is located and the adjacent superior suture limb is brought underneath other sutures and up through the loop as before. The nonlooped ends of the passing suture are identified medially and laterally and then those ends are pulled to pass and secure the locking sutures.

In a similar fashion, the process of guide or jig placement, suture placement, and suture management is repeated for the distal Achilles stump; with the except that now the Keith needles with sutures are directed from a medial to lateral direction through the targeting holes in the jig (i.e. in a right Achilles tendon rupture).

The foot is placed in slight plantarflexion (to match the resting position of the normal side) using towels to support the dorsum of the foot. Suture pairs are then tied as per protocol. Initial sutures nearest to the tear are tied first. For simple sutures, one side (i.e. medial) suture pair is selected to be tied first as a stay suture. The other side (i.e. lateral) suture pair then is tied and the proper tension and tissue advancement is established (Fig. 7). As the

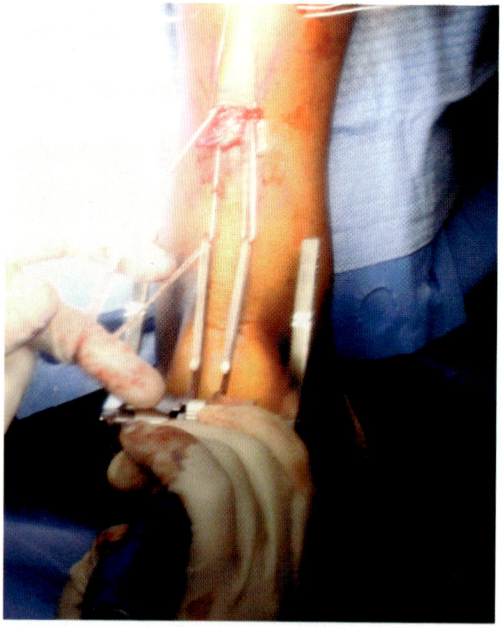

Fig. 6: The percutaneous repair jig is removed from the proximal Achilles tendon stump as the stitches are taken out of the outer limbs of the jig. Medial and lateral stitches are kept separate

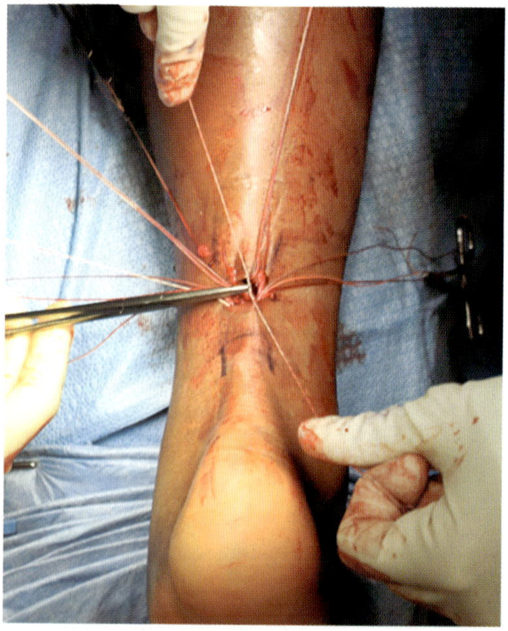

Fig. 7: The sutures from the proximal and distal stumps are organized. The ankle is placed in the proper position. The nonlocking loop sutures are tied first by placing a stay stitch on one side and tying the other pair of colored sutures on the other side to tension the repair

locked suture pairs are identified in the proximal and distal stumps, tension should be applied prior to tying in order to seat the locked suture (Krackow-type) loop. Those locking sutures then are tied in place and secured.

The adequacy of the repair is then evaluated (Fig. 8) (The ankle should not be plantarflexed more than 30° and plantarflexion angle should match the resting tension of the normal side). Thompson test is also performed confirming continuity. The repair can be augmented with careful placement of epitenon sutures with absorbable suture (2-0 vicryl).

Copious irrigation of the wound is then performed. A multilayered closure with absorbable suture is performed for the paratenon (2-0 or 4-0 vicryl) and subcutaneous tissue (4-0 vicryl). Finally, the skin is closed with nonabsorbable suture (4-0 nylon).

After dressings are placed, the tourniquet is released. The patient is placed in a well-padded posterior splint and sugar tong splint with the foot in slight equinus.

Postoperatively, patients are released the same day, non-weight bearing on the operative extremity with crutches or with a knee walker. Patients are given narcotic pain medication initially and are started on DVT prophylaxis on postoperative day 1 that continues for 3–4 weeks.

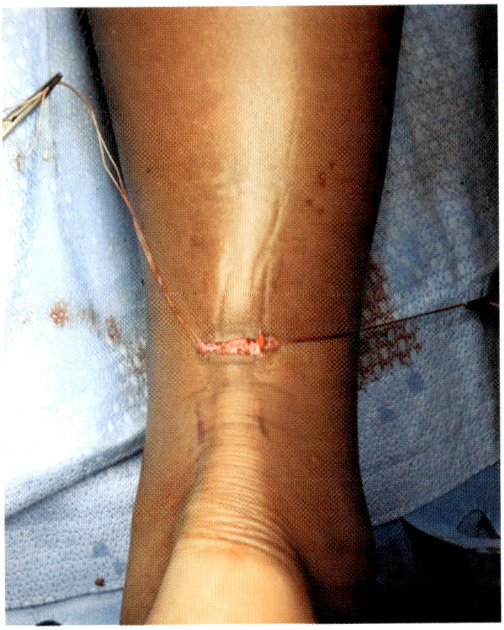

Fig. 8: The repair is finished and direct tendon apposition is appreciated. Tag sutures have been placed in the paratenon

During the initial phases of healing (1–2 weeks), patients are kept immobilized and non-weight bearing. Typically, patients are seen in the office 7–10 days post surgery and placed in a non-weight-bearing short leg cast in slight equinus. They are instructed to perform quadricep sets, supine hip and core exercises, and toe range of motion daily. The second phase (2–4 weeks) focuses on edema control and protected range of motion. Sutures are removed in the office and patients are transitioned into a tall cam walker boot with a heel lift to maintain slight plantarflexion. Patients remain non-weight bearing and must keep the boot on at all times, except to bathe or when doing supervised physical therapy. Outpatient physical therapy involves active-assisted plantarflexion, dorsiflexion (not past neutral dorsiflexion position), inversion, and eversion. Additionally, electrical stimulation, edema control, scar massage, and passive non-weight bearing calf stretches are performed. In the third phase (4–6 weeks), motion is advanced and weight-bearing on the operative extremity is allowed. One portion of the heel lift is removed weekly for 2–3 weeks until neutral dorsiflexion is achieved in the boot comfortably. Ankle range of motion can be advanced with the therapist's help. Depending on patient's progress, Thera Band exercises are introduced around 5th week along with stationary bike use (out of boot in athletic shoe, low resistance). The fourth phase (6–8 weeks) focuses on full weight-bearing and starting strength development. Therapy is continued and weaning of the boot is begun as strength, balance, and gait improve. Once patients are out of the boot, a pool program can be considered. After 8–10 weeks, balance exercises, seated and standing toe raises, and treadmill walking are further introduced depending on patient progress and comfort. The therapeutic exercise program is continued over the next few months and advanced with respect to agility, walking program, and walk-jog program. Sports-specific exercises generally start at 3 months and progress to a jump-land neuromuscular training program and conditioning program including running. Return to sports usually occurs 4–6 months after injury at the earliest.

In general, patients with medical co-morbidities such as diabetes, inflammatory arthritis, or other conditions which are detrimental or slow down soft tissue healing are advanced at a slower pace during physical therapy and are kept non-weight bearing 1–2 weeks longer than young, healthy patients.

Open Repair Techniques

Open repair of Achilles tendon ruptures is used in the majority of patients. Its advantages include an incision that can be easily extended if need be to improve exposure or perform additional procedures such as FHL tendon transfer, proximal V-Y lengthening, turn-down fasical flaps, or plantaris augmentation. Also, the exposure allows for direct visualization of the ruptured tendon ends and for confirmation that proper tendon length and apposition is accomplished with the repair. The repair also is stronger as compared to percutaneous repairs, particularly utilizing the modified augmented Krackow technique with epitenon repair or gift box suture technique.

However, to minimize wound healing complications postoperatively, it is important that soft tissue swelling has resolved sufficiently before surgery. Skin wrinkling over the posterior calf and ankle is an easy sign to look for on physical exam which means that the soft tissues are healed enough to safely tolerate a skin incision. Recommendations would be to wait at least a few days and up to 2 weeks before repairing the tendon.

Surgical Technique of end-to-end Repair of Proximal (Noninsertional) Achilles Rupture

Anesthesia, tourniquet placement, and patient positioning are the same as that described for the percutaneous repair technique.

Surgical Technique Steps and Details

The rupture site is identified. A longitudinal incision centered over the rupture is performed slightly medial to the midline (Fig. 9). (The incision is not placed too far medially as the blood supply to the skin is less robust). A direct midline incision is also not used either due to problems with shoewear rubbing the previous incision site. Lateral incisions are not recommended due to concern for injury to the sural nerve or inadvertent entry into the peroneal tendon sheath.

The paratenon is identified and split longitudinally. Medial and lateral flaps of the paratenon are mobilized to expose the rupture site. No touch skin technique is used throughout the case to prevent iatrogenic damage to the skin from forceps. Stay sutures can be placed in the paratenon to aid in retraction and in paratenon closure later.

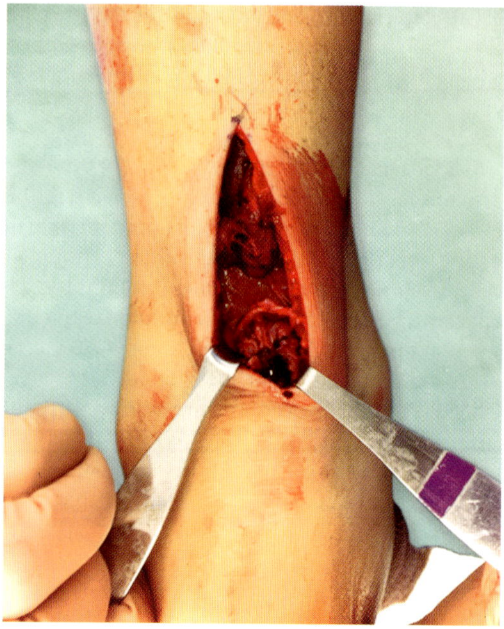

Fig. 9: The longitudinal incision for open Achilles tendon repair is placed just medial to midline

The rupture site is seen and the stump ends are debrided. Any intervening hematoma or unhealthy appearing tissue is removed. Soft tissue adhesions proximally and distally are released with blunt dissection to allow for mobilization of the tendon stumps.

A Kocher clamp is gently placed on the central, distal aspect of the proximal stump. A Krackow stitch utilizing no. 2 Fiberwire (Arthex, Naples, FL) is performed around the periphery of the tendon. A second Krackow stitch is placed in the central portion of the tendon. Four core sutures are then available to increase the strength of the repair. Each throw of the Krackow stitch is placed approximately 5 mm from the previous suture loop in order to not damage the vascularity of the tendon. Three or four throws are done before proceeding across the tendon and going down the other side.

The process is repeated for the distal stump with the Krackow suture technique. Figure 10 demonstrates the suture technique. (# 5 suture, used in this figure, is currently superseded by # 2 suture).

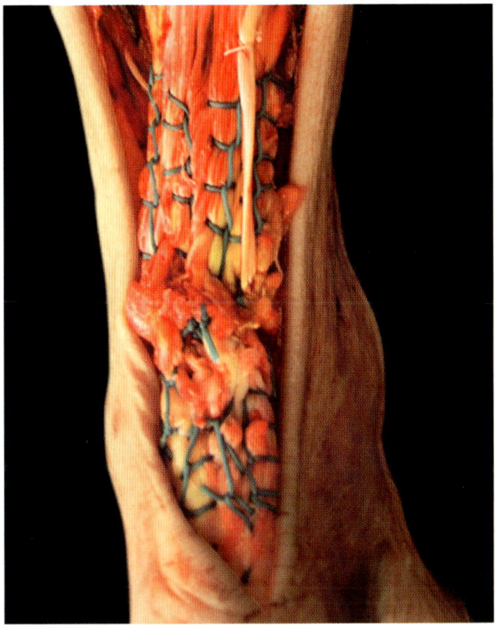

Fig. 10: An example of Krackow suture technique is demonstrated resulting in four core stitches

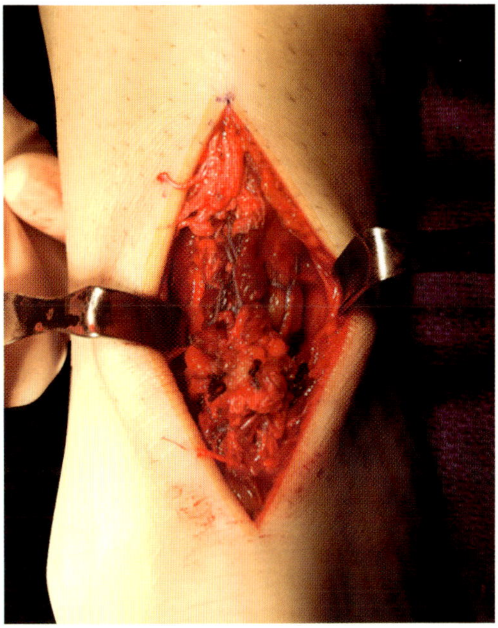

Fig. 11: Completed open repair of proximal (non-insertional) Achilles tendon rupture is shown including epitenon repair

Epitenon stitches are then placed with 0 vicryl or 2-0 vicryl and then tagged with hemostats for tying later. Figure of eight stitches are placed over the anterior surface of the tendon since access to that area for repair is not feasible after the Krackow stitches are tied into place.

Ankle dorsiflexion is set to match the uninjured side (usually 15–20° of plantarflexion). Sterile towels are placed to support the dorsum of the foot to hold position. The sutures are pulled to advance the tendon ends together to evaluate the tightness of the repair to make sure that it will not be under undue tension.

The Achilles tendon is then repaired and the sutures are tied in sequence. While the surgical assistant holds tension on the Krackow stitches to have the tendon ends approximated, the surgeon ties and secures the first series of Krackow stitches. This is repeated until all of the four core sutures are tied. Then, the anterior epitenon stitches are tied and secured. No anterior gapping of the tendon is present. Finally, the posterior epitenon stitches are placed in a figure of eight fashion, simultaneously burying the fiberwire knots so that they are not prominent. The epitenon stitches also help to contour the tendon's shape. The final repair is shown (Fig. 11).

Copious irrigation of the wound is then performed followed by a layered closure with careful technique. The paratenon is repaired with interrupted 2-0 vicryl and 4-0 vicryl absorbable stitches. The wound is irrigated again. The subdermal tissue is repaired with 4-0 vicryl subcutaneous sutures. Finally, the skin is closed with 4-0 nylon simple and mattress sutures to make sure that the skin edges are properly everted to aid in wound healing.

The dressing is placed and tourniquet is released. Then, a well-padded short leg posterior and sugar tong splint is applied in slight plantarflexion.

Surgical Technique of Repair of Insertional Achilles Rupture

Insertional Achilles ruptures are repaired via an open incision to ensure that the tendon is repaired back down to its footprint on the posterior calcaneus. Additionally, there may be insertional tendinopathy with calcaneal spur formation through which the rupture occurred. To maximize tendon healing and minimize residual posterior heel pain in the future, all degenerative tissue and ossifications should be removed so that healthy Achilles tendon tissue can be repaired to healthy calcaneal bone.

Surgical Technique Steps for Repair of Insertional Rupture

Anesthesia, tourniquet placement, and patient positioning are the same as that described for the percutaneous repair technique.

An L-shaped incision is made to allow for a thick skin flap that can be retracted to expose the entire posterior tuberosity of the calcaneus and the distal Achilles tendon. The longitudinal portion of the incision is placed slightly medial to midline and progresses distally toward the medial border of calcaneus. The transverse limb of the incision is made at the glaborous skin junction (just inferior to any posterior calcaneal spur that may be present).

After the skin incision is made, the paratenon is identified and incised. Using no touch skin technique where only the subdermal tissue is grasped with the forceps, a thick flap including the paratenon is elevated off of the Achilles tendon and calcaneus. A 2-0 suture is temporarily placed in the thick skin flap to keep it retracted laterally to allow for surgical exposure during the case. Moistened sponges are placed over the flap during the procedure.

The remaining distal Achilles tendon stump is identified and evaluated. Degenerative tissue or unhealthy appearing tissue is debrided with a rongeur.

The posterior calcaneus is inspected for insertional tendinopathy spur formation. If present, the posterior spur is removed via a sagittal sawblade placed parallel to the normal posterior surface of the calcaneus aiming distally. Once the cut is made, it is completed with an osteotome and the bone fragments are mobilized and removed. If a Haglund deformity is also present, it is also removed. The posterior calcaneus is prepared with the saw to create a normal contour and a healthy, bleeding bone surface to which the tendon will be reattached.

A suture-bridge technique is utilized to restore the footprint of the Achilles tendon attachment and provide a high strength repair. Two suture anchors that are double-loaded are placed in the upper left and right corner of the posterior calcaneal surface (Fig. 12).

One set of sutures from each anchor will be placed to restore the proximal attachment point of the Achilles. With the ankle slightly plantarflexed (preferably matching the normal resting position of the uninjured side or about 15°), a Kocher clamp is used to gently grab the tendon end and advance it toward its insertion. This gives the surgeon an idea of where the initial mattress stitches should be placed. One set of sutures are selected from each anchor (The second set of sutures are clamped and put to the side). A mattress stitch with the tendon reduced is performed with stitches from each anchor. Then, a Krackow stitch is done proximally up the left half of the tendon and the right half of the tendon with those sutures. Knots then are tied to secure each suture limb to the other on the anterior surface of the tendon (Fig. 13).

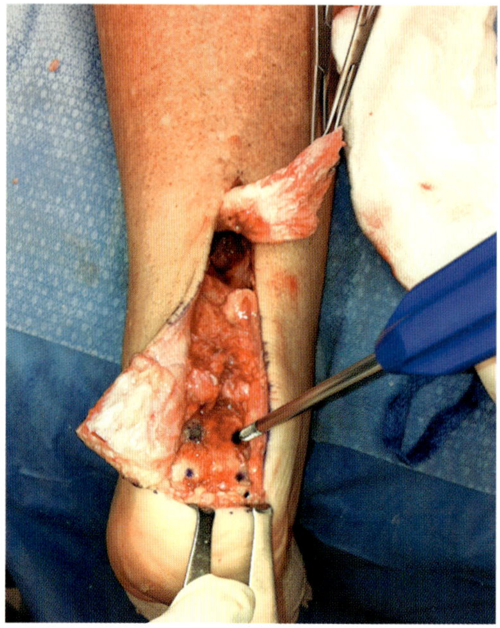

Fig. 12: Repair of insertional rupture utilizing a suture-bridge technique. Two double-loaded suture anchors are placed superiorly in the calcaneus after the calcaneal bone bed is prepared

The second set of sutures from each anchor will aid in coaptating the distal Achilles tendon to its central and distal footprint, much like a double row arthroscopic rotator cuff repair. The clamps are removed on the second set of sutures from the left and right suture anchors. The needles are passed from inferior to superior through the Achilles to allow for separation of the suture limbs. Once those four sutures are passed through the tendon, the needles are cut off and one limb from each anchor is selected and tagged with a hemostat (Fig. 14). Drill holes now are made with a drill bit designed for a knotless suture anchor system in the lower left and lower right corner of the prepared calcaneal surface. The tagged sutures are released and the two limbs are threaded through the knotless suture anchor's

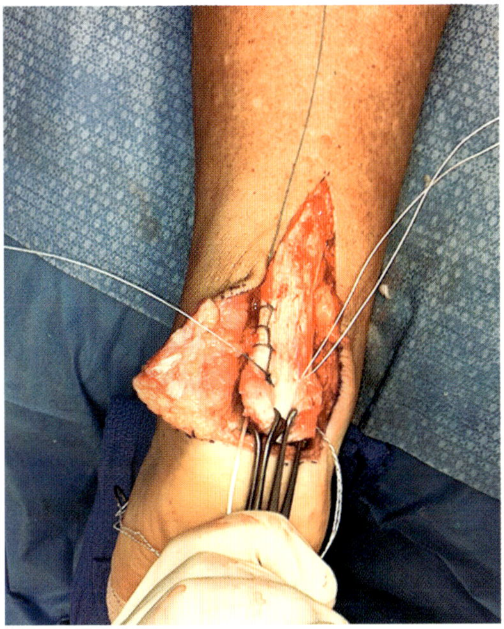

Fig. 13: Repair of insertional rupture. Mattress sutures are placed to recreate the superior footprint of the Achilles tendon. The left side is complete with placement of Krackow stitches. The right side would then be sutured similarly

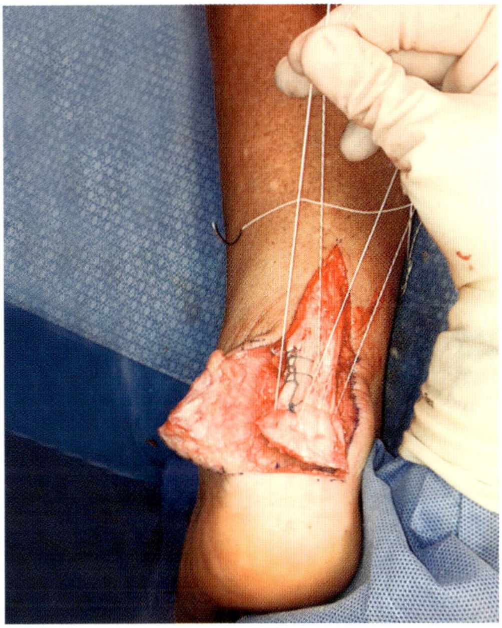

Fig. 14: Repair of insertional rupture. The second set of sutures from the double-loaded suture anchors are passed through the tendon. One suture from each anchor is paired with the other as shown

eyelet (Fig. 15). The tendon tissue is properly tensioned by pulling on the sutures as the knotless anchor is advanced and seated into the bone using a mallet. The process is repeated with a second knotless anchor to complete the repair. This creates a criss-cross pattern of suture and restoration of the Achilles footprint (Fig. 16).

The repair is evaluated and Thompson test is performed. If satisfactory, copious irrigation of the wound is performed. Wound closure, dressings, and splinting are done as described for the open repair previously.

Postoperatively, the management is similar to that described for the percutaneous and open repairs. Careful heel wound protection and monitoring is required. Sutures are usually removed later at 3–4 weeks post surgery to ensure healing. Depending on the patient's health and body habitus, weight-bearing is initiated at 4 or 6 weeks, postoperatively. A functional rehabilitation program is utilized.

OTHER SURGICAL OPTIONS

In the setting of acute Achilles tendon ruptures, additional techniques have been described to augment the primary end-to-end repair. It is felt

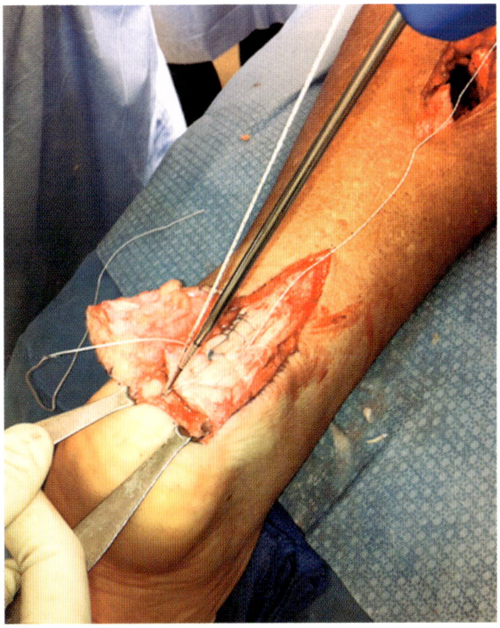

Fig. 15: Repair of insertional rupture. The paired sutures are passed through the eyelet of a knotless suture anchor and the anchor is seated after proper tensioning of the suture limbs. Another anchor on the lower right side would then be placed

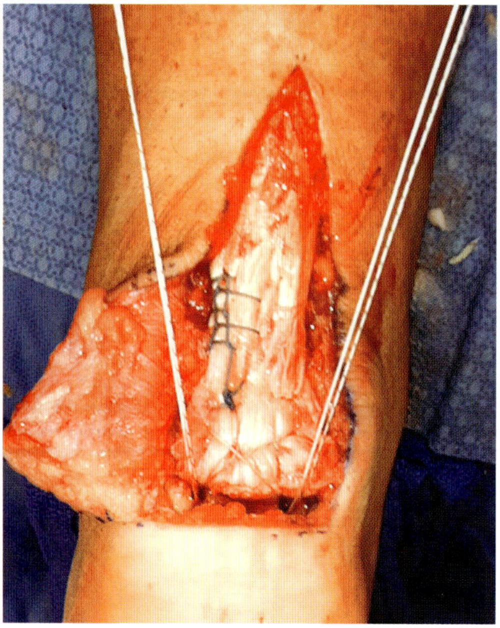

Fig. 16: Completed repair of insertional rupture. The Achilles footprint is reestablished and the sutures from the knotless anchors are trimmed flush with the bone

that augmentation techniques may yield higher tensile strength of the repair, enable a more aggressive rehabilitation program, and decrease re-rupture rates. Unfortunately, these augmentation techniques have lead to increases in incision length, surgical time, bulkiness of the repair, infection rates (up to 4%), and wound complications as compared to nonaugmented repairs. Augmentation techniques include turn down gastrocnemius flaps, polypropylene braid, polyethylene mesh, and local tendon transfers [fascia lata, plantaris, FHL, flexor digitorium longus (FDL), peroneals]. In one recent prospective randomized study comparing augmented (10 mm wide central gastrocnemius aponeurosis turn-down flap) vs nonaugmented fresh Achilles ruptures, there was no difference in outcomes, thus routine augmentation of acute rupture repairs is not supported and offers no advantage over simple end-to-end repairs with Krackow locking loop technique.[49]

Surgical Complications and Salvage

As discussed earlier in the management section, complications can occur from surgical repair of the ruptured Achilles tendon and the surgeon should be familiar with salvage techniques or algorithms that can be applied intraoperatively or postoperatively.

Intraoperative

Problem 1

To repair the Achilles tendon stumps end-to-end or to reattach a distal Achilles tendon rupture, due to tissue quality or loss, the ankle has to be excessively plantarflexed at or past 30°. The surgeon does not want to repair the tear under undue tension.

Potential Solution to Problem 1

The surgeon can perform a proximal V-Y Achilles tendon lengthening.

Surgical Steps

The surgeon measures the gap between tendon ends with proper positioning of the ankle (Gaps greater than 3 cm usually require a tendon transfer but such large gaps are rare in the setting of acute Achilles tendon ruptures. Tendon transfers will be discussed later in this and other chapters).

An additional longitudinal incision is made proximally over the musculotendinous junction. Dissection through the soft tissues is performed and the medial sural cutaneous branch is identified and protected. Occasionally, there may be additional fasical or fatty tissue layers that the dissection has to proceed through to reach the aponeurosis.

Deeper retractors are inserted medially and laterally to visualize the aponeurosis and its tendinous margins (Fig. 17).

The 'V' is outlined on the aponeurosis with the apex of the 'V' pointing cephald. The length of each limb of the 'V' has to be 1.5 times that of the measured gap (i.e. a 2 cm gap requires a 3 cm length for each limb).

Using a no. 11-blade, a sawing motion is used to make an angled cut in the aponeurosis only along the limbs of the 'V,' leaving the underlying muscle intact (Fig. 17). There are generally deeper fascial bands that can be visualized by applying distal traction on the proximal tendon stump. These bands have to be sharply released with a no. 11-blade or tenotomy scissors in order to get maximum tissue advancement.

By pulling distal traction on the newly created intermediate segment, the proximal Achilles stump can now be mobilized so that direct end-to-end

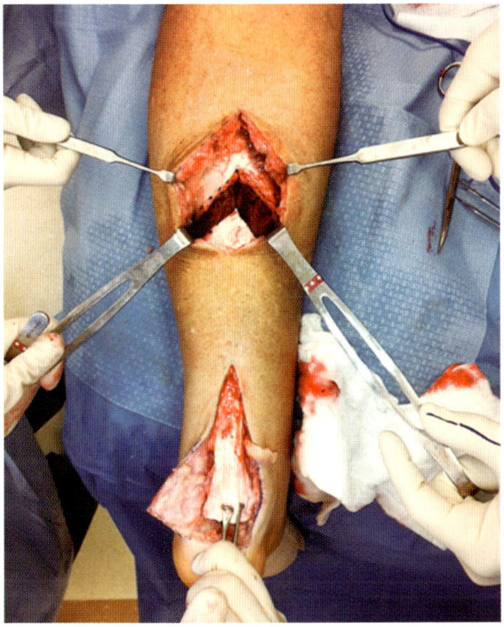

Fig. 17: Proximal V-Y lengthening procedure. The aponeurosis is identified after dissecting through adipose tissue and sometimes a few fascial layers. The 'V' cut is completed after the deep fascial bands are released. Traction is placed on distal stump to determine amount of advancement available

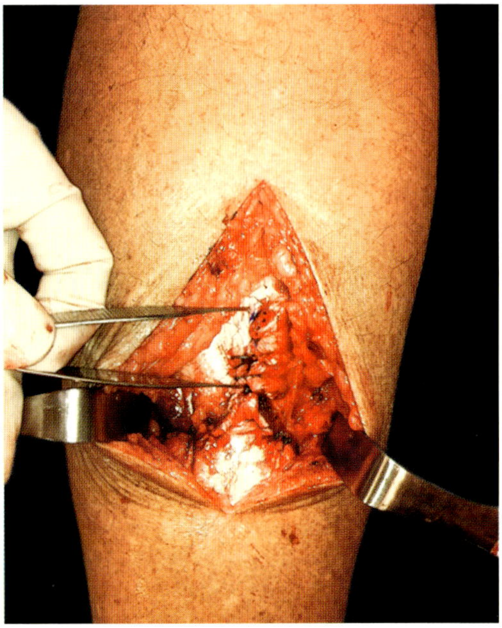

Fig. 18: Proximal V-Y lengthening procedure. The repair and lengthening are completed. The tips of the forceps mark the vertical portion of the 'Y' which indicates the amount of distal advancement

repair or distal tendon to calcaneus repair can be performed. The position of the ankle is set and the tendon is repaired as discussed previously in this chapter.

While maintaining the desired slight plantar-flexion or neutral dorsiflexion position, the 'V' now becomes a 'Y.' The vertical component of the 'Y' represents the amount of lengthening achieved. The aponeurosis is now repaired with no. 2 fiberwire stitches (Arthrex, Naples, FL) utilizing mattress and simple sutures, with the completed repair (Fig. 18).

Problem 2

The surgeon finds that the remaining tendon tissue is poor in quality and repair is not felt to be substantial.

Potential Solutions to Problem 2

The surgeon can utilize augmentation techniques to reinforce the repair.

Surgical Steps

If the surgeon elects to perform a turn down gastrocnemius aponeurosis flap,[50] a 10 mm wide segment is outlined in the central aspect of the proximal stump. The length of this central tongue of tissue was determined by the need to overlap with the distal Achilles stump by 2–3 cm. The depth of the flap is 1/3 to 1/2 of the tendon thickness from anterior to posterior. The flap is harvested with a no. 11-blade, keeping the distal portion of the proximal stump intact by a few centimeters. Then, the flap is flipped backwards 180° on itself and is sutured to the proximal and distal stumps utilizing simple sutures as originally described (mattress or Krackow sutures could also be used). The proximal rent in the tissue created by the turn down flap is repaired side to side.

If the surgeon elects to use the plantaris tendon as a local graft, it is better with respect to repair strength to weave the plantaris through the Achilles tendon, rather than just trying to fan out a very small structure and wrap it around the repair. The plantaris tendon can be released proximally with an open-ended tendon stripper. A whipstitch with 2-0 vicryl is placed in the plantaris tendon stump to help with passage and final tensioning. The tendon then is woven through the proximal stump first from medial to lateral. A curved tendon transfer clamp can be used to make passage through the Achilles tendon easier. The plantaris tendon then is passed through the distal stump from laterally to medially. At each entrance and exit point from the Achilles tendon, the plantaris tendon is secured into place with suture. If there is still tendon length left, the plantaris end is then either sutured to itself or fanned out and wrapped around the repair.

If the Achilles tendon tissue is diffusely degenerative, the surgeon may elect to perform an FHL tendon transfer to bring a better blood supply to the tendon and suture the tendon transfer into the repair. The fascia deep to the Achilles is released longitudinally with tenotomy scissors and the muscle belly of the FHL is readily seen (Fig. 19). The tendinous portion travelling medially toward the posterior medial talus is identified and the retinaculum is released. A retractor is placed underneath the FHL muscle belly to pull tension and visualize the tendinous portion. If there is not a large gap to reconstruct, the FHL tendon can be harvested at this point at the sustentacular tunnel sharply with a knife. The muscle belly of the FHL is brought to the anterior surface of the Achilles and sutured into place and around the repair site. After placement of a whipstitch in the stump of the FHL tendon with 2-0 vicryl, the FHL tendinous portion can be either passed through a tunnel in the calcaneus from medial to lateral and secured with a biotenodesis screw, or it can be woven through the distal stump of the Achilles using a curved tendon transfer clamp or curved hemostat or Kelly clamp. The FHL tendon is secured and sutured into place after tensioning (Fig. 20).

Postoperative

Problem 3

The patient has wound healing problems after open repair of an Achilles tendon rupture.

Potential Solutions for Problem 3

First the surgeon should determine the size of the wound and whether the wound involvement is superficial or deep or if there is any evidence of infection that would require antibiotics and/or surgical irrigation and debridement. If there is any retained suture material causing a granuloma or suture abscess, it should be removed in the office. If the wound base is red and healthy appearing and

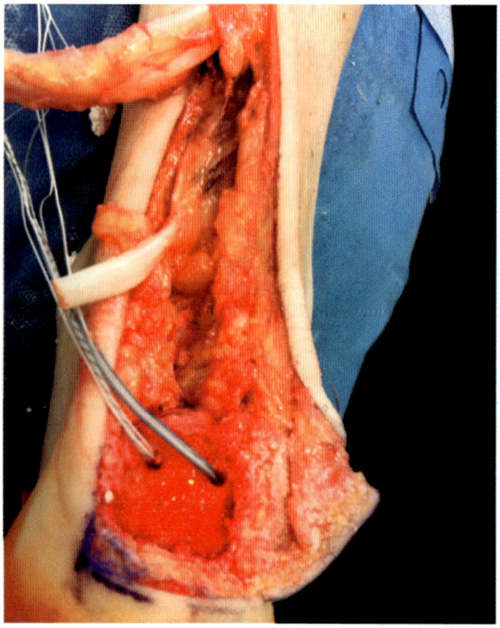

Fig. 19: Flexor hallucis longus (FHL) tendon transfer. After the deep fascia beneath or anterior to the Achilles is released the muscle belly of the FHL is seen and the tendon can be followed distally and transected for tendon transfer. FHL tendon for transfer is seen just anterior to the Achilles tendon stump

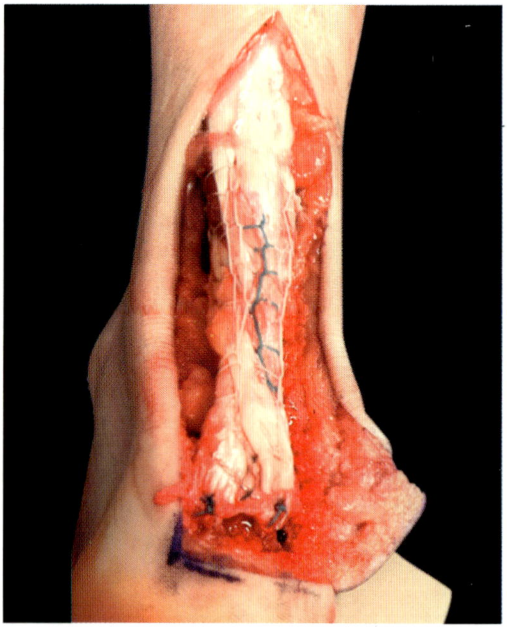

Fig. 20: FHL tendon transfer. The FHL tendon is sutured to the distal Achilles stump to augment the repair and the muscle belly is sutured around the proximal Achilles tendon to improve vascularity to the tendon

the tendon is not exposed, then simple dressings paratenon level, a vacuum assisted closure, skin grafting, or both may be needed. In some instances, a local rotational or vascularized flap may be needed.

Problem 4

The patient sustains acute re-rupture of their Achilles tendon after repair.

Potential Solutions to Problem 4

The surgeon should try to identify the cause or mode of failure, biological or biomechanical. If it was a reinjury, then was the patient fully rehabilitated or was the postoperative rehabilitation protocol too aggressive? Was the repair strong enough, biomechanically, and did failure occur from suture pullout or knot rupture? Was the repair placed under too much tension and was the ankle hyperplantarflexed at the time of repair? If there is poor quality of the healing tissue, are there patient-related factors that contribute and could be neutralized with treatment or other interventions? Was there any infectious process that contributed?

Treatment options at this point include conservative vs revision surgery. If tendon ends can be coaptated, then nonoperative treatment can be instituted in lower demand patients who have medical conditions that raise the risks of surgery. In higher demand patients and athletes, revision surgery utilizing a tendon transfer is considered and generally recommended. Reconstruction with an Achilles allograft with the bone plug inserted into the calcaneus may also be an option but there are concerns regarding time for graft incorporation, graft strength, and rare disease transmission.

Surgical Steps for Flexor Hallucis Longus Tendon Transfer

Previous steps are outlined as part of Problem 2.

To gain extra length of the FHL graft, a second longitudinal incision is made starting distal to the navicular and proceeding just inferior to the border of the first metatarsal along the superior border of the abductor hallucis.

Careful hemostasis with bipolar cautery is performed as the dissection plane in between the abductor and the first metatarsal is deepened and a venous plexus is encountered.

Self-retaining retractors are placed in the wound. The FHL and FDL tendons are identified (FHL is deeper and lateral to the FDL). The knot of Henry is visualized. The medial plantar artery and plantar nerve run deep and lateral to the FHL tendon and so a retractor or freer elevator is passed underneath the FHL tendon. The FHL tendon is carefully transected under direct visualization as distal as needed to gain appropriate graft length. Soft tissue connections between the harvested FHL and the FDL are released and the FHL tendon is pulled into the posterior wound by pulling on the muscle belly.

Tenodesis of FHL stump to the FDL can be performed but rarely is done as enough residual plantarflexion strength in the great toe is maintained. The literature has not shown any significant clinical morbidity as a consequence of FHL transfer.

Utilizing a drill bit of similar size as the FHL tendon graft, a bony tunnel is drilled transversely in the posterior tuberosity of the calcaneus, making sure that adequate bony bridges are present so that the tunnel is secure. A whipstitch with 2-0 vicryl suture is placed in the FHL tendon stump to tubularize the stump and facilitate graft passage through the tunnel. The entry and exit points of the tunnel are cleared of debris with a currette. A Hewson suture passer is placed from lateral to medial and the FHL stump suture is placed through the loop and pulled out of the tunnel laterally.

The ankle is placed in 15–20° of dorsiflexion and the graft is pulled through the tunnel and out the lateral side. If the surgeon wishes to use biotenodesis screws, then the appropriately sized biotenodesis screw which corresponds to the drill bit used to create the tunnel is inserted while tension is maintained on the graft. One screw or two screws (one medially and one laterally) can be used. The final repair is shown in Figure 21. Otherwise, the graft can be tied onto itself with no. 2 fiberwire and incorporated via suturing into the remaining proximal and distal Achilles tendon tissue to fill the gap.

Problem 5

Tendon elongation has occurred after repair with decreased push-off strength and increased passive dorsiflexion.

Potential Solutions to Problem 5

Tendon elongation has been shown to be associated with poorer functional results after rupture repair.

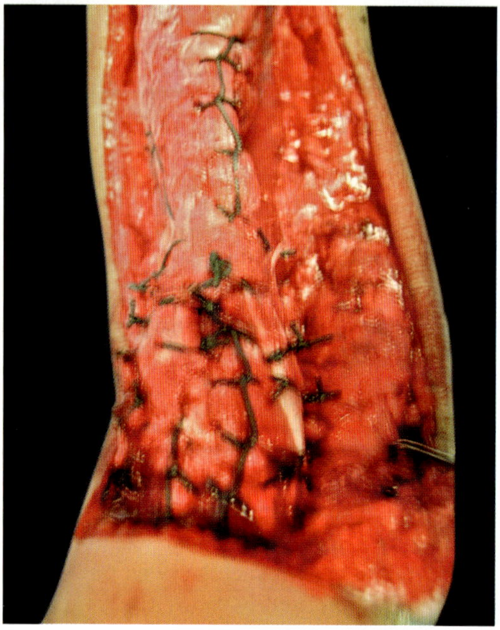

Fig. 21: Flexor hallucis longus tendon transfer. The FHL transfer is passed medially to laterally through a bone tunnel in the calcaneus. The remaining length of the FHL tendon is seen laterally (on right side) as it is sutured to itself and the Achilles tendon

Tendon elongation can be addressed by focusing on rehabilitation of the primary and secondary plantar flexors and working on ankle proprioception and neuromuscular facilitation. In an attempt to reestablish normal length of the muscle, so called 'inner range' exercises that utilize contractions of the triceps surae in its shortest position, combined with eccentric exercises may lead to improved sarcomere adaptation. These muscular adaptations essentially result in the re-establishment of proper sarcomere length by altering the serial sarcomere number. Also, tendons in subjects with more muscle strength have been found to be stiffer. Building muscle mass may aid in force generation and energy storage capacity of the tendon. Finally, with the sparse information available, surgical shortening of the tendon does not appear to be a feasible option.

CONCLUSION

Treatment of Achilles tendon ruptures is challenging. The optimal treatment and rehabilitation methods are elusive. During the decision-making process regarding a treatment option for an individual patient, the surgeon should have a long discussion with the patient regarding expectations, previous activity level, co-morbid health conditions, compliance ability with an intensive rehabilitation program, and risks and benefits of nonoperative vs surgical treatment. Success can be achieved with or without surgery. A functional accelerated rehabilitation protocol after rupture leads to improved outcomes in both nonoperative and operative patients. Nonoperative treatment has a lower overall complication rate and outcomes are approaching those of surgical repair in a few more recent studies. But, surgical repair has the advantages of a lower re-rupture rate, improved push-off strength, and a higher rate of return to sports activities. However, it is associated with a higher complication rate. If surgery is performed, attention to careful patient selection, soft tissue handling, surgical timing, and postoperative management is essential to avoid wound healing and other complications. When complications do occur, the surgeon should have knowledge of additional salvage procedures that can be employed.

REFERENCES

1. Leppilahti J, Puranen J, Orava S. Incidence of Achilles tendon rupture. Acta Orthop Scand 1996;67:277-9.
2. Lea RB, Smith L. Nonsurgical treatment of tendo achillis rupture. J Bone Joint Surg Am 1972;54; 1398-1407.
3. Sode J, Obel N, Hallas J, et al. Use of fluoroquinolone and risk of achilles tendon rupture: A population-based cohort study. Eur J Clin Pharmacol 2007;63(5): 499-503.
4. Casparian JM, Luchi M, Moffat RE, et al. Quinolones and tendon ruptures. South Med J. 2000;93(5): 488-91.
5. Burdett RG. Forces predicted at the ankle during running. Med Sci Sports Exerc 1982;14:308-16.
6. Cummins JE, Anson JB, Carr WB, et al. The structure of the calcaneal tendon (of Achilles) in relation to orthopaedic surgery with additional observations on the plantaris muscle. Surg Gynecol Obstet 1946;83: 107-16.
7. Schepsis AA, Jones H, Hass AL. Achilles tendon disorders in athletes. Am J Sports Med 2002;30 (2):287-305.
8. Barfred T. Experimental rupture of the Achilles tendon. Comparison of various types of experimental ruptures in rats. Acta Orthop Scand 1971;42:528-43.
9. O'Brien M. The anatomy of the Achilles tendon. Foot Ankle Clin. 2005;10:225-38.
10. Carr AJ, Norris SH. The blood supply of the calcaneal tendon J Bone Joint Surg Br 1989;71(1);100-1.

11. Lagergren C, Lindholm A. Vascular distribution in the Achilles tendon: An angiographic and microangiographic study. Acta Chir Scand 1959;116:491-5.
12. O'Brien T. The needle test for complete rupture of the Achilles tendon. J Bone Joint Surg Am 1984;66: 1099-1101.
13. Maffulli N. The clinical diagnosis of subcutaneous tear of the Achilles tendon. A prospective study in 174 patients. Am J Sports Med 1998;26:266-70.
14. Thompson TC. A test for rupture of the tendo Achillis. Acta Orthop Scand 1962;32:461-5.
15. Copeland SA. Rupture of the Achilles tendon: a new clinical test. Ann R Coll Surg Engl 1990;72:270-1.
16. Hartgerink P, Fessell DP, Jacobson JA, et al. Full versus partial thickness Achilles tendon tears: Sonographic accuracy and characterization in 26 cases with surgical correlation. Radiology 2001;220: 406-12.
17. Willits K, Amendola A, Bryant D, et al. Operative versus nonoperative treatment of acute Achilles tendon ruptures: a multicenter randomized trial using accelerated functional rehabilitation. J Bone Joint Surg Am. 2010;92(17):2767-75.
18. Khan RJ, Carey Smith RL. Surgical interventions for treating acute Achilles tendon ruptures. Cochrane Database Syst Rev 2010;8:CD003674.
19. Wong J, Barrass V, Maffulli N. Quantitative review of operative and nonoperative management of achilles tendon ruptures. Am J Sports Med 2002; 30(4):565-75.
20. Cetti R, Steen-Erik C, Ejsted R, et al. Operative versus nonoperative treatment of Achilles tendon rupture: A prospective randomized study and review of the literature. Am J Sports Med 1993;21:791-9.
21. Khan RJ, Fick D, Keogh A, et al. Treatment of acute Achilles tendon ruptures. A meta-analysis of randomized, controlled trials. J Bone Joint Surg Am 2005;87:2202-10.
22. Kotnis R, David S, Handley R, et al. Dynamic ultrasound as a selection tool reducing achilles tendon reruptures. Am J Sports Med 2006;34: 1395-1400.
23. Poynton AR, O'Rourke K. An analysis of skin perfusion over the achilles tendon in varying degrees of plantarflexion. Foot Ankle Int 2001:22:572-4.
24. Akizuki KH, Gartman EJ, Nisonson B, et al. The relative stress on the Achilles tendon during ambulation in an ankle immobiliser: Implications for rehabilitation after Achilles tendon repair. Br J Sports Med 2001;35:329-33.
25. Enwemeka CS, Speilholz NI, Nelson AJ. The effect of early functional activities on experimentally tenotomized Achilles tendons in rats. Am J Phys Med Rehabil 1988;67:264-9.
26. Saleh M, Marshall PD, Senior R, et al. The Sheffield splint for controlled early mobilization after rupture of the calcaneal tendon. A prospective, randomized comparison with plaster treatment. J Bone Joint Surg Br 1992;74:206-9.
27. Wallace RG, Traynor IE, Kernohan WG, et al. Combined conservative and orthotic management of acute ruptures of the Achilles tendon. J Bone Joint Surg Am 2004;86:1198-1202.
28. Twaddle BC, Poon P. Early motion for Achilles tendon ruptures: Is surgery important? A randomized, prospective study. Am J Sports Med 2007;35: 2033-8.
29. Hufner TM, Brandes DB, Thermann H, et al. Long term results after functional nonoperative treatment of Achilles tendon rupture. Foot Ankle Int 2006;27:167-71.
30. Paoloni J, De Vos RJ, Hamilton B, et al. Platelet-rich plasma treatment for ligament and tendon injuries. Clin J Sports Med 2011;21(1):37-45.
31. Gabel S, Manoli A. Neglected rupture of the Achilles tendon. Foot Ankle Int 1994;15:512-7.
32. Bruggeman N, Turner N, Dahm DL, et al. Wound complications after open Achilles tendon repair: An analysis of risk factors. Clin Orthop Relat Res. 2004;427:63-6.
33. Olsson N, Nilsson-Helander K, Karlsson J, et al. Major functional deficits persists 2 years after acute Achilles tendon rupture. Knee Surg Sports Traumatol Arthroscopy. 2011;19(8):1385-93.
34. Garrick JG. Does accelerated functional rehabilitation after surgery improve outcomes in patients with acute achilles tendon ruptures? Clin J Sport Med. 2012;22(4):379-80.
35. Labib SA, Rolf R, Dacus R, et al. The 'Giftbox' repair of the Achilles tendon: A modification of the Krackow technique. Foot Ankle Int 2009;30(5): 410-4.
36. Magnussen RA, Glisson RR, Mooreman CT. Augmentation of Achilles tendon repair with extracellular matrix xenograft: a biomechanical analysis. Am J Sports Med 2011;39(7):1522-7.
37. Fukashiro S, Komi PV, Järvinen M, et al. In vivo Achilles tendon loading during jumping in humands. Eur J Appl Physiol Occup Physiol 1995;71(5): 453-8.
38. Lee SJ, Sileo MJ, Kremenic IJ, et al. Cyclic loading of 3 Achilles tendon repairs simulating early postoperative forces. Am J Sports Med 2009;37(4):786-90.
39. Kangas J, Pajala A, Ohtonen P, et al. Achilles tendon elongation after rupture repair: A randomized comparison of 2 postoperative regimens. Am J Sports Med. 2007;35(1):59-64.
40. Suchak AA, Bostick GP, Beaupré LA, et al. The influence of early weight-bearing compared with nonweightbearing after surgical repair of the Achilles tendon. J Bone Joint Surg Am 2008;90(9):1876-83.

41. Cretnik A, Kosanovic M, Smorkolj V. Percutaneous versus open repair of the ruptured Achilles tendon: A comparative study. Am J Sports Med. 2005;33(9): 1369-79.
42. Klein W, Lang DM, Saleh M. The use of the Ma Griffith technique for percutaneous repair of fresh ruptured tendo Achillis. Chir Organi Mov. 1991; 76(3):223-8.
43. Assal M, Jung M, Stern R, et al. Limited open repair of Achilles tendon ruptures: A technique with a new instrument and findings of a prospective multicenter study. J Bone Joint Surg Am. 2002;84(2):161-70.
44. Ismail M, Karim A, Shulman R, et al. The Achillon Achilles tendon repair: Is it strong enough? Foot Ankle Int. 2008;29(8):808-13.
45. Hockenbury RT, Johns JC. A biomechanical in vitro comparison of open versus percutaneous repair fo tendon Achilles. Foot Ankle 1990;11(2):67-72.
46. Web JM, Bannister GC. Percutaneous repair of the ruptured tendo Achillis. J Bone Joint Surg Br. 1999;81(5):877-80.
47. Majewski M, Rohrbach M, Czaja S, et al. Avoiding sural nerve injuries during percutaneous Achilles tendon repair. Am J Sports Med 2006;34(5):793-8.
48. McMahon SE, Smith TO, Hing CB. A meta-analysis of randomised controllled trials comparing conventional to minimally invasive approaches for repair of an Achilles tendon rupture. Foot Ankle Surg. 2011;17(4):211-7.
49. Pajala A, Kangas J, Siira P, et al. Augmented compared with nonaugmented surgical repair of fresh total achilles tendon rupture. A prospective randomized study. J Bone Joint Surg Am. 2009;91:1092-100.
50. Gerdes MH, Brown TD, Bell AL, et al. A flap augmentation technique for Achilles tendon repair. Postoperative strength and functional outcome. Clin Orthop Relat Res 1992;280:241-6.

33

Haglund Deformity, Retrocalcaneal Bursitis, and "Pump Bumps"

John S Gould

INTRODUCTION

Pain in the region of the posterior heel, particularly near on or involving the insertion of the tendo-Achilles may have several causes and requires an accurate diagnosis for appropriate treatment. Confusion concerning the actual diagnosis has led to spurious diagnoses, nomenclature, and often empiric and inadequate treatment. The differential diagnosis with posterior heel pain include the titles in this section, which pertain to the tendo-Achilles, and posterior ankle impingement secondary to soft tissue, a symptomatic os trigonum, and afflictions of the flexor hallucis longus behind the subtalar joint. Posterior impingement is seen most commonly in dancers, particularly in ballet, and will be discussed elsewhere. This also includes tenosynovitis of the flexor hallucis, the "jumping toe" phenomenon seen with triggering of the flexor as it passes through the fibro-osseous tunnel behind the medial posterior ankle and subtalar joints.

Diagnosis of these various conditions requires attention to the history, careful examination, plain X-rays, and on occasion, use of the magnetic resonance imaging (MRI) and ultrasound. The history of insidious onset is common to all these conditions, with the exception of ruptures which usually occur as a sudden painful event. A recent increase in the extent of physical activity may be an inciting cause. The appearance of a swelling or prominence and the exact location of this finding are helpful. Finally, palpation for the exact location of the painful structure and crepitus under the examining finger can make the diagnosis obvious. X-rays can demonstrate bony deformities and soft tissue swelling. MRIs can be supportive, particularly for surgical planning.

HAGLUND DEFORMITY AND RETROCALCANEAL BURSITIS

Prominence of the posterior superior aspect of the calcaneal tuberosity, when it is excessive, has been implicated as a source of pain behind the ankle (Fig. 1).[1] There has been no consensus, however, concerning when the angle of the bone is excessive or on how much to remove of it at surgery. Clinically, there may be prominence or swelling on both sides of the tendo-Achilles, but not over the tendon itself. There may also be tenderness directly over the tendon insertion distal to the ankle joint and on either or both sides of the tendon. The patient may complain of aching up the leg, but the tendon above the insertion is not tender, has a smooth feel and no crepitus. The sagittal X-ray shows soft tissue swelling anterior to the tendon, but no changes of the tendon contour or bone within the substance of the tendon. An MRI will confirm a soft tissue swelling anterior to the tendon which could be interpreted as fluid or an amorphous soft tissue mass. The flexor hallucis will be normal and there should be no reaction in the bone.

The use of an elevated heel on the shoe, a lift inside the heel of the shoe, and a padded sleeve or over-the-counter appliance which combines padding around the posterior heel and a lift are available for conservative treatment (Fig. 2) along with oral anti-inflammatories.[2] Aspiration and injection with steroids is done, but is of concern due to the potential of tendon injection and inciting of a rupture.[3] Advocates for an ultrasound-guided injection for accurate placement of the steroid support this approach.

For recalcitrant cases, a surgical approach can be considered. A longitudinal incision just medial to

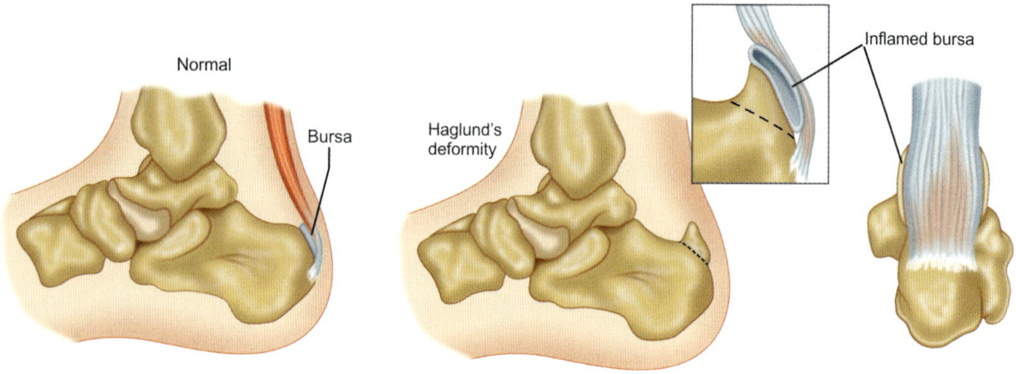

Fig. 1: The Haglund deformity and retrocalcaneal bursitis

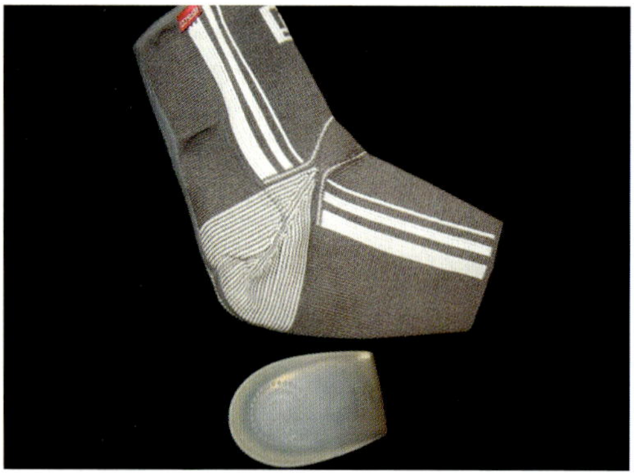

Fig. 2: Posterior heel cushion and lift for retrocalcaneal bursitis and insertional tendinosis of the tendo-Achilles

the tendo-Achilles is posterior to the neurovascular bundle and avoids the sural nerve on the lateral side. The deep dissection anterior to the tendon, at the insertion, allows debridement of the retrocalcaneal space and an ostectomy of the posterior superior angle of the calcaneal tubercle. Granulation anterior to the tendon insertion or bursal material has been found in the space. A soft bulky dressing is utilized postoperatively and mobilization begun as soon as the wound allows.

In recent years, an endoscopic approach to the posterior retrocalcaneal space has been advocated and used successfully by the author for this condition. Under general anesthesia, with the patient in the prone position and without traction on the foot, arthroscopic portals are placed on either side of the tendo-Achilles aimed at the insertion area, anterior to the tendon. A Keith needle is placed through the tendon, from posterior to anterior, directed at the midpoint of the insertion for orientation. A 2.7 mm 30-degree-angle arthroscope is placed in one portal and a 4.0 mm shaver in the other. A tourniquet is used initially and the saline inflow rate is placed on gravity to avoid flooding the soft tissues. The retrocalcaneal space is a potential one which is realized by special orientation and creation by the shaver. Prolonging the procedure can create significant edema and a "whiteout effect". The needle used for orientation is a helpful adjunct initially. Release of the tourniquet will actually clear the field if the "whiteout" occurs. Once the soft tissue debridement is done, one works proximally up the slope of the calcaneus to the Haglund angle. Use of a burr is added to the initial work with the shaver. The blunting of the angle with the burr is a maneuver of questionable value but has been done traditionally and continues. No matter how much or little of the angle is taken, patients respond positively to the procedure as long as "insertional tendinosis" is not the proper diagnosis. Debridement of the tendon with the arthroscopic technique seems to be a risky maneuver and is not done by most surgeons. The outcomes of this surgery when retrocalcaneal bursitis is the appropriate procedure seem to be universally good with few if any complications. Relief of symptoms and a very prompt recovery and mobilization appear to be the rule.[4]

PUMP BUMPS

The Haglund deformity is frequently confused with the term, "pump bump". The Haglund deformity is seen on X-ray and other than swelling around the tendo-Achilles, is not visualized clinically. The "pump bump" is an exostosis located eccentrically on the posterolateral, sometimes medial, calcaneus. It is irritated by the posterior heel counter of a shoe, or lady's pump, but not caused by it. It becomes irritated with the formation of a swollen bursa over the bone. Lowering or eliminating the heel counter or wearing a sleeve with an inner layer of silicone padding, can ameliorate symptoms. Injection with steroids are painful, but can help, at least temporarily. Incision and ostectomy is the treatment of choice in recalcitrant patients.

REFERENCES

1. Stephens MM. Haglund's deformity and retrocalcaneal bursitis. Orthop Clin North Am. 1994;25(1):41-6.
2. Nicholson CW, Berlet GC, Lee TH. Prediction of the success of nonoperative treatment of insertional Achilles tendinosis based on MRI. Foot Ankle Int. 2007;28(4):472-7.
3. Jones JG. Achilles tendon rupture following steroid injection. J Bone Joint Surg Am. 1985;67(1):170.
4. Ortmann FW, McBryde AM. Endoscopic bony and soft-tissue decompression of the retrocalcaneal space for the treatment of Haglund deformity and retrocalcaneal bursitis. Foot Ankle Int. 2007;28(2):149-53.

34

Insertional Tendinosis of the Tendo-Achilles

John S Gould

INTRODUCTION

Insertional tendinosis of the tendo-Achilles is a disease of the tendon at the insertion occurring in middle age patients. It begins insidiously with swelling of the tendon and typically flares and recedes, often for years. The observation of swelling of the tendon at the insertion and with palpation, the tenderness, fullness, and irregularity of the tendon in this location makes the diagnosis fairly obvious (Fig. 1). On X-ray, the thickness of the tendon can be seen. As the condition persists or recurs, tendon deterioration occurs with the formation of vacuoles, and metaplasia (Fig. 2). Heterotopic bone, not calcium, forms in the tendon at the insertion. Initially it appears with what seems to be a spur into the tendon, usually referred to an enthesiophyte by radiologists (Fig. 3). As the condition progresses, more bone is formed, increasingly larger and more proximally.

Use of a heel protection device with padding and elevation of the heel (Fig. 4), as described above is helpful in relieving symptoms, as well as stretching exercises for the tendo-Achilles. Injection with steroids seems likely to provoke a rupture at the insertion, and some spontaneous ruptures have been reported to occur without injection. Although this condition may respond to conservative treatment early in its course, once tendon metaplasia has occurred, a chronic condition seems to be inevitable. Debridement of the retrocalcaneal bursa is not successful.

SURGICAL TREATMENT FOR INSERTIONAL TENDINOSIS

There are several approaches recommended for debridement of the tendo-Achilles insertion with advocates for accessing the tendon from the medial, lateral, and midline incisions. The consensus is to debride the diseased tendon from the anterior side either medially or laterally or to split the tendon in the midline and work to both directions from this starting point.[1-3] The author contends that the medial approach is preferable for the following reasons: (i) The medial side avoids damage to the branch of the sural nerve which runs alongside the lateral border of the tendon. (We have observed painful neuromas in patients in which the lateral approach

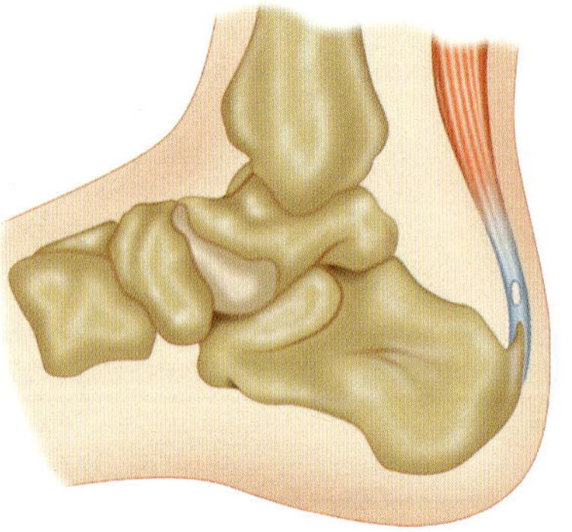

Fig. 1: Insertional tendinosis of the tendo-Achilles (artist's rendition)

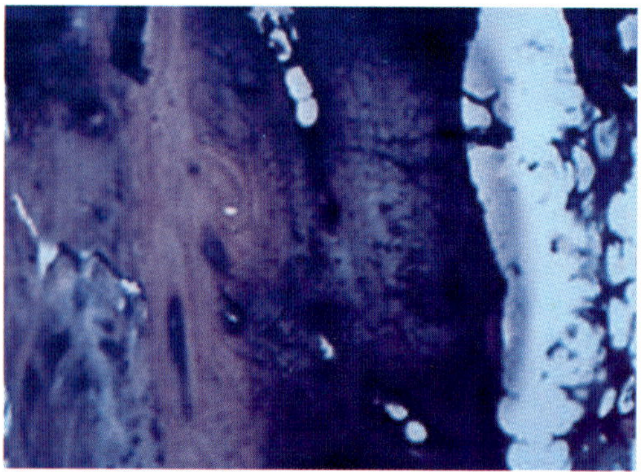

Fig. 2: Heterotopic bone in the insertion of the tendo-Achilles photomicrograph

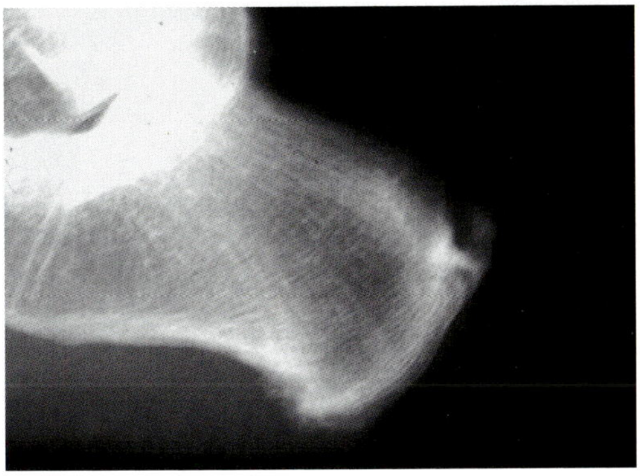

Fig. 3: Insertional tendinosis of the tendo-Achilles. The "enthesiophyte" at the insertion

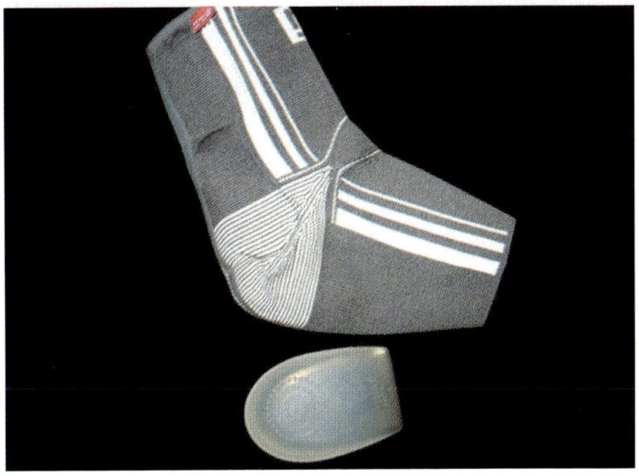

Fig. 4: Posterior heel cushion and lift for retrocalcaneal bursitis and insertional tendinosis of the tendo-Achilles

was taken. When we have to do salvage surgery on these patients, we go through the old incision and excised the sural nerve as part of the procedure); (ii) If a hypertrophic scar occurs with a longitudinal incision, it is less prominent and problematic than one developing in the midline; (iii) As the flap is raised over the medial to lateral side, venous drainage to the lesser saphenous vein is not impaired and at least theoretically, a wound slough seems to be less likely with this approach. In addition, the author believes that thorough debridement of the distal diseased tendon is important for the complete resolution of symptomatology. Consequently, with complete distal excision, the entire tendon will require proximal lengthening and distal reinsertion. It is altogether possible to achieve this without the need for a tendon transfer. Following the ostectomy of the hypertrophic bone at the insertion of the tendon and the posterosuperior angle of the calcaneal tubercle (Haglund's deformity), a new bed is prepared and a wide bone contact insertion is created.[4] Placing the insertion slightly more anteriorly led to a prediction of a 4% loss of power plantarflexion; whereas, in fact, none was observed in the clinical study.[5] The technique follows.

Technique for Debridement, Proximal Lengthening, and Reinsertion of the Tendo-Achilles for Insertional Tendinosis[3]

With the patient in the prone position, the tendon is approached, under tourniquet, with a medial incision along the course of the tendon and the medial gastrocsoleus muscle complex. Distally, a transverse limb made in the horizontal crease distal to the bony prominence within the underlying tendon. This component of the incision is carried down to the tendon and connects to the longitudinal incision. The medial edge of the paratenon is divided and this structure along with the subcutaneous tissue and skin is lifted off the tendon and muscle as a flap (Fig. 5). At the diseased insertion area of the tendon, the paratenon has become very adherent and it is debrided down to diseased but native tendon fibers and discarded. At this point, some surgeons and the author in the early stages of developing the current technique would attempt to debride the diseased tendon, attempting to preserve the insertion without having to reinsert. Nunley et al.[6] stated, following a bench cadaver study that if a third of the tendon at the insertion remained, the attachment was secure. The debridement, clinically, however, frequently led to a tenuous attachment. The current technique includes total detachment of the tendon from the bone. Under the tendon, a patch of granulation tissue is frequently found adjacent to the tendon and the insertion. The tendon is debrided easily with a #10 blade, shaving the layers of the anterior diseased tendon and also creating a bevel for later reattachment. Flecks of heterotopic bone are also sharply excised (Fig. 6).

The "enthesiophyte" is planed off with a micro-sagittal saw along with the prominence of the Haglund's deformity, creating a beveled broad bed of exposed cancellous bone for reattachment of the tendon (Fig. 7). Proximally, a V-Y lengthening is done of the gastrocnemius aponeurosis. The apex of the cut is proximal and the two limbs of the V extend distally to the musculotendinous junction. In order to stay on the marked incision line, the surgeon needs a fresh blade and the cut is performed

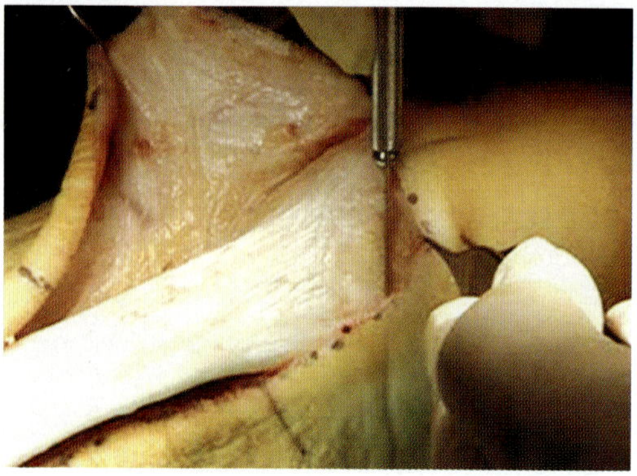

Fig. 5: The exposed tendon prior to release from its insertion

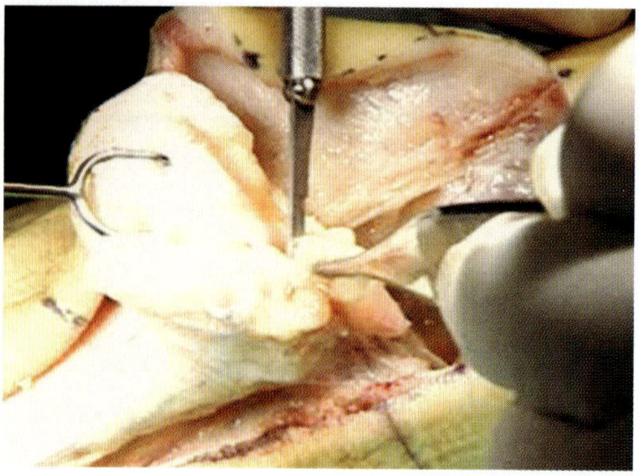

Fig. 6: Debridement of the tendon

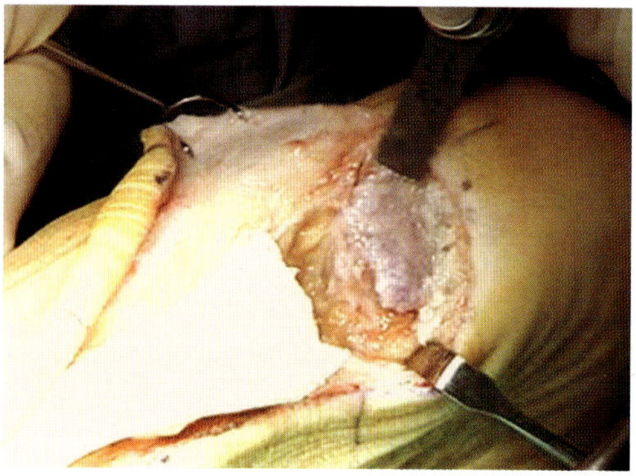

Fig. 7: Ostectomy of the calcaneus enthesiophyte and Haglund's prominence

in a sawing manner to cross the longitudinal fibers on the bias (Figs 8 and 9). In order to achieve a 1 cm lengthening, the limbs need to be at least 2 cm. The author makes the limbs as long as possible to maximize overlap during the repair of the Y. The soleus is left intact but deep longitudinal tendinous fibers are severed. An Allis or Kocher clamp grasps the end of the tendon and the assistant applies traction to gain the lengthening and bring the tendon to the new insertion area.

On the rare occasion where there is insufficient lengthening achieved by the V-Y, a Z lengthening may be done as well in the tendon and the repair described below is supplemented with a transfer of the flexor hallucis longus (FHL). This transfer requires a length of tendon which is marginally sufficient with a release behind the ankle joint. The tendon is found plantar and deep to the abductor hallucis in the arch and is released; the distal end sutured to the flexor digitorum. The medial plantar nerve is protected. The fascia of the FHL is incised anterior to the Achilles and the tendon withdrawn from the arch. [A slip between the FHL and flexor digitorum longus (FDL) may exist at the knot of Henry and has to be released to allow the tendon to be withdrawn proximally]. The tendon is included in the repair of the tendon and the distal end of the FHL is inserted into the calcaneus through a transverse tunnel distal to the reinsertion site of the tendo-Achilles. It can be secured with a bone anchor or an interference screw.

Three large bone anchors with size #2 braided polyethylene or orthocord (TM) suture are inserted in the new bed for the tendon attachment. The first is placed centrally and distally and the other two are placed medially and laterally and proximally to form an equilateral triangle formation on the base (Figs 10A and B). The distal sutures are brought through the distal tendon centrally and distally and secured with a surgeon's knot. Each suture is then brought through the tendon a little more proximally and centrally and tied again. The side sutures are brought through the tendon on either side and tied in a like manner. These sutures securely hold the broad part of the tendon against the wide cancellous footprint. The central suture ends are cut, but the side sutures are advanced proximally up the tendon. With one strand on each side, a ½ Krakow locking stitch is applied and the other strand is simply threaded proximally through the tendon to emerge anteriorly at the musculotendinous junction. Traction is placed on the strand which was simply threaded and the knot is tied. After both side sutures are completed and tied with the ankle plantarflexed, the V-Y is repaired with 2-0 braided polyethylene with the ankle placed in neutral position. Relaxing the ankle, the edges of the distal tendon are sutured to remnants of the old insertion tendon and the paratenon is repaired with

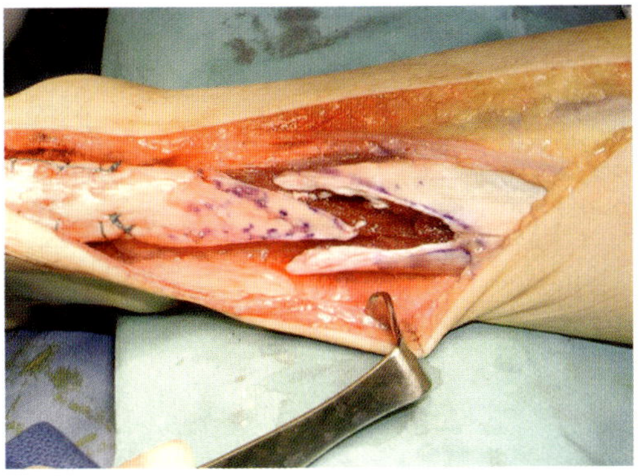

Fig. 8: V-Y lengthening of the gastrocnemius aponeurosis

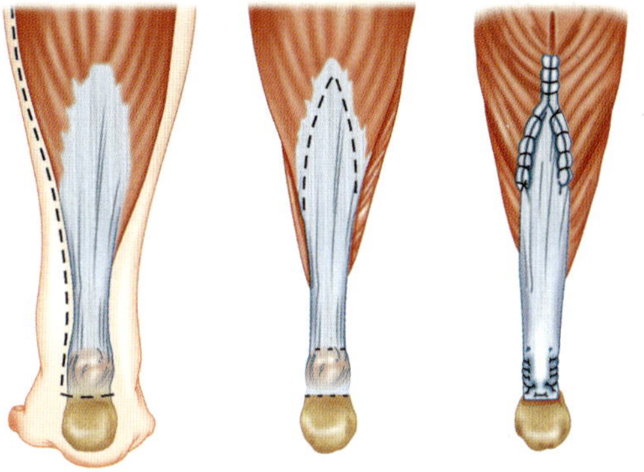

Fig. 9: Summary of the technique for tendon debridement, proximal V-Y lengthening and reattachment of the tendon

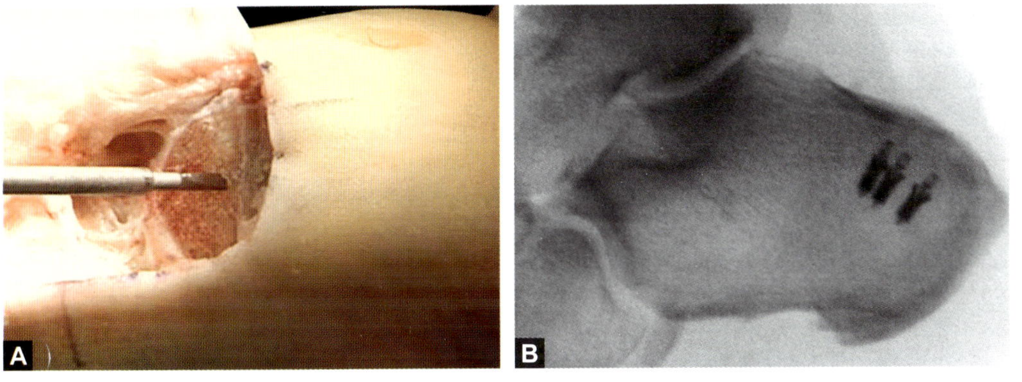

Figs 10A and B: Suture anchors place in the new bed for insertion on the calcaneus. (A) Clinical photograph; (B) Lateral X-ray

4-0 dissolving suture. The length of the transverse component of the skin incision is measured and an equal length is measured and marked from the apex of this flap to the appropriate point along the longitudinal limb. This corner of the flap is the most vulnerable to slough and will be closed with a special suture technique to protect the blood supply to this corner. The subcutaneous tissue proximal to the 1 × 1 distal flap is closed with 4-0 Monocryl™ and the skin closed with staples. The distal corner of the flap is closed with 4-0 nylon flap sutures, using the skin to subcuticular to skin method popularized by Gillie and Allgower. There are no knots placed on the flap side. A bulky dressing is applied with the ankle in plantarflexion and the tourniquet released unless this was done prior to skin closure. A fiberglass shell is applied and bivalved. The patient is non-weight bearing and sutures are removed at 2 weeks. A cast is applied for an additional 2 weeks and at 4 weeks; the ankle is gently brought to or toward neutral. At 6 weeks, the ankle is brought to neutral and a walking cast is applied for 6 weeks. At 3 months, the patient is placed in a walking boot which can be removed for bathing and for sleep. At 4 months, physical therapy begins to strengthen the gastrocsoleus complex and this is continued for 6 weeks for most patients; and for 3 or more months in athletes. Patients will have a limp or will experience muscle fatigue up to 9 months. Return to high performance may take up to 18 months (Figs 11A and B). Recurrences are extremely rare and complications, with this technique are minimal. There are occasionally minor incision problems and in the author's series, there was a probable rupture at the lengthening site which healed with 6 weeks immobilization. One partial rupture at the insertion early in the series occurred, and healed with conservative care.[3]

Reported complications for other surgery techniques at the insertion include recurrent

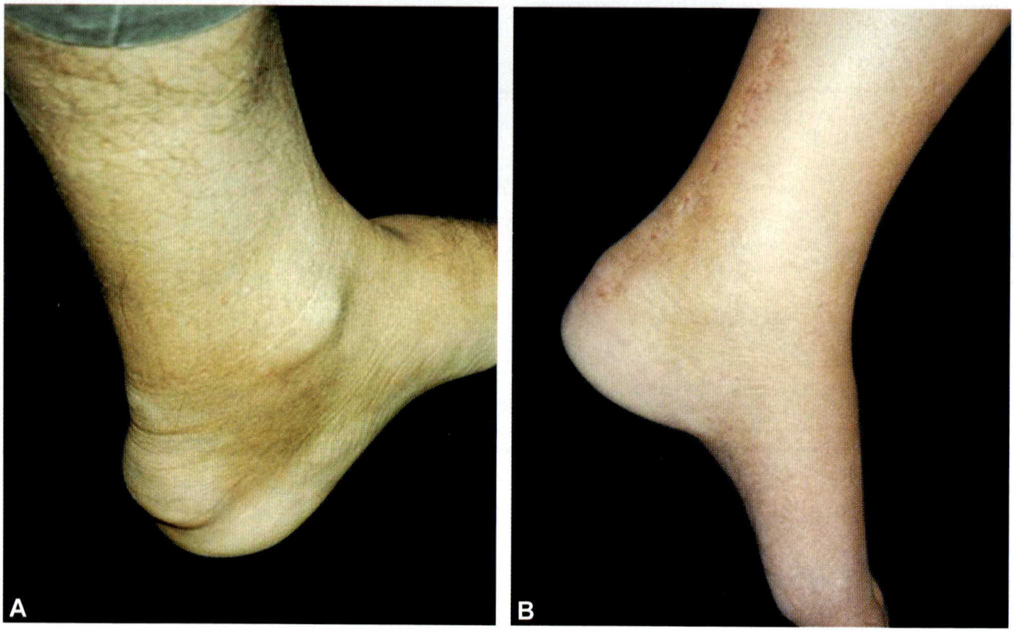

Figs 11A and B: Clinical photographs of patient with insertional tendinosis. (A) Preoperative; (B) Postoperative

symptoms and wound sloughs, pain, and tendon rupture. Salvage includes excision of the sural nerve and carrying out the procedure, secondarily, described above.

REFERENCES

1. McGarvey WC, Palumbo RC, Baxter DE, et al. Insertional Achilles tendinosis: surgical treatment through a central tendon splitting approach. Foot Ankle Int. 2002;23(1):19-25.
2. Wilcox DK, Bohay DR, Anderson JG. Treatment of chronic achilles tendon disorders with flexor hallucis longus tendon transfer/augmentation. Foot Ankle Int. 2000;21(12):1004-10.
3. Wagner E, Gould JS, Kneidel M, et al. Technique and results of Achilles tendon detachment and reconstruction for insertional Achilles tendinosis. Foot Ankle Int. 2006;27(9):677-84.
4. Gould JS. Insertional tendonitis of the tendo Achilles. Tech Foot Ankle Surgery. 2005;4:222-9.
5. Wagner E, Gould JS, Bilen E, et al. Change in plantar flexion strength after complete detachment and reconstruction of the Achilles tendon. Foot Ankle Int 2004;25:800-4.
6. Nunley JA, Ruskin G, Horst F. Clinical outcomes following the central incision technique for insertional Achilles tendinopathy Foot Ankle Int. 2011; 32(9):850-5.

35 Noninsertional Tendinosis and Paratendinitis of the Tendo-Achilles

John S Gould

INTRODUCTION

Tendinosis in the more proximal tendon occurs in younger athletic patients and may take the form of paratendinitis, tendinosis, and a combination of the two (Fig. 1). A history of trauma to the tendon, including probably micro-or mini-ruptures is typically found to have occurred. The tenderness is 7–8 cm from the insertion, often near the site of actual ruptures. An X-ray will confirm increased thickening of the soft tissue shadow of the tendon. With paratendinitis (paratenonosis, or peritendinitis), the tendon feels lumpy and there is palpable crepitus. Magnetic resonance imaging (MRI) is useful to distinguish between thickening and disease of the paratenon and tendinosis within the tendon proper. Ultrasound (US) can also be used for this purpose. Conservative treatment consists of stretching exercises for the muscle-tendon unit and oral anti-inflammatories. A 6–12 week trial of this approach is warranted and may be successful in early cases.

SURGICAL APPROACHES FOR PARATENDINITIS AND NON-INSERTIONAL TENDINOSIS

The involved area of the tendon is approached through a medial longitudinal incision with the patient prone. When there is paratendinitis only, stripping or debridement of the paratenon is all that is needed for resolution of the symptoms (Fig. 2). The subcutaneous tissue and skin are closed and mobilization begun as soon as the wound allows at 2–3 weeks. The patient is treated with a soft tissue dressing and allowed partial weight bearing with crutches using a three point gait.

When tendinosis is involved, the medial longitudinal incision is used and the paratenon is incised if it is healthy and repaired later during the closure or debrided if it is diseased. What to do to the tendon is a matter of debate. All agree to debride the tendon with longitudinal incisions in the tendon and excision of diseased tissue and vacuoles with repair of the tendon using permanent suture. The author, however, supplements this maneuver with a muscle transfer using the flexor hallucis longus (FHL).[1] The concept is to provide a muscle bed for the tendon rather than the subcutaneous tissue alone to improve the tendon nutrition and healing potential. In this circumstance, the muscle belly is being used as a vascular flap and only a short segment of tendon is needed. If a longer tendon is needed as in a rupture with tendinosis, then the tendon is taken in the arch. The fascia over the FHL is incised, the FHL tendon is divided behind the ankle, and the muscle is moved posteriorly. The distal tendon is inserted

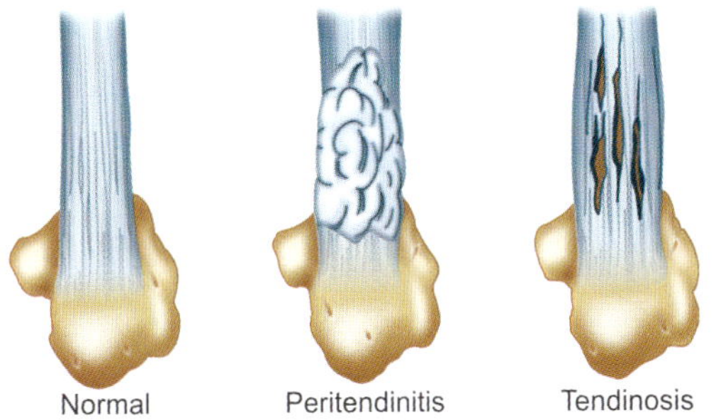

Fig. 1: Non-insertional tendinosis and paratendinitis

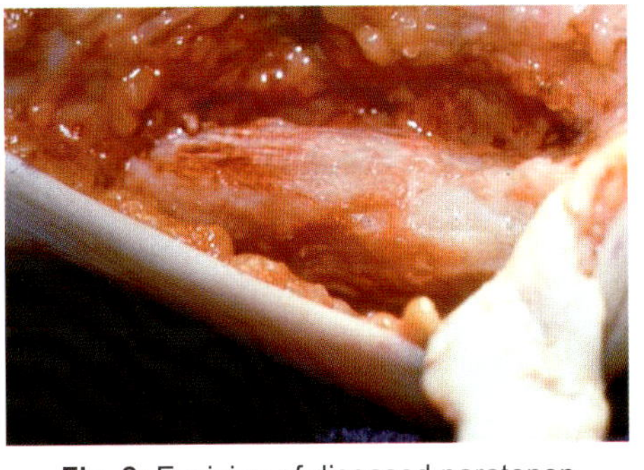
Fig. 2: Excision of diseased paratenon

into the distal healthy tendon of the Achilles through a simple slit in the recipient, sutured with 2-0 or 3-0 braided polyethylene at the entry and exit of the tendon; and the muscle is tacked around the diseased tendo-Achilles with 4-0 dissolving sutures. The paratenon is closed if it was not debrided; the subcutaneous and skin closed with dissolving and permanent suture respectively. Immobilization in a well-padded fiberglass shell is continued for 6 weeks and the patient is then mobilized. Physical therapy is used for 6 more weeks. In the author's series, the procedure has been successful, but only historic controls have been used.

REFERENCE

1. Wilcox DK, Bohay DR, Anderson JG. Treatment of chronic Achilles tendon disorders with flexor hallucis longus tendon transfer/augmentation. Foot Ankle Int. 2000;21(12):1004-10.

36

Peroneal Tendon Pathology

John S Gould

INTRODUCTION

The problems with the peroneal tendons include tenosynovitis, tears, ruptures of the peroneus longus and brevis, and subluxation of the tendons from their normal location behind the fibula. The pathology may be due to traumatic incidents such as lateral ankle sprains and as such have to be considered as concomitant pathology to the other and be recognized and managed with the perhaps more dominant lesion.[1] The tendon pathology may also result from developmental conditions which place more stress on the lateral tendons and bone, such as the cavus foot. In this case, the peroneal pathology may be predominant in terms of symptomatology, but without addressing the underlying problem, the repair is doomed to fail.[2] As noted in Chapter 26, in the cavus foot, there can be multiple concomitant pathologies and everything needs to be noted and managed. Physical examination includes observation of swelling over the tendons, or of their subluxated position; tenderness and crepitus to palpation over the tendons; or palpation of the tendons during maneuvers in which the patient notes subluxation. Magnetic resonance imaging (MRI) is valuable for recognizing tenosynovitis and fluid around the tendons and longitudinal tears and ruptures of the tendons. When the structures lie outside their normal position, subluxation can be recognized and elevation of the peroneal sheath from the anterior edge of the fibula akin to the Bankart lesion in the shoulder can also be visualized. Unfortunately, as the tendon curves around the tip of the fibula, one may encounter "magic angle" artifacts on the MRI which can mimic ruptures. In addition, folds in the peroneus brevis can also be misinterpreted as tears. Finally, the MRI does not provide dynamic images which would be helpful in subtle subluxation including peroneus longus intertendinous subluxation through a tear in the peroneus brevis. A peroneus quartus within the sheath of the other tendons can be confusing, suggesting a tear in the larger tendons.[3] The ultrasound testing (USK) can reveal otherwise unseen tears and demonstrate dynamically subluxation. It is also not infallible, however, and if the USK head is not perpendicular to a tendon, a tendon in continuity can also be misinterpreted.[4] To summarize, the history and physical examination are paramount in the evaluation. The USK should be done by the surgeon or in his presence to assure everyone that the findings of the study are compatible with the basic examination. The findings on the MRI must also be compatible, and not interpreted in a void. Tenoscopy with very small arthroscopes have been used for interpretation, but have not gained wide acceptance, as treatment with the arthroscopic tools is very limited.

PERONEUS BREVIS TEARS

Split tears in the brevis tendon tend to occur just distal to the tip of the lateral malleolus and occur on the underside of the tendon. They may be multiple with loose strands and fronds developed on the tendon and do not heal spontaneously. Conservative treatment is really not of particular value, although the reactive tenosynovitis can be ameliorated by rest and anti-inflammatories. At surgery, an incision is made over the sheath, the tendon explored and subsequently debrided and repaired. Loose strands, fronds and the tenosynovium are removed and the splits repaired usually with a running 3-0 or 4-0 polypropylene monofilament suture. The tendon may be tubularized, when indicated to create a more tidy and stronger structure. The sheath is repaired over the tendon (Fig. 1).

PERONEUS LONGUS TEARS AND RUPTURES

The peroneus longus is more apt to rupture than to split, but longitudinal tears do occur and can be repaired in a similar manner to the brevis injuries. The longus tears occur just distal to the malleolus as well and over a calcaneal bony process which may contribute to the injury. The ruptures often occur more distally, as the tendon makes an abrupt turn and passes under the cuboid through its groove prior to passing under the foot to the base of the first metatarsal (Figs 2A and B). Not infrequently, the longus has a sesamoid, the os peroneum, incorporated in the tendon with an articular surface in contact with the underside of the cuboid (Fig. 3). This bone may fracture and a retracted portion of the bone may be visualized separate from the distal component and more proximal than usual. The bone may be bipartite, but greater separation and irregularity of the fracture edges is typical of the pathologic appearance. It is ideal to repair the peroneus longus, as it depresses the first metatarsal. When this becomes elevated a "dorsal bunion" of the metatarsophalangeal (MTP) joint can occur. Arthrodesis of the first tarsometatarsal joint in a reduced position could be used as a late reconstruction. In the chronic situation of a rupture, retraction of the proximal muscle-tendon with myofibrosis of the muscle obviates repair as the structure has no elasticity, but if repair is possible, at least the first metatarsal is stabilized. The proximal portion of the tendon can be lengthened with a Z-plasty and a straight forward tendon repair then can be accomplished. With a distal rupture at the cuboid level, the distal tendon may be difficult to find and the repair is difficult to accomplish. Many surgeons will then attach the proximal tendon to the brevis and ignore stabilization of the first metatarsal unless it becomes a problem, at which point, they do the fusion noted above. When the os peroneum is fractured, it is excised, preserving the tendon which is then tubularized and repaired. The proximal component of the tendon can be lengthened with a Z-technique, if need be.[5]

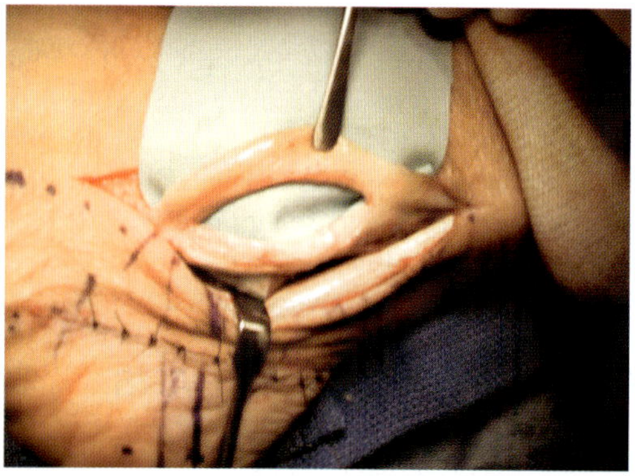

Fig. 1: Longitudinal tear of the peroneus brevis

RUPTURE OF BOTH THE PERONEUS LONGUS AND BREVIS

When both tendons are ruptured, eversion is lost and the patient may develop an inversion deformity. If the distal ends can be found and the muscles have elasticity, a direct repair may be accomplished. If length is an issue, a proximal Z-lengthening can be done or an intercalary graft can be done with

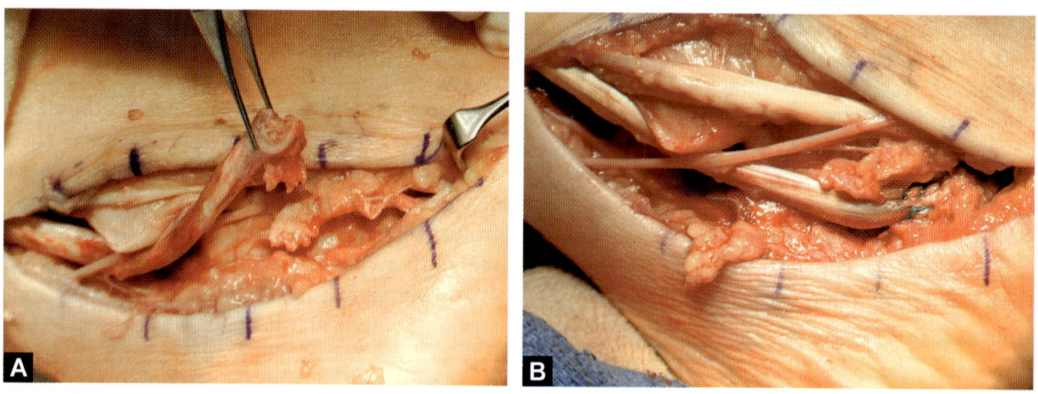

Figs 2A and B: (A) Rupture of the peroneus longus just proximal to the turn under the cuboid; (B) Repair of the ruptured tendon

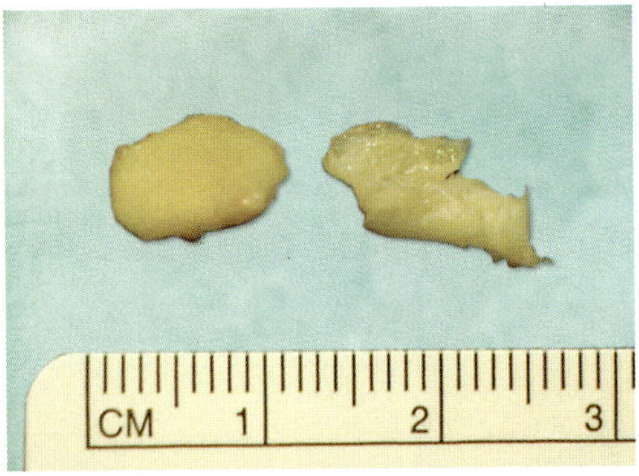

Fig. 3: The os peroneum after excision from a ruptured peroneus longus

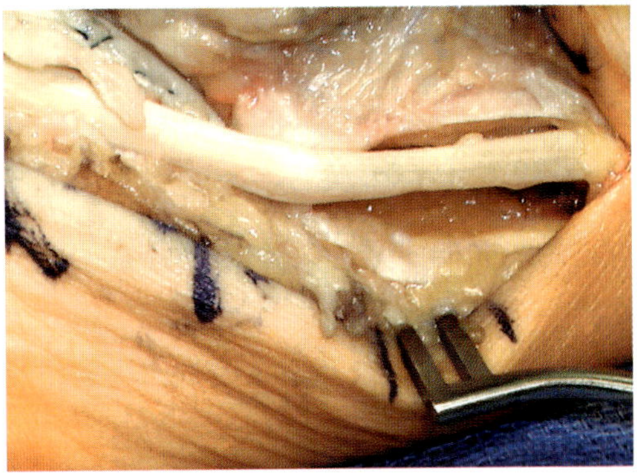

Fig. 4: Subluxated peroneal tendons

autograft, such as the plantaris or a hamstring, or even allograft has been used, although the author prefers the autograft. When the bed for the tendon is badly scarred, various synthetic materials of bovine and porcine origin have been advocated to promote gliding. There are no studies which prove the efficacy of these materials. Silicone rods (Hunter) have been used as well to create a tube-bed through which an intercalary graft has been placed.[6] When the peroneal muscles have no elasticity, the need to balance the foot inversion/eversion is approached by tendon balancing. One option is to transfer the flexor hallucis longus behind the tendo-Achilles into the distal peroneal tendons.[6,7] The posterior tibial may be Z-lengthened to decrease its inversion power and the medial portion of the anterior tibial tendon is released from the medial first metatarsal and moved to the lateral side of the remaining slip on the dorsum. On occasion, a subtalar fusion may be needed for balance, but lengthening of the posterior tibial and dorsalization of the anterior tibial should still accompany the fusion.

SUBLUXATION OF THE PERONEAL TENDONS

This condition occurs for various and sundry reasons such as the cavus foot, from trauma due to a strong inversion thrust, and for developmental reasons such as a shallow fibular groove for the tendons. A supernumerary tendon, such as the peroneus quartus has also been implicated as well as a low lying peroneus brevis muscle.[8] Whatever the cause, the subluxation can be annoying and even painful to patients (Fig. 4). After the diagnostic studies noted above confirm this diagnosis and an underlying cavus, for example, is managed, surgical repair is the treatment of choice for subluxation. The fundamentals of treatment include tightening of the sheath, correction of the Bankart type lesion if it exists, deepening of the fibular groove, or the use of various constricting bone blocks or pseudo ligaments to prevent the displacement. The groove may be deepened either directly or indirectly (Figs 5A to C).

In the immature patient, simple imbrication of the ligament is done, reserving a bone procedure if there is a recurrence after growth is complete. If there is a pocket under the periosteum of the anterior fibula (the Bankart type lesion), the excess edge of the sheath is released and drill holes made in the edge of the fibula for attachment of the sheath edge to the proper place. Deepening of the groove may be done directly with a gouge[9] or by excavating the bone under the groove and collapsing the groove into a deeper position.[10] Creating a slot in the fibula and sliding the slot bone distally and securing it is a bone block technique of recent description.[11]

With the patient in the lateral position, either with a beanbag or with a large bump under the hip to facilitate access to the fibula, an incision is made over the distal 5 cm of this bone. The sheath is incised along the anterior edge of the fibular groove. If the plan is to directly deepen the groove, the periosteum is incised on the far or posterior side of the groove and carefully lifted from the bone with a knife or sharp periosteum elevator making every attempt to preserve it in its entirety. The groove is deepened with a gouge and the periosteum flap replaced and sewn in place under the tendons. Where there may be bare bone, bone wax is used to

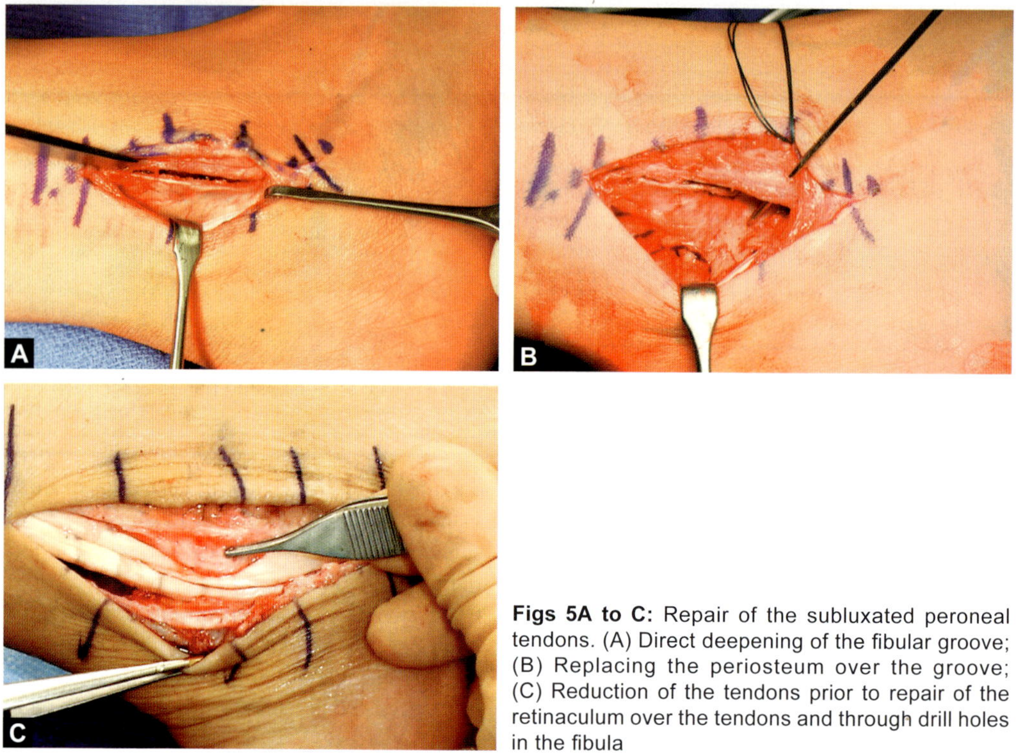

Figs 5A to C: Repair of the subluxated peroneal tendons. (A) Direct deepening of the fibular groove; (B) Replacing the periosteum over the groove; (C) Reduction of the tendons prior to repair of the retinaculum over the tendons and through drill holes in the fibula

prevent overgrowth and adherence to the tendons. Drill holes are made from the outside of the anterior edge to the inside for reattachment and tightening of the flap over the tendons to the edge of the groove. If indirect deepening is planned, a drill is inserted through the tip of the malleolus and the bone under the groove is drilled out. The author will use a guide pin and assess its central placement under the groove with fluoroscopy. Cannulated drills of increasing diameter are used for more precise drilling. The floor of the groove is then tamped down to create the deepening. The periosteum has not been raised as in the other technique. The remainder of the procedure is identical. Immobilization in a cast is used for 6 weeks.

REFERENCES

1. Brandes CB, Smith RW. Characterization of patients with primary peroneus longus tendonopathy: A review of twenty-two cases. Foot Ankle Int. 2000;21:462-8.
2. Manoli A, Graham B. The subtle cavus foot, "the underpronator". Foot Ankle Int. 2005;26:256-63.
3. Khoury NJ, El-Khoury GY, Saltzman CL, et al. Peroneus longus and brevis tears: MR imaging evaluation. Radiology. 1996;200:833-41.
4. Grant TH, Kelikian AS, Jereb SE, et al. Ultrasound diagnosis of peroneal tendon tears: a surgical correlation. J Bone Joint Surg. 2005;87-A:1788-94.
5. Peacock KC, Resnick EJ, Thoder JT. Fracture of the os peroneum with rupture of the peroneus longus tendon. A case report and review of the literature. Clin Orthop Relat Res. 1986;(202):223-6.
6. Wapner KL, Taras JS, Lin SS, et al. Staged reconstruction for chronic rupture of both peroneal tendons using Hunter rod and flexor hallucis longus tendon transfer: a long term followup study. Foot Ankle Int. 2006;27:591-7.
7. Hansen ST (Ed). Transfer of the flexor hallucis longus to peroneus brevis. Functional Reconstruction of the Foot and Ankle. Philadelphia: Lippincott Williams & Wilkins; 2000. pp. 462-6.
8. Zammit J, Singh D. The peroneus quartus muscle. Anatomy and clinical relevance. J Bone Joint Surg Br. 2003;85:1134-7.
9. Zoellner G, Clancy W. Recurrent dislocation of the peroneal tendon. J Bone Joint Surg. 1979;61:292-4.
10. Kollias S, Ferkel R. Fibular grooving for recurrent peroneal tendon subluxation. Am J Sports Med. 1997;25:329-35.
11. Micheli KJ, Waters PM, Sanders DP. Sliding fibular graft repair for chronic dislocation of the peroneal tendons. Am J Sports Med. 1989;17:68-71.

37

Anterior Tibial Ruptures

John S Gould

INTRODUCTION

Ruptures of the anterior tibial tendon are seen in trauma and spontaneously in older, middle-aged patients[1] with diabetes, gout and rarely in patients taking fluoroquinolones (ciprofloxacin, levofloxacin etc.).[2] Many patients do not present acutely and direct repair may be problematic. Foot drop is present and must be differentiated from a nerve lesion. Palpation and imaging with magnetic resonance imaging (MRI) or ultrasound can aid in the diagnosis as well as the determination that there is no concomitant loss of the peroneals or sensory deficit (Fig. 1). If there is any elasticity in the muscle, a direct repair, perhaps with a proximal lengthening or an intercalary graft may be considered (Figs 2 and 3). If the muscle is too fibrotic for use, a tendon transfer should be done. With intact peroneals, dorsal transfer of the posterior tibial may lead to an eversion deformity. The peroneus brevis transfer alone, with an intact peroneus longus and posterior tibial may be a better choice. Balance with a subtalar fusion may be desirable or necessary.

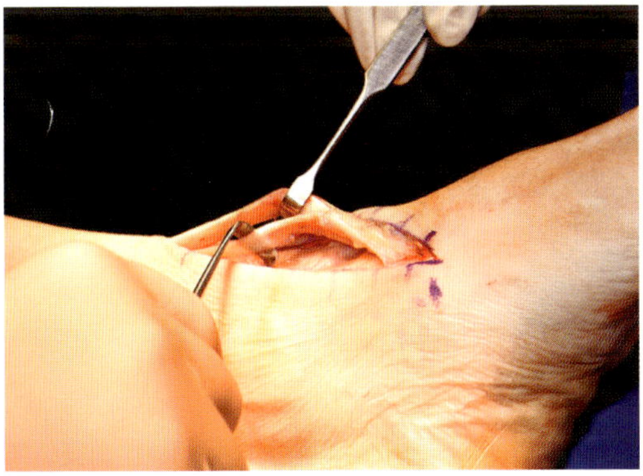

Fig. 1: A split tear in the anterior tibial tendon

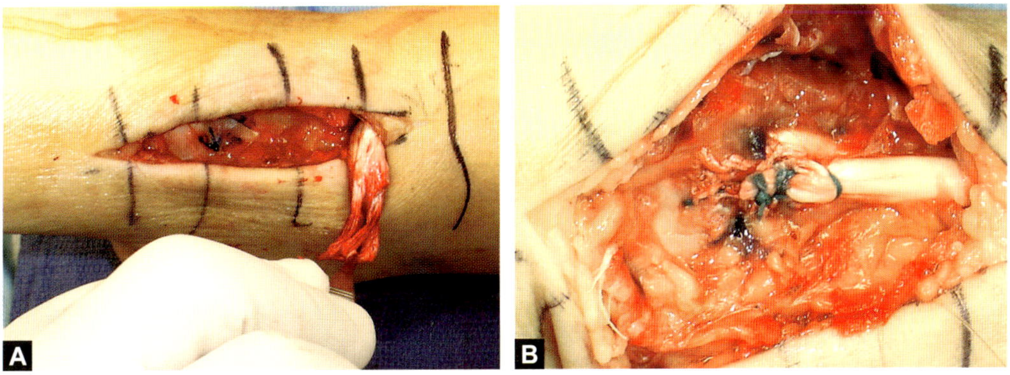

Figs 2A and B: (A) Acute rupture of an anterior tibial tendon; (B) Direct repair

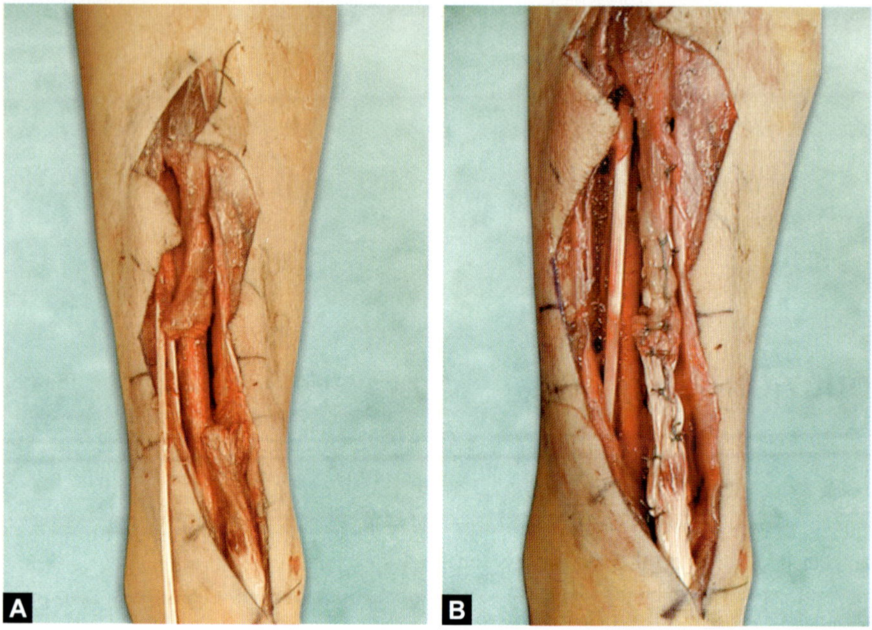

Figs 3A and B: (A) Old rupture in an anterior tibial tendon with notable gap, but with elasticity of the muscle; (B) Repair with intercalary graft

REFERENCES

1. Stuart MJ. Traumatic disruption of the anterior tibial tendon while cross-country skiing. A case report. Clin Orthop Relat Res. 1992;(281):193-4.
2. Kim GK. The Risk of Fluoroquinolone-induced Tendinopathy and Tendon Rupture: What Does The Clinician Need To Know? J Clin Aesthet Dermatol. 2010;3(4):49-54.

38 Arthritis of the Ankle Including Adjacent and Pantalar Arthritis

John S Gould

ETIOLOGY

Arthritis in the ankle is most commonly of post-traumatic origin. In addition to fractures, dislocations, and penetrating wounds, chronic ligament instability is also a major cause of degenerative arthritis (Figs 1A and B). Primary osteoarthritis is relatively uncommon in this joint. Rheumatoid arthritis and various other collagen disorders including gout are also causes. Deterioration of the joint occurs in old club feet and hemophilia as well.[1-3]

DIAGNOSIS

Examination reveals swelling, erythema, pain, and loss of motion. Tenderness is noted along the joint margins anteriorly, and along both recesses of the joint. When the disease is mainly in the anterior joint with spurring, impingement symptoms are noted with walking uphill or upstairs.

CONSERVATIVE TREATMENT

Conservative treatment may begin with oral anti-inflammatories and a simple wrap around ankle support. Many brands are available over the counter which marginally restrict motion. Some more rigid ankle supports allow flexion and extension while blocking inversion and eversion, assisting patients with both ankle and subtalar inflammation. A molded reinforced leather brace may be custom fitted and will block all motion (Arizona™ brace). Such braces for this purpose are generally the 6" variety. As the disease progresses, axial loading becomes a source of pain and bracing has to include various degrees of off-loading of the joint. The molded leather type can be obtained in a 9" variety or a "high unweighting" variety which extends just below the knee and popliteal space when the patient sits (Fig. 2). Other options include articulated and nonarticulated varieties at the ankle which fit inside

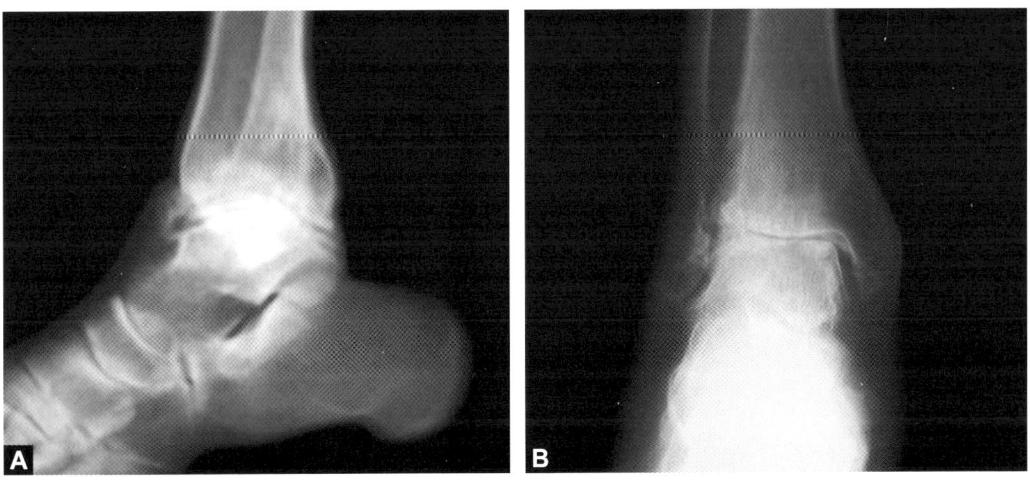

Figs 1A and B: Osteoarthritis of the ankle. (A) Lateral X-ray; (B) Anteroposterior X-ray

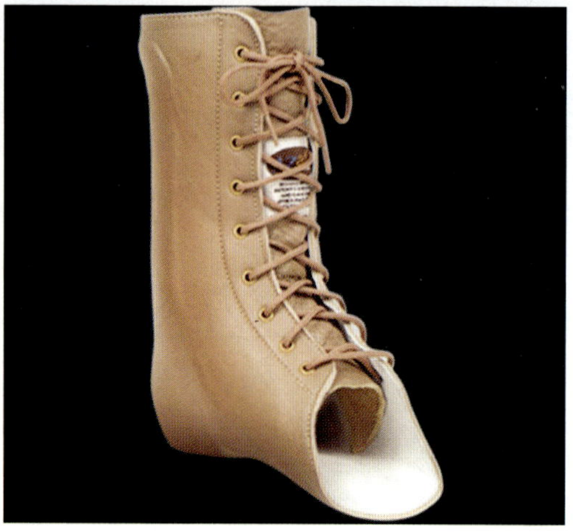

Fig. 2: The Arizona™ brace—"High unweighting type"

the shoe or are attached to it. Polypropylene braces can be hinged or not and fit into a shoe. Double upright braces which attach to a shoe depend on a bridle which fits through a channel in the center of the heel and is reinforced by a steel shank in the midsole. The metal piece attaches to a hinge at the ankle axis and may be locked or free. Proximally, off-loading is accomplished either by a calf lacer attached to the uprights or by an attached patellar weight-bearing polypropylene cuff. If off-loading provides pain relief, the ankle hinge may be free; if not, it can be locked; or with a drop lock, motion can be optional and left for the patient to determine. The shoe must have a rocker sole to walk if the hinge is locked. Patients tend to favor the high Arizona™ brace as it is more comfortable, sleeker, and more trouble free.

Anti-inflammatory regimens can be escalated as needed and tolerated. Intra-articular lubricants have been tried in the ankle but without the universal success found in the knee (albeit temporary).[4] In end stage disease, steroid injections can help periodically. Their use in early stages of arthritis is thought to accelerate the deterioration.

SURGERY

Surgical options include debridement, arthrodesis, or arthroplasty. Arthroscopic debridement is used, often indiscriminately. In early stages with anterior impingement or minimal disease, open or closed excision of the spurs may relieve symptoms successfully and arthroscopic debridement with drilling or "microfracture" of small lesions may have some value. Often such treatment is not of much help and in more advanced disease of minimal to no value at all.

REFERENCES

1. Saltzman CL, Salamon ML, Blanchard GM, et al. Epidemiology of ankle arthritis: report of a consecutive series of 639 patients from a tertiary orthopaedic center. Iowa Orthop J. 2005;25:44-6.
2. Coester LM, Saltzman CL, Leupold J, et al. Long-term results following ankle arthrodesis for posttraumatic arthritis. J Bone Joint Surg Am. 2001;83-A:219-28.
3. Spiegel TM, Spiegel JS. Rheumatoid arthritis in the foot and ankle—diagnosis, pathology, and treatment. The relationship between foot and ankle deformity and disease duration in 50 patients. Foot Ankle.1982;2:318-24.
4. Pleimann JH, Davis WH, Cohen BE, et al. Viscosupplementation for the arthritic ankle. Foot Ankle Clin. 2002;7:489-94.

39

Arthrodesis of the Ankle

John S Gould

INTRODUCTION

Arthrodesis of the ankle is the salvage procedure of choice for pain relief and stability from ankle arthritis secondary to old infections, fractures with significant deformity, young patients, under 50 years of age, with work requiring long periods of walking, standing, lifting heavy objects and carrying them.[1] It is often the best salvage from other failed procedures. As an ankle fusion is compatible with a functional, albeit not normal gait, it is durable, and as such is the "gold standard" for ankle salvage operations. Even in patients with a compromised soft tissue envelope; one with flaps and skin graft from prior post-traumatic procedures, there is usually a way to achieve an ankle fusion. It has several drawbacks:[2,3] lack of motion which is incompatible with activities requiring flexibility; it increases the symptoms and the speed of deterioration of adjacent joints with arthritis (e.g. the subtalar); and as noted by Saltzman et al.[4] results in radiologic and often symptomatic arthritis is adjacent joints after periods of 20 years or more. Despite these issues, it remains the most frequently performed salvage for this joint. The most common early complication of the procedure is delayed or nonunion.[5] The other is malunion, typically with positioning in calcaneus, occasionally too much equinus or in varus or valgus.[6] Despite these events, either shoe modifications or revision is still compatible with a good result.

ARTHROSCOPIC ANKLE FUSION

In recent years, arthroscopic fusion of the ankle has become popular. As long as the ankle does not require significant correction of deformity, less wound problems, rapid healing of the soft tissues and joint, and a more benign postoperative course provides significant advantages over the open techniques.[7,8] The author has utilized this technique whenever possible, and in acquired immunodeficiency syndrome (AIDS) and Hepatitis C patients, along with other typical precautions for benefit of the patient and for the protection of OR personnel and surgeons.

Using the standard ankle arthroscopy setup, the ankle is approached through anteromedial and anterolateral portals. A posterolateral portal is utilized as necessary. There is the option to use either the 2.7, 3.0 or 4.0 scope for visualization but the larger shavers and burrs are always used for this procedure (4.0–4.5). After initial shaving of the joint debris arthroscopically, narrow curved osteotomes, curettes, and gouges are used to grossly denude all the remaining cartilage and fibrous tissue and to penetrate the subchondral bone. A 4.0 or 4.5 burr is then used to complete the preparation of all the surfaces. With this visualization, it is relatively easy to thoroughly prepare both the talus and overlying tibial mortise and both "gutters". Finally, under fluoroscopic control and direct visualization, a 7.3 guide pin is placed from above the medial malleolus, percutaneously, through the medial tibia into the lateral anterior talus body. With such excellent visualization, a second guide pin is placed from lateral to medial, through the tibia anterior to the fibula, and more posteriorly into the talar body. If the positioning is good in all planes, the scope is withdrawn, the joint is compressed manually as the lateral pin is withdrawn into the tibia, the medial pin is backed out a bit and then advanced to confirm compression. The lateral pin is then advanced and positioning is checked for alignment in all plains. The joint should be fixed in neutral without equinus or calcaneus (a bit of equinus is satisfactory; no calcaneus is tolerated); no varus or valgus, and the foot is externally rotated about 15°. The length of the medial screw is determined, the tibia and the entrance into the talus is over drilled and the lag screw, usually the 16 mm threaded 7.3 cannulated cancellous screw is inserted. With compression, the medial side of the talus should be snugged against the inner medial malleolus. The lateral pin is advanced to depth, over drilled, and the screw inserted. If excellent compression was achieved with the first screw, the second can be a 32 mm threaded one as the compression has already been achieved and the increased thread length may be more stabilizing and controls rotatory forces. No adjuncts are used with this technique such as bone graft or bone graft substitutes. The portals are closed, the tourniquet released and a bulky dressing applied, covered with a bivalved fiberglass shell. Sutures are removed at 2 weeks; and casting is continued up to 6 weeks. The patient is then placed in a rocker soled walking boot, which can be removed for bathing and bed. At some interval between this time and 12 weeks, the fusion is deemed healed clinically and radiologically and the patient mobilized (Figs 1A and B). The patient is fitted with a shoe with a rear apex rocker sole which aids easier roll off with walking. What is frequently seem with arthroscopic fusions is that the bone contact at the fusion site is not as impressive as with open techniques, but the area fills in with bone rapidly and homogenous solid bony fusions are almost always achieved. The most common error with this technique is to use it when significant deformity exists, which is not addressed. The salvage can be an open osteotomy, often through the fusion site.

OPEN ANKLE FUSION

The literature is replete with technique and fixation devices for ankle fusion. Anterior, posterior, medial, and lateral approaches have been used and advocated. Among the early standards were the Royal Air Force (RAF) technique in which the ankle was approached through a fibular osteotomy; the inner surface of the fibula removed, and after joint preparation, the fibula was reapplied to the tibia and talus with screws. The "Hat" technique was an anterior approach with an anterior tibial slot created with the slot bone advanced distally into the neck of the talus and secured as well. One of the earlier advances was the use of a Charnley external compression device to provide compression forces across the fusion site. Calandruccio designed a three dimensional clamp for the same purpose and this became a popular device.[9]

At this point in history, an anterior or lateral approach is used. With the lateral approach, the fibular osteotomy is performed and it is often used as autogenous bone graft by morselizing it with a bone mill. The surfaces are prepared with curved and straight osteotomes, curettes, and gouges, as well as small saws to correct alignment issues. A short vertical incision is made over the medial gutter and it is prepared to a close fit of the medial talus and the inner surface of the medial malleolus. Adjunct autogenous bone graft from the iliac crest, or the morselized fibula or bone graft substitutes are often

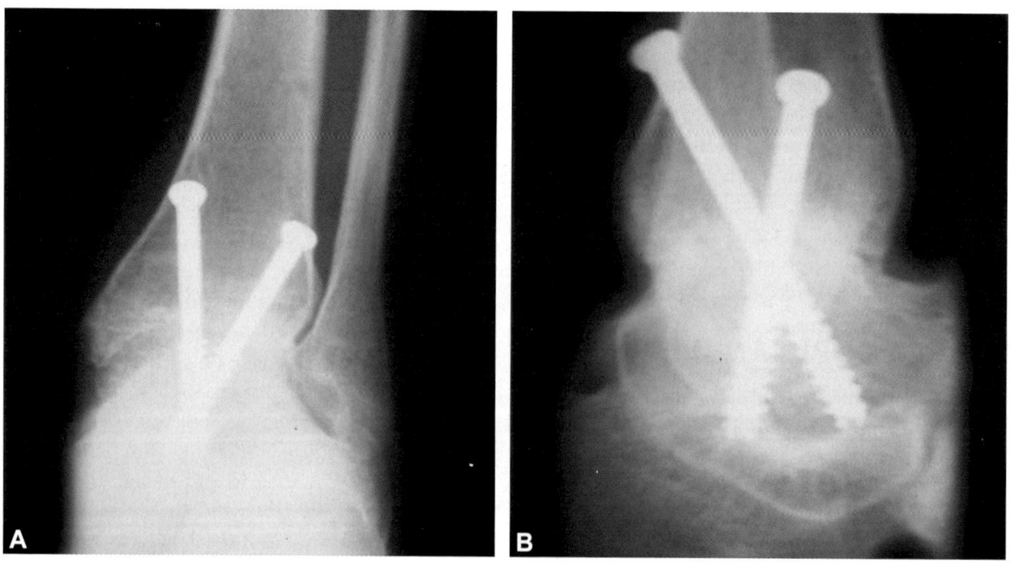

Figs 1A and B: Arthroscopic fusion of the ankle: (A) anteroposterior (AP); (B) Lateral X-ray

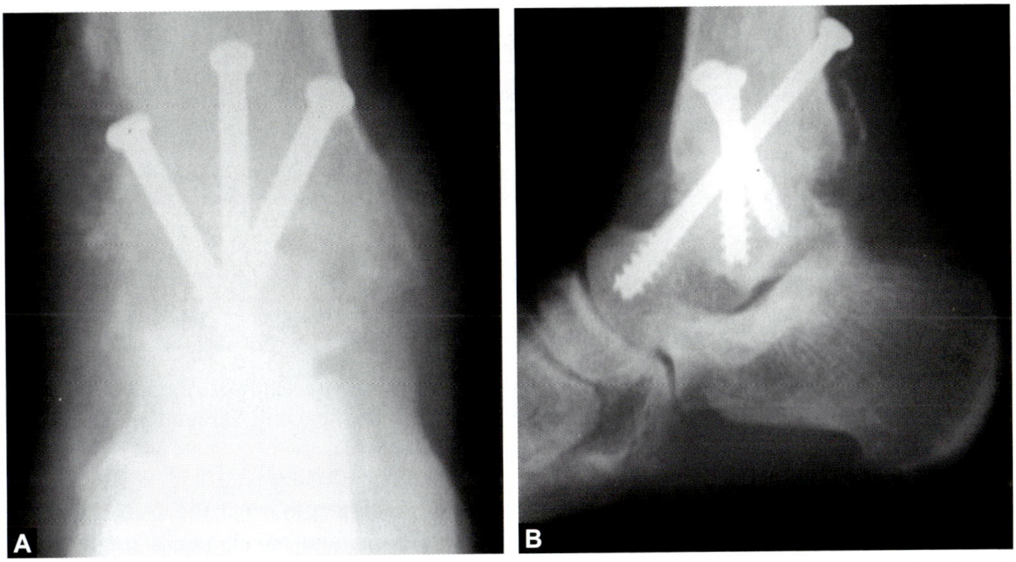

Figs 2A and B: (A) Anteroposterior; (B) Lateral X-rays of an open ankle fusion using a three screw fixation technique

used. Alignment fixation is often used with large K-wires or Steinman pins for temporary fixation. Final fixation is achieved with 2–3 cannulated cancellous screws. The medial one above the medial malleolus is inserted first, extending distal, lateral, and into the posterior talar body. The lateral pin and subsequent screw are placed anterior to the fibula and is aimed distally, medially and essentially toward the center of the talar body on the sagittal view. The third screw with the "Michigan technique" is started higher or more proximal than the others and is placed from the posterior tibia, between the other two crisscrossing screws into the neck of the talus anteriorly "(The Home Run Screw)". On the mortise view of the ankle, the screws extend from medial to center to lateral; on the sagittal view, they fan from anterior to central to posterior, affording ideal control (Figs 2A and B).

The anterior approach to the ankle has become increasingly popular primarily because patients have been promised that at some point in time they may become eligible for total ankle replacement and the fusion could be taken down. With hardware easily accessible on the anterior tibia and with preservation of the fibula, such a revision is potentially more feasible. An approach is made in the anterior tibial/extensor hallucis longus interval. Preparation of the ankle is carried out without removal of the fibula. Fixation with medial and lateral percutaneous screws is done as in the lateral approach. The final screw is placed through the anterior tibia into the posterior talar body. The lateral screw is directed centrally and medially and the medial screw is begun more posteriorly and aimed laterally and anteriorly. Alternatively, compression plating between the anterior tibia and the neck of the talus may be done and several commercial devices have been designed for this very purpose.

REFERENCES

1. Abidi NA, Gruen GS, Conti SF. Ankle Arthrodesis: indications and techniques. J Am Acad Orthop Surg. 2000;8:200-9.
2. Mann RA, Rongstad KM. Arthrodesis of the ankle: a critical analysis. Foot Ankle Int. 1998;19:3-9.
3. Astion D, Deland J, Otis J, et al. Motion of the hindfoot after simulated arthrodesis. J Bone Joint Surg Am. 1997;79:241-6.
4. Coester LM, Saltzman CL, Leupold J, et al. Long-term results following ankle arthrodesis for post-traumatic arthritis. J Bone Joint Surg Am. 2001;83:219-28.
5. Katsenis D. Bhave A, Paley D, et al. Treatment of malunion and nonunion at the site of ankle fusion with the Ilizarov apparatus. J Bone Joint Surg Am. 2005; 87:302-9.
6. Kitaoka HB, Anderson PJ, Morrey BF. Revision of ankle arthrodesis with external fixation for non-union. J Bone Joint Surg Am. 1992;74:1191-200.
7. Corso S.J., Zimmer TJ. Technique and clinical evaluation of arthroscopic ankle arthrodesis. Arthroscopy. 1995;11:585-90.
8. Gougoulias NE, Agathangelidis FG, Parsons SW. Arthroscopic ankle arthrodesis. Foot Ankle Int. 2007;28(6):695-706.
9. Dohm MP, Benjamin JB, Harrison J, et al. A biomechanical evaluation of three forms of internal fixation used in ankle arthrodesis. Foot Ankle Int. 1994; 15(6):297-300.

40 Total Ankle Arthroplasty Including Combinations with Osteotomies and Arthrodesis of Surrounding Bones and Joints

Sonya Ahmed, William McGarvey, John S Gould

INTRODUCTION

Perhaps some of the most rewarding procedures in orthopedic surgery are joint replacements. While ankle arthrodesis has been the mainstay of treatment and even the gold standard for ankle arthritis, there is a rising trend toward total ankle arthroplasty. Ankle arthrodesis has had its success, but leaves the patient with a nonmobile joint, gait abnormalities, and increased wear and stress on the adjacent joints. As shown previously, at an average of 22 years, the majority of patients had substantial, accelerated arthritic changes in the joints of the ipsilateral foot but not the knee.[1]

Due to these concerns, total ankle arthroplasty has become a rising trend. There are frequent adjustments and refinements made to current prostheses and the addition of new and improved prostheses, all to increase the survival of the total ankle replacement. In a recent meta-analysis of total ankle replacement, 10 years survivorship was 78%[2] with another publication revealing a risk of revision surgery at 9% at 1 year and 23% at 5 years.[3]

Relatively, the absolute indications for total ankle arthroplasty are few but the extended indications have become many; among these are primary ankle osteoarthritis, post-traumatic ankle arthritis, post-traumatic secondary to chronic instability, adjacent midfoot/hindfoot arthrodesis or arthritis and rheumatoid arthritis. Extensions of these indications have applied to patients with bilateral ankle arthritis, previous ankle arthrodesis and ipsilateral total knee or hip arthroplasty. However, due to the many complications that can occur with total ankle arthroplasty, especially in the inexperienced hand, the contraindications are many. Among these are extensive talar avascular necrosis, active or deep infection, extreme malalignment of the hindfoot (varus/valgus > 15°), peripheral neuropathy with charcot arthropathy, severe osteoporosis, extreme proximal limb malalignment, high activity demand, skeletal immaturity and morbid obesity.

Due to the rising tendency to maintain joint motion and function and the increasing desire among the patient population, a single, primary total ankle arthroplasty may not be possible and may require other procedures concurrently or concomitantly. Such procedures may be tibial or hindfoot realignment osteotomies, subtalar or triple arthrodesis (Figs 1A to E), deltoid ligament release or imbrication, lateral ligament reconstruction and tendo-achilles lengthening. It is important to remember to regain proper realignment of the hindfoot prior to the ankle arthroplasty either through supramalleolar osteotomy or calcaneal osteotomy. In our experience it is thought that this is best performed in a staged fashion. In contrast, soft tissue procedures and balancing, such as tendo-achilles lengthening, deltoid release and lateral ligament reconstruction can be done simultaneously with the total ankle arthroplasty.

Currently, Food and Drug Administration (FDA) approved total ankle arthroplasties for use in the United States are the Scandinavian total ankle replacement (STAR) [Small bone innovations (SBI)] (Fig. 2), Salto-Talaris (Tornier, Inc.) (Fig. 3), Agility (Depuy) (Fig. 4) and the InBone (Wright Medical) (Fig. 5). In Europe, Canada, and in South America the Belgian-Swiss Hintegra prosthesis (Intregra Life Sciences) is very popular (Fig. 6). All of the companies and their advocates are making modifications in the prostheses and insertion technology at a rate exceeding the likelihood that any print media can remain current. For example, the Zimmer TM prosthesis, which removes minimal bone from each surface, using a milling device, and is inserted through a lateral transfibular approach, has been introduced within the last three months.

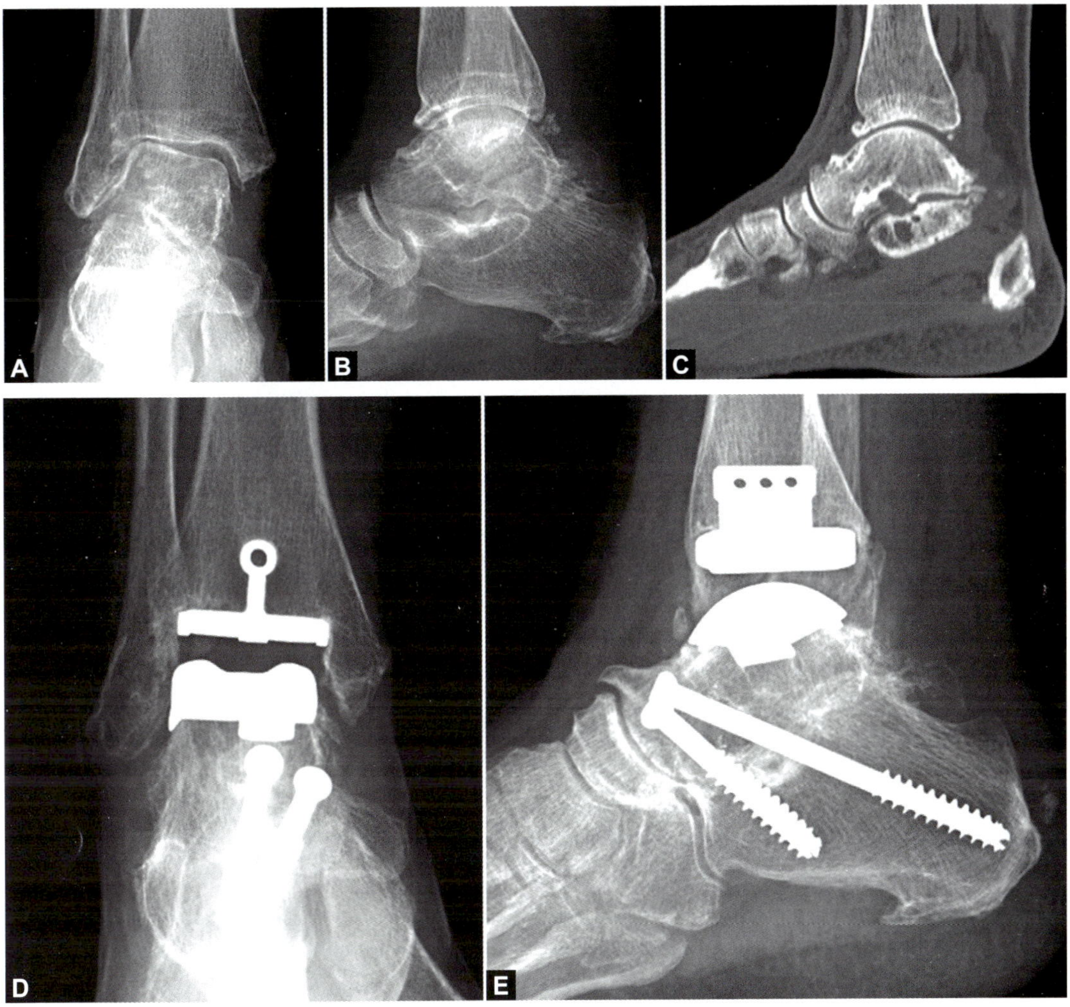

Figs 1A to E: (A to C) Degenerative arthritis of the ankle and subtalar joint with calcaneonavicular bar; X-rays and sagittal computed tomography (CT); (D and E) Two years postoperative Salto talaris total ankle, subtalar fusion, and excision of calcaneonavicular bar. *Note*: the development of exostosis at talonavicular joint. Patient had a postoperative peroneal palsy 2° to pressure at upper edge of cast during a long acting nerve block anesthetic given to control postoperative pain. Complete recovery resulted after neurolysis of nerve at neck of fibula and collagen wrapping of nerve

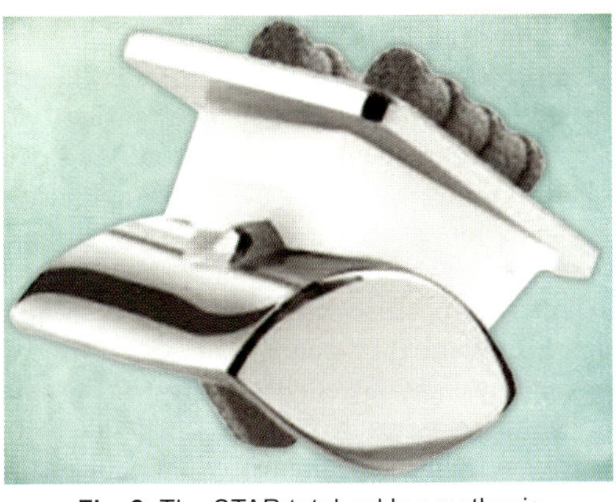

Fig. 2: The STAR total ankle prosthesis

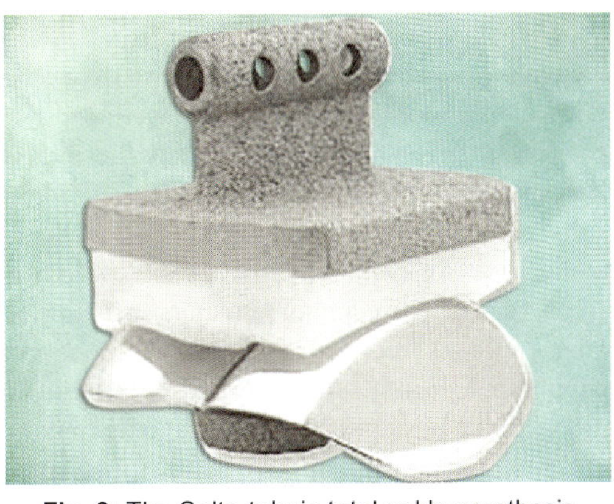

Fig. 3: The Salto talaris total ankle prosthesis

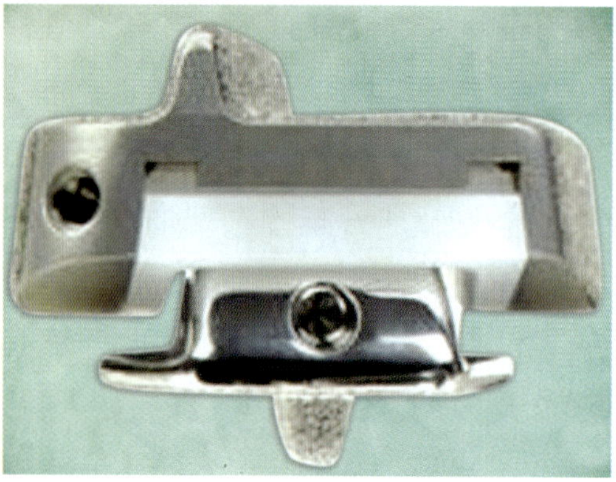

Fig. 4: The LP Agility total ankle

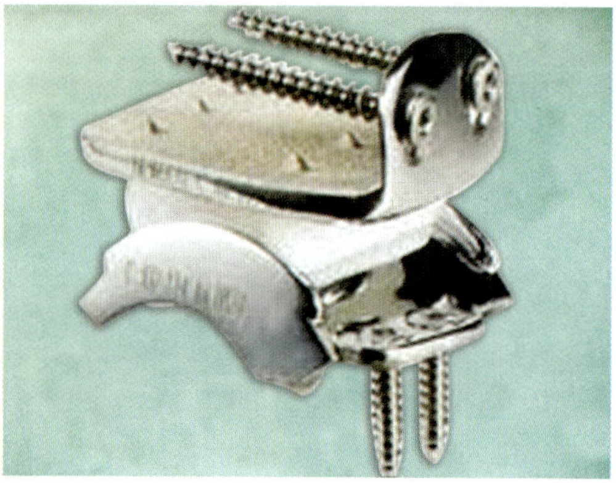

Fig. 6: The Hintegra total ankle

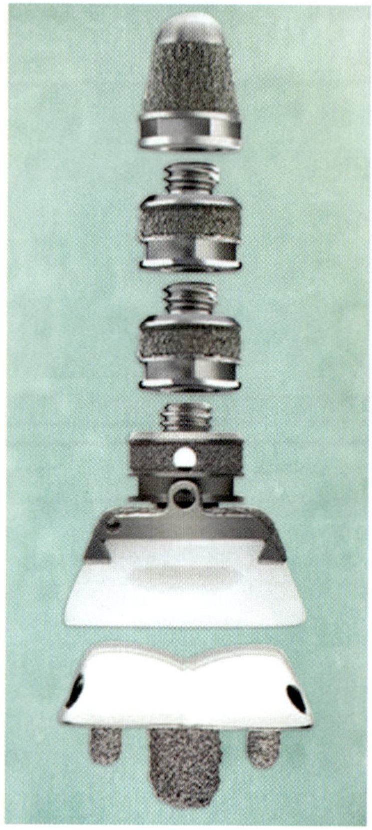

Fig. 5: The InBone II total ankle

All of the other most popular prostheses are inserted through a standard anterior approach to the ankle with the exception of the InBone. While the other prostheses require alignment guides for the tibial and talar cuts the InBone requires the use of an external alignment device and entry through the heel and subsequently the medullary canal. Although the utility of the extensile anterior approach is apparent, it is laden with difficulties with wound closure and wound complications. Wound complications have extended from inconsequential suture abscesses major sloughs requiring flap coverage, and on occasion, eventual amputation. Due to these risks, it is imperative for the surgeon to be meticulous in dissection, protect the anterior neurovascular bundle, maintain the tibialis anterior in its sheath, be cautious using self-retaining retractors and carry out an anatomic layered closure. Other complications encountered during total ankle replacement are intraoperative/postoperative periprosthetic fracture, continued instability or soft tissue imbalance, Polyethylene wear with bone osteolysis and component loosening are long-term concerns.

The STAR total ankle arthroplasty (SBI), approved by the FDA in 2009, is the only FDA approved ankle prosthesis for uncemented use, although most American surgeons do not routinely use polymethylmethacrylate with the other devices as well. It is a mobile bearing, nonconstrained design, and the first of the mobile bearing devices to be approved for use in the United States. For the most part, all of the international devices outside the USA are of the mobile bearing type. The tibial component is a highly polished, flat, cobalt chrome component with two cylindrical bars and a porous plasma spray covering. The talar component has a polished, gliding surface with a central, anteroposterior ridge made to guide the poly core. Lastly, the third component is an ultra-high molecular weight polyethylene core that has a flat surface that articulates with the tibial side and a concave side meant to articulate with the talar side.

As a result, there are two bearing surfaces in the STAR. These two surfaces are the interface between the upper side of the mobile bearing and the tibial component and the lower side of the mobile bearing and the talar component. The tibial component also bears two anteroposterior projecting cylinders which serve to aid in fixation of the device into the distal tibia. As with all mobile bearing devices, this device too is intended to reduce shear and rotational forces on the bearing which can decrease stress at the metal/bone interface and lead to loosening of either of the components. As a result, in the first US long-term prospective study for the STAR prosthesis, the probability of implant survival was 96% at 5 years and 90% at 10 years.[4]

The Salto-Talaris (Tornier), FDA approved in 2006 is a fixed bearing derivation of the original French origin mobile bearing design. The instrumentation was improved from the original mobile bearing design to reproduce near anatomic tibiotalar alignment and thus allowing the fixed bearing design. The mobile bearing concept was moved to the instrumentation and is determined at the trialing phase of the procedure after resections have been completed to the talus and tibia. The trial tibial base plate is placed and as the ankle is taken through a trial range of motion, the highly polished back surface remains mobile against the tibia and is able to rotate into proper position. Once this key step is completed, the tibial keel slot can be cut to accommodate the final, titanium plasma sprayed tibial component. The talar component offers matched articular geometry to the native talus with two separate radii of curvature medially and laterally allowing more anatomic ankle kinematics, thus decreasing stresses on the surrounding ligaments (Figs 7A to C).

The InBone (Wright Medical), FDA approved in 2005 is a fixed bearing prosthesis which is the only modular system on the market. It requires an intramedullary alignment system with a highly polished, cobalt chrome talar component and stemmed tibial and talar components. This system is unique in that it offers modularity which allows a bit of patient customization and stem customization on the tibial side. It also offers intramedullary alignment which may allow for more precise, anatomic implant positioning (Figs 8A and B).

The Agility (Depuy), FDA approved in 2002, is a semiconstrained prosthesis with a talar component that is wider anteriorly than posteriorly and allows translation medially and laterally. The talar component (cobalt chrome alloy) is placed in 20° of external rotation at the joint line and perpendicular to the tibial component. It is also tapered posteriorly. The tibial component (titanium alloy) is obliquely rectangular and intended to allow for 20° of external rotation at the joint line. The tibial component and polyethylene component are fixed and supported by the required distal tibiofibular syndesmosis fusion. Syndesmotic fusion is required and unique to this prosthesis in order to allow an increased contact surface area and a better force distribution. In two prospective studies in 2004, survivorship rates were 80% at 5 years[5] and 63% at 10 years.[6]

Complications may occur during and early after the index procedure (Figs 9A to E). Longer term problems include: Failure of ingrowth to secure the prosthesis, loosening, subsidence, component migration, failure and late infection. With the newer design prostheses, failure of ingrowth, particularly for the talar component has become far less common. This is also true of metal and polyethylene component fractures. Polyethylene wear debris and resultant ballooning osteolysis continues to be a problem, but occurs much later in well-aligned and well-secured components. Consequently, the surgeon should be prepared for salvage procedures that exist for limb preservation in this population and also the consideration of limb sacrifice. Such options for limb preservation include bone grafting to cystic lesions surrounding the prostheses (Figs 10 and 11), polyethylene exchange, revision prosthesis with custom implants when necessary (Figs 12A to G), and a hindfoot arthrodesis with an interpositional bulk allograft. It has been portrayed that most complications surrounding total ankle arthroplasty can be successfully treated with revision and in other instances require arthrodesis. In a recent meta-analysis, implant failure at an average of 5.2 years was reported as 9.8% with 62% of these managed with revision and 36% requiring conversion to arthrodesis. Also, in the same meta-analysis, less than 1% required transtibial ampulation.[7] In specific instances not amenable to revision, failed total ankle arthroplasty can be converted to a successful hindfoot or tibiotalar fusion by using structural allograft with rigid fixation, either angled blade plate or an intramedullary rod.[8] As with most surgeries, outcomes require careful postoperative management. Immediately postoperative, the ankles are usually splinted and

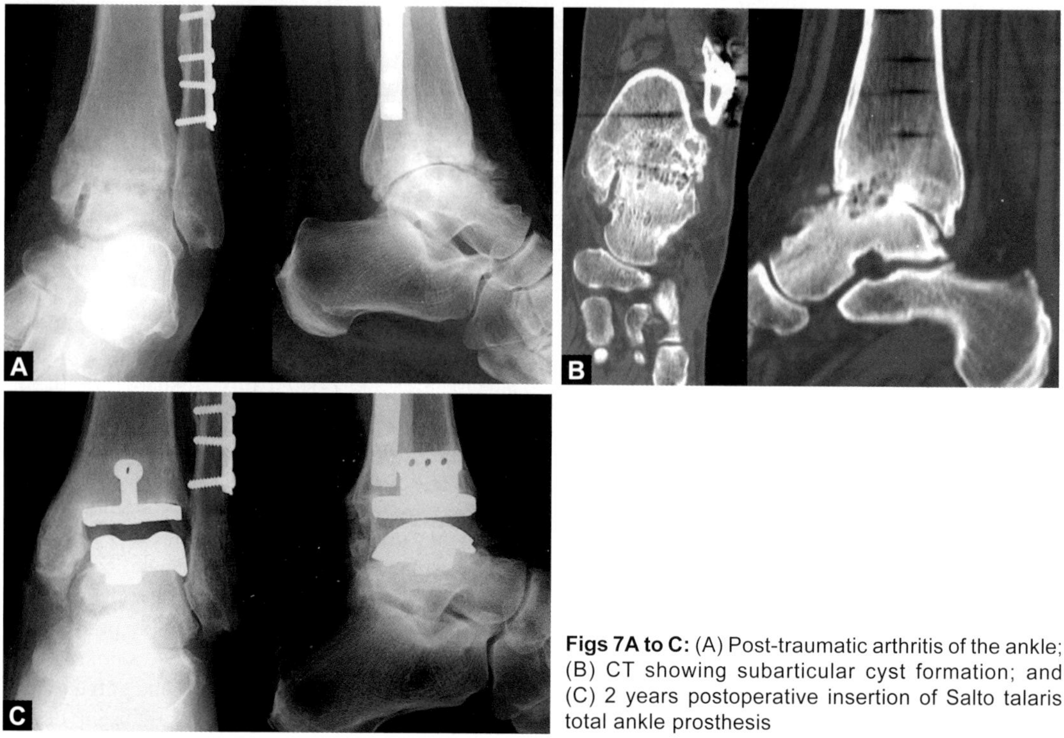

Figs 7A to C: (A) Post-traumatic arthritis of the ankle; (B) CT showing subarticular cyst formation; and (C) 2 years postoperative insertion of Salto talaris total ankle prosthesis

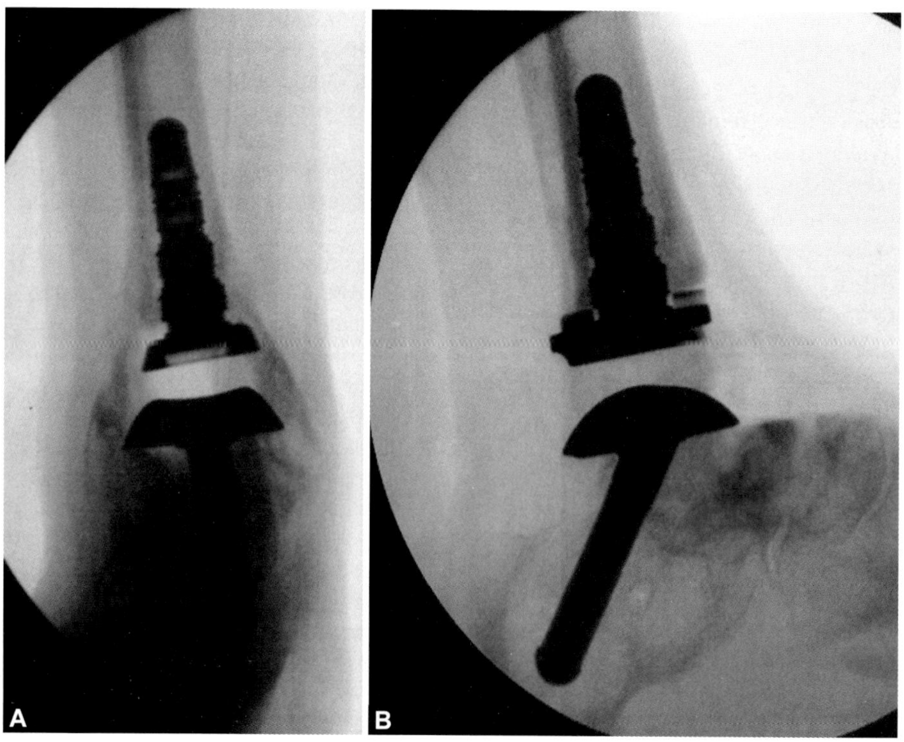

Figs 8A and B: The InBone prosthesis

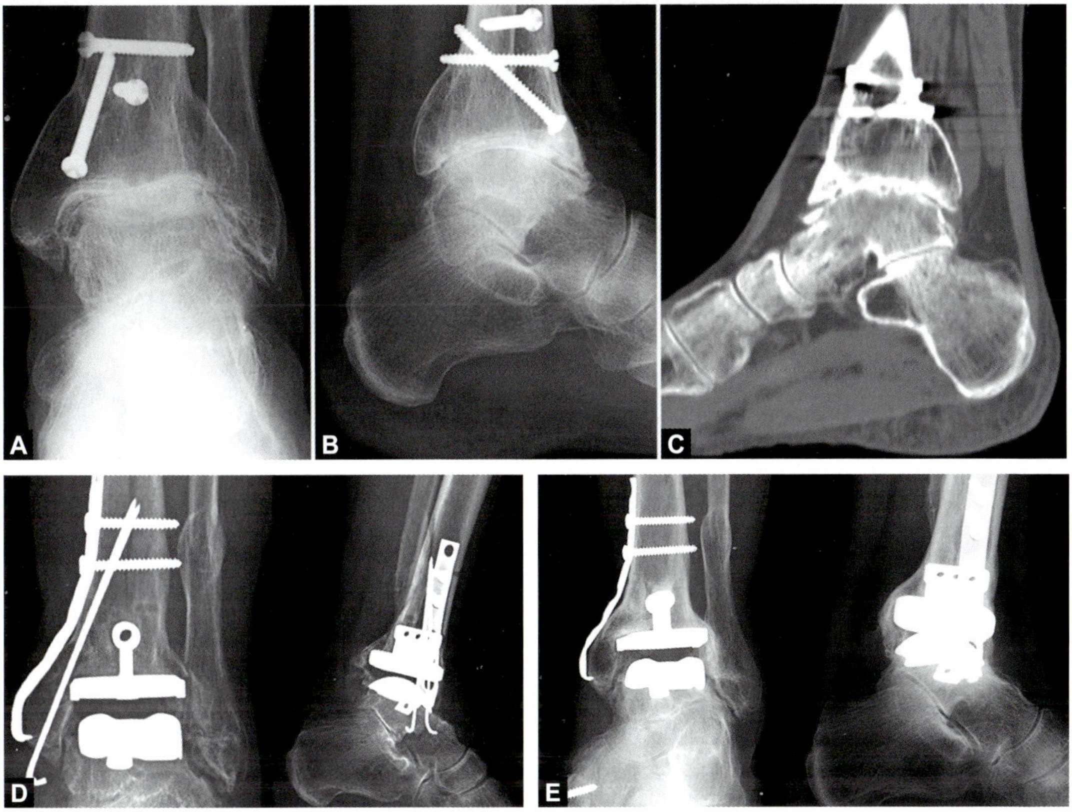

Figs 9A to E: (A to C) Degenerative arthritis of the ankle 2° to old pilon fracture: X-rays and lateral CT scan; (D) 15 days postoperative total ankle with repair of medial malleolar fracture with 2 K-wires and medial hook plate; and (E) 2 years postoperative with K-wires removed

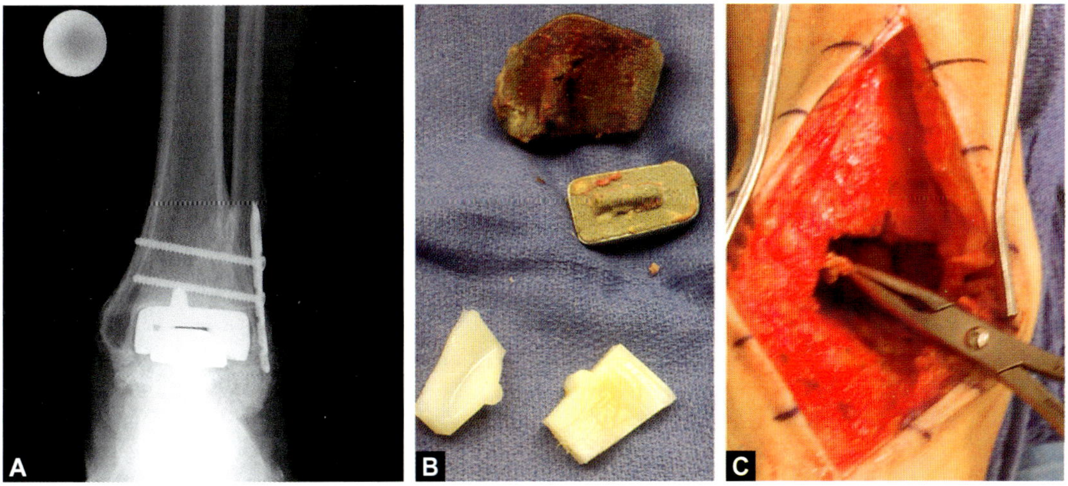

Figs 10A to C

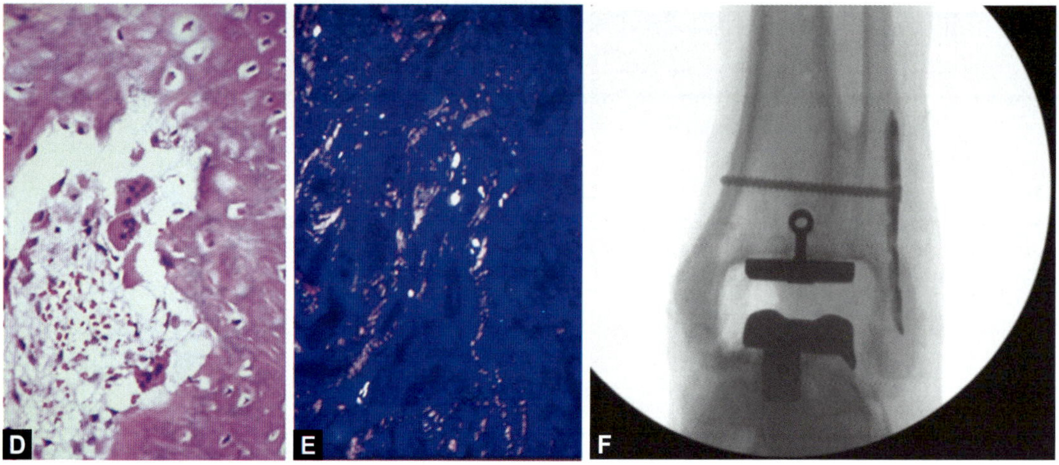

Figs 10A to F: (A) A 10-year-old standard Agility total ankle prosthesis with enlarging medial malleolar cyst. The patient had mild pain after exertion, but regularly played golf; (B and C) The prosthesis has been removed; the talus had only fibrous ingrowth; minimal wear is noted on the polyethylene component (the component was split by the surgeon for ease in removal); the rongeur is removing the cyst lining; (D and E) Photomicrographs showing giant macrophages and osteoclast tunneling creating the cysts; and polyethylene particles on adjacent plate using poly refringence; (F) Revision to a Salto talaris prosthesis with a custom talar component 20 mm stem to promote a better opportunity for bone ingrowth. The cyst has been packed with hydroxyapatite with silicate to promote bone regeneration

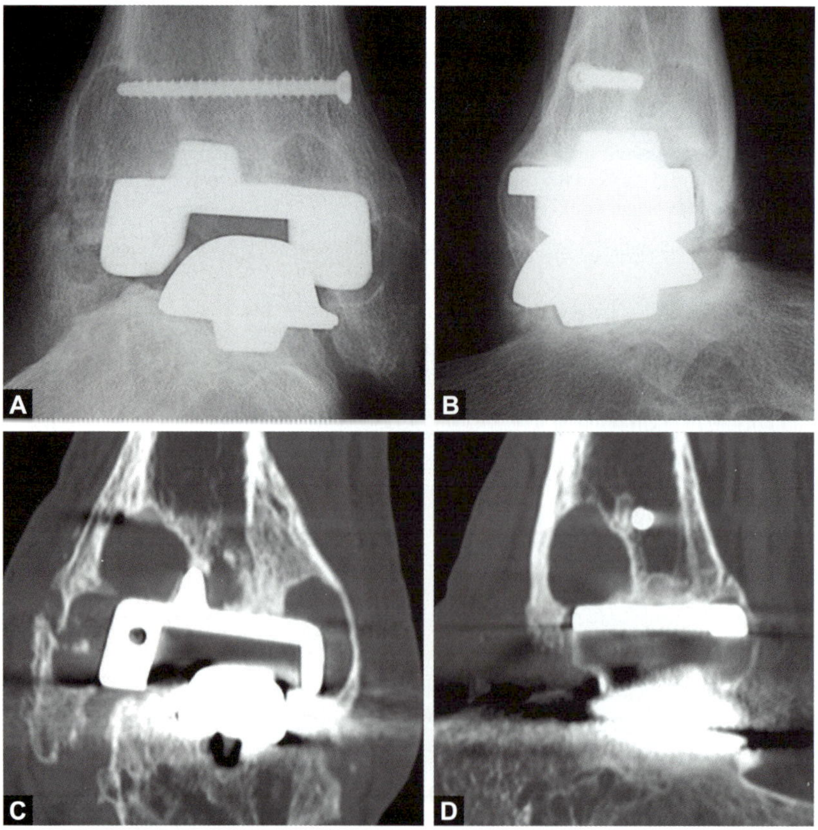

Figs 11A to D

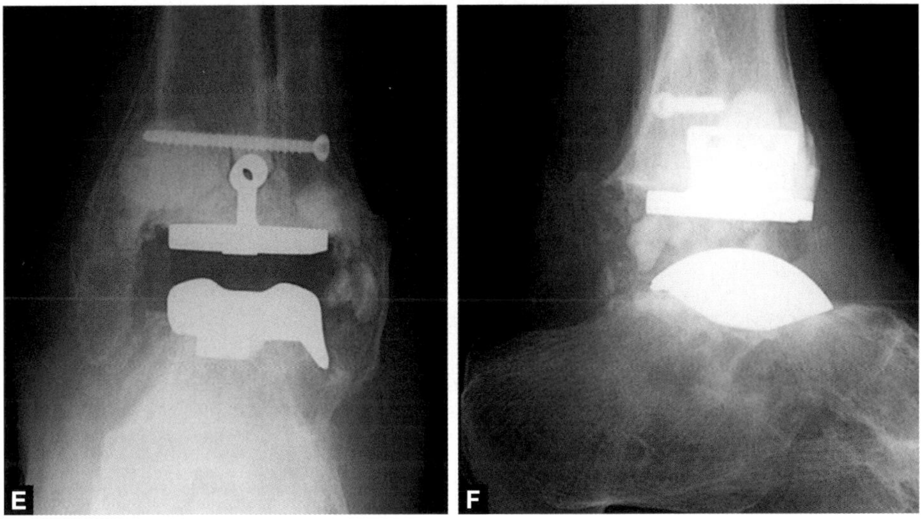

Figs 11A to F: (A and B) A 10-year-old Agility prosthesis with polyethylene particle cysts and a loose talar component; (C and D) CT scan of ankle with ballooning osteolysis; (E and F) Revision to a Salto talaris with packing of the cysts with calcium sulfate with silicate

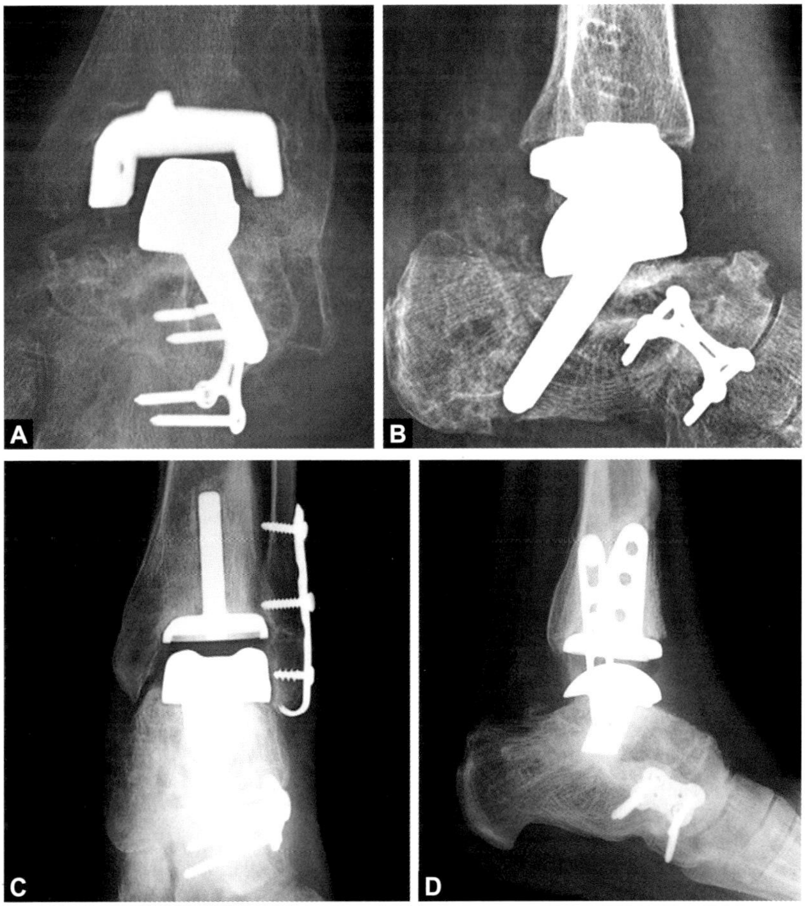

Figs 12A to D

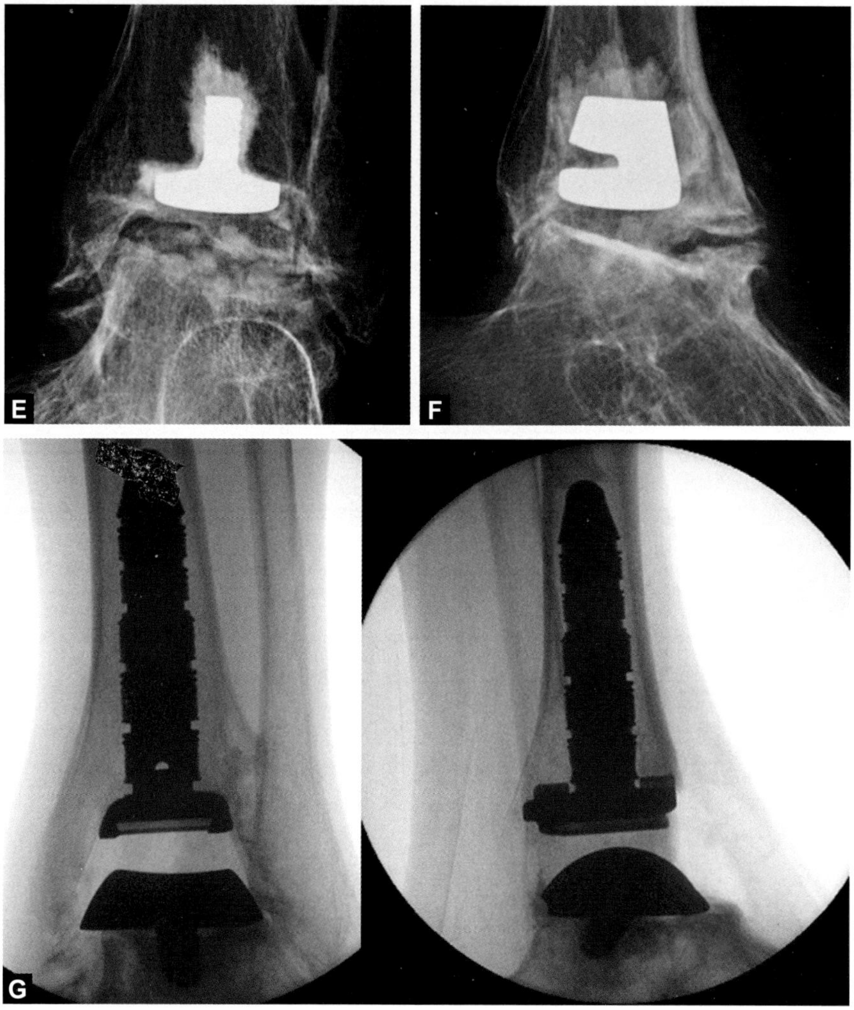

Figs 12A to G: Revision custom components: (A and B) Long stem LP Agility (for loose talar component); (C and D) Salto talaris with "shark fin" tibial component and 20 mm. talar stem components (for a patient with bone infarcts in tibia and talus 2° to long-term steroid use for lupus; (E and F) Smith prosthesis implanted 01 years prior; (G and H) Revised with InBone prosthesis using multiple tibial components for vertical stabilization

remain splinted until follow-up about 2 weeks afterward at which time radiographs and wound evaluation are completed. In general, if a primary, uncomplicated total ankle was completed, suture removal can occur at this visit and range of motion can be initiated along with protected weight-bearing in a boot. If the wound exhibits any complications or drainage, sutures should remain and motion/weight-bearing should not be initiated until wound stability. Full weight bearing typically protected in a boot commences at 2–6 weeks according to the prostheses used and surgeon preference. It continues to remain controversial among surgeons about the accepted use of a physical therapist in the postoperative course or to allow the patient to rehabilitate themselves. In general, 80% of total motion obtained in the operating room should be present by 3 months and 100% by 6 months.[9] Subsequent follow-up should at least take place 6 weeks, 3 months, 6 months and yearly thereafter.

REFERENCES

1. Coester LM, Saltzman CL, Leupold J, et al. Long-term results following ankle arthrodesis for post-traumatic arthritis. J Bone Joint Surg Am 2001;83(2):219-28.

2. Haddad SL, Coetzee JC, Estok R, et al. Intermediate and long-term outcomes of total ankle arthroplasty and ankle arthrodesis: A systematic review of the literature. J Bone Joint Surg Am 2007:89(9): 1899-905.
3. SooHoo NF, Zingmond DS, Ko CY. Comparison of reoperation rates following ankle arthrodesis and total ankle arthroplasty. J Bone Joint Surg Am 2007;89(10):2143-9.
4. Mann JA, Mann RA, Horton E. STAR ankle: long-term results. Foot Ankle Int 2011;32(5):S473-84.
5. Spirt AA, Assal M, Hansen ST. Complications and failure after total ankle arthroplasty. J Bone Joint Surg Am 2004;86(6):1172-8.
6. Knecht SI, Estin M, Callaghan JJ, et al. The Agility total ankle arthroplasty. Seven to sixteen-year follow-up. J Bone Joint Surg Am 2004;86(6):1161-71.
7. Gougoulias N, Khanna A, Maffulli N. How successful are current ankle replacements? A systematic review of the literature. Clin Orthop Relat Res 2010;468:199-208.
8. Berkowitz MJ, Clare MP, Walling AK, et al. Salvage of failed total ankle arthroplasty with fusion using structural allograft and internal fixation. Foot Ankle Int 2011;32(5):S493-502.
9. Saltzman CL, McIff TE, Buckwalter JA, et al. Total ankle replacement revisited. J Orthop Sports Phys Ther 2000:30(2):56-67.

41 Combined Ankle and Subtalar Arthrodesis (Pantalar), Ankle and Triple Combined Arthrodesis

John S Gould

INTRODUCTION

Arthrodesis of the ankle and subtalar joint severely limits motion in the ankle region, but leaves some dorsi and plantarflexion and adduction/abduction through the transverse tarsal joint.[1] This is a reasonable alternative in the younger patient and when total ankle replacement is contraindicated. Use of a shoe with a rocker sole with the apex of the rocker toward the heel makes a smooth walking gait feasible. The surgical technique is to either use ankle and subtalar fusion hardware technique in combination or to plan a technique which utilizes a single device. Attempting to achieve an ankle fusion with the subtalar joint already fused or vice versa results in a higher incidence of delayed and nonunions. When the ankle is already fused, the author places the typical two screws across the subtalar joint and then adds a third screw across the subtalar joint beginning in the anterior tibia and placing the screw in parallel to the first one across the tibiotalar joint. When the subtalar joint is already fused, the ankle screws continue into the calcaneus from the talus rather than stopping proximal to the joint.

TIBIOTALOCALCANEAL ARTHRODESIS

Preferentially, when the joints are to be fused concomitantly or even when there is a fusion present in one joint and the original hardware has been removed, an intramedullary compression device is used for fixation. In order to remain oriented for the proper alignment of the ankle, the patient is placed in the supine position with a bump under the ipsilateral hip which aligns the foot in neutral. A transfibular approach is used which provides access to both the ankle and subtalar joint. The medial incision over the medial gutter is also used. With large deformities, it may be necessary to remove the medial malleolus for reshaping of the mortise. If the malleolus can be preserved, this provides better orientation for alignment. Once preparation is finished, the author uses a large Steinmann pin from the heel into the tibia for temporary alignment relative to varus, valgus, equinus, calcaneus, and tibiotalar translation. Prior to final fixation, proper rotation is added. Various intramedullary devices are available, each with an individual technique. The factors in common include the preparation and that all the devices provide external compression of both joints prior to final fixation and some add internal compression for the subtalar joint as well. The guide pin is placed through the heel, across the subtalar joint and ankle joint and into the tibia. Fluoroscopy is used to assist placement. The pin, once in place, is over drilled and the tibia reamed at least to the level of the isthmus or even proximal to it. One attempts to obtain a good fill of the tibial intramedullary canal. The nails provide options of diameter and length. The nail is inserted with a targeting device attached distally. Using the targeting device, screws are placed through the distal nail and across the calcaneus, with one typically in the direction of the cuboid. A transverse pin is placed through the tibia and through the nail proximally and compression provided. Screws are then placed, across the talus through the nail and with two screws across the tibia and through the intramedullary nail. The screws are locked into the nail (Figs 1A and B). Some nails have a targeting device which allows supplementary screws to be placed alongside the intramedullary nail for additional support. Adjunct bone graft or bone graft substitutes are used between the prepared joint surfaces and around the fusion sites (Figs 2 and 3). Postoperative management is

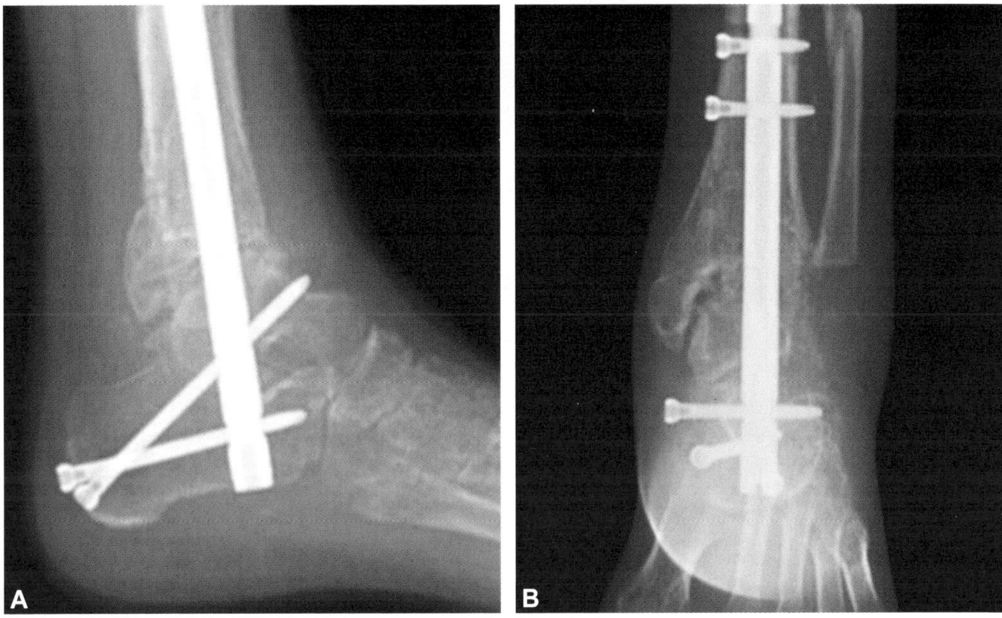

Figs 1A and B: Tibiotalocalcaneal fusion with locked intramedullary nail: (A) Lateral X-ray; (B) Anteroposterior (AP) view

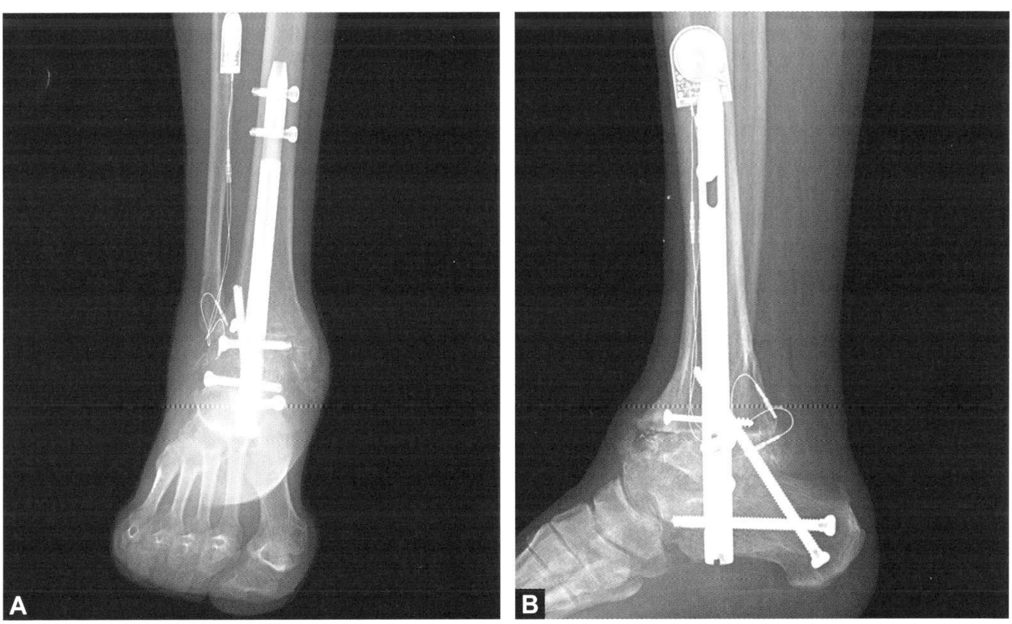

Figs 2A and B: Tibiotalocalcaneal fusion with locked compression nail and implanted bone stimulator (A) AP view; (B) Lateral view

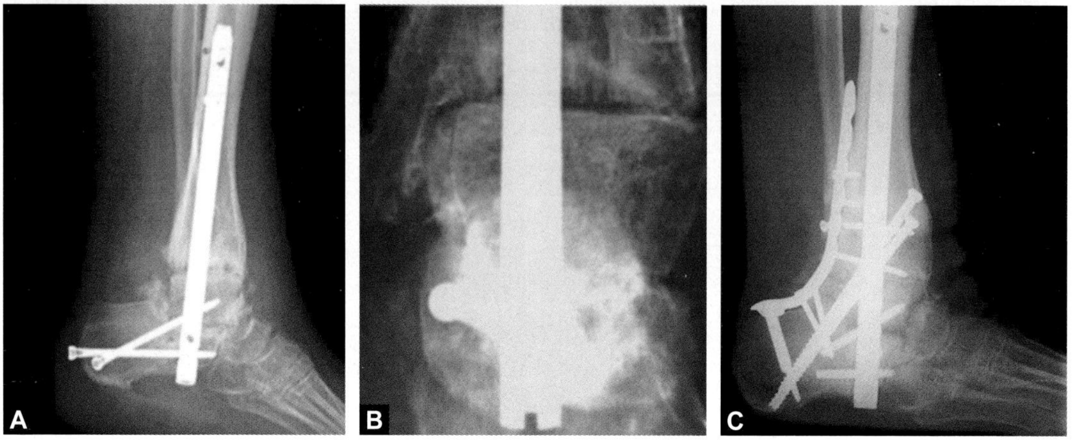

Figs 3A to C: Tibiocalcaneal fusion with locked nail with interposing allograft as salvage of total ankle: (A) Lateral ankle; (B) AP ankle; (C) Salvage of nonunion with posterior tibial-calcaneal plate and supplemental screws

similar to the other ankle and hindfoot fusions with 6 weeks of non-weight bearing followed by 6 weeks of protected weight bearing. The primary complications are delayed and nonunions.

ANKLE AND TRIPLE ARTHRODESIS

Fusion of the ankle over a triple arthrodesis or a combined procedure is done as infrequently as possible. Severe trauma is the usual indication. Although a heel rocker sole shoe is usually provided to assist gait, the stiffness with this construct often leads to significant problems with gait and complaints of pressure areas over bony prominences in the mid and forefoot. The base of the 5th metatarsal often is problematic. A total contact insert is added to the shoe with relief wells placed under problem areas. Patients complain of bone pain with ambulation and stress fractures of the tibia are not uncommon. Despite the added stress on a prosthetic joint, maintaining a mobile segment over a triple arthrodesis is definitely desirable if it is not contraindicated by other factors. The various ankle fusion techniques cited above are added to the triple fused joints, or after removing the necessary hardware, an intramedullary rod is used for the ankle fusion. Although fusing an ankle over a triple is not technically difficult, the incidence of nonunions is higher than when the fusion is done as an isolated joint. The author prefers to stage the procedures and to remove the hardware after the triple is fused. An intramedullary rod is then used for the ankle fusion component.

REFERENCE

1. Papa JA, Myerson MS. Pantalar and tibiotalocalcaneal arthrodesis for post-traumatic osteoarthritis of the ankle and hindfoot. J Bone Joint Surg Am. 1992;74:1042-49.

SECTION 6

Nerve Problems of the Foot and Ankle

Chapters Outline

42

Nerve Problems of the Foot and Ankle

John S Gould

THE PAINFUL NERVE

Making the diagnosis of neurogenic pain vs mechanical pain is not always as easy as one might assume. The characteristics of the pain are that it occurs at rest and nocturnally, waking one from his/her sleep. Nerve pain may be characterized as aching, burning, itching, stabbing, and with parenthesis, numbness, and autonomic complaints (sweating, dryness), and motor weakness or paralysis. It is to be differentiated from pain of infectious or oncologic etiologies. When infection markers are not present locally or systemically, and tumor has been ruled out with appropriate studies [X-ray, magnetic resonance imaging (MRI)], mechanical pain should be differentiated. Typically, mechanical pain is increased by activity and relieved by rest. An enthesiopathic pain typically occurs during the first step in the morning or after rest and is momentary, relieved by further movement. Some nerve pains are increased by activity and lessened by rest, and are known as *quasimechanical*. If the mechanical activity causes more irritation of the nerve, this finding is understandable. What differentiates mechanical from neurogenic pain may be the speed of recovery. With a mechanical etiology, offloading usually results in immediate or rapid relief. Activation of an inflamed tendon or bursa may take a few moments to recover, but a stimulated painful nerve recovers very slowly, taking far more time than any mechanical source.

Although a damaged nerve is often classified, anatomically, as a neurapraxia, axonotmesis, or neurotmesis, a painful nerve may be constricted by external tissue, have an area of fibrosis, or intraneural neuromas of various fasciculi. When there is external constriction, a neurolysis may be sufficient for relief, but barriers to prevent reconstriction have to be considered. If a nerve is dysvascular, replacement into a better vascularized bed may be helpful. Intraneural neuromas may respond to barrier wrapping, but may need resection of the neuromas and repair or resection of expendable nerves. Details of the options for treatment are covered in the chapter on the recurrent tarsal tunnel and on painful neuromas.

43

Neuromas—Acute and Chronic or Recurrent

John S Gould

ETIOLOGY AND PATHODYNAMICS

Neuromas of the foot and ankle are a frequent source of pain in the foot. The etiology may be spontaneous, the result of both sharp and blunt trauma, or iatrogenic. The neuroma itself is found on the end of a nerve, a so called "stump neuroma" or within the substance of an intact nerve, a "neuroma in continuity". The stump neuroma is typically due to division of the nerve by a sharp object and the neuroma in continuity due to blunt trauma or entrapment. The natural history varies. Some neuromas spontaneously become less painful or even asymptomatic; others become increasingly painful, recruit a sympathetic nervous system response and overflow, and may progress to a more global pain response known as a sympathetically mediated pain syndrome or even classic causalgia.

MAKING THE DIAGNOSIS

The history of the inciting incident may make the diagnosis obvious. Secondly, the history should be of neurogenic pain; typically not brought on by activity, but occurring at rest and particularly at night. Nerve pain, at times, may be continuous, but lessen during periods of activity or distraction, and increase during rest or nocturnally. Finally, some nerve pain may be ongoing but aggravated by certain movements, particularly when a neuroma is further mechanically disturbed. The author refers to this as "quasimechanical" pain, as activity such as direct pressure or a moving tendon to which the neuroma is attached increases the otherwise neurogenic type pain.

On physical examination, point tenderness or a Tinel's sign (paresthesias) may be present directly over the neuroma and the course of the nerve. Hypersensitivity or hyperesthesia is specifically within the distribution of the involved nerve. The findings are usually most acute over the neuroma and involved nerve, but there may be referred pain and tenderness proximally and distally along the course of the nerve and at times, in other branches of the nerve. Autonomic effects may also be present, including a feeling of localized swelling, when it cannot actually be observed; temperature exaggerations (heat, burning, coldness); and color changes (red, blue, purple, pale) compared to the adjacent skin. With further autonomic involvement, the dystrophic effect may become more global, and a pain syndrome occurs. It is essential to realize that nerve pain may not include all these changes and be very subtle. Consequently, the initial findings that this pain may not have a mechanical etiology, is subtly neurogenic, and has a history compatible with a nerve injury, with supportive physical findings may be all you have to go on to make this diagnosis.

TREATMENT

The initial treatment for neuromas, particularly the more superficial ones, is to use mechanical desensitization, a therapy modality. This involves stroking the hypersensitive area with increasingly coarse materials, crossing the site in various directions in a prescribed numerical series. Simply having the patient stroke or rub the area frequently with the hand, may be sufficient to make the area less sensitive, adding formal therapy when needed. This treatment, combined with sufficient elapsed time may be sufficient to provide relief.

Transcutaneous electrical nerve stimulation (a TENS unit) may be added if necessary. Initially, the author would often use systemic medications which help with peripheral nerve pain, such as gabapentin, and other alternatives in this category (Topamax, Lyrica). For night pain, amitryptyline can be helpful. The author has also used topical salves and ointments containing gabapentin, anti-inflammatories, and local anesthetics as supplemental therapy when manual desensitization is not enough.

Finally, physical therapists will often use iontophoresis (electrolysis) to drive surface cortisone preparations under the skin to depths of a millimeter or two. Phonophoresis, or the use of an ultrasound head, to drive the medications to a subdermal location is not advantageous as the heat generated by the device aggravates a hypersensitive nerve. Heat, cold, and vibration all aggravate nerves and should not be used.

Local anesthetic injections may be helpful in some instances. The author dislikes the use of cortisone injections, as the substance causes subcutaneous fat dissolution, with local atrophy of the tissues, occasional vitiligo, and loss of the fat, the natural cushion and protection of the nerve. The author particularly dislikes the use of subcutaneous alcohol due to the denaturation of the surrounding tissues. The nerve bed is destroyed and finding a good new home for the nerve is made more difficult. In addition, not only is the neuroma damaged but also more of the nerve proximally, which complicates reconstructive procedures.[1,2]

SURGICAL OPTIONS

Goals of Surgery and Basic Technique

The primary goal of this surgery is to relieve pain permanently. If this cannot be achieved, at least we attempt to lessen the extent of the pain to a manageable level. The approach is biologic and traditional, attempting to remove the source and prevent recurrence. The sensory nerves of the foot are multiple and the autonomous area for each nerve is relatively small and clinically insignificant. Peripheral sprouting of the adjacent sensory nerves assists in further dampening the patient's awareness of the insensitive area. In terms of the surgical options, the simplest maneuver is usually the primary procedure. This also may result in the most benign postoperative course. When a patient presents with a history of failed prior procedures, the technique used is reviewed to determine the reason for failure. At the time of surgery, the findings may explain the problem.

Knowledge of the nerve anatomy and known variations in the anatomy of this nerve are essential, as well an understanding of anticipated nerve physiologic behavior. Good visualization at surgery is needed so that magnification in the form of surgical loupes or a microscope are utilized; meticulous hemostasis is required to limit postoperative scarring which requires fine tipped bipolar cautery; and gentle tissue handling, particularly of the nerve, is essential to minimize postoperative pain.

If the primary approach by the author or another surgeon was to simply excise the neuroma, the next maneuver is to redirect the end of the nerve or to utilize a conduit. Postoperatively, conservative modalities, as described above are included in the regimen.

Simple Excision of the Neuroma

Many neuromas of the foot become attached to surrounding superficial tissues and become painful either because they are so easily contacted from the surface or have traction applied to them when the surrounding tissue moves with an activity. If they are simply excised by cutting the nerve at a more proximal normal appearing nerve level, the end retracts under deeper tissue, particularly fascia or muscle. Here it is better protected from the surface. A new neuroma "always" forms on the end, but unless it becomes attached to a moving part such as a tendon, it becomes less sensitive or at more amenable to desensitization. "This is the primary surgical approach to use with most neuromas."[3] Specific recommendations for individual nerves entrapped or with neuromas will be discussed under "entrapments".

Excision of a Neuroma with Redirection

After excision of a nerve, the end may be redirected into a less vulnerable location if it does not naturally retract to such a place. A dissolving suture may be placed on the end of the nerve to guide it into the area and a generous opening is made into a muscle or fascia. One uses a hemostat from the far side of the host tissue and tunnels through it to the opening, grasping the needle on the suture. The nerve is guided into the muscle or fascia and then the suture is tied without tension at a more remote site. This maintains the nerve in the new position until healing is complete. A technique which was popular in the past would be to drill a hole in bone and pass the end of the nerve into the medullary canal with a small hole beyond for the guide suture. The author has not seen good results with this, finding a neuroma in continuity just proximal to the nerve's entrance into the bone.

Excision of a Neuroma with Placement into a Conduit

Over the years, nerves, after excision of a neuroma, have been placed into numerous natural and synthetic materials.[4,5] In addition, they have been manipulated many other ways including cauterization electrically, with phenol, and with alcohol. None of these methods have been dependably successful and the pain often was increased. More recently, a technique was devised to suture the extruding fascicles together at the end of the nerve or to suture two cut digital nerves together. These results have also been highly variable.

Of the natural tissue into which a nerve might be placed, a large, relatively immobile muscle has usually been the preferred site.[6] Unfortunately, these do not exist in the hand or foot. As an alternative, closed end silicone nerve caps were devised, but again, a neuroma at the entrance to the cap tube was the frequent result. In the 1980s, several specialists in nerve problems independently came upon the concept of using nerve grafts. These were sutured only proximally to a nerve, after removal of a neuroma, to lead the nerve away from a site without an inadequate hiding place, to a better environment. This concept was initiated in the hand, leading the graft back into the forearm where a larger muscle cover exists. Susan MacKinnon of St Louis called this a "wandering nerve graft". The author deemed it a "nerve graft to nowhere".[7] Robert Strauch of New York studied these grafts further and found that the nerve regenerated only a centimeter or so and then did not form a neuroma.[8] We had similar findings in our studies and hypothesized that the lack of neurotropic effect from the distal unconnected nerve may be the responsible factor for this behavior. Our only problem with this technique was that some patients with long-standing neuromas had such hypersensitive nerves, systemically, that the donor site for the grafts sometimes became hypersensitive.

We then began using veins as conduits instead of nerves and our results were still highly satisfactory. Typically, the author would use a segment of the greater saphenous nerve, which lacks many distal branches and valves. The opening could be narrowed or enlarged to accommodate the diameter of the nerve to be sutured into it. In the last few years, synthetic smooth or corrugated collagen conduits have been introduced into the market. Corrugation was added to avoid kinking when tunneling the conduit. Several different lengths and multiple diameters of lumen are now available. In the last 2 years, the author has used these devices in preference to the veins as this avoids the use of a donor graft and the potential morbidity of the site. Their use also shortens surgical time, and they are available in multiple lengths and diameters. The cost of the product is its current drawback. Our results to date are still as good as with the veins, but more time must elapse to assure their efficacy.[9] The techniques for vein and collagen conduits are described below. When the end of the conduit can be hidden under a protective tissue, this alone is done; in other instances, the conduit is redirected with a guide suture. We found, with the veins, that regeneration distance was also no more than a centimeter and that a neuroma was also not formed. The collagen conduit is gradually resorbed and we have not had the opportunity to re-explore these surgical sites to determine the behavior of the nerves within them.

Technique for Attachment of Vein and Collagen Conduits

The author used 3.5 or 4.5 wide angle surgical loupes for this procedure. After dissection of the nerve and neuroma, the nerve is palpated proximally to where it feels normal and is no longer firm and fibrous. The neuroma is excised with a sharp knife over a firm cutting surface, often a sterile tongue blade. The nerve end is inspected to note exposed fascicles. If scar is still present, the nerve is cut back farther.

If a vein is to be taken, an incision is made anteromedially just above the malleolus over the greater saphenous vein. About a 4–5 cm segment is exposed of the vein, carefully dissecting off the saphenous nerve. Damage to this nerve can be another source of pain. Metal LigaClips™ are placed on the vein at either end, with a third clip placed proximally and left on the graft to mark the direction of blood flow (toward the clip). Alternatively, suture may be used instead of the

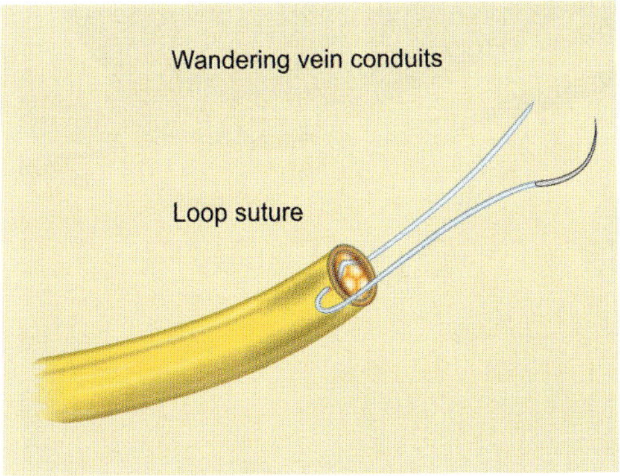

Fig. 1: A 4-0 nylon suture is placed through the end of the nerve and the needle is removed

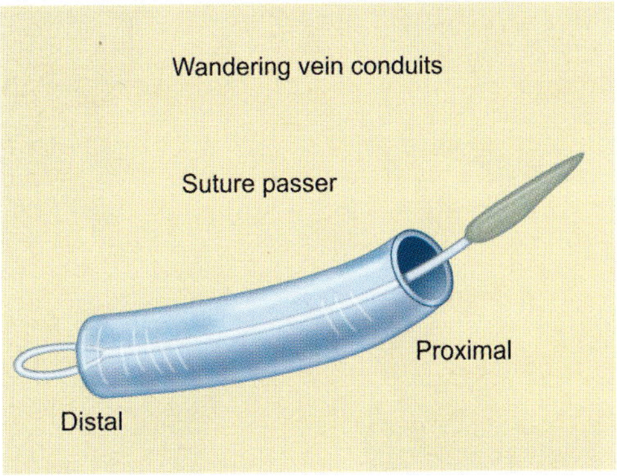

Fig. 2: A suture passer (plastic and metallic handle with a plastic loop attached) is placed through the vein from the clipped end distally

clips. In this distal segment of the vein there are few valves, but in other veins which may be used or in the more proximal vein, it is essential to know the direction of flow. The distal end of the vein is attached to the nerve and the regenerating axons are not blocked by a valve, leading to a neuroma at this site. The saphenous nerve has few branches in this area, but if one is encountered, it is clipped or sutured. It should also be noted that in the operative site, there may be a large tributary to the saphenous, which could be used, but length, valves, and branches can be problematic. To assure that one has found the saphenous itself, one should note the accompanying saphenous nerve.

A 4-0 nylon suture is placed through the end of the nerve and the needle is removed. The two ends of the suture are placed in a hemostat (Fig. 1). A suture passer (plastic and metallic handle with a plastic loop attached) is placed through the vein from the clipped end distally (Fig. 2). If there is a marked discrepancy between the lumen size of the vein and the nerve, the lumen of the vein is enlarged by cutting across it at an angle; or it is narrowed by suturing it partially closed with 8-0 sutures. It is very important that the lumen of the vein not be too tight, for, if it is, a neuroma will form at the entrance. If it is too wide open, the end of the nerve may slip out of the vein. The rule of thumb is that the nerve should slide into the vein easily without a big gap at the entrance.

The 4-0 nylon suture from the nerve is placed through the loop on the suture passer and the nerve is slid into the vein to a distance of 1 cm. The hemostat, which was temporarily detached to carry out the last maneuver, is reapplied to provide a little tension and hold the nerve in the vein. The edge of the vein is sutured to the epineurium of the nerve with 8-0 monofilament suture usually on a BV-130 needle. Typically, two sutures are placed 180° apart. The 4-0 nylon suture is withdrawn (Fig. 3).

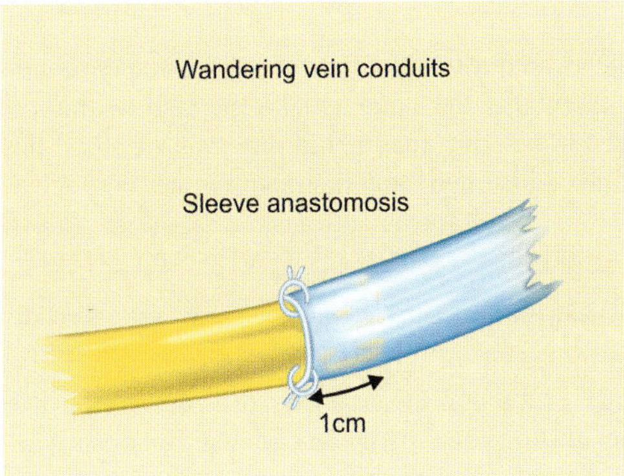

Fig. 3: The 4-0 nylon suture from the nerve is placed through the loop on the suture passer and the nerve is slid into the vein to a distance of 1 cm. The hemostat, which was temporarily detached to carry out the last maneuver, is reapplied to provide a little tension and hold the nerve in the vein. The edge of the vein is sutured to the epineurium of the nerve with 8-0 monofilament suture usually on a BV-130 needle

The nerve and its conduit are placed in their new bed or a dissolving suture is placed on the end of the conduit and it is directed into a new site as described above (Figs 4A and B).

When a collagen conduit is used, the diameter of the nerve is measured with a device provided and a conduit is selected with a slightly larger diameter. A length of 2–4 cm is used. The author prefers the corrugated conduits when redirection is contemplated.

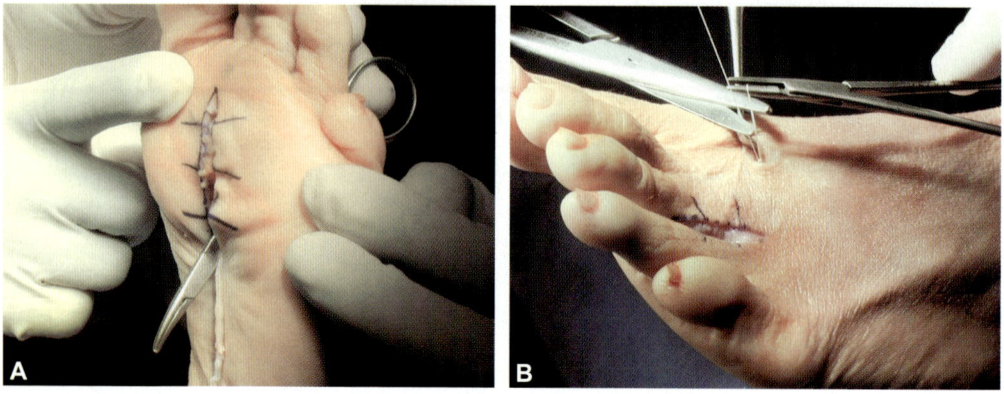

Figs 4A and B: After the conduit is attached to the nerve, a suture is added to the end of the conduit. The suture is grasped by a hemostat and the conduit is drawn into a silent area (in this instance, between the metatarsal heads for a recurrent intermetatarsal neuroma). The conduit is secured to superficial fascia on the dorsum of the foot

The technique used to insert the nerve into the conduit is essentially the same as with the vein, without the need to be concerned about direction of blood flow, lumen adjustment, and donor site issues.

COMPLICATIONS AND SALVAGE

A recurrent painful neuroma is the primary complication of any of these procedures. If, after simple excision or excision with redirection fails, the author then proceeds to use a conduit and recently, the collagen conduits.

If a conduit fails, and we have experience with failed vein conduits, it has either been due to the formation of a neuroma at the entrance of the conduit lumen or at a valve within a conduit, or that the nerve somehow slipped out of a conduit, presumably due to a wide opening in the conduit with the end of the nerve curling back out of the lumen. In any case, we have simply redone the procedure using the careful technique described above. The author has not encountered a failed collagen conduit, but presumably the approach would be to use a longer conduit with a more appropriate lumen size.

REFERENCES

1. Wu J, Chui D. Painful neuromas: a review of treatment modalities. Ann Plast Surg. 1999;43(6): 661-7.
2. Glazebrook M, Paletz J. Treatment of post-traumatic injuries to the nerves in the foot and ankle. Foot Ankle Clin. 2006;11:183-90.
3. Friscia DA, Strom DE, Parr JW, et al. Surgical treatment for primary interdigital neuroma. Orthopedics 1991;14(6):669-72.
4. Dellon AL, Mackinnon SE. Treatment of the painful neuroma by neuroma resection and muscle implantation. Plast Reconstr Surg. 1986;77:427-38.
5. Dellon AL, Mackinnon SE, Pestronk A. Implantation of sensory nerve into muscle: preliminary clinical and experimental observations on neuroma formation. Ann Plast Surg. 1984;12:30-40.
6. Robbins TH. Nerve capping in the treatment of troublesome terminal neuromata. Br J Plast Surg. 1986;39:239-40.
7. Mackinnon SE. Wandering nerve graft technique for management of the recalcitrant painful neuroma in the hand: a case report. Microsurgery. 1988;9: 95-102.
8. Strauch B, Ferder M, Lovelle-Allen S, Moore K, Kim DJ, Llena J. Determining the maximal length of a vein conduit used as an interposition graft for nerve regeneration. J Reconstr Microsurg. 1996;12:521-7.
9. Gould JS, Florence MN, Naranje SM, McGwin G. Use of collagen conduits in management of painful neuromas of foot and ankle: A retrospective study of 69 nerves in 50 patients. Foot and Ankle International. Forthcoming 2013.

44

Entrapment Syndromes

John S Gould

INTERMETATARSAL NEURITIS AND NEUROMAS (MORTON'S NEUROMA)

Irritation of the intermetatarsal nerve at the distal edge of the intermetatarsal ligament, particularly of the two-third and three-fourth interspaces is a common entity of middle age and at times in young adults. As the nerve passes under the distal edge of the ligament, it glides distally and proximally with toe off and subsequent heel strike and foot flat during gait. The nerve divides at or just distal to this point into the digital nerves. In time, in some patients, the nerve gradually develops increasing fibrosis within the nerve structure and increases in size. The enlargement of the nerve increases the developing problem. The "intraneural fibrosis" at this site probably occurs in many if not most people with the aging process, but in some patients becomes a source of pain and dysfunction. A painful bursa may also develop between the neurovascular structures and the intermetatarsal ligament which extends between the metatarsophalangeal (MTP) plantar plates. There may or may not be a history of trauma, although a distal metatarsal fracture with a more dorsal position of the metatarsal may be a precursor for this problem.[1,2]

The patient presents with "metatarsalgia", or pain in the metatarsal area, which is often difficult to pinpoint and seems to involve several metatarsals and often the third or fourth toes. Patients often complain of numbness of the toes and the feeling of their sock or stocking being "wadded up" under the toe creases. The patient may also complain of increased pain in closed shoes with relief when barefooted or wearing sandals. Some patients do better in high heels which maintain the toes in dorsiflexion without the reciprocal motion allowed in a flat shoe.

The diagnosis is typically made clinically. The intermetatarsal space between the heads is palpated from dorsal to plantar using the thumb and long finger (Fig. 1). Medial-lateral compression with the other hand while palpating dorsal-plantar may accentuate the positive finding of significant tenderness (Figs 2 and 3). A click may be noted with side to side compression as the nerve is pushed back into the space from the dorsal to plantar action and

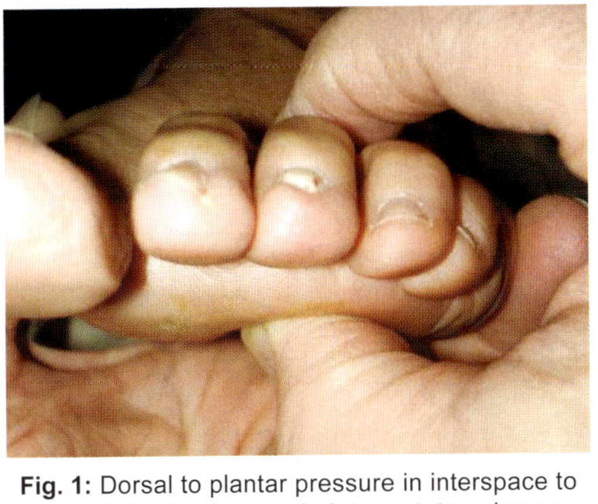

Fig. 1: Dorsal to plantar pressure in interspace to evaluate for tenderness in intermetatarsal nerve

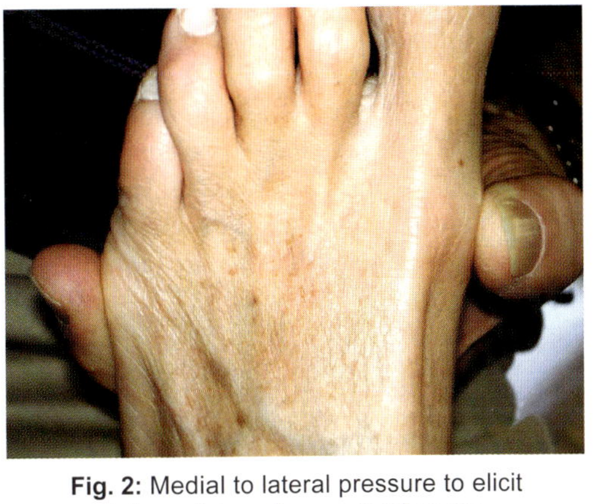

Fig. 2: Medial to lateral pressure to elicit intermetatarsal nerve tenderness

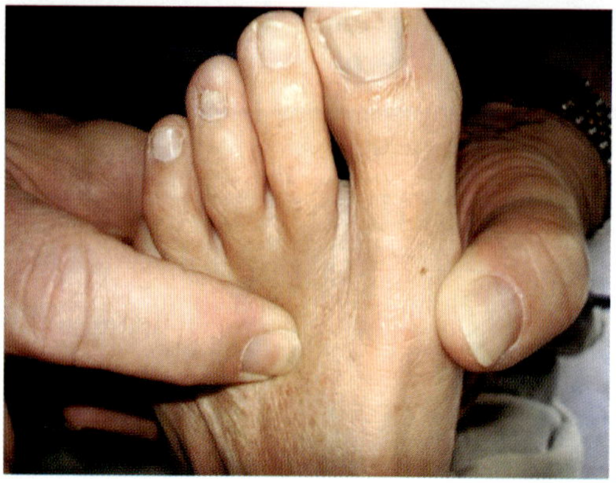

Fig. 3: Medial to lateral and dorsal to plantar pressure to elicit intermetatarsal nerve tenderness and Mulder's click

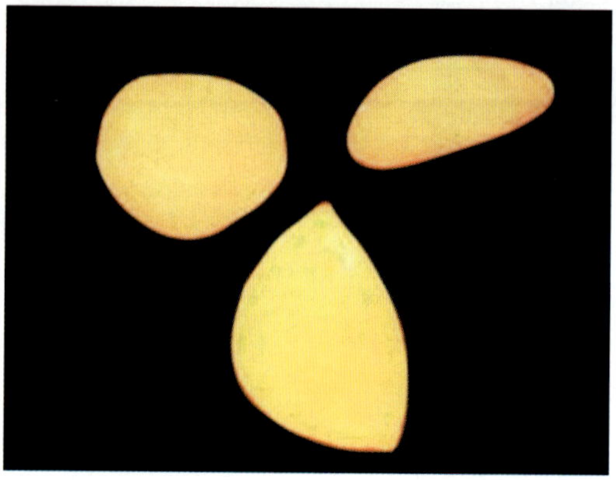

Fig. 4: Metatarsal pads to be placed behind metatarsal heads for relief of intermetatarsal neuralgia

then is squeezed or pushed out (Mulder's click). When there is a swollen bursa, the fullness and induration may be palpated in the interspace.

A "diagnostic injection" of a local anesthetic into the space is often used to aid the diagnosis, but anything causing pain in the space including an adventitial bursa as seen in rheumatoid arthritis, is relieved by the injection, so it is not a specific enough test to be conclusive.[3] Plain X-rays are needed to rule out a metatarsal fracture or foreign body. Magnetic resonance imaging (MRI) can show the enlarged thickened nerve and other soft tissue masses, and an ultrasound exam can be very helpful for the same information. It is essential to utilize the history and physical findings[4] in the involved interspace to make the diagnosis, as simple enlargement of a nerve, which, as noted, may occur in many older patients, may not be the actual cause of pain. The spontaneous development of interspace pain occurs almost invariably in the three-fourth and two-third interspaces, so that findings in the one-two and/or four-five interspaces should be viewed with a skeptical eye. It is also important to be aware that all the interspaces may be tender with nerve compression more proximally at the tarsal tunnel, but the complaint then is in the heel, arch or medial ankle, not the metatarsals. Both the location of the pain and the physical findings have to be considered in making the diagnosis.[5]

CONSERVATIVE TREATMENT

The use of a metatarsal pad proximal to the two-three or three-four interspace or both tends to provide relief in many patients (Fig. 4). This pad may be attached to the sock liner over the insole of the shoe or built into a shoe insert (orthotic), either over the counter or custom, if there may be an indication for that as well. Positioning of the pad is critical and a certified pedorthist and a cooperative patient may best accomplish this.

Injection of an anesthetic with steroid into the interspace may be helpful in some cases, but there is a risk of a patch of vitiligo with a superficial steroid injection and atrophy of the tissue in the web from the steroid effect on the local fat. Injection with alcohol is used by some practitioners,[6] particularly podiatrists, with reported good results.[7] The author is skeptical about this practice due to the extensive denaturing of the soft tissue protein. When pain is not relieved, exploration of the injection site has revealed extensive tissue damage including a large segment of the nerve and surrounding intrinsic muscle and protective fat when this agent has been used.

SURGICAL MANAGEMENT

It is often difficult to determine which interspace is more tender, indicating one to be the primary pathologic site and the other to be referred pain into the adjacent branches of the nerve. Both spaces may be involved. Although bilateral nerve involvement may not be the rule, it does occur in either of the spaces as well. Consequently, the author may explore both spaces on a given foot.

A dorsal longitudinal incision is made from the midline of the dorsal edge of the web space commissure to just proximal to the involved metatarsal heads (Fig. 5). The incision is deepened to the level of the intermetatarsal ligament. Small

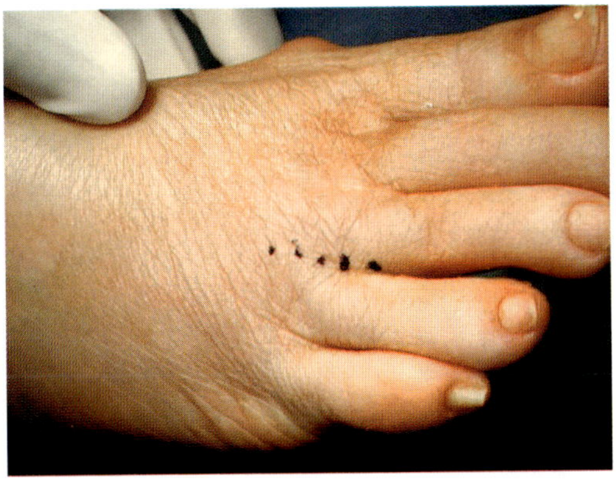

Fig. 5: The linear incision in the interspace

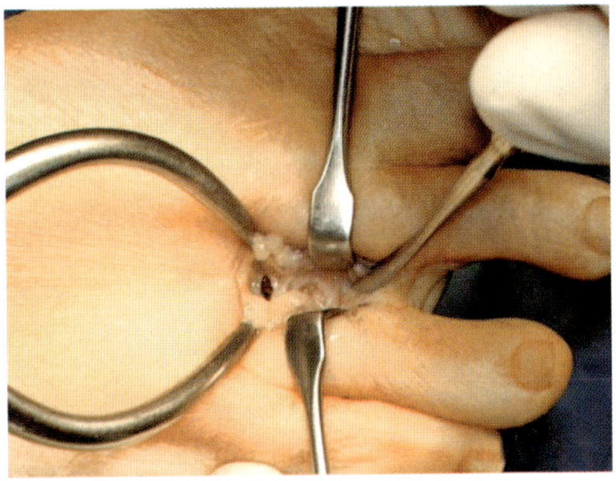

Fig. 6: Insertion of the reverse Gelpi retractor; the Freer elevator demonstrates the distal edge of the intermetatarsal ligament

vessels are cauterized and thin fascial bands are divided to get to the proper level where the stout ligament is located extending between the adjacent plantar plates. The use of loupes for the surgery is helpful to identify the anatomy. A reverse Gelpi retractor (Johnson's neuroma retractor) is placed between the metatarsal heads, rotated and opened, separating the heads and placing the ligament on stretch (Fig. 6). The surgeon repositions himself from the side of the table to the end, to look directly into the interspace from the end of the toes. The distal edge of the ligament is exposed by palpating it with the tips of the scissors and spreading above and below the structure. The ligament is divided carefully staying on the structure from distal to proximal. If the knife or scissors strays plantarward, the neurovascular structures and the intrinsic tendon in the space may be damaged. The use of magnification and careful spreading and cutting under direct vision should avoid any difficulties. *If the tendon is cut, it should be repaired prior to closure to avoid postoperative splaying of the toes.*

Returning to the side position, the surgeon dissects in the space to identify the intermetatarsal nerve and the distal digital nerve branches. In most cases of a Morton's neuroma, the lesion will be easily visualized before or immediately after dividing the ligament, and pops into the wound. In some cases a watery bursa may be encountered just under the ligament. The metatarsal artery and distal branches are dorsal to the nerve and may be intertwined with it. They should be carefully dissected apart and preserved, if possible. In some cases, the artery and nerve are so intimately connected, it is impossible to separate them, and the vessel has to be sacrificed. When the intermetatarsal nerve is difficult to find, dissecting distally into the toe where the digital nerve is more normal in appearance and in location may be done and then the nerve is followed proximally to the intermetatarsal branching. Excellent tourniquet control and a bloodless field allows easier identification of the structures. The yellowish white color of the nerve and its normal striations differentiate it from the tubular and smoother artery. In the pathological state, the identification is more difficult but with the distal nerve identified, the proximal dissection is significantly assisted. The nerve is inspected for size and appearance and palpated with the tips of a delicate Adson forceps to determine the extent of fibrosis. The nerve is gently grasped with the forceps and then pulled off the nerve to determine if it is soft or hard and scratchy. In the case of the latter, one can even hear the roughness of the nerve when fibrosis is significant (Fig. 7).

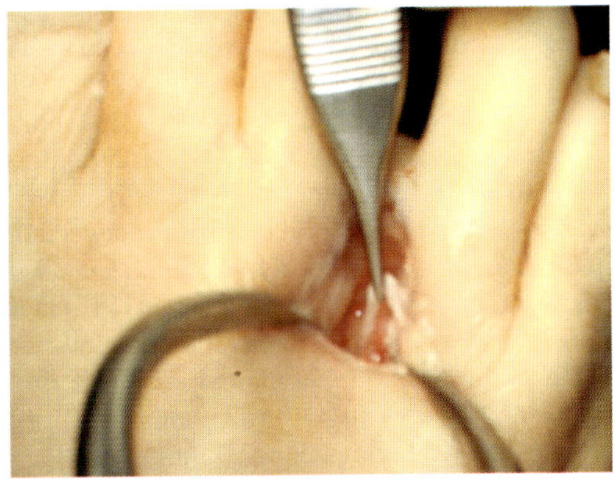

Fig. 7: The nerve is palpated for coarseness indicating fibrosis

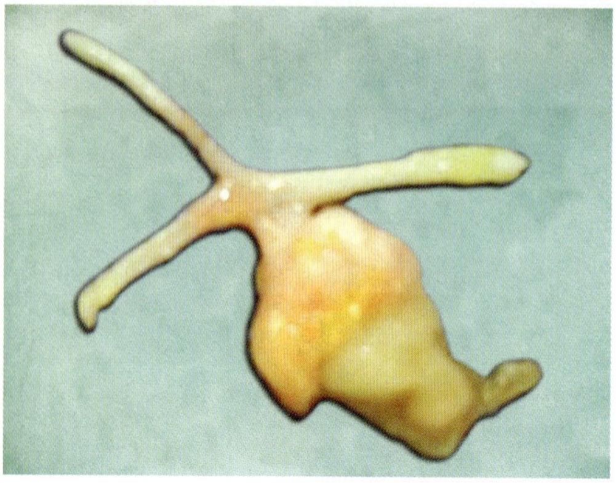

Fig. 8: The intermetatarsal nerve is found to have a neurolemmoma

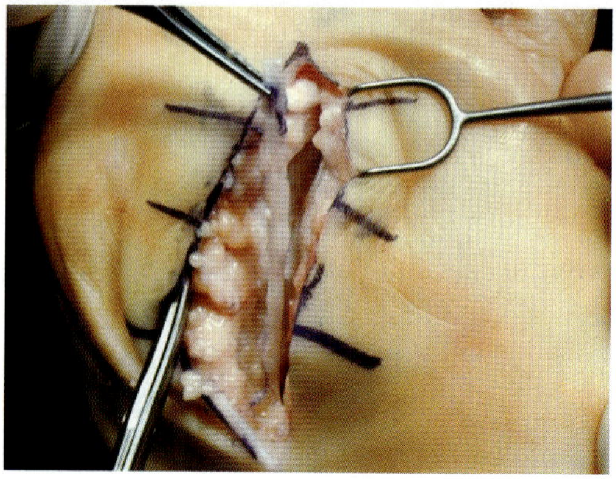

Fig. 9: Plantar approach to a recurrent intermetatarsal neuroma

If two spaces are to be explored, one proceeds in both spaces to reach this point in the procedure. The surgeon would prefer to leave one of the two nerves intact. The removal of one leaves only numbness in the involved web space sides, as the contralateral nerve provides overlapping sensibility for the entire toe. If both nerves are removed, the toe between the spaces becomes significantly numb except on its dorsum to the proximal interphalangeal (PIP) level and slightly beyond, with innervation coming from the dorsal nerves. The periungual area as well as the plantar toe loses all sensibility and trimming of the nail should be relegated to a family member or a pedicurist to avoid the possibility of cutting the toe during such a maneuver.

An enlarged fibrotic nerve should usually be excised; an enlarged but not fibrotic nerve may well recover after the neurolysis (division the intermetatarsal ligament). Removal is done by dividing the distal digital nerves, unwinding of the nerve from the vessels, applying traction distally, and then dividing the nerve sharply and allowing it to retract behind the metatarsal heads (Fig. 8). If the nerve is divided prematurely (more distal than intended), a longitudinal plantar incision should be made and the end of the nerve found and a proper level resection carried out immediately.

Recurrent Intermetatarsal Neuroma

A recurrent intermetatarsal neuroma should be approached plantarward. Re-entering a dorsal incision is fraught with difficulty. There is significant scarring and identification of tissues can be difficult. In addition, the plantar approach is through normal territory and the neuroma is found in the interspace, directly under the plantar fascia.[8] Further resection is helpful if the nerve has become attached to a metatarsal head or a moving tendon. Redirection to a point midway between dorsal and plantar or placement into a muscle are options (Fig. 9). Use of a collagen or vein conduit (as described in Chapter 43 on the treatment of neuromas) may be the best option.

DEEP PERONEAL NERVE ENTRAPMENT[9]

The deep peroneal nerve enters the ankle just beneath the tendon of the extensor hallucis longus, accompanied by the anterior tibial artery and subsequently the dorsalis pedis artery. It passes under, and innervates the extensor hallucis brevis muscle and distal facial edge and then accompanies the first dorsal metatarsal artery into the interval between the first and second metatarsals, after the deep communicating branch descends from the dorsalis pedis at the proximal end of the intermetatarsal space. It continues with the artery into the first web innervating the webspace and the adjacent sides of the great and second toes. Above the ankle joint, the nerve lies between the extensor digitorum communis and the extensor hallucis longus. A centimeter above the ankle, a mixed motor/sensory branch exits the deep nerve and passes laterally to supply the extensor digitorum brevis and the tarsal joints. This nerve has been implicated in sinus tarsi pain conditions (Fig. 10).

The deep peroneal is most commonly injured during surgery in the first web space in the course of bunion surgery. It may also be irritated by an

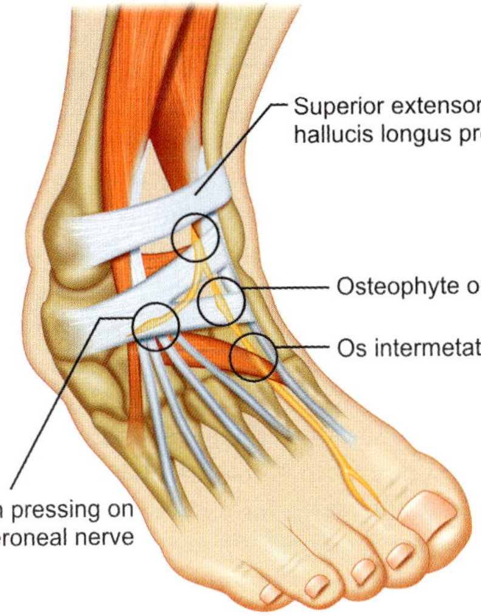

Fig. 10: Deep peroneal nerve compression sites

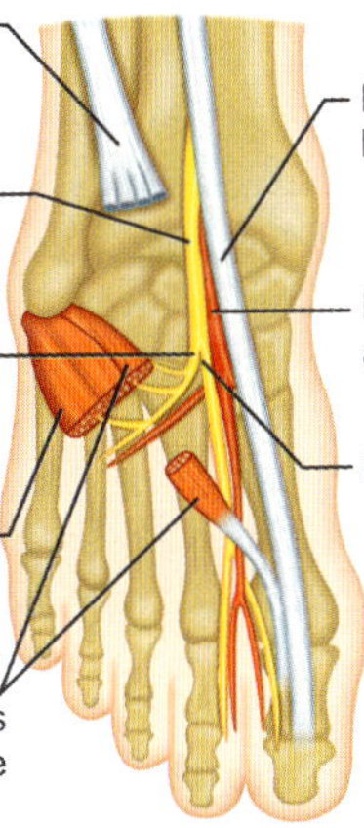

Fig. 11: Deep peroneal compression under the distal border of the extensor hallucis brevis

osteophyte from a joint adjacent to its path and by the distal edge of the extensor hallucis brevis. Finally, a thrombosis of the dorsalis pedis in cases of arteritis occurring in certain collagen diseases may cause pain from the proximity of the swollen adjacent structure.

Excision of the neuroma in the first web space may be sufficient treatment when this occurs. Use of a conduit attached to the neuroma, as described earlier, may be a needed option. Where a neuroma in continuity has been found under the distal edge of the extensor hallucis brevis, the tendon has been divided and placed under the nerve (Fig. 11). In the case of the thrombosed artery, excision of thrombotic segment of the artery has been curative.

An entrapment syndrome of the nerve, known as the "anterior tarsal tunnel"[10] sometimes occurring in diabetics, has been described. This occurs under the fascia between the extensor hallucis longus and anterior tibial tendons and is relieved by a release of the distal extensor retinaculum. It is manifested by dorsal foot pain with paresthesias into the first web; also diagnosed by localized tenderness and a Tinel sign. Forced plantarflexion and inversion may exacerbate the symptoms. It is not typically recognized by electrodiagnostic testing, although there may be abnormal signals in the extensor hallucis brevis with electromyography.

SUPERFICIAL PERONEAL NERVE

The superficial peroneal nerve is the most commonly injured or entrapped nerve in the foot and ankle due to it vulnerable location on the top of the foot. The nerve becomes superficial as it enters the subcutaneous area through a small opening in the fascia overlying the anterior musculature on the anterolateral leg at the junction of the middle and distal third of the leg. As it travels distally over the extensor retinaculum it divides, above the ankle, into the medial cutaneous nerve of the foot and the intermediate cutaneous nerve of the foot.[11] The medial crosses the dorsal foot obliquely in a medial direction, passing over the distal medial cuneiform and follows the dorsomedial side of the first metatarsal, crosses the MTP joint and ends in the medial skin of the great toe. It may be joined by branches of the saphenous nerve. The intermediate supplies the center of the dorsum of the foot, dividing into two main branches which supply the first web, lateral side of the second toe, medial side of the third toe and usually the lateral side of that toe as well (fourth and fifth toes are supplied by the lateral cutaneous nerve of the foot, the dorsal branch of the sural nerve) (Fig. 12).

In its superficial vulnerable position, this nerve is subject to injury with every contusion of the foot, including crushes, fractures, and sprains.[12] When patients have persistent pain in the foot despite negative X-rays after an injury, one should suspect nerve injury! The nerve is also vulnerable to pressure from underlying joint osteophytes, particularly with closed shoes. Finally, iatrogenic injury can occur from surgical interventions, injections, and even with attempts at starting an intravenous (IV).

As with the superficial radial nerve in the wrist and hand, injury to the superficial peroneal is not only difficult to manage, but also may be the inciting cause of a sympathetic overflow reaction and subsequent chronic regional pain syndrome (CRPS). Consequently, it behooves the surgeon to make the diagnosis of nerve injury rapidly and to treat the patient aggressively for it.

The superficial peroneal nerve may be entrapped at the point where it emerges from the fascia by a muscle hernia at this window. In this location, simple enlargement of the window may provide relief. The medial cutaneous branch is notoriously injured

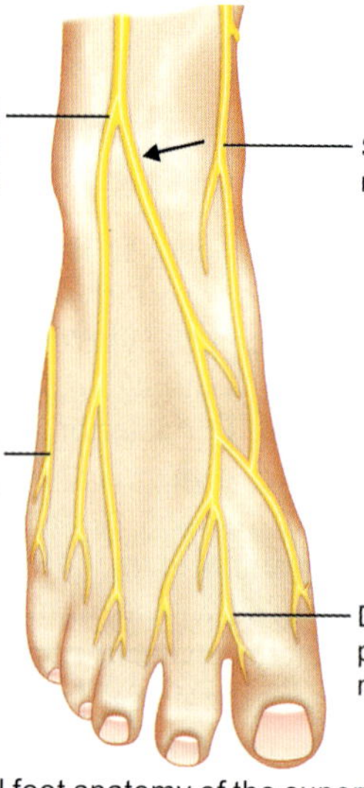

Fig. 12: Dorsal foot anatomy of the superficial peroneal nerve: distally, the medial cutaneous nerve of the foot takes off and the anastomosis of the saphenous nerve

during bunion surgery or during an osteotomy of the medial cuneiform. The intermediate branch may be injured during lateral ligament of the ankle reconstruction, or during ankle arthroscopy, particularly involving the lateral portal. More distally, it is vulnerable during an anteromedial ankle surgery approach or during approaches to the midtarsals and tarsometatarsal joints. Furthermore, it may be injured along with midfoot and metatarsal fractures. As the distal branches of the nerve extend to the PIP level of the toes supplied by these nerves, injury or surgery to these areas may injure the nerves. A ganglion of these various joints may also involve the nerves and be the primary source of pain when these occur. The most frequent cause of injury is, however, blunt trauma to the top of the foot; and this may be the most subtle presentation.

A significant source of pain in the intermediate cutaneous branch is a stretch injury, occurring with an inversion sprain of the lateral ligaments of the ankle. These can be recalcitrant to conservative measures.[12]

The diagnosis is made by appreciating the history of the injury, the characteristics of neurogenic pain, and knowledge of the nerves location. Palpation for tenderness of the nerve and the finding of a Tinel's sign clarifies the diagnosis. As an adjunct to diagnosis, an ultrasound exam may show a change in the characteristic nerve signal and an enlargement or narrowing of the nerve may be recognized, as well as the appreciation of increased fibrous tissue around the nerve.

Conservatively, mechanical desensitization and topical medications are the hallmark of treatment. Transcutaneous electrical nerve stimulator (TENS) units, anti-inflammatories, systemic medications for nerve pain, and even steroids injections have been used. In the end, persistence of the symptoms, or the development of sympathetic overflow, indicate the need for surgical intervention to relieve the ongoing irritant. When there is a concurrent, sympathetic response, systemic medications for nerve pain and sympathetic blocks may also be needed.

Surgically, neurolysis has been the hallmark of treatment and excision of neuromas has frequently been attempted and has been often unsuccessful. Wrapping of this hypersensitive nerve has also not been singularly rewarding. When a neuroma or segment of the damaged nerve has been excised, the proximal end has been purposely drawn under the superficial fascia for protection. A resorbable suture is attached to the end of the nerve; the nerve is led into its new location, and the suture is tied into adjacent fascia to maintain the location while healing occurs. When this has been unsuccessful, the entire nerve has been excised at the level of the fascial opening at the junction of the distal and middle third of the leg and the nerve end is allowed to retract under the fascia. The resultant deficit of sensibility becomes increasingly smaller with peripheral sprouting of the surrounding nerves and is usually well tolerated.

SURAL NERVE[9]

The sural nerve emerges between the heads of the gastrocnemius muscle in the proximal posterior leg receiving branches of the tibial and peroneal nerves after they divide from the sciatic. The sural continues down the midline of the posterior leg with the lesser saphenous vein. From the mid-calf, it veers laterally, to pass midway between the lateral edge of the tendo-Achilles and the posterior edge of the lateral malleolus. It gives off a branch which follows the lateral border of the Achilles tendon. It continues distally plantar to the peroneal sheath to the level of the base of the fifth metatarsal where it splits into a dorsal and plantar branch, supplying the lateral border of the foot and lateral fifth toe and the dorsal fifth and fibular half or the entire fourth toe to the PIP level (Figs 13A and B). The distal portion is known as the "lateral cutaneous nerve of the foot."

Unfortunately, the anatomy of the sural nerve is highly variable and accessory branches of the nerve may emerge proximally and run down the mid and lateral aspects of the calf. Resection of the entire sural nerve may therefore be difficult due to confusion about which and how much of the nerve should be resected.

Injury to the nerve occurs frequently with calcaneal fractures with scarring around and entrapment of the nerve. In addition, iatrogenic injury occurs proximally with gastrocnemius slide procedures, surgery on the tendo-Achilles, open surgery for calcaneal fractures, calcaneal osteotomy, peroneal tendon surgery, surgery at the calcaneo-cuboid and at the base of the fifth metatarsal.

If manual desensitization, time or other conservative measures fail, surgical intervention is indicated. Neurolysis is rarely successful and resection leaves only a small lateral border of the foot insensitive area which is well tolerated. In fact, the sural nerve is frequently used as a nerve graft for this very reason. The problem is leaving a residual painful neuroma. The proximal nerve end may be buried into peroneal or gastrocnemius muscle or resected high in the calf and allowed to retract under

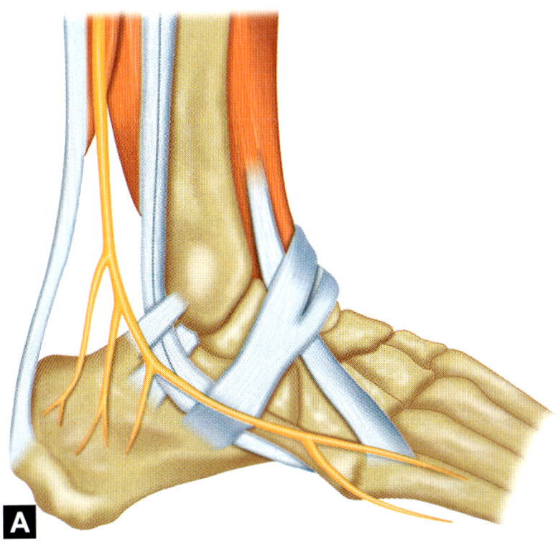

A

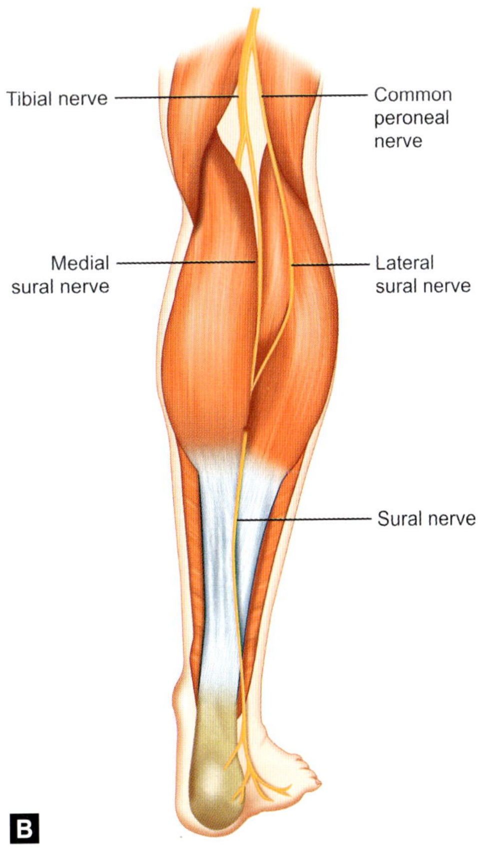

B

Figs 13A and B: The sural nerve: (A) Lateral foot; (B) Posterior calf perspective the head of the gastrocnemius. It is important to find the site of the neuroma and make certain that the nerve being resected proximally is connected to it and is not an accessory nerve. Finding the lesser saphenous vein accompanying the nerve is a reliable reference marker.

SAPHENOUS NERVE

Entrapment or damage to this nerve is not particularly frequent in foot and ankle surgery, although surgery around the medial malleolus in somewhat apt to cause injury in its position adjacent to the greater saphenous vein. The two most common sites for damage to this nerve are the infrapatellar branch of the nerve which may be injured with an incision just distal to the medial joint line of the knee anteriorly or with a medial parapatellar incision carried distally;[13] and along the greater saphenous vein during harvest for its use for coronary artery bypasses surgery. Distally, the nerve passes between the anterior tibial tendon and the medial malleolus, may communicate with branches of the superficial peroneal nerve, and supplies the medial dorsal foot and medial first metatarsal (Figs 12 and 14).

Patients with lesions of this nerve complain of pain, paresthesias and numbness in the distribution of the nerve. Although sensory nerve conduction studies may be helpful, the diagnosis is usually made by clinical examination. The usual conservative treatment includes manual desensitization, topical anti-inflammatories and antineuritic medications,

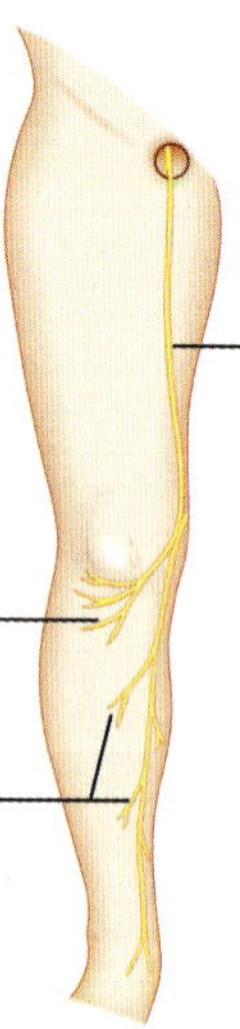

Fig. 14: Saphenous nerve

systemic nerve pain medications, and transcutaneous electrical nerve stimulation. Simple neurectomy, however, is successful in most cases.[9]

TIBIAL NERVE (TARSAL TUNNEL SYNDROME)

Introduction

Tarsal tunnel syndrome, unlike its similar sounding counterpart in the hand, is a significantly misunderstood clinical entity in every respect. The confusion concerning the anatomy involved, the presenting symptomatology, the appropriateness and significance of various diagnostic tests, conservative and surgical management, and finally, the variability of reported results of surgical intervention all attest to the confusion surrounding this condition. The terminology involved in various diagnoses for chronic heel pain is also a hodgepodge of poorly understood entities, many of which are probably variants of the tarsal tunnel syndrome. Because the diagnosis of carpal tunnel syndrome and its usual etiologies is well understood, and the name sounds similar to tarsal tunnel, the diagnostic tools used and the expectations for successful management of the tarsal tunnel problem have not been realized. In fact, the entities have very little in common. In the carpal tunnel, the median nerve lies within a fibro-osseous tunnel surrounded by nine tendons, all of which are subject to various inflammatory conditions, as well as underlying carpal bones subject to synovitis and traumatic dislocations, which create space-occupying lesions. These and hormonal factors result in increased pressure in the tunnel, and effects on the nerve which are easily measurable with delays in nerve conduction and electromyography (EMG) changes found in the thenar eminence. These entities do not exist per se in the tarsal tunnel.

Classic Tarsal Tunnel Syndrome

Classic or proximal tarsal tunnel syndrome is the entity to which many clinicians refer, when the term, "tarsal tunnel", is used. It is an entrapment syndrome of the entire tibial nerve behind the medial malleolus and under the flexor retinaculum or laciniate ligament. The deep and superficial aponeuroses of the leg form the ligament which is closely attached also to the sheaths of the three adjacent flexor tendons, the posterior tibial, the flexor digitorum, and the flexor hallucis. The syndrome was described by Kopell and Thompson in 1960[14] and then named by both Keck[15] and Lam[16] in 1962.

The clinical presentation is typically of posteromedial pain, tenderness posteromedially over the nerve, a positive Tinel's sign in some instances, and in some cases bulging of the retinaculum. In some patients, there may be bonafide neurogenic signs including both the sensation of numbness and actual hypoesthesia and clawing of the toes. X-rays and particularly a CT scan may reveal a lesion, but an MRI and/or ultrasound imaging may be more helpful. A nerve conduction study may demonstrate slowing of conduction of the nerve, and an EMG of the intrinsic muscles: abductor hallucis, abductor digiti quinti, and interossei may also be positive.

Space occupying lesions have been commonly cited for the etiology of this problem. These include ganglia from the subtalar joint or tendon sheaths, lipomas, accessory muscles, tenosynovitis of the adjacent flexors, even though they are within independent sheaths, varicose veins, a bone spicule from an adjacent fracture, foreign bodies, and iatrogenic causes including osteotomies of the os calcis with inadvertent deep penetration medially, or pressure from or penetration by fixation hardware. Classic presentations include the following: a middle-aged physician presented with posteromedial ankle pain, no tenderness, and no neurological deficits. X-rays and an initial MRI were obtained. Both were interpreted as negative for pathology. The author was uncertain of the diagnosis and had little evidence for posteromedial tenosynovitis. For over 2 years, the patient treated himself with analgesics and anti-inflammatories, assuming this to be some form of tendon problem. Although mention was made of tarsal tunnel syndrome, the physical findings were too vague to suggest surgical intervention. Two years later, with symptoms now interfering with his work, and some complaints of rest pain, another MRI, with greater sensitivity, was done. Again, this was interpreted as normal. With increased interest in ultrasound imaging for assessing nerves, a study with this methodology was done and was interpreted as showing a lipoma lying under the nerve (Fig. 15A). Surgical decompression and excision of the lipoma confirmed the diagnosis and the patient obtained full relief (Figs 15B to E). Further review of the MRI revealed that the now obvious lesion had been interpreted as normal fat. A woman in her early twenties presented with a similar history. She was found on MRI and ultrasound to have an accessory muscle, the flexor digitorum accessorius, and had a decompression, excision of the muscle and had slow, but complete relief. The author has also removed a small number of ganglions from the tunnel, but these have presented typically more distally.

Surgical management for the classic tarsal tunnel and its various etiologies requires a release of the laciniate ligament and appropriate management of the underlying lesion. Throughout the literature, there are reports of variable outcomes of the surgical procedure, unlike the results of carpal tunnel release, which, although reliable in the classic postmenopausal female with the entity, gives variable results in occupational etiologies. My opinion and experience with the classic tarsal tunnel outcomes is that when the space occupying lesion is discrete, as in the cases described above, and damage to the nerve does not appear grossly to be anatomic, the anticipation should be for full relief and recovery. When there is obvious damage to the nerve from a fracture or osteotomy, the nerve recovers in a variable manner. When the diagnosis is made without good objective data and the source of compression is not clear, the outcomes are not favorable.

Distal Tarsal Tunnel Syndrome

Distal tarsal tunnel syndrome was first described by Heimkes et al.[17] in 1987 and is a fairly common entity, especially combined with chronic plantar fasciitis[18] and on occasion with posterior tibial tendon dysfunction.[19] This condition involves irritation to the terminal branches of the tibial nerve: typically the medial plantar, lateral plantar, and medial calcaneal nerve. It may involve combinations of these or only the first branch of the lateral plantar, the nerve to the abductor digiti quinti. The most commonly involved of the branches is the lateral plantar.

Anatomy

As the tibial nerve travels distally with the posterior tibial artery and venous comitans, it lies plantar to these structures and slightly deeper. The vessels are easily seen just under the laciniate with a darker blue

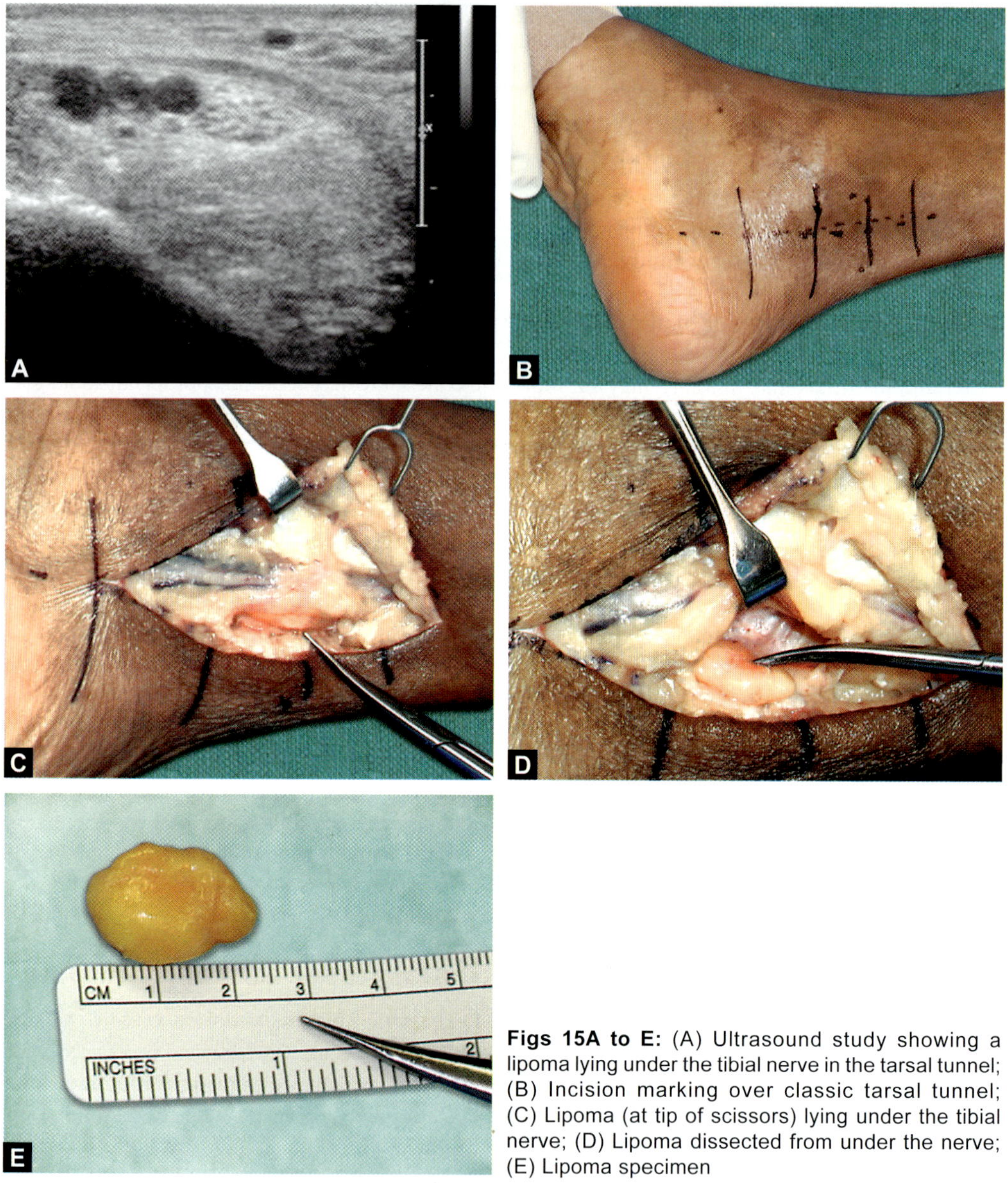

Figs 15A to E: (A) Ultrasound study showing a lipoma lying under the tibial nerve in the tarsal tunnel; (B) Incision marking over classic tarsal tunnel; (C) Lipoma (at tip of scissors) lying under the tibial nerve; (D) Lipoma dissected from under the nerve; (E) Lipoma specimen

appearance of the veins and a paler blue appearance of the thicker walled artery, lying between the veins. The nerve has a whitish appearance with striations. At variable locations, but typically just under the upper edge of the abductor hallucis muscle, the nerve gives off its various branches (Figs 16A and B).

Calcaneal branch: Just prior to passing under the upper edge of the abductor hallucis, the nerve gives off the calcaneal branch or branches which pass posteriorly, then distally in the subcutaneous tissue to the skin of the heel. On occasion, the calcaneal branch may emerge under the upper edge of the muscle and then pierce the muscle and its fascia to enter the subcutaneous tissue.

First branch of the lateral plantar: Just under the upper edge of the abductor, the first branch of the lateral plantar is given off posteriorly. On occasion, it may branch from the lateral plantar portion of the main tibial nerve prior to the upper edge of the abductor, but still travels under the muscle with the lateral plantar. The first branch travels

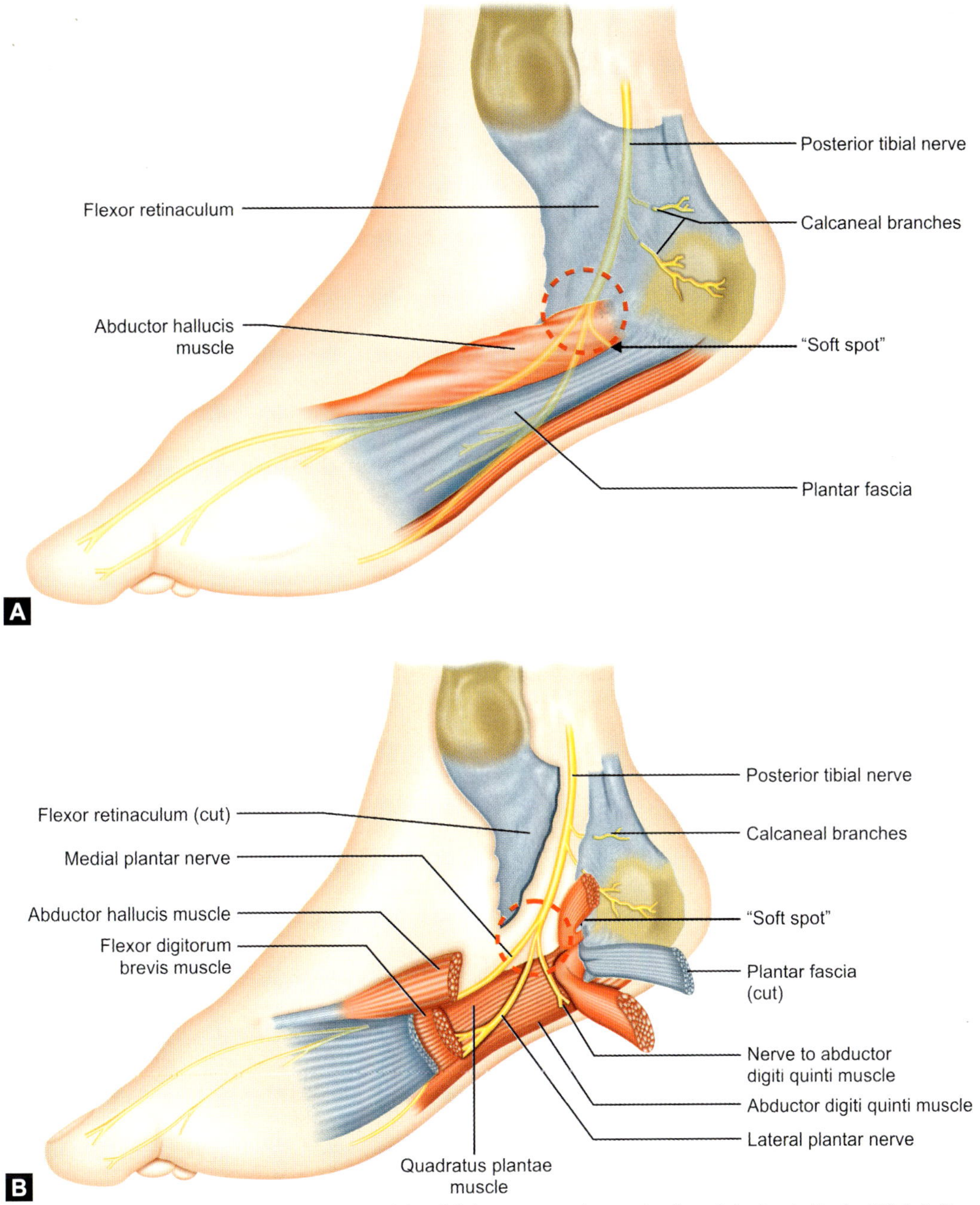

Figs 16A and B: (A) Artist's depiction of the tibial nerve passing under the abductor hallucis; (B) Artist's depiction of the tibial nerve and branches in the distal tarsal tunnel. Note the "soft spot"

under the abductor hallucis and its deep fascia and over the medial fascia of the quadratus plantae. It passes over the edge of the quadratus fascia, under the medial edge of the plantar fascia and then continues transversely across the heel under the flexor digitorum brevis muscle, sends a sensory branch to the central heel skin, and terminates in the muscle of the abductor digiti quinti.

Lateral plantar nerve: The lateral plantar nerve continues distally in the tunnel but is more anterior than its first branch, passing under the deep fascia of the abductor hallucis, under the medial edge of the plantar fascia, over the quadratus plantae and its overlying fascia and then turns distally under the flexor digitorum brevis muscle emerging under the plantar fascia to form the intermetatarsal nerve to the four-fifth interspace and a branch to the three-four intermetatarsal nerve. It also gives off motor branches to the intrinsics as well.

Medial plantar nerve: The medial plantar nerve emerges typically from the tibial under the abductor hallucis muscle and travels under it with the medial plantar artery and veins, innervating the abductor and then terminating under the plantar fascia into the intermetatarsal nerves to the one-two, two-three, and three-four interspaces and motor branches to the interossei and lumbricals. In the longitudinal arch subcutaneous tissue, the nerve lies medial to but adjacent to the flexor digitorum and flexor hallucis tendons.

Pathophysiology

Several etiologies and mechanisms may create compression of the distal tibial nerve and its branches. A space occupying lesion such as a ganglion, may involve the lateral and medial plantar nerves with the lesion emerging from the subtalar or talonavicular joints. A fracture of the medial wall of the calcaneus may cause compression. Neurolemmomas and neurofibromas have been noted to affect these nerves. Direct trauma to the heel and surgical misadventures may affect the calcaneal branches. Inflammatory conditions leading to tenosynovitis of the flexor hallucis and/or flexor digitorum may affect the medial plantar nerve, as well as harvesting of the flexor hallucis in this area of the longitudinal arch for a tendon transfer. However, the more typical etiology is traction neuritis of the lateral plantar and first branch of the lateral plantar nerve.

Baxter and Thigpen[20] in 1984 attributed "central heel pad syndrome" in runners to involvement of this nerve branch and suggested release of the deep fascia of the abductor hallucis and medial edge of the plantar fascia to relieve this problem. In the United States, this nerve branch is commonly known as "Baxter's nerve". Rondhuis and Huson[21] in 1986 described what they considered compression of the first branch of the lateral plantar nerve and its association with heel pain.

Lau and Daniels,[22] in a cadaver study, demonstrated with selective division of the supporting structures of the longitudinal arch: the plantar fascia, posterior tibial tendon, and the interosseous ligaments, increased traction would occur to the tibial nerve and branches and suggested traction neuritis as a possible etiology for distal tarsal tunnel symptoms in conditions which resulted in arch lowering or collapse. Labib et al.[19] in 2002 reported the association with posterior tibial tendon dysfunction. DiGiovanni and Gould, in a number of reports and publications,[18,23] described the association of distal tarsal tunnel with chronic plantar fasciitis; their approach for decompression and the outcome of the procedures. The concept for the release is based on the above literature suggesting the traction etiology.

History and Physical Findings

The typical patient complaint is pain in the plantar heel, often in the posteromedial aspect of the heel and ankle, and sometimes in the longitudinal arch. The history seems very similar to plantar fasciitis and is often wrongly diagnosed and treated.

Plantar fasciitis is a very distinct entity involving the origin of the plantar fascia on the calcaneus, is an enthesopathy, and presents as such. Pain is experienced in the plantar heel with the first step in the morning or when arising during the day from a resting position. The pain remits after a few steps and does not recur with continued walking. The physical finding is discrete tenderness on the medial tubercle of the calcaneus and essentially there alone. The natural course of that disease is that it is self-limited and that it particularly resolves with stretching exercises, with or without simple over the counter arch support.

Tarsal tunnel syndrome, as indicated above, has a broader area of pain involvement and usually begins with prolonged walking, becoming worse the longer one walks. Unlike plantar fasciitis, the pain does not remit spontaneously or immediately with rest. The pain more gradually remits after non-weight bearing. This more gradual resolution of the pain was described by the author as "afterburn." The symptoms may also be even more typically neurogenic, with paresthesias and rest or night pain. It should be emphasized, however, that these more typical neurogenic symptoms are not always present, although the "afterburn" typically is. It should also be noted that more severe neurological deficits, such as numbness and/or motor deficits as

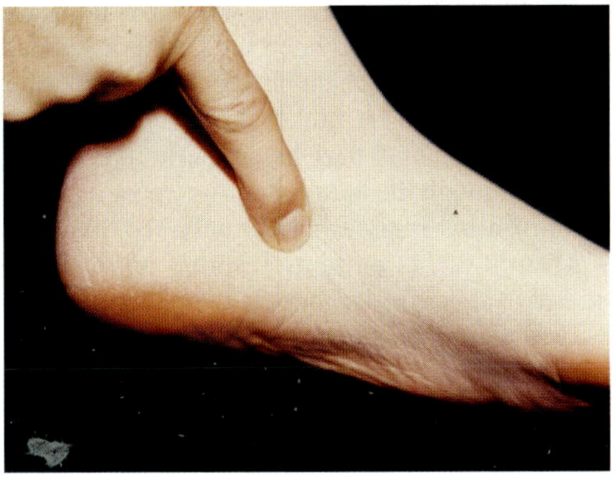

Fig. 17: The clinical "soft spot" where the tibial nerve passes from the ankle to the foot

manifested by clawing of the toes are not common with tarsal tunnel syndrome and should bring to mind other diagnoses, including generalized neuropathy, radiculopathy, or central lesions such as multiple sclerosis.

The physical findings in tarsal tunnel syndrome include point tenderness on the posteromedial heel in the "soft spot" (Fig. 17) at the lower edge of the abductor hallucis where the neurovascular structures enter the foot. As one palpates the medial border of the heel from posteriorly and proximal to distal, the probing finger falls into the soft area described above. There may even be a Tinel's sign over this area and pain may radiate proximally and distally. Palpation of the nerve proximally and in the longitudinal arch may also produce tenderness. In addition, there may be tenderness in each of the intermetatarsal spaces distally, suggesting intermetatarsal neuritis or a Morton's neuroma. However, when the history is of heel pain, this distal tenderness represents nerve irritability, not an accompanying distal lesion. If the complaint is of metatarsal pain and the tenderness is also distal, then the lesion is distal as well. It should be noted that with intermetatarsal neuritis or Morton's neuroma that the complaint and tenderness is distal, but the nerve may also be sensitive proximally or over the "soft spot" but the lesion is distal and the patient does not complain of heel pain. This emphasizes the mandatory correlation of the history and the physical findings.

Distal tarsal tunnel with chronic plantar fasciitis[24] is an extremely common entity and is often extraordinarily confusing to the clinician. In truth, it is simpler than it seems. The history and the physical findings combine both entities. The typical history is of plantar fasciitis which remitted either with standard noninterventional care or more typically, with steroid injections to the origin of the plantar fascia. The earlier treatment was successful, but now there is a recurrence. The recurrence now may not respond to stretching, injections, or simple inserts.

When the history is carefully obtained, one may find that it has changed since the earlier episode. While there may still be first step in the morning pain, it may not remit with continued walking or immediately with rest. The "afterburn," noted above, may now exist. Another presentation is pain with the first step, remission with walking, and then recurrence with prolonged walking and very slow remission of pain afterwards. Finally, there may now be rest or night pain, accentuated by first step pain, or walking in general. *The physical findings include tenderness over the nerve, over the "soft spot," and at the origin of the plantar fascia on the medial tubercle.*

Another finding, which validates the impression that this is a "traction" phenomenon, is that the plantar fascia is found to be attenuated or ruptured. When the ankle is dorsiflexed to neutral or beyond and the great toe is also dorsiflexed, the plantar fascia is placed on stretch. One can palpate the medial border of the fascia from the MTP joint of the great toe to the heel with the opposite hand. When the fascia is attenuated, it becomes less distinct, particularly compared to the normal side; and, in the event of frank rupture, it cannot be felt at all or minimally at best.

Additional Diagnostic Studies

Imaging studies should be obtained to rule out fractures, particularly stress fractures, or other bone lesions. Computed tomography (CT) can demonstrate such pathology in more detail. Radioactive isotope bone scanning is very nonspecific, leading to a variety of diagnoses such as stress fractures or osteomyelitis which need correlation with the history and physical findings and more specific objective testing. MRI is extremely sensitive and will show a space occupying lesion, or a subtle stress fracture, which needs to be confirmed with CT. It may also show a defect or thickening in the plantar fascia suggesting a new or chronic rupture, or simply signal changes at the origin of the plantar fascia, often wrongly interpreted as osteomyelitis or stress fracture, but which may only represent the inflammatory reaction of an enthesiopathy. There has been the suggestion that signal changes may be found in nerves with traction neuritis as well, but this has not been a consistent finding.[25]

Electrodiagnostic studies will not confirm conduction delays anywhere near as frequently as with the carpal tunnel syndrome, and a positive testing is not considered as mandatory for surgical intervention as it is for the upper extremity condition. However, electromyography will often show changes in the abductor hallucis muscle and, when tested, in the abductor digiti quinti.[26] Moreover, the testing is absolutely essential when there is any suggestion of generalized neuropathy or radiculopathy. It is important to point out that with a strong history and physical findings which correlate with distal tarsal tunnel and the failure of the patient to respond to conservative therapy, a negative electrodiagnostic testing does not provide a contraindication for surgery.

Nonoperative Treatment

The author uses the term nonoperative treatment, rather than conservative treatment, to suggest that there are indications where surgery, rather than a nonoperative approach, may be indicated and be the more conservative approach.

For nonoperative treatment, we use a custom total contact insert with a posteromedial nerve relief channel[27] (Figs 18A and B). The channel is placed in the medial wall of the heel component and to the midline in the plantar area. The channel corresponds to the anatomy of the lateral plantar nerve and its first branch and is placed within the cork which is used for posting the heel and longitudinal arch. The channel is filled with a viscoelastic polymer. When the patient's diagnosis is "central heel pad syndrome" or the tenderness is also found in the central heel pad in distal tarsal tunnel, the channel is extended more posteriorly both medially and plantarward. When the medial plantar nerve seems to be involved, the distal edge of the channel is feathered and the channel may be continued along the medial longitudinal arch. When a patient with distal tarsal tunnel is treated with a more standard insert, without the channel, he or she will often state that the insert makes his problem worse. Adding the channel may be dramatic in providing relief. Although the author does not have hard data to confirm his impression, he believes that about two-thirds of his patients respond positively to the use of this insert, alone. If the patient also has residual plantar fasciitis symptoms, we recommend stretching exercises as described by DiGiovanni et al.[28]

Systemic nonsteroidal anti-inflammatories are used for fascia component; oral gabapentin and other drugs to ameliorate neurogenic symptoms with some success as well as topical anti-inflammatories and nerve pain relievers, and iontophoresis as administered by physical therapy. Patients are urged to avoid modalities which are irritating to nerves such as heat, cold, and vibration. This negates the use of hot packs, whirlpool, and ultrasound including phonophoresis.

Operative Intervention

Operative intervention is based on two concepts: that of treating the residuals of chronic plantar fasciitis, and the effort to decompress the tibial nerve and its branches, with emphasis on the lateral plantar and its first branch, and the medial calcaneal and the medial plantar when indicated. Medial calcaneal decompression is usually done in recurrent surgery and is covered in that chapter. Medial plantar decompression is not routinely done, but will be discussed. Treatment of the chronic plantar fasciitis component is based on the observation that chronic ruptures of this tissue tend to remain painful with chronic tenderness of the fascia at its origin, or, with the development of neurogenic symptoms. Complete release of this fascia, as with partial ruptures of other collagen structures such as tendons, (e.g. long head of the biceps, flexor carpi radialis), will provide relief.

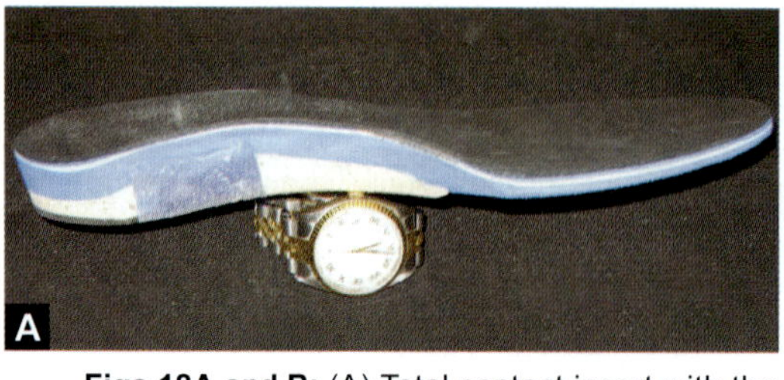

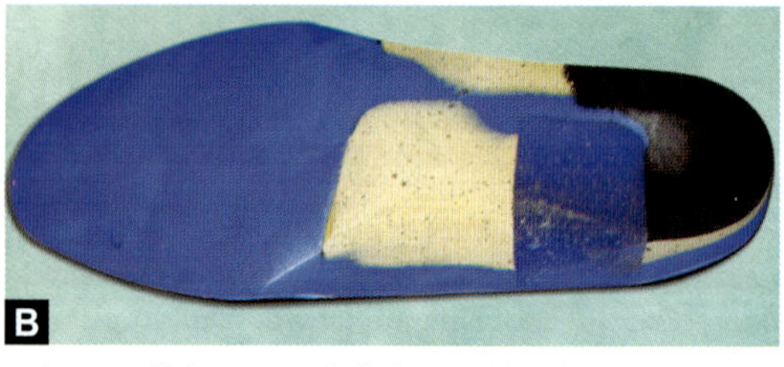

Figs 18A and B: (A) Total contact insert with the posteromedial nerve relief channel (medial view); (B) Total contact insert with nerve relief channel extending around plantar medial side

The decompression of the nerve is based on the concept of traction of the nerve with the fulcrum of pressure as it passes under the distal edge of the deep fascia of the abductor hallucis and medial edge of the plantar fascia, and over the fibers of the quadratus plantae fascia. The nerve can be observed to be "tented" under and over these structures at the "soft spot," as it makes a significant turn from the ankle into the foot. The releases of the structures allow the nerve to lie freely at this angle.

Since partial rupture of the plantar fascia seems to remain symptomatic, if it is necessary to release some of the plantar fascia to relieve the nerve, the author has been hesitant to not release it all. Concern over dorsal arch and lateral border pain after release of the entire plantar fascia has lead to our postoperative regimen of non-weight bearing for 4 weeks and the use of the insert postoperatively during the first year. Our experience has shown that to be successful in avoiding the dorsal and lateral foot pain after this procedure.

Operative Indications

Most patients with a diagnosis of distal tarsal tunnel syndrome with or without chronic plantar fasciitis deserve a trial of nonoperative treatment. If the history and physical are compatible with the diagnosis and there is either no indication of radiculopathy or generalized neuropathy, or that and other possible diagnoses have been appropriately ruled out, a 6 week trial of treatment with the total contact insert, as described, is indicated.

If, at 6 weeks, the patient is somewhat improved, the author continues with this approach for another 6 weeks. As long as improvement is seen, the author continues nonoperatively.

If the patient is not improved at 6 weeks, initially, the orthotic device is examined to be certain it has been properly made and fits well. The patient is asked if he or she is using it constantly when up and about. If the patient has been compliant and the device is appropriate, diagnostic points are reviewed, and if still consistent with the initial impression, surgery is recommended.

If the patient was improving with the insert and has reached a plateau, the same ritual is followed, and the patient is asked if he is satisfied to continue to use the insert rather than to have surgery.

Some patients present with a history and physical findings totally compatible with the distal tarsal tunnel diagnosis and a significant period of nonoperative treatment, which may be similar to but not an exact replica of the author's regiment. A new insert is prescribed, or if possible, the existing insert is modified to include the nerve relief channel. The surgery is scheduled and the patient is asked to begin wearing the new insert. If the patient improves, he or she is given the option to delay the surgery; or, if the improvement is not significant, the surgical option is available.

Operative Technique[29]

The surgery is performed under general or regional anesthesia, but not local, which obscures the anatomy. It is usually an outpatient procedure. A thigh or high calf tourniquet is used along with good lighting and magnifying loupes (3.5X or 4.5X). With the patient in the supine position and the leg externally rotated, a curvilinear incision is begun midway between the posterior edge of the medial malleolus and the medial border of the tendo-Achilles. The incision continues distally curving gently forward to cross the "soft spot" and then continue across the plantar skin just distal to the heel pad about three-fourth of the distance across the plantar surface (Fig. 19A).

The vascular bundle is noted under the laciniate ligament. The ligament is divided over the bundle distally to the abductor hallucis superficial fascia which is also divided, watching for the occasional calcaneal branch which may pierce it in its proximal substance (Fig. 19B). The subcutaneous fat over the plantar fascia is divided and deeper retractors, such as Senns, are inserted. The convex shape of the plantar fascia is noted and a small angled retractor is placed at the medial edge of the abductor digiti quinti. The entire plantar fascia is divided from the abductor hallucis to the abductor digiti quinti (Fig. 19C).

Dissecting under the abductor hallucis, the muscle is teased away from its deep fascia, approaching the muscle from either proximally or distally. A small right angle is inserted into the space between the muscle and fascia, the deep fascia is divided with a tenotomy scissors (Fig. 19D). The division is begun either proximally or distally and then completed from the other direction.

Across from the plantar edge of the abductor hallucis the muscle of the flexor digitorum brevis is lifted and a deep fascia of variable thickness is also divided. Care is taken throughout this process to avoid lacerating any of the small branches of the posterior tibial artery or veins. If visibility is obscured, particularly with bleeding, the entire muscle of the abductor hallucis is divided and even the medial edge of the flexor brevis with a cutting cautery to gain good access to the bleeder. To stop this bleeding, a bipolar cautery or a small ligaclip is used.

Assuming that the incision is properly placed, and the abductor hallucis is intact, the interval between the abductor and the flexor digitorum brevis is exposed with a small self-retaining retractor (Weitlaner) (Fig. 19E). Within this interval are the vascular structures, the first branch of the lateral plantar nerve and the lateral plantar nerve. The first branch lies closer to the posterior heel, the veins with the artery in the middle lie more anteriorly, followed by the lateral plantar nerve which lies even more anteriorly and a little deeper than the vascular structures. Filmy fascia and fat may be found over the nerve which, with dissection, becomes very distinct as a white serrated tubular structure (Fig. 19F).

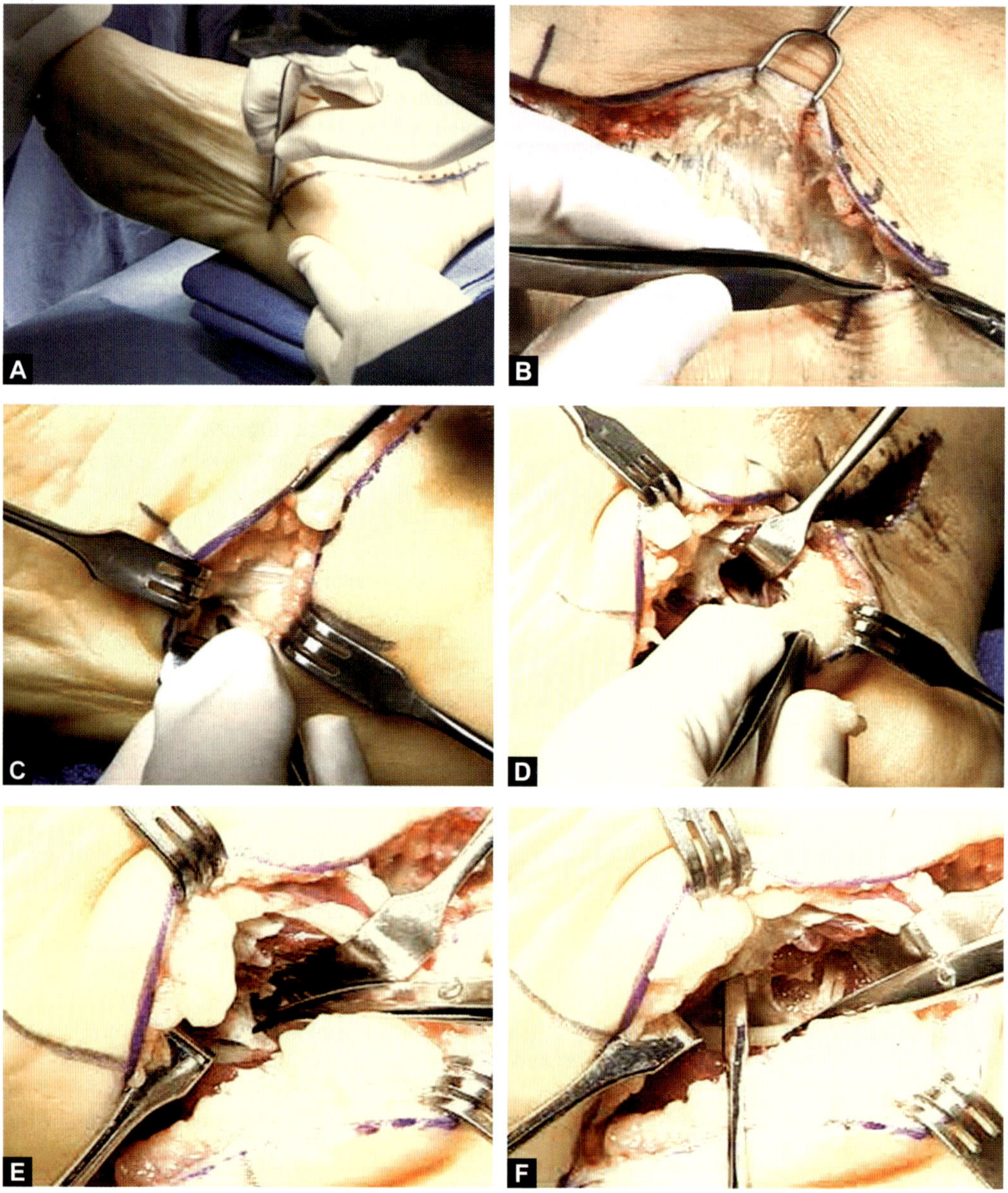

Figs 19A to F: (A) The posteromedial incision used for the tarsal tunnel release; (B) The laciniate ligament; (C) The convex plantar fascia; (D) Release of the deep fascia of the abductor hallucis; (E) The interval between the abductor hallucis and the flexor digitorum brevis; (F) The lateral plantar nerve

At this point, the medial plantar nerve has divided off more proximally and is traveling anteriorly under the abductor muscle. Moving the lateral plantar nerve aside with the tip of the tenotomy scissors and a fine forceps, the underlying fibers of the quadratus plantae are visualized and divided.

Unless access to stop bleeding is needed; one is doing a recurrent case which requires full visualization of the nerve; decompression of the medial plantar nerve is required; or one is disoriented and better visualization of the neurovascular anatomy is required, the abductor muscle is not released, as this adds to the morbidity of potentially more scarring.

Additional decompression is done when there is a septum between the vessels and the lateral plantar nerve. This may be seen by looking under the abductor muscle and is suspected when seen distally in the interval between the abductor and flexor. The muscle may have to be divided when this is present.

When the medial plantar nerve is involved, the same initial approach is used, dividing the muscle and then, noting exactly where the medial neurovascular bundle is running, making a skin incision over this pathway and decompressing the vessels and nerve along this route through the muscle.

The closure consists of dissolving suture (4-0 monocryl) for the subcutaneous skin of the ankle with 4-0 nylon on the skin, and skin only closure with 3-0 nylon for the glabrous skin area plantarly and distally medially.

Postoperatively, the patient is placed in a soft bulky dressing and kept non-weight bearing for the first 2 weeks. Sutures are removed at this time and non-weight bearing is continued for 2 more weeks. No dressing is needed and the patient can bathe the foot. Motion of the foot and toes is encouraged to maintain the gliding of the nerve. At 4 weeks, the patient is allowed to walk with the total contact insert in a shoe or sandal, which is continued for 9 months.

Outcomes

DiGiovanni and Gould[16] reported an 82% rate of total recovery in a group of primary releases done and followed for at least 2 years, with no recurrences and no patients made worse. In a group of 104 feet in 92 patients operated at the American Sports Medicine Institute, between 1996 and 2000, Hollis et al.[30] found that the average time for patients to reach a plateau of recovery was 19.6 months with a range from 6 months to 2.5 years. A further report from Gould and DiGiovanni[31,32] has confirmed continued success with this operative approach with excellent long-term outcomes. The approaches and outcomes related to relapsed, recurrent or failed procedures are reported in the next segment.

THE FAILED TARSAL TUNNEL RELEASE

Introduction

As noted in the previous section on the "Tarsal Tunnel Release," the literature on the tarsal tunnel syndrome presents a confusing picture of the entity itself, the anatomy involved, and the etiology of the condition. While the failure rate ranges from numbers as high as 40–60%[33] to the author's data which suggests numbers as low as less than 5%,[2] this is based on a variety of recommended surgical releases and multiple other factors, to be discussed below. In the practices of the author and his associates, large numbers of patients with heel pain with failure to respond to standard conservative and surgical approaches are seen. As a result of this, extensive exposure to the problem over 24 years, a series of reasons for surgical failures and potential solutions for these problems have evolved.[24] Painful nerves respond to treatment in a variable manner and patients with these problems also have a variety of responses, highly dependent on their own reaction to ongoing painful stimuli. The central perception of pain is a complex process, dependent on multiple factors and various psychological issues which make management of these patients difficult. Nonetheless, an algorithm has developed for management based on what seem to be logical interpretations of why the nerves remain painful after a surgical release.[35,36]

Why the Surgical Release Fails

The following are the usual reason for failure of the surgical release:[5]

- Inadequate release due to a lack of understanding of the anatomy involved.
- The failure to execute the release properly.
- The bleeding with subsequent scarring.
- The damage to the nerve or its branches in the course of the release.

- The persistent hypersensitivity of the irritated nerve.
- The intrinsic damage to the nerve initially.

Inadequate Release due to the Lack of Understanding of the Anatomy

It is essential to appreciate that although there are space occupying lesions involved in the classic tarsal tunnel, as described in the prior section, in the so-called "distal tarsal tunnel," which is the more common entity, adequate release of the confluence of the superficial and deep fascias of the abductor hallucis and the proximal medial edge of the plantar fascia is essential, as well as the underlying fascia of the quadratus plantae, in some cases. As noted in the description of the complete release, the laciniate ligament and the entire plantar fascia is also released. In chronic heel pain, the partial rupture of the plantar fascia is likely a pain generator with persistent symptoms in chronic plantar fasciitis. As nerve pain is also a factor in this entity, the distal, plantar edge of the abductor fascia and medial edge of the plantar fascia appears to be the site where the nerve sustains the traction irritation.

Failure to Execute the Release Properly

Landmarks are essential. The "soft spot" on the posteromedial heel is a distinct location where the neurovascular bundle enters the foot. It marks the exact location of the lateral plantar and where the traction point occurs. The skin incision is made in the midline about halfway between the posterior edge of the medial malleolus and the medial edge of the tendo-Achilles. It crosses into the foot over the "soft spot" (Fig. 17) and then extends across the sole of the foot about three quarters of the width just distal to the heel pad. As one enters the laciniate ligament, the neurovascular bundle is easily visualized. In the interval between the abductor hallucis muscle and the flexor digitorum brevis, after the fascias have been released, the lateral plantar nerve is found in the distal potion of the tunnel making a 45° turn into the plantar foot (Figs 16A and B). The first branch of the nerve is more proximal and posterior. If the incision does not follow the surface landmarks, the anatomy is confusing and the structures do not lie is this relationship. The release may be inadequate and not include the critical structures.

Bleeding with Subsequent Scarring

Bleeding not only obscures the visualization of the anatomy, but also leads to increased postoperative scarring and potential traction on the nerve with foot and ankle movement. To avoid this, it is important to use loupe magnification, good lighting, delicate instruments, and careful bipolar cautery. When a vessel is lacerated or torn, and the venous comitans are very vulnerable, the abductor hallucis and/or flexor digitorum brevis are divided with a unipolar cutting cautery, and small "ligaclips" to halt the bleeding are used. Careful hemostasis is essential.

Persistent Hypersensitivity

This problem occurs with neuropathy and also in some diabetics without neuropathy *per se*. With longstanding compression/traction and consequent high grades of nerve injury, pain and hypersensitivity may persist. During regeneration of nerves, following release, painful dysesthesia is also not uncommon.

Potential Solutions to the Causes of Failed Releases

Inadequate Releases

Carrying out an adequate release involves a release of all the structures indicated in the primary release. However, in the revision surgery, the abductor hallucis, and possibly the flexor digitorum brevis, are released with a cutting mode unipolar cautery, and the tibial nerve and its branches are fully exposed. This is not done in a primary release where the philosophy is minimal nerve handing, as is recommended with carpal tunnel release. The calcaneal branches are examined for possible injury, as well as looking for iatrogenic scar bands potentially compressing the nerve. If there are symptoms involving the medial plantar nerve, the release is carried into the abductor hallucis muscle until the source of compression or irritation is found. Release or external neurolysis alone is done unless damage has occurred to portions of the nerve. If this is found, further measures are taken as described and illustrated below.

External Scarring of the Nerve(s)

Adherence of the nerve to surrounding tissues prevents movement or gliding of the nerve within the tissues as adjacent joints move. As for the tibial nerve, flexion/extension, inversion/eversion of the ankle and subtalar joints requires that the nerve moves with these motions. When gliding fails to occur, due to scarring of the nerve, traction neuritis and pain results. In the natural state, nerves are frequently surrounded by loose adipose tissue. Efforts to replace this gliding tissue have included placing free fat around the nerve and the use of various materials to "wrap" the nerve. Attempts to wrap rabbit nerves with free fat (Unpublished data from St Vincent's Microsurgical Unit, Melbourne, Australia, 1982) resulted in the formation of dense adherent fibrous tissue. Free vascularized adipose tissue, muscle and fascia have all been used successfully. Allograft and autograft veins and bovine collagen tubes have also been used in this effort.

The technique for autogenous veins usually involves the use of the greater saphenous vein. The technique involves harvesting the vein, carefully ligating or cauterizing the branches, dissecting free the saphenous nerve, and ligating the ends of the vein on either side of the harvested portion. The vein is soaked in 1% lidocaine to relax the smooth muscle and then it is slit longitudinally. The nerve is wrapped barber pole fashion with the intima of the vein against the nerve. The end of the coil is attached to surrounding tissue and not to the vein itself, to avoid a constricting end. The wrapping is done loosely but without redundancy in order to have enough tissue. The length of graft necessary to wrap a tibial nerve with the greater saphenous is usually about three times the length of vein for the length of nerve needing to be wrapped. Each loop is sewn to the adjacent one with one or two sutures of 6-0 nylon (Fig. 20). Gliding seems to occur between the outside of the vein and the surrounding tissues although there is definitely a tissue plane and some movement between the vein and the nerve (Figs 21A and B).

Collagen tubes are also available for this purpose and are far more convenient (Figs 22A and B). They come in up to 5 cm segments, split

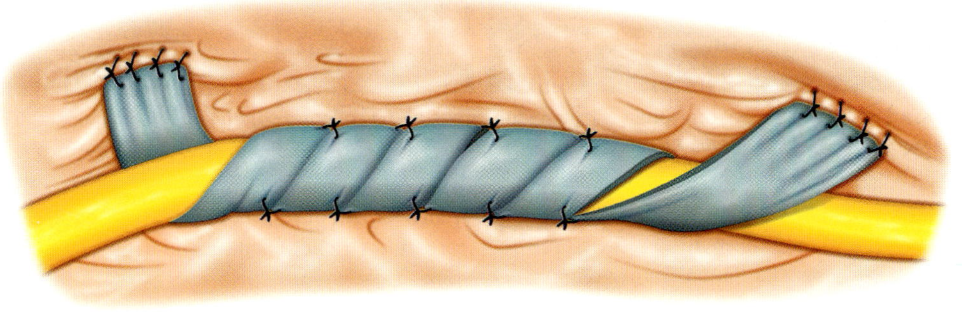

Fig. 20: Vein wrapping a nerve (Artist's rendition)

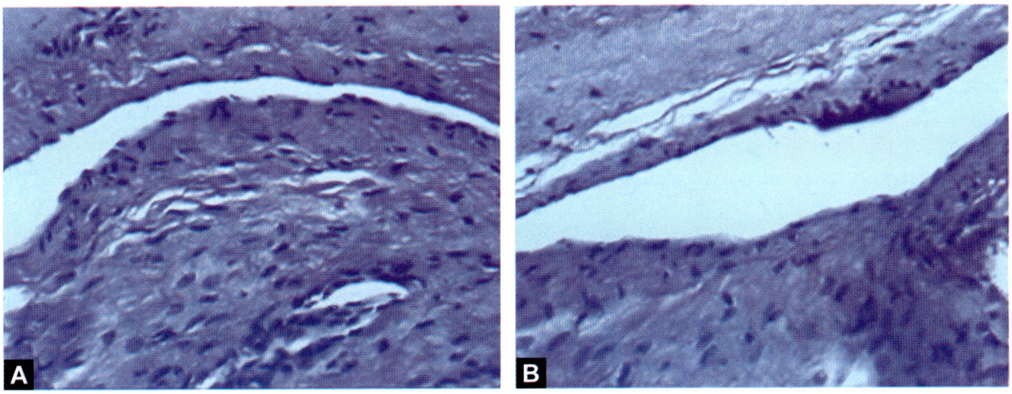

Figs 21A and B: The cleavage plane between the nerve and vein

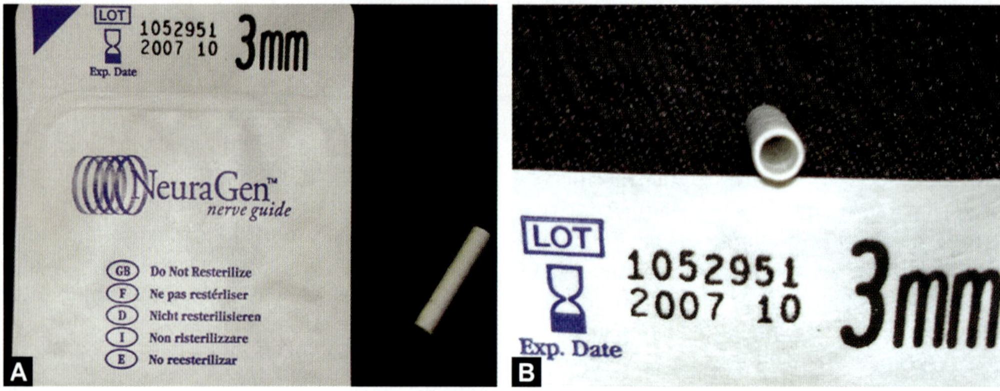

Figs 22A and B: Collagen wraps

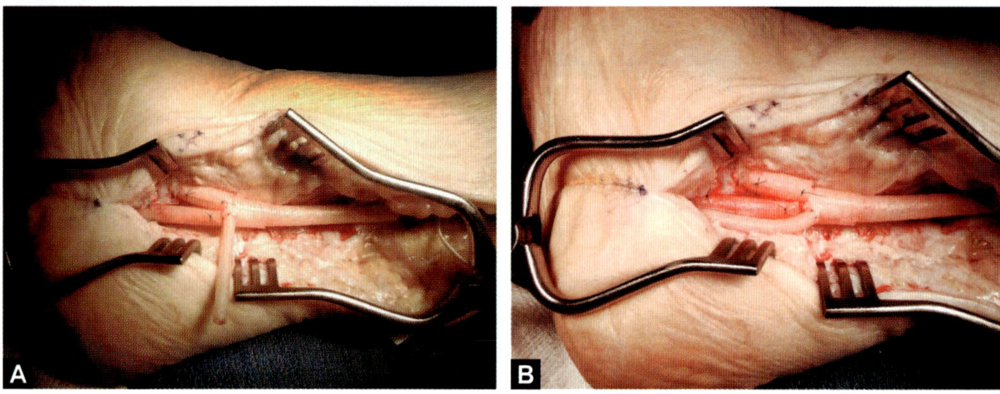

Figs 23A and B: The tibial nerve wrapped with collagen wraps and a collagen conduit on the cut calcaneal nerve. (A) The conduit projecting from the nerve; (B) the corrugated conduit laid alongside the rest of the wrapped nerve

longitudinally, and a variety of diameters, ranging from 2 mm to 12 mm. This allows the nerve to be simply laid within the lumen, rather than to be wrapped. Some brands require a few sutures of 6-0 to close the tube loosely, while other brands open up longitudinally to admit the nerve and wrap around it more than one and half times so that no sutures are required to close the loop. Segments of various diameters can be applied and then sutured to each other. For example, one might use a larger diameter segment for the tibial nerve and smaller diameters for the lateral and medial plantars. The tube material may also be corrugated to prevent kinking as the nerve goes around a corner. The advantage of the prepared tubes is the availability in various diameters, quantities, and avoidance of donor site morbidity and scarring. Our results to date show no difference or advantage of the veins over the commercial products. The bell shaped curve of outcomes suggests at least 70% significant improvement or relief of pain for all patients in this category with none without some improvement and none made worse.

Intrinsic Damage to the Nerve

For areas of the nerve with obvious severe internal scar and/or neuromas in continuity, several solutions have been attempted. When the nerve essentially provides good plantar sensibility, nerve wrapping, as described above, has been done with some success. Neuromas of the calcaneal branches have been placed in vein and collagen conduits (Figs 23A and B). Damaged segments of the nerve have been resected under the microscope and grafted with contralateral sural nerve grafts. When the entire tibial or a plantar nerve has been intrinsically damaged and there is no sensibility in its distribution, the entire segment has been excised and repaired with sural graft or when the

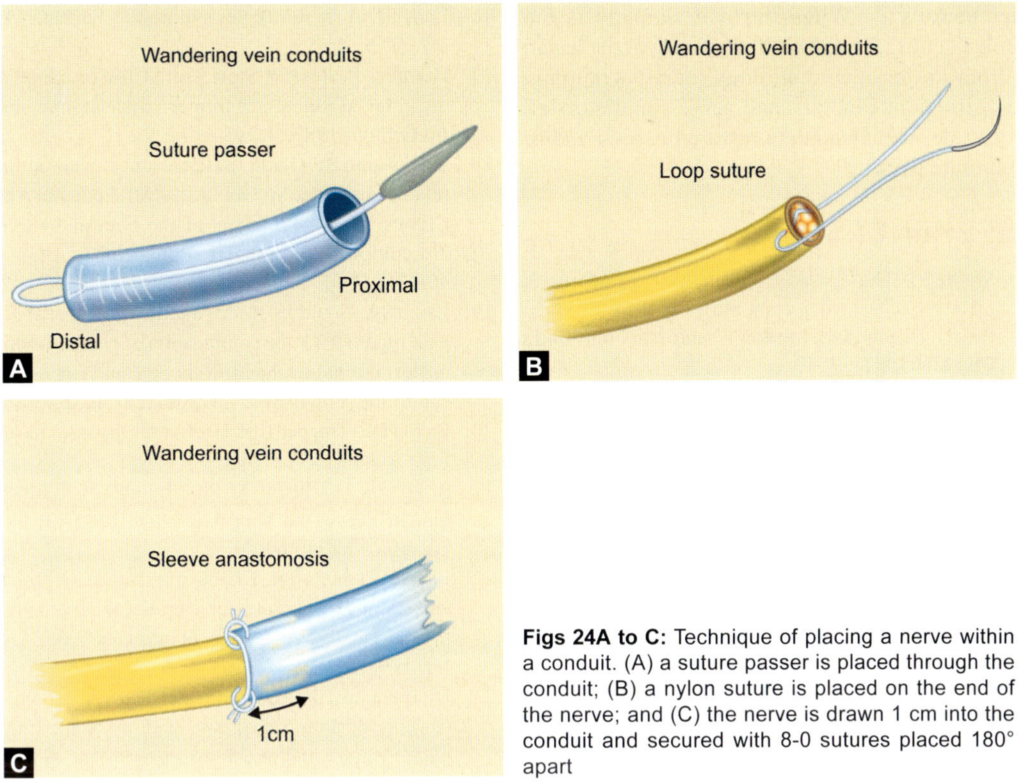

Figs 24A to C: Technique of placing a nerve within a conduit. (A) a suture passer is placed through the conduit; (B) a nylon suture is placed on the end of the nerve; and (C) the nerve is drawn 1 cm into the conduit and secured with 8-0 sutures placed 180° apart

distal segment is remote or not found, the end of the nerve has been placed within a vein or collagen conduit (Figs 24A to C). The nerve is drawn into the conduit about 1 cm. A nylon suture is placed on the end of the nerve. A Hewson suture passer is placed through the conduit with the nylon ends placed through its loop. The nerve is drawn into the conduit as noted and the edge of the conduit sutured to the epineurium of the nerve with 8-0 monofilament suture using surgical loupes for magnification.

Collagen conduits are particularly advantageous as they are available in various diameters, e.g. 2, 2.5, 3, 4, 5 mm in diameter and 2.5 cm in length. The end of the conduit may be laid next to the parent nerve, or led into a quiet area such as the retrocalcaneal space. The concept of the conduit is that the nerve will regenerate only 1 cm and then fails to form a neuroma with the lack of neurotropic effect of a distal segment of nerve.

Additionally, peripheral nerve and dorsal column stimulators were used. At one point in time, the author was fairly enthusiastic about the peripheral nerve stimulators. However, failure to maintain contact of the stimulator electrodes with the nerve, electrical leaks at the stimulator connectors, and other issues including patient complaints of shocking when passing through electronic metal detectors has led to the discontinuation of implantation. Patients are still referred to pain clinic specialists (anesthesiologists) and neurosurgeons that implant dorsal column stimulators. Trial implantations are done routinely prior to permanent implants. There are many patients with good pain control with these devices, but good studies with reliable data are scanty.

CONCLUSION

Failed surgical releases of the tarsal tunnel may be due to numerous causes including inaccurate diagnosis. Many of the failures are due to lack of appreciation of the involved anatomy or inadequate technique. When an insufficient release is done, a revision simply completes the necessary steps. When external scarring is the problem, barrier materials may be used to help and protect the nerve after neurolysis. When intrinsic damage is the problem, either from the primary cause of the lesion or from an iatrogenic etiology, nerve wrapping, reconstruction, conduits, and nerve stimulators all play a role, as indicated, to restore function and/or ameliorate pain.

REFERENCES

1. Mulder J. The causative mechanism in Morton's metatarsalgia. J Bone Joint Surg Br. 1951;33:94-5.
2. Kay D, Bennett GL. Morton's neuroma. Foot Ankle Clin. 2003;8(1):49-59.
3. Younger AS, Claridge RJ. The role of diagnostic block in the management of Morton's neuroma. Can J Surg. 1998;41(2):127-30.
4. Sharp RJ, Wade CM, Hennessy MS, et al. The role of MRI and ultrasound imaging in Morton's neuroma and the effect of size of lesion on symptoms. J Bone Joint Surg Br. 2003;85(7):999-1005.
5. Weinfeld SB, Myerson MS. Interdigital neuritis: diagnosis and treatment. J Am Acad Orthop Surg. 1996;4(6):328-35.
6. Peters PG, Adams Jr SB, Schon LC. Interdigital neuralgia. In: Gould JS, Myerson MS (Editors). Foot and Ankle Clinics. Philadelphi (PA); WB Saunders Co;2011.
7. Mozena JD, Clifford JT. Efficacy of chemical neurolysis for the treatment of interdigital nerve compression of the foot: a retrospective study. J Am Podiatr Med Assoc. 2007;97(3):203-6.
8. Beskin JL, Baxter DE. Recurrent pain following interdigita lneurectomy—a plantar approach. Foot Ankle. 1988;9(1):34-9.
9. Flanigan RM, DiGiovanni BF. Peripheral nerve entrapments of the lower leg, ankle, and foot. Foot Ankle Clin. 2011;16:255-74.
10. Borges LF, Hallett HM, Selkoe DJ, et al. The anterior tarsal tunnel syndrome: report of two cases. J Neurosurg. 1981;54:89-92.
11. Adkison DP, Bosse MJ, Gaccione DR, et al. Anatomical variation in the course of the superficial peroneal nerve. J bone Joint Surg Am. 1991;73:112-4.
12. O'Neill PJ, Prks BG, Walsh R, et al. Excursion and strain of the superficial peroneal nerve during inversion ankle sprain. J Bone Joint Surg Am. 2007; 89:979-86.
13. Kopell HP, Thompson WA. Knee Pain due to saphenous nerve entrapment. N Engl J Med. 1960;263:351-3.
14. Kopell HP, Thompson WA. Peripheral entrapment neuropathies of the lower extremity. N Eng J Med. 1960;262:56-60.
15. Keck C. The tarsal tunnel syndrome. J Bone Joint Surg. 1962;44:180-2.
16. Lam SJ. A tarsal-tunnel syndrome. Lancet. 1962; 2:1354-5.
17. Heimkes B, Posel P, Stots S, et al The proximal and distal tarsal tunnel syndromes. An anatomic study. Int Orthop. 1987;11:193-6.
18. DiGiovanni BF, Gould JS. Tarsal tunnel syndrome and related entities I. In: Gould JS (Ed). Foot and Ankle Clinics "Nerve Problems of the Foot and Ankle," 3rd edition. WB Saunders; Philadelphia: 1998. pp. 405-26.
19. Labib SA, Gould JS, Rodriguez del Rio FA, et al. Heel pain triad (HPT): the combination of plantar fasciitis, posterior tibial tendon dysfunction, and tarsal tunnel syndrome. Foot Ankle Int. 2002;23:212-20.
20. Baxter DE, Thigpen CM. Heel pain: Operative Results. Foot Ankle. 1984;5:16-25.
21. Rondhuis JJ, Huson A. First branch of the lateral plantar nerve and heel pain. Acta Morphol Neerl Scand. 1986;24:269-79.
22. Lau JT, Daniels TR. Effects of tarsal tunnel release and stabilization procedures on tibial nerve tension in a surgically created pes planus foot. Foot Ankle Int. 1998;19:770-7.
23. DiGiovanni BF, Rodriguez del Rio FA, Gould JS. Chronic disabling heel pain with associated nerve pain: primary and revision surgery results. Podium presentation and abstract at the 17th Annual Summer meeting of the American Orthopaedic Foot and Ankle Society. San Diego, July 2001
24. Gould JS. Chronic plantar fasciitis. Am J Orthop. 2003;32:11-3.
25. Lopez-Ben R. Department of Radiology, Division of Orthopaedic Surgery, University of Alabama at Birmingham Personal Communication, 2010.
26. Schon LC, Glennon TC, Baxter DE. Heel pain syndrome: electrodiagnostic support for nerve entrapment. Foot Ankle. 1993;14:129-35.
27. Gould JS, Ford D. Orthoses and insert management of common foot and ankle problems. In: Schon LC, Porter DA (Eds). Baxter's the Foot and Ankle in Sport. Mosby Elsevier; Philadelphia: 2008. pp. 585-93.
28. DiGiovanni BF, Nawoczenski DA, Lintal ME, et al. Tissue-antar fascia stretching exercise enhances outcomes in patients with chronic heel pain. A prospective randomized study. J Bone Joint Surg Am. 2003;85(7):1270-7.
29. DiGiovanni BF, Abuzzahab FS, Gould JS. Plantar fascia release with proximal and distal tarsal tunnel release: surgical approach to chronic disabling plantar fasciitis with associated nerve pain. Tech Foot Ankle Surg. 2003;2:254-61.

30. Hollis M, Ferguson A, Gould JS, et al. American Sports Medicine Institute review of 104 feet (92 patients) following the complete plantar fascia and tarsal tunnel release between 1996-2000. Unpublished.
31. Gould JS, DiGiovanni BF. "Plantar fascia release in combination with proximal and distal tarsal tunnel release." In: Wiesel SW (Ed). Operative Techniques in Orthopaedic Surgery, 4th Edition, Wolters Kluwer/ Lippincott, Williams and Wilkins; Philadelphia: 2011. pp. 3911-9.
32. Gould JS. "Tarsal tunnel syndrome." In: Nerve Problems of the Lower Extremity Foot and Ankle Clinics. WB Saunders/Elsevier; Philadelphia: 2011. pp. 275-86.
33. Davies MS, Weiss GA, Saxby TS. Plantar fasciitis: how successful is surgical intervention? Foot Ankle Int. 1999;20:803-7.
34. DiGiovanni BF, Abuzzahab FS, Gould JS. Plantar fasciitis release with proximal and distal tarsal tunnel release: surgical approach to chronic disabling plantar fasciitis with associated nerve pain. Tech Foot Ankle Surg. 2003;2:254-61.
35. Gould JS, DiGiovanni BF. "Plantar fascia release in combination with proximal and distal tarsal tunnel release" in Operative Techniques in Orthopaedic Surgery, Wiesel, SW Ed. Vol 4, Chap 57 p 3911-3919. Wolters Kluwer/ Lippincott Williams and Wilkins; Philadelphia: 2011.
36. Gould JS. "The Failed Tarsal Tunnel Release" in Nerve Problems of the Lower Extremity Foot and Ankle Clinics. Myerson (Ed). MS16(2) 287-93 WB Saunders/ Elsevier Philadelphia. 2011.

SECTION 7

Neuromuscular Problems

Chapters Outline

45

Cerebral Palsy

Michael Conklin, Stephen F Pehler

ETIOLOGY

Cerebral palsy (CP) is a catch-all term for brain injuries that occur in the prenatal, perinatal or postnatal period and involve motor dysfunction. The motor dysfunction may manifest as spasticity, athetosis, hypotonia, ataxia or mixed. Classification can be based on the type of movement disorder or the geographic pattern of involvement. The most common patterns of involvement include hemiplegia, diplegia and quadriplegia.

PATHOPHYSIOLOGY AND NATURAL HISTORY

Lower extremity and foot deformities occur in CP because of abnormal muscle forces. The imbalance between agonist and antagonist leads to predictable deformities such as equinus contracture. Muscles that are contracted add less sarcomeres with growth and contractures become rigid. Bone deformities and gait deviations eventually develop due to abnormal muscle forces. Gait patterns have generally developed by age of 7 years but are still alterable with treatment. As the patient further matures, particularly in adolescence or young adulthood, gait becomes harder to improve with treatment.

DIAGNOSIS

Patients with CP may present to the orthopedist without an established diagnosis, with developmental delay or abnormal gait. The diagnosis of CP at this age requires a careful birth and developmental history and physical examination. A suspicious birth history [prematurity, low birth weight, extended neonatal intensive care unit (NICU) stay] and motor developmental delay are usually sufficient to establish the diagnosis, but neurology consultation can be useful in confusing cases. Generally, surgical treatment decisions are not being made in the first few years of life so a "watch and see" strategy can be adopted with enrollment in early intervention therapy. For those patients presenting with an established diagnosis, a history is obtained regarding previous treatment such as physical therapy, bracing, tone modifying medication or surgery. Inquire as to perceived deformities or gait abnormalities to establish a chief complaint. Physical examination should include the spine, upper and lower extremities and observational gait analysis. In a patient who is not yet ambulatory, effort should be made to evaluate the potential for ambulation as it will be relevant for goal setting. The ability to sit independently by 2 years of age is a reasonable predictor of ambulation. Persistence of two or more primitive reflexes past 15 months is a negative predictor.[1] Lower extremity examination includes evaluation for hip flexor tightness (Thomas test), hamstring tightness (popliteal angle), rectus femoris spasticity (Ely test) and gastrocsoleus tightness (Silfverskiold test). Neurologic examination for tone, reflexes and clonus is performed. Evaluation of the foot in a weight-bearing position is imperative. Equinus is the most common foot and ankle deformity but equinovarus, planovalgus and hallux valgus deformities are also common. Deformities should be evaluated for severity and flexibility. Foot dorsiflexion is evaluated with the knee flexed and extended, the Silfverskiold test. Inability to dorsiflex the foot with knee extended but adequate dorsiflexion with knee flexed is indicative of gastrocnemius rather than soleus tightness. This test may be somewhat unreliable in CP due to the hypersensitive stretch reflex. Evaluate hindfoot varus or valgus for flexibility. For the planovalgus foot, note if the arch reconstitutes when non-weight bearing and evaluate ankle dorsiflexion with the hindfoot corrected. Also, the clinician should evaluate for forefoot supination with hindfoot correction.

Gait is observed both with and without ankle-foot orthotics (AFOs) where possible. Parameters such as velocity, cadence, step length and stride length are assessed. Kinematics are evaluated in the sagittal, coronal and transverse planes. Evaluate hip, knee and ankle position at initial contact. Does the patient achieve heel strike or land on the forefoot? Does the ankle excessively dorsiflex in stance leading to crouch at the knee? This may be seen after overlengthening of the Achilles tendon. A flexed knee at initial contact may indicate hamstring tightness. Knee hyperextension at mid-stance is usually secondary to equinus. Knee hyperflexion during swing may signify steppage gait to clear an equinus foot. Decreased knee flexion during swing may be present due to rectus femoris spasticity. The coronal and transverse planes are also assessed. Is the ankle or hindfoot in excessive varus or valgus? Is the forefoot excessively supinated or pronated? The foot progression angle is evaluated and correlated with a rotational examination (hip internal and external rotation in a prone position and thigh-foot angle) if abnormal.

One of the more difficult aspects of observational gait analysis is differentiating primary from compensatory gait deviations. Correlation of observational gait analysis with the static examination (e.g. foot dorsiflexion, popliteal angle) is imperative. Treatment of the compensatory problem without recognizing the primary cause may make the patient worse.

MANAGEMENT

General Principles

Goal Setting

Treatment decisions are based on goal setting which in turn is based on prognosis for ambulation. If a child is not ambulatory by 7 years of age, they probably will not be an ambulator. Candid communication with the family regarding goal setting and family expectations is paramount. Families need to understand that while deformities can be corrected, the patient will still have CP postoperatively. Postoperative follow through by the family is necessary to achieve and maintain a good result, so they should understand their role "going in". Multiple orthopedic surgeries during childhood should be avoided in favor of comprehensive surgery at a single setting. Temporizing measures are employed until the child's gait has matured. The ideal time is between 6 years and 9 years of age as gait is mature, but not so ingrained as to be unalterable. Also, tendon lengthenings performed too early (before age of 6 years) may need to be performed again due to recurrence. Some exceptions occur. Hips at risk for dislocation are best treated when identified. Hemiplegics may have significant contracture of the Achilles at a young age requiring early surgery. Surgery, particularly soft tissue procedures such as tendon lengthening or transfer is more predictable in spastic than athetoid patients. Surgical decisions should not be made on the basis of one visit since tone and patient cooperation may vary from visit to visit.

Conservative

There is a significant role for conservative treatment. This includes physical therapy, orthotics, casting and medical management.

Physical Therapy

Physical therapy is initiated in the first few years of life when motor developmental delay is noted. Stretching plays a role for specific deformities, i.e. heel cord stretching for equinus, and in the postoperative period. Therapists can serve in an advisory role regarding wheelchairs and adaptive equipment.

Orthotics

Orthotics, particularly ankle foot orthoses (AFOs) play a pivotal role in the treatment of ambulatory patients with CP. In patients with flexible equinus, the AFO provides swing phase clearance of the foot and prepositioning for heel strike. This also decreases the stance phase genu recurvatum caused by the plantarflexion-knee extension couple. An AFO used in this setting can be either solid or hinged with a plantarflexion stop at neutral. The solid AFO is less bulky while the hinged AFO may facilitate rising from a seated position. Also, hinged AFOs allow for greater power generation during toe-off. In patients with crouch due to an overlenthened Achilles, a solid AFO or ground reaction AFO may be useful if there is not significant hamstring or knee flexion contracture.

Casting

When equinus becomes fixed, or when tone is such that keeping the heel in the AFO is problematic, casting or botulinum injection can be considered. Serial casting for mild equinus may be helpful, but overly aggressive casting in the face of significant Achilles contracture may lead to midfoot break (hyperextension). Inhibitory casting can be considered to manage dynamic equinus. This technique involves placement of a short leg cast with toe-plate and mold beneath the metatarsal heads and above the heel. Casting is generally carried out for 6 weeks. When used as a temporizing measure in the young child, casting can be successful.[2]

Botulinum Toxin

Botulinum toxin is produced by the bacterium *Clostridium botulinum* and acts by irreversibly binding to the presynaptic nerve ending at the neuromuscular junction. The muscle is denervated until new nerve endings sprout. There are limitations to botulinum toxin injection. Since the result is not lasting (approximately 3 months), it may be a good temporizing measure, but not definitive treatment. There are dosage range issues so it is ideal for a few muscles, but not sound management for overall spasticity.[3]

Medical Management

Tone reducing medication such as baclofen can be useful, but side effects include somnolence. It is not a good treatment strategy for isolated foot and ankle deformities. Intrathecal baclofen through an implantable pump can be used for tone management in severely involved patients, usually non-ambulators. These medications are best managed by a physiatrist or neurologist.

Selective Dorsal Rhizotomy

This may be useful for ambulatory diplegics.

SURGICAL MANAGEMENT

Equinus

One of the most common gait abnormalities in CP is equinus. It is important to differentiate between primary equinus and compensatory equinus (Figs 1A and B). If the patient manifests equinus and good knee extension, at initial contact, with recurvatum during mid-stance, then the equinus is almost certainly primary. Gastrocnemius recession (GR) or tendo-Achilles lengthening (TAL) is

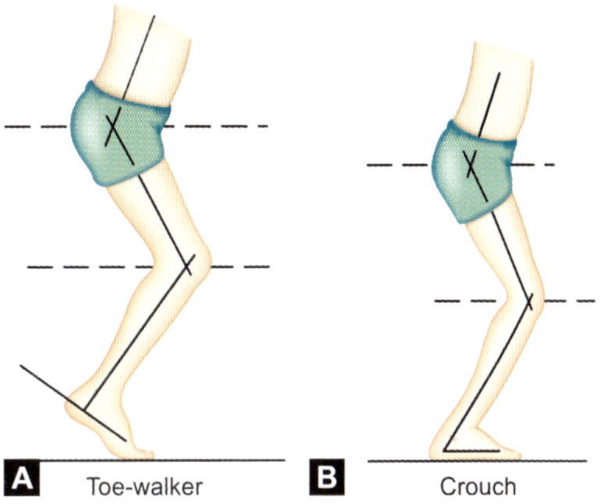

Figs 1A and B: Compensatory toe walking. (A) Patient is toe walking due to knee flexion; (B) Heel cord lengthening results in crouched gait

indicated. However, if the patient manifests equinus during stance phase but the knee remains flexed, the equinus may be compensatory for hamstring tightness or quadriceps weakness. Evaluate ankle dorsiflexion and the popliteal angle. If ankle dorsiflexion is less than neutral and the hamstrings are tight, the patient will likely benefit from a TAL or GR plus hamstring lengthening. If ankle dorsiflexion is well above neutral but hamstrings are tight, then hamstring lengthening is indicated. If neither hamstrings nor gastrocsoleus are tight, the patient may be in crouch due to weak quadriceps and/or an overlengthened Achilles, and ground reaction AFOs are indicated. Some patients, particularly young diplegics, may have dorsiflexion above neutral but significant tone leading to dynamic equinus. If the heel will not stay in the AFO, then a procedure (botulinum toxin injection or lengthening) may be indicated.

Once the decision is made to surgically intervene for equinus, three basic options are available: (1) GR, (2) percutaneous TAL and (3) open TAL. Some authors believe that GR better preserves power and carries less risk of overlengthening. Others use the Silfverskiold test under anesthesia to determine which procedure to perform. If ankle dorsiflexion is less than neutral with knee extended but above neutral with knee flexed (positive Silfverskiold), GR is performed. There may be a higher rate of recurrent equinus with GR versus TAL. It has been authors' experience that if the patient has significant equinus contracture, recession may not gain enough length and TAL should be chosen. In severe equinus, open Achilles Z-lengthening with posterior ankle capsulotomy may be necessary. After TAL or GR, a short leg cast and knee immobilizers (or long leg cast) are worn because the gastrocnemius crosses both the knee and ankle joint.

Gastrocnemius Recession

The authors prefer the Vulpius recession (Fig. 2).[4] With the patient pron, a midline longitudinal incision is made in the calf at midleg. Dissection is deepened to fascia which is incised and the sural nerve protected. An inverted V-shaped incision is made in the aponeurosis of the gastrocnemius just distal to the muscle. The midline fibrous septum of the soleus is divided. A short leg cast plus knee immobilizer is applied with the foot dorsiflexed 5–10° above neutral for 4 weeks postoperatively with weight bearing to tolerance.

Percutaneous Tendo-Achilles Lengthening

For percutaneous TAL, the authors prefer the three incision technique (Fig. 3).[5] With the patient supine or prone and the assistant holding a dorsiflexion force on the foot, the Achilles is palpated and a # 15 blade is inserted in the center of the tendon posteriorly. The blade is oriented longitudinally on insertion then turned transversly tenotomizing 60% of the tendon with each cut. The proximal and distal cuts are medial, and the middle cut is lateral. The distal cut is immediately proximal to the tendon insertion, the proximal cut is at the proximal extent of the tendon, and the middle cut is midway between. The foot is slowly dorsiflexed 5–10° above neutral with knee extended. Occasionally a distinct "pop" is felt when the tendon lengthens. This is generally not a cause for alarm but necessitates a Thompson test to verify tendon continuity. A short leg cast and knee immobilizer is worn for 6 weeks. Weight bearing to tolerance is allowed.

Open Tendo-Achilles Lengthening

The authors prefer this operation for patients with severe equinus who may also need a posterior ankle capsulotomy. Disadvantages include the open nature of the procedure and the need for tendon healing before weight bearing is allowed. There is a tendency for the tendon to "bunch up" with suturing which occasionally leads to a local prominence. With the patient prone or supine, a longitudinal incision is made over the posteromedial aspect of the ankle along the medial border of the

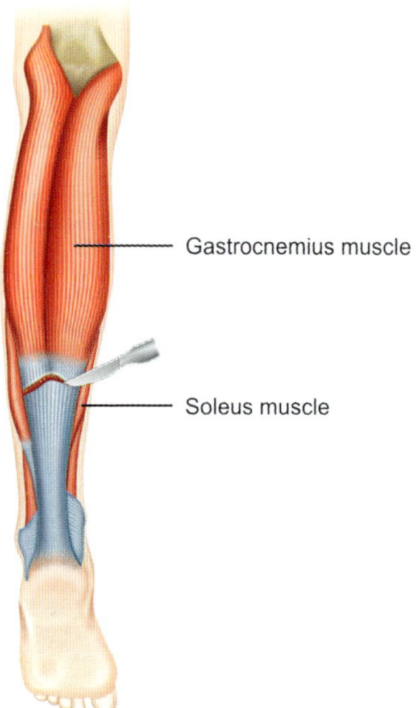

Fig. 2: Vulpius gastrocnemius recession

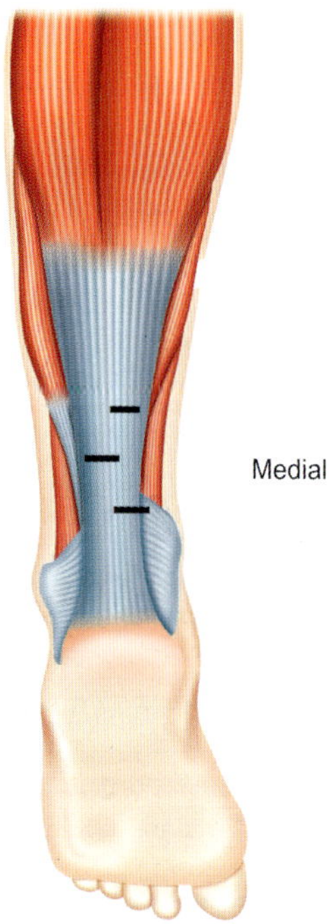

Fig. 3: Three incision percutaneous Achilles tendon lengthening. The proximal and distal incisions are medial, and the middle incision is lateral

Achilles. Do not place the incision straight posterior where the shoe will irritate the scar. The incision is deepened through tendon sheath and a longitudinal incision made through the center of the tendon in the coronal plane. The distal aspect is divided medially and the proximal aspect laterally. The foot is dorsiflexed and the tendon repaired under tension with the knee fully extended and the foot 5–10° above neutral. Remember, an overlengthened Achilles is worse than a tight Achilles! A short leg cast and knee immobilizer is worn for 6 weeks non-weight bearing.

Equinovarus

General Considerations

Equinovarus deformities are common in hemiplegia. There is an imbalance in tone between the invertors (tibialis posterior, tibialis anterior) and the peroneals. Tightness or increased tone in the gastrocsoleus is also a contributing factor since plantarflexion of the foot is coupled with inversion. Equinovarus deformities may be tight early and temporizing is problematic.

Diagnosis

It may be difficult to differentiate between the tibialis anterior and tibialis posterior as the primary deforming force. Differentiation can be made by clinical evaluation or electromyography (EMG). The tendons are palpated for tightness. Foot position is observed during gait. If the tibialis posterior is the main culprit, hindfoot inversion or varus is seen with no additional supination of the forefoot. When the tibialis anterior is the main deforming force, more forefoot supination than hindfoot varus is seen. Also, one may be able to visualize bowstringing of the tight tendon during gait. The "confusion test" is performed. With the patient sitting, he is asked to flex the hip against resistance while observing the foot. Foot dorsiflexion in this scenario is known as a positive confusion test. If the foot supinates during dorsiflexion, the tibialis anterior is a deforming force. Further evaluation involves computerized gait analysis with EMG. Tibialis anterior activity persisting through second and third rocker of stance phase is considered abnormal. The tibialis posterior is abnormal if active during swing phase. Most centers do not have access to a gait analysis and, therefore, decisions can be made on clinical grounds.

Treatment

In young patients with flexible deformities, nonoperative treatment can be attempted. An AFO with a plantarflexion stop at neutral is prescribed. If the deformity is flexible, but significant tone issues are interfering with brace wear, botulinum toxin injection can be performed with injection of the gastrocsoleus and either the tibialis anterior or posterior. It would be useful if injection of the anterior versus the posterior tibialis could be used as a diagnostic tool for surgical planning, but there is no hard data to support this. Serial casting can be tried for moderately rigid deformities. If there are no compelling reasons to temporize, or if the deformity is becoming rigid, then tendon lengthening and/or transfers are indicated. Fixed deformities may, in addition, require posterior ankle capsulotomy or osteotomies.

- *Tibialis posterior lengthening*: The authors prefer this option when an equinovarus foot that is unbraceable is forcing the surgeon's hand at a young age. This is because split tendon transfers in very small tendons may not adequately hold suture. The equinus is addressed with TAL. The tibialis posterior can be Z-lengthened or fractionally lengthened. The authors' preference is for an open Z-lengthening of both tendons using one posteromedial incision.
- *Split posterior tibial tendon transfer*: This is the mainstay of treatment for the equinovarus foot. Splitting rather than transferring the tendon makes overcorrection unlikely. When dynamic EMG is not available and the tibialis anterior is not obviously a deforming force, this is a "safe bet". If there is significant heel varus, the tendon lengthening may need to be combined with a Dwyer osteotomy of the calcaneus. The technique is as described by Green (Figs 4A to D).[6] With the patient supine, a 2 cm incision is made starting at the posterior tibialis tendon (PTT) insertion and extending proximally. The sheath is split to the flexor retinaculum. The plantar half of the tendon is released from the navicular and split to the level of the preserved retinaculum. A second longitudinal incision is made midway between the medial malleolus and tendo-Achilles extending proximally for 6 cm. The PTT sheath is incised above the flexor retinaculum. A tendon passer is delivered through the flexor retinaculum, the free end of tendon is

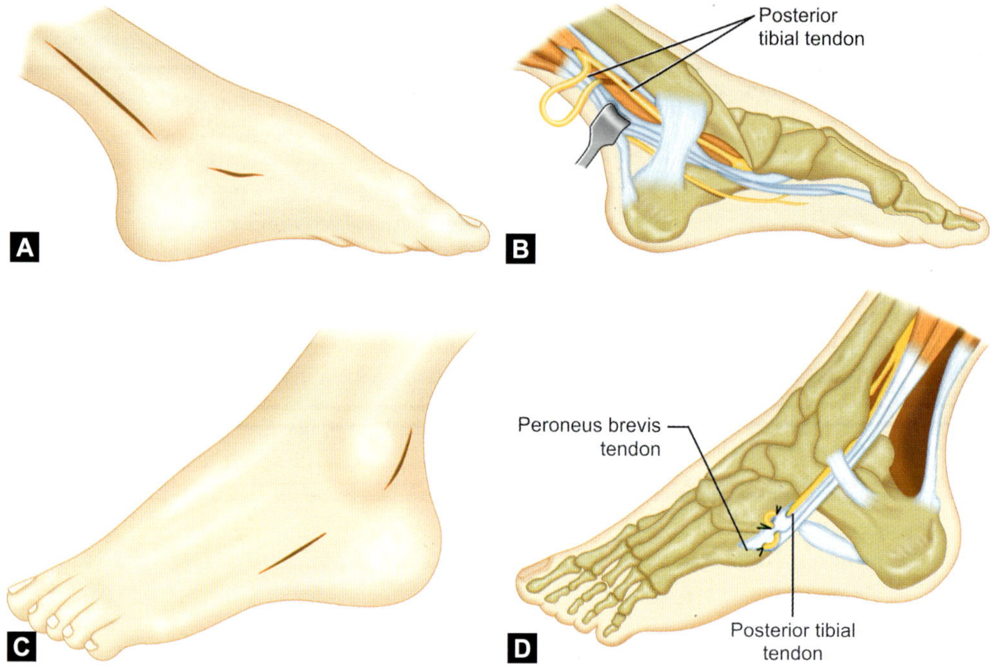

Figs 4A to D: Split posterior tibial tendon transfer. (A) Location of medial incisions; (B) Split is propagated to musculotendinous junction. Tendon is delivered into proximal wound; (C) Location of lateral incisions; (D) Tendon stump is woven through peroneus brevis

grasped and delivered above the retinaculum where the split is carried as far proximal as the musculotendinous junction. A heavy suture is sewn into the tendon stump. The Achilles tendon is lengthened. A third lateral incision is made above the lateral malleolus along its posterior margin. The peroneus brevis sheath is incised above the peroneal retinaculum. From the medial incision, a plane is developed staying directly on the tibia passing posterolateral deep to the flexor digitorum, neurovascular bundle and flexor hallucis. The suture and tendon are passed to the lateral incision immediately posterior to the fibula. The tendon stump is passed into the peroneus tendon sheath. A fourth incision is made over the course of the peroneus brevis just distal to the lateral malleolus ending near the base of the fifth metatarsal. The sheath is split and the suture grasped to deliver the stump through the peroneal retinaculum into the distal wound. The split portion of the posterior tibial tendon is woven through the peroneus brevis and sutured under tension to hold the hindfoot in neutral. If residual calcaneal varus is present, a lateral calcaneal slide or closing wedge osteotomy is performed. Postoperatively a knee immobilizer and short leg cast with the hindfoot in neutral to slight valgus and the ankle in 5–10° of dorsiflexion is applied. The patient is non-weight bearing for 6 weeks. The cast is worn for 6–8 weeks followed by an AFO for 3–6 months. If the patient then demonstrates a plantigrade foot with adequate dorsiflexion during swing phase, the AFO can be discontinued.

- *Split anterior tibial tendon transfer*: This transfer can be considered for the equinovarus foot when the patient manifests supination of the foot on confusion test or stance phase activity of the tibialis anterior on dynamic EMG.[7] A TAL is performed to manage equinus. With the patient supine, an incision is made over the dorsal aspect of the first metatarsal base (Figs 5A to F). The lateral half of the anterior tibial tendon is detached and the split propagated proximally. A suture is woven through the tendon stump. A second incision is made over the anterior ankle immediately proximal to the extensor retinaculum. A tendon passer is advanced deep to the retinaculum and used to

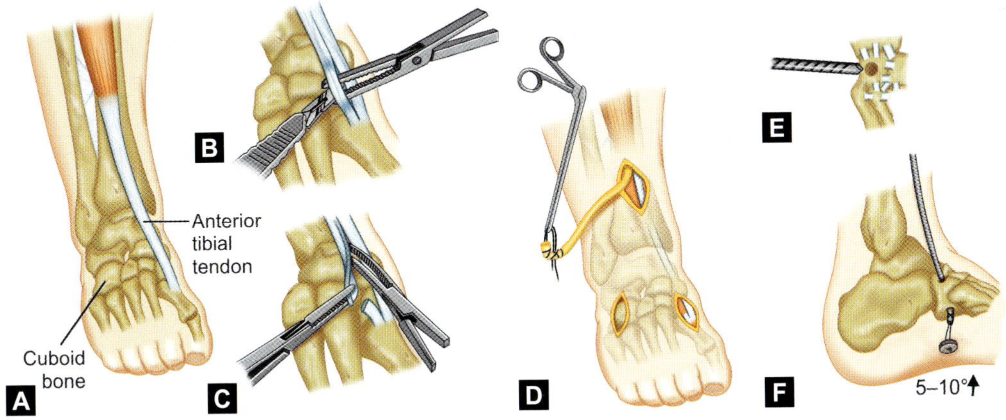

Figs 5A to F: Split anterior tibial tendon transfer. (A) Anterior tibial tendon; (B) Lateral half of anterior tibial tendon is released from first metatarsal; (C) Split is propagated; (D) Tendon stump is delivered into proximal wound; (E) Drill hole in cuboid; (F) Tendon is passed through cuboid and sewn over a button

grasp the suture delivering the split tendon into the proximal wound. A third incision is made over the dorsum of the cuboid and a drill hole is made from dorsal to plantar. The Achilles is lengthened with a three incision percutaneous technique. The split tendon is passed deep to the retinaculum and into the lateral wound. The passing suture is removed and a Keith needle is used to weave a large suture through the tendon stump. The Keith needle is passed through the cuboid and out the plantar aspect of the foot. It is tied over a felt pad and button under tension with the foot at neutral. A short leg cast, non-weight bearing is worn for 6 weeks followed by an AFO.

Planovalgus

General

Planovalgus deformity of the foot is extremely common in patients with CP, particularly in diplegia or quadriplegia.

Clinical Evaluation

The prominence of the talar head and weight bearing on the inside border of the foot leads to callosities over the plantar medial aspect of the talar head which may be symptomatic. The foot is inspected in a weight bearing and non-weight bearing position. The Achilles is carefully examined for contracture by inverting the hindfoot, thus preventing spurious dorsiflexion at the midfoot. The relative flexibility of the deformity is noted by inverting and everting the hindfoot. Care is taken to evaluate the forefoot for fixed supination when the hindfoot is in a corrected position. Patients will usually have an externally rotated foot progression angle during gait.

Treatment

Often, significant amounts of deformity are well tolerated, so the presence of this deformity alone is not an indication for surgical treatment. In patients who are symptomatic, the mainstay of nonoperative treatment is orthotics, whether shoe inserts or AFOs. Radiographs are not helpful in determining when to proceed with surgery, but they are necessary in planning surgery. Standing foot X-rays as well as ankle films to evaluate for ankle valgus are necessary. On the standing lateral foot radiograph, the talus is noted to be in significant equinus and a markedly divergent lateral talo-calcaneal angle is noted (Fig. 6A). On the anteroposterior (AP) view, the navicular is lateralized on the talar head (Fig. 6B). Ankle X-rays may show valgus of the tibial plafond and proximal migration of the distal fibular physis.

Once surgery is decided upon, three basic options exist: (1) calcaneal osteotomy, (2) subtalar arthrodesis and (3) triple arthrodesis. In most cases TAL is also necessary. Flexible deformities can be treated with a calcaneal osteotomy or subtalar fusion. Rigid and severe deformities will require triple arthrodesis. Because of the concerns about degeneration of joints proximal or distal to fusions, the authors feel that calcaneal osteotomy should

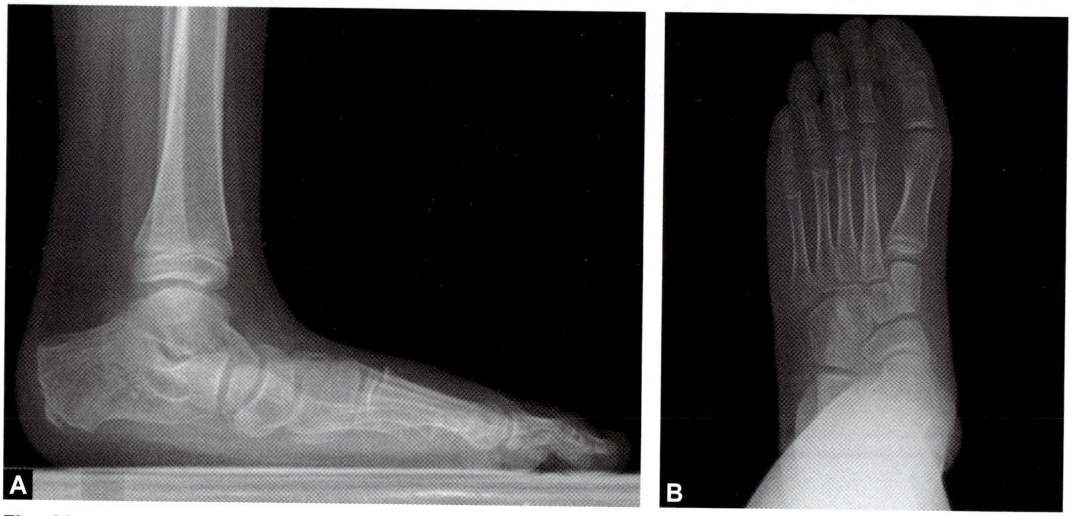

Figs 6A and B: Standing radiographs of planovalgus foot. (A) Lateral radiograph. Note the excessive divergence of the lateral talo-calcaneal angle; (B) Anteroposterior radiograph. The navicular is lateralized on the talar head

be chosen over subtalar fusion. The decision to do a medial calcaneal slide versus a lateral column lengthening is decided as follows: when valgus of the calcaneal tuberosity is the most marked clinical feature, the authors prefer the calcaneal slide. When there is a significant convexity of the medial border of the foot and lateralization of the navicular on the talar head is noted on the standing AP radiograph, the authors prefer lateral column lengthening.

- *Extra-articular subtalar arthrodesis*: This operation, first described by Grice,[8] involves placement of a structural bone graft in the sinus tarsi with correction of subtalar valgus (Fig. 7). Dennyson and Fulford added internal fixation to maintain position and used cancellous iliac crest graft.[9] The Ferguson modification involves internal fixation and local bone graft technique by turning down "trap doors" of opposing bone from the talus and calcaneus.[10] Whatever the technique, Achilles lengthening is generally necessary to prevent failure due to midfoot break. In the authors' practice, lateral column lengthening and calcaneal tuberosity osteotomy have supplanted extra-articular arthrodesis.
- *Lateral column lengthening* (Figs 8 and 9):[11] This operation is appropriate for the symptomatic planovalgus foot when the hindfoot is correctable and forefoot supination is not severe or rigid. It will generally need to be combined with TAL or midfoot break will lead to failure. With the patient supine, a lateral longitudinal incision is made over the calcaneus. Superficial dissection is blunt to avoid injury to the sural and superficial peroneal nerves. The calcaneus is exposed subperiosteally at the junction of the beak with the sinus tarsi and the calcaneocuboid joint visualized dorsally, but the capsule is left intact. A small Homan retractor is placed over the dorsum of the calcaneus 1.5 cm proximal to the calcaneocuboid joint and pulled proximally until the resistance of the sustentaculum tali is felt. An AP fluoroscopic image will confirm the location of the retractor immediately distal to the sustentaculum. A pin is advanced percutaneously into the cuboid, then retrograde across the calcaneocuboid joint and barely into the calcaneus. A transverse osteotomy of the calcaneus is made just distal to the sustentaculum and opened cautiously with a laminar spreader as the calcaneus is soft and

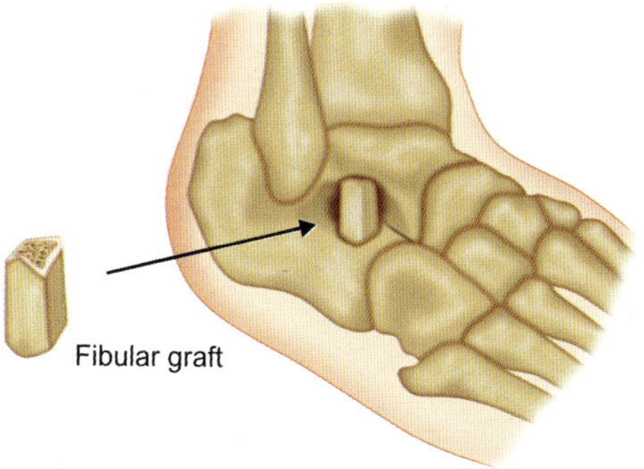

Fig. 7: Grice extra-articular subtalar arthrodesis

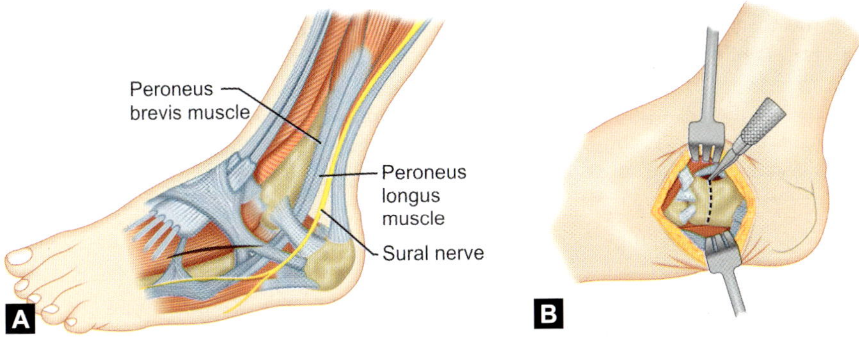

Figs 8A and B: Lateral column lengthening. (A) Location of incision; (B) Location of osteotomy 1.5 cm proximal to calcaneo-cuboid joint

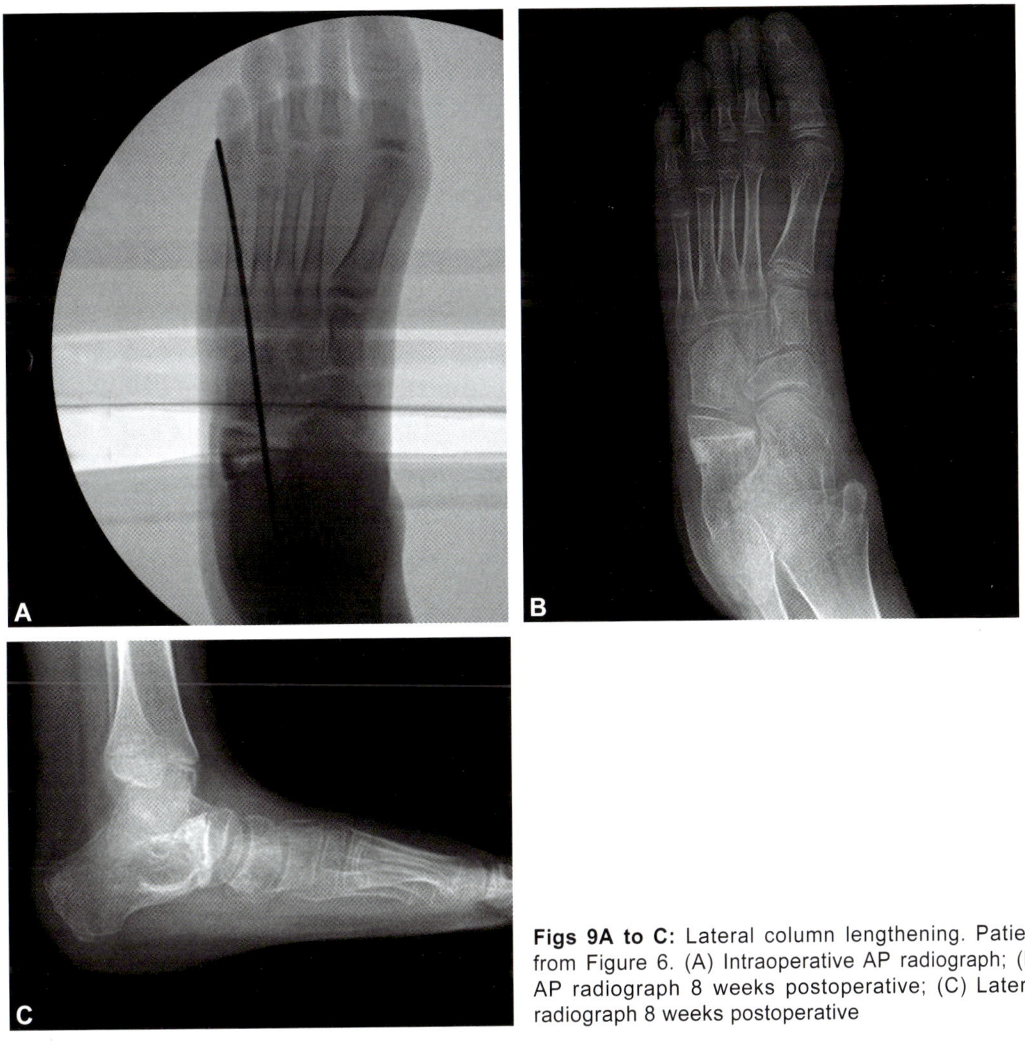

Figs 9A to C: Lateral column lengthening. Patient from Figure 6. (A) Intraoperative AP radiograph; (B) AP radiograph 8 weeks postoperative; (C) Lateral radiograph 8 weeks postoperative

can be crushed. A tricortical iliac crest graft is inserted into the osteotomy site. The authors use allograft unless other procedures at the hip (iliacus recession) would facilitate autograft harvest. The pin is advanced into the proximal calcaneus. The calcaneocuboid joint and distal calcaneal fragment are inspected clinically and radiographically to ensure against dorsal subluxation. Alternatively, a single staple may be used to span the osteotomy or no fixation if the osteotomy is stable and no tendency towards dorsal subluxation is noted. The peroneals are Z-lengthened or fractionally lengthened if tight. Skin is closed with interrupted suture. A short leg cast is applied with an inversion force on the hindfoot, pronation force on forefoot and ankle above neutral. A knee immobilizer is also used if a TAL was performed. The pin is removed in clinic at 3–4 weeks, weight bearing allowed in the cast at 6 weeks with a total cast time of 6–8 weeks, followed by an AFO.

- *Calcaneal tuberosity medialization* (Figs 10A to D):[12] The authors prefer the medial calcaneal slide when the hindfoot valgus is more marked than the abduction at Chopart's joint. The osteotomy will reliably improve heel valgus, but often also improves the planus and abduction aspects of the deformity. This procedure provides rapid healing without the need for bone graft. A lateral oblique or curvilinear incision is made

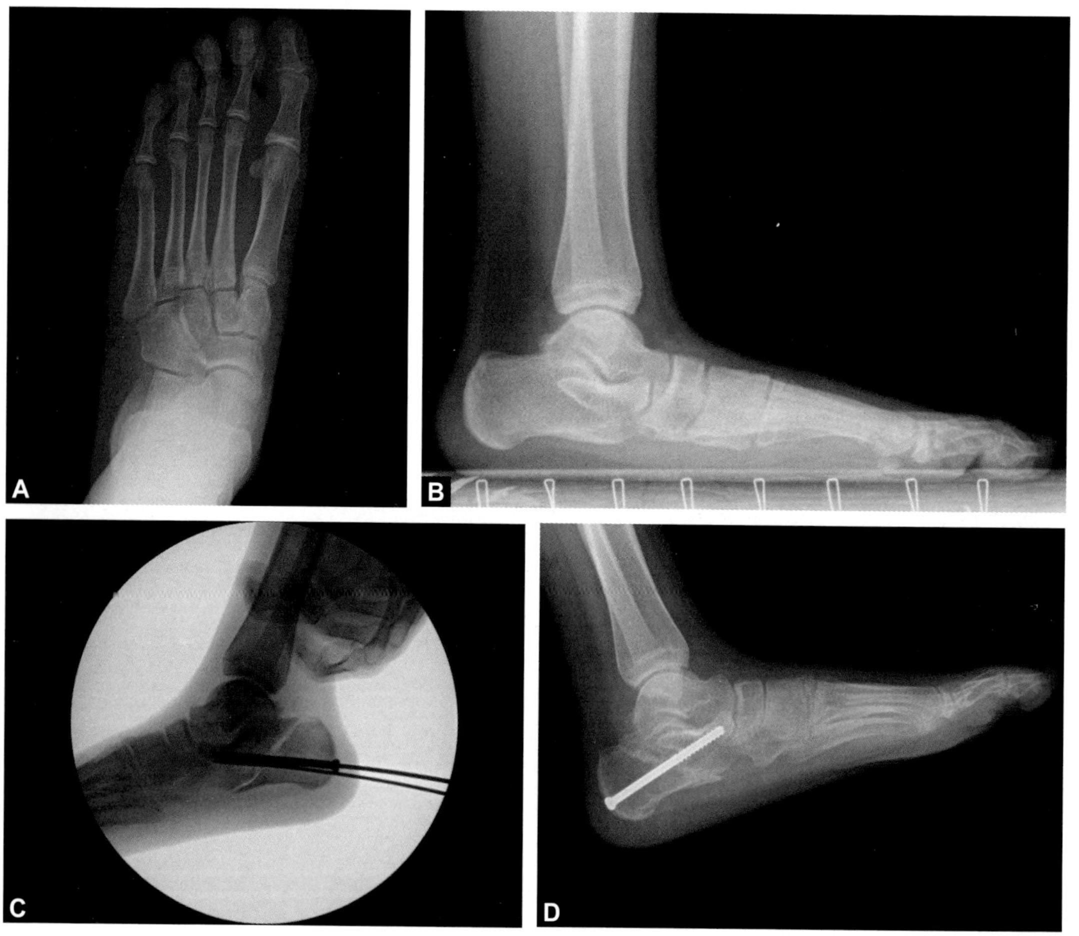

Figs 10A to D: Medial calcaneal slide. (A) Preoperative anteroposterior (AP) radiograph of a 15-year-old patient. Because of concerns about forefoot supination if lateral column lengthening were performed a calcaneal slide was chosen; (B) Lateral radiograph; (C) Intraoperative lateral radiograph; (D) Lateral radiograph 8 weeks postoperative over the calcaneal tuberosity and deepened to bone immediately plantar to the peroneal tendons, with observation and protection of the sural nerve. The lateral periosteum is incised and Chandler retractors placed dorsal and plantar wrapping around to the medial side of the tuberosity. A lateral X-ray is obtained to confirm the location of the planned osteotomy. The dorsal, plantar and lateral cortices are cut with a saw. The osteotomy is opened with a lamina spreader and the medial cortex and periosteum removed with a Kerrison rongeur. Adequate mobilization of the medial periosteum is necessary to achieve medial slide. The osteotomy must be made perpendicular to the bone, as well as, to allow medial translation. The authors have found that at least 1 cm of medial translation is easily achievable, but more may be necessary in severe valgus deformities. Alternately, a medial closing wedge can also be removed. The osteotomy is stabilized with two smooth K-wires or a cannulated screw. The Achilles tendon is lengthened using the three incision percutaneous technique. A short leg non-weight bearing cast is worn for 6–8 weeks, followed by an AFO. For cases with more severe abduction and planus, the calcaneal-cuboid-cuneiform osteotomy described by Rathjen and Mubarak[13] should be considered before proceeding to triple arthrodesis.

- *Triple arthrodesis*: Triple arthrodesis should be reserved for the significantly symptomatic severe and rigid planovalgus foot in the adolescent or young adult. The technique is as described in previous chapters.

Ankle Valgus

As previously stated, any neuromuscular patient in whom consideration is being given to surgery for hindfoot valgus should have ankle radiographs to rule out ankle valgus. Normally the distal fibular physis is at the level of the ankle joint. When it lies above the distal tibial articular surface and there is valgus tilt of the plafond, surgery can be considered for the symptomatic patient. Generally, the authors have not seen the severe ankle valgus in patients with CP, that have noticed this in those with myelomeningocele. Ankle valgus in growing patients can be treated with medial malleolar hemiepiphyseodesis. The authors prefer using a single cannulated medial malleolar screw. Screw removal after correction will generally result in resumption of growth.[14] In severe deformity or if immediate correction is desired then supramalleolar osteotomy is performed. Care is taken to shift the distal fragment laterally with varus angulation to avoid medial prominence.

Hallux Valgus

Hallux valgus is extremely common in CP, particularly in those with planovalgus and is often well tolerated. However, the medial prominence of the first metatarsal may lead to symptomatology, particularly with AFO wear. AFO modification or discontinuance may lead to improved symptoms, but many of these patients require the AFO for swing phase clearance or to prevent crouch. In patients unresponsive to conservative measures, surgery can be considered. The recurrence rate is extremely high in patients treated with soft tissue realignment and osteotomy, particularly if the planovalgus foot is not also corrected. Metatarsophalangeal (MTP) joint fusion is the most reliable and durable procedure for CP hallux valgus. This can be performed as described by McKeever with the ideal position being 15–25° of dorsiflexion and slight valgus.

REFERENCES

1. Bleck EE. Locomotor prognosis in cerebral palsy. Dev Med Child Neurol. 1975;17(1):18.
2. Cottalorda J, Gautheron V, Metton G. Toe-walking in children younger than six years with cerebral palsy. The contribution of serial corrective casts. J Bone Joint Surg Br. 2000;82(4):541-4.
3. Koman LA, Mooney JF, Smith BP, et al. Botulinum toxin type A neuromuscular blockade in the treatment of lower extremity spasticity in cerebral palsy: a randomized, double-blind, placebo-controlled trial. BOTOX Study Group. J Pediatr Orthop. 2000;20(1):108-15.
4. Javors JR, Klaaren HE. The Vulpius procedure for correction of equinus deformity in cerebral palsy. J Pediatr Orthop. 1987;7(2):191-3.
5. Hoke M. An operation for stabilizing paralytic feet. Am J Orthop Surg. 1921;3:494-507.
6. Green NE, Griffin PP, Shiavi R. Split posterior tibial-tendon transfer in spastic cerebral palsy. J Bone Joint Surg Am. 1983;65(6):748-54.

7. Hoffer MM, Barakat G, Koffman M. 10-year follow-up of split anterior tibial tendon transfer in cerebral palsied patients with spastic equinovarus deformity. J Pediatr Orthop. 1985;5(4):432-4.
8. Grice DS. An extra-articular arthrodesis of the sub-astragalar joint for correction of paralytic flat feet in children. J Bone Joint Surg Am. 1952;34A(4): 927-40.
9. Dennyson WG, Fulford GE. Subtalar arthrodesis by cancellous grafts and metallic internal fixation. J Bone Joint Surg. 1976;58-B(4):507-10.
10. Jeray KJ, Rentz J, Ferguson RL. Local bone-graft technique for subtalar extraarticular arthrodesis in cerebral palsy. J Pediatr Orthop. 1998;18(1): 75-80.
11. Mosca VS. Calcaneal lengthening for valgus deformity of the hindfoot. Results in children who had severe, symptomatic flatfoot and skewfoot. J Bone Joint Surg Am. 1995;77(4):500-12.
12. Koman LA, Mooney JF, Goodman A. Management of valgus hindfoot deformity in pediatric cerebral palsy patients by medial displacement osteotomy. J Pediatr Orthop. 1993;13(2):180-3.
13. Rathjen KE, Mubarak SJ. Calcaneal-cuboid-cuneiform osteotomy for the correction of valgus foot deformities in children. J Pediatr Orthop. 1998;18(6):775-82.
14. Davids JR, Valadie AL, Ferguson RL, et al. Surgical management of ankle valgus in children: use of a transphyseal medical malleolar screw. J Pediatr Orthop. 1197;17(1):3-8.

46

Acquired Brain Injury

Michael Conklin

ETIOLOGY

Acquired brain injury (ABI) is frequently used to describe traumatic brain injury but can also include injury from intracranial sources such as cerebral vascular accident or tumor. Damage to pyramidal or extrapyramidal tracts can lead to movement disorders, most commonly spasticity. There is development of imbalance between agonist and antagonist muscles. The imbalance usually favors the antigravity muscles such as the gastrocsoleus. Muscle imbalance leads to abnormal joint posture. With persistence of the abnormal posture, adaptive shortening of muscle occurs and deformities gain rigidity. Equinovarus is the most common foot deformity in ABI.

TREATMENT

Conservative

Physiotherapy

Physiotherapy is the first line of treatment for acquired foot deformities in ABI. In one study of patients with moderate to severe ABI admitted to a rehabilitation facility, physiotherapy remediated equinovarus contracture in over half of the cases. This involved daily therapy with weight-bearing in a standing frame and muscle re-education.[1]

Orthotics

Ankle-foot orthotics (AFOs) is the mainstay of orthotic management for equinus or equinovarus after ABI. AFOs is suitable when the foot is passively correctable to neutral. In more rigid deformities, serial casting or surgery will be necessary to achieve a braceable foot. Patients with severe tone such as decerebrate posturing will need the rigidity of solid AFOs while those with milder involvement, particularly ambulators after tendon transfer can gain advantage from hinged AFOs.

Serial Casting

Serial casting in ABI can be useful in preventing loss of joint range, restoring range of motion and inhibiting reflex hyperexcitability. The patient is placed prone and the knee is flexed to reduce stretch reflex hyperexcitability. Gel pads are placed over the bony prominences of the malleoli. A short leg cast is applied with dorsiflexion force. When clawing of the toes is present a toe plate is incorporated with the toes in neutral to slight extension. Casts are changed weekly until adequate dorsiflexion achieved, generally about 10°. Casting is discontinued if no measurable gains are made over three successive casts and consideration given to surgical treatment.[2] Aggressive stretching, weight bearing and AFO bracing will be necessary to consolidate gains. Recurrence is more common in patients with brain stem lesions, i.e. decerebrate posturing.

Medical

Oral antispasticity medication has previously been discussed under cerebral palsy (CP). This is managed by a physiatrist or neurologist.

Denervation

Denervation includes temporary and permanent techniques. A classic technique is nerve phenolization. Side effects include neuropathic pain and the permanent nature of the denervation. Botulinum toxin injection in the gastrocsoleus and posterior tibial tendon (PTT) has been shown to be effective in reducing tone, improving range of motion and improving gait after ABI. It is less effective in patients with longer duration of spasticity. The effect is short lived, lasting as little as 4 weeks in some subjects.

Surgical Treatment

In equinovarus deformities unresponsive to the above treatments, surgery can be considered. Goal setting is important at this time. Patients who are ambulatory or expected to be ambulatory have a more compelling need for a plantigrade foot. In contrast, it is not inappropriate to stop short of surgical treatment in severely involved patients with no hope of recovery. Communication with the physiatrist and the family can be helpful in these cases. A reasonable treatment algorithm is Achilles tendon lengthening (ATL), PTT lengthening, split anterior tibial tendon transfer and toe flexor tenotomies.[3]

REFERENCES

1. Singer BJ, Dunne JW, Singer KP, et al. Non-surgical management of ankle contracture following acquired brain injury. Disabil Rehabil. 2004;26(6):335-45.
2. Singer BJ, Jegasothy GM, Singer KP, et al. Evaluation of serial casting to correct equinovarus deformity of the ankle after acquired brain injury in adults. Arch Phys Med Rehabil. 2003;84(4):483-91.
3. Reddy S, Kusuma S, Hosalker H, et al. Surgery can reduce the nonoperative care associated with an equinovarus foot deformity. Clin Orthop Relat Res. 2008;466(7):1683-7.

47

Muscular Dystrophy

Michael Conklin

DESCRIPTION

The muscular dystrophies are a group of inherited disorders characterized by progressive weakness due to pathologic changes within skeletal muscle. The severity varies from Duchenne's muscular dystrophy (DMD) which leads to early loss of ambulation and death to the relatively mild involvement seen in Becker's muscular dystrophy. Patterns of muscle involvement also vary between diseases.

ETIOLOGY

The dystrophies are genetic disorders. Both Duchenne's and Becker's muscular dystrophy are caused by a mutation of the gene coding for dystrophin, a protein found in muscle cell membrane. This gene is recessive and found on the X chromosome, so only males are affected except in rare scenarios such as Turner's syndrome. Boys with DMD make no dystrophin while those with Becker's muscular dystrophy make either abnormal dystrophin or reduced amounts of dystrophin. A separate gene on the X chromosome is responsible for Emery-Dreifuss dystrophy with abnormalities in the muscle protein, emerin.

NATURAL HISTORY

The clinical course varies for the dystrophies with DMD being the most rapid and debilitating. Boys with DMD will manifest toe walking and ankle equinus at an early age. From a weakness standpoint, hip extensors, abductors and quadriceps are most affected early. This results in a typical ambulatory posture keeping the ground reaction force posterior to the hip joint and anterior to the knee (Fig. 1). Ankle equinus facilitates this through the plantarflexion/knee extension couple. Trendelenburg gait is present due to hip abductor weakness. Worsening muscle weakness and lower extremity contractures eventually lead to loss of ambulation at around 10–12 years of age. When the patient becomes wheelchair dependent, pulmonary function plummets and scoliosis develops. Death is generally in the 3rd decade due to cardiopulmonary disease. The natural history of foot and ankle deformities follows a predictable pattern with gastrocsoleus tightness leading to equinus gait at about 3 years of age. The dynamic equinus becomes fixed and eventually rigid equinovarus develops, rapidly progressing when the patient becomes nonambulatory.

DIAGNOSIS

Duchenne's muscular dystrophy should be considered in the differential diagnosis of young boys

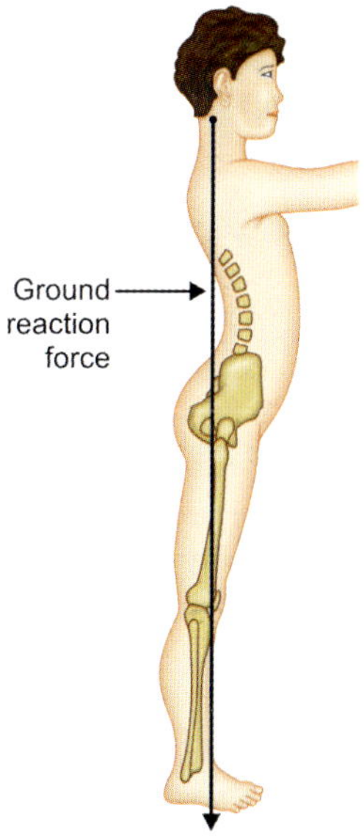

Fig. 1: Gait adaptations in Duchenne's muscular dystrophy (DMD). Hyperlordosis keeps ground reaction force posterior to hip joints. Knee hyperextension keeps ground reaction force anterior to knee joint

presenting with toe walking. Boys with DMD will usually manifest normal motor development early with insidious onset of weakness between 3 years and 6 years of age. Ankle equinus develops due to contracture. Though the calf muscles are relatively spared until later in the disease, fibrofatty infiltration results in enlargement or "pseudohypertrophy". Proximal muscles are more involved than distal muscles, and lower extremity involvement develops earlier than upper extremity. Therefore, hip extensor weakness develops early, resulting in a positive Gower's sign. To evaluate for this, ask the child to get up while sitting on the floor. A patient with hip extensor weakness will walk his hands up his thighs to get up. Laboratory testing is useful in making the diagnosis. Serum creatine kinase (CK) and aldolase are elevated nonspecifically in patients with muscle disease. Genetic testing can make the diagnosis in the majority of cases but occasionally muscle biopsy is still necessary. The author recommends referral to pediatric neurology for any patient who is suspected of having muscular dystrophy or other progressive neurologic conditions.

TREATMENT

The primary goal of orthopedic treatment in DMD is to facilitate or maintain ambulation in the younger patient. Once ambulation ceases, then the focus is on scoliosis and palliative treatment of lower extremity deformities.

Conservative

Home stretching programs and night-time bracing can forestall the development of contractures. Serial casting can be valuable for equinus or equinovarus as the deformities gain rigidity.

Surgical

Shapiro and Specht classified the timing of lower extremity surgery.[1] Lower extremity surgery can be thought of as early, to prolong ambulation; rehabilitative, to re-establish ambulation; or palliative, to correct equinovarus deformity and facilitate shoe wear in the nonambulatory patient. Surgery to prolong ambulation can either be comprehensive with releases at the hips, knees, and ankles or a more minimalist approach involving surgical management of the equinovarus alone: the tendo-Achilles lengthening (TAL) and posterior tibial tendon transfer (PTTT) through the interosseous membrane. Smith and colleagues noted that ambulation could be prolonged an average of 2 years with comprehensive releases performed at an average age of 10 years.[2] Surgery done to re-establish ambulation must be done soon after ambulatory function is lost, with aggressive mobilization and physical therapy postoperatively. Palliative surgery on significantly deformed feet in the nonambulator is more likely to require posterior ankle capsulotomy and toe flexor tenotomies, in addition to TAL and PTTT.

Anterior Transfer of the Posterior Tibial Tendon

The author prefers the modification described by Scher and Mubarak.[3] Four incisions are used (Figs 2A to G). The first incision is made over the navicular tuberosity to release the posterior tibial tendon (PTT). A second incision is made over the medial leg at the junction of the middle and distal thirds into which the stump is delivered. The Achilles is lengthened. A third incision is made just lateral to the tibial crest at the same level. The fascia is incised over the anterior compartment and the anterior compartment contents are retracted medially. A large window is excised from the interosseous membrane and enlarged proximally. A clamp is passed through the window and into the medial wound, the PTT stump is grasped and delivered into the anterior wound. The tendon is split longitudinally thus doubling its length. A fourth incision is made over the dorsum of the second metatarsal base. The tendon is passed subcutaneously into the dorsal foot wound and passed around the base of the second metatarsal. Toe flexor tenotomies are performed at the base of each toe and all incisions except the dorsal foot incision are closed. Lastly, the tendon is sutured to itself under appropriate tension with the foot at neutral. A short leg cast is applied and ambulation is begun on the first postoperative day. *Note that the postoperative protocol on ambulatory patients undergoing lower extremity surgery is aimed at early mobilization. Down time rapidly leads to irreversible loss of strength.* Weight bearing is begun on the first postoperative day, short leg casts are used whenever possible, and ankle-foot orthoses (AFOs) or knee-ankle-foot orthoses (KAFOs) are molded prospectively and ready for use when casts are removed. For a further discussion of the

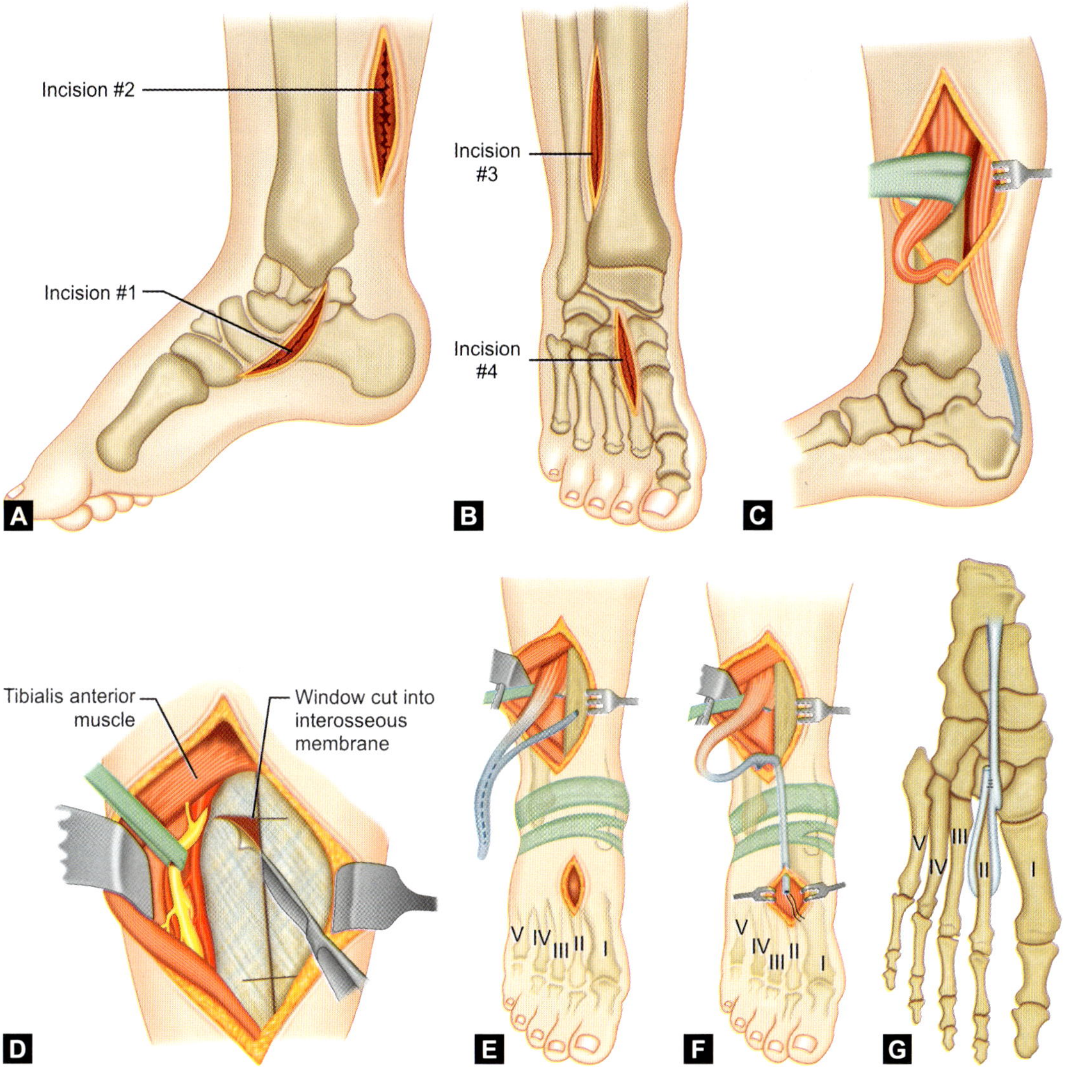

Figs 2A to G: Posterior tibial tendon transfer (PTTT) through interosseous membrane. (A and B) Location of incisions; (C) Released posterior tibial tendon (PTT) is delivered into proximal wound; (D) Window excised from interosseous membrane; (E) Tendon is delivered through interosseous membrane, split and turned down to double its length; (F) Tendon is delivered subcutaneously into distal wound; (G) Tendon is passed around base of second metatarsal and sutured to itself

diagnosis and treatment of muscular dystrophy, the reader is encouraged to consult the comprehensive review by Shapiro and Specht.[1]

REFERENCES

1. Shapiro F, Specht L. The diagnosis and orthopaedic treatment of inherited muscular diseases of childhood. J Bone Joint Surg Am. 1993;75(3):439-54.
2. Smith SE, Green NE, Cole RJ, et al. Prolongation of ambulation in children with Duchenne muscular dystrophy by subcutaneous lower limb tenotomy. J Pediatr Orthop. 1993;13(3):336-40.
3. Scher DM, Mubarak SJ. Surgical prevention of foot deformity in patients with Duchenne muscular dystrophy. J Pediatr Orthop. 2002;22(3):384-91.

SECTION 8

The Rheumatoid Foot

Chapter Outline

48

Rheumatoid Pathology

Katherine C Ma, Judith F Baumhauer

INTRODUCTION

Rheumatoid arthritis (RA) is a chronic systemic inflammatory illness that attacks multiple organ systems, most specifically, the synovial joints. There is a chronic synovitis leading to erosive changes to the joints with progressive destruction and subsequent deformity. Extra-articular manifestations include bursitis, pericarditis, tendonitis, fasciitis, rheumatoid nodules, neuritis and vasculitis.[1,17]

ETIOLOGY

The cause of RA remains unknown, however; it is believed to be mediated by interactions between the various cell types within the autoimmune system. RA has been associated with the class II major histocompatibility complex, specifically HLA DR4.[2,3] It is hypothesized that the disease is triggered in genetically susceptible individuals by an infectious process. The T-cell and B-cell response to these inciting antigens begins the inflammatory cascade which includes activation of various pro-inflammatory cytokines. This leads to upregulation of endothelial adhesion molecules which cause an influx of monocytes and leukocytes into the synovial tissue. Macrophages within the synovium produce interleukin-1, tumor necrosis factor (TNF)-alpha, and other growth factors, which causes the release of proteases by chondrocytes and fibroblasts, ultimately leading to the destruction of the joint.[3] There is synovial tissue angiogenesis resulting in synovial hyperplasia and pannus formation.[12] In the patient with RA, the fibroblastoid cells exhibit a transformed phenotype allowing them to adhere to and degrade cartilage in the absence of T-cells through the expression of metalloproteinases.[8]

EPIDEMIOLOGY

The prevalence of RA is 0.6% in the United States,[4] with an overall worldwide prevalence of about 1%. Women are affected at least twice as often as men, and the incidence increases with age.[10] Recently, it is felt that there has been a decline in the overall incidence of RA with a later age of onset.[3] According to Grondal's survey of patients in 2005, 75% of those surveyed were women with an average age of 60 years old and a median duration of disease of 10 years.[5] In the United States, there is a correlation between lack of formal education and lower socioeconomic class with both the incidence and a poorer prognosis of the disease. Patients affected by RA are more likely to be disabled within 10 years of onset of the disease. This leads to a decrease in their earnings coupled with an estimated three times the healthcare costs, four times the number of ambulatory visits to a physician and twice the number of hospitalizations when compared with an age- and gender-matched population.[6]

Hormonal influences can help explain the increased prevalence in women. There has been an association of use of oral contraceptives prior to the onset of RA with decreased severity of the disease.[13] The majority of woman may have remission of their symptoms during pregnancy, however; these patients usually relapse during the postpartum period.[14]

It is estimated that 20–50% of patients present with problems related to the foot or ankle[5,9] and the foot is involved in 80–89% of patients at some point over the course of the disease.[7] The forefoot is involved with the greatest frequency at the start of the disease (45%) with the hindfoot or ankle being present initially only 17% of the time. Involvement of both the forefoot and hindfoot/ankle at the debut of the disease is 9%. The hand is the only other joint complex involved more frequently than the foot and ankle. Eighty percent of patients surveyed by Grondal had current foot/ankle involvement, with 86% of people symptomatic in the forefoot and 52% symptomatic in the hindfoot/ankle. There were no differences in patients treated with or without anti-TNF agents. Difficulty with walking was present in 17% of patients, and this was found to correlate with disease duration, with the foot and ankle being the most common joint affecting their gait.[5] After 6 years of disease duration, almost half of the patients have considerable radiologic destruction of the ankle and tarsus.[11]

PATHOPHYSIOLOGY AND NATURAL HISTORY

The inflammatory cascade in RA eventually leads to articular changes. It begins with a chronic, erosive synovitis, followed by capsular and ligamentous laxity, cartilage destruction, and finally osseous erosion. The classic structural changes that are seen within the forefoot include dorsally dislocated metatarsal phalangeal joints of the lesser toes and hallux valgus. These deformities are due to the capsular and ligamentous laxity of the metatarsophalangeal (MTP) joints. As the patients bear weight on their foot, there is a dorsiflexion stress to the joints causing subluxation of the proximal phalanx on the metatarsal through the already weakened capsule. The intrinsic muscles to the lesser toes now lie in a dorsal position resulting in a loss of flexion at the MTP joint and a loss of extension at the interphalangeal (IP) joints. Continued dorsiflexion leads to frank dislocation of the lesser MTP joints with the proximal phalanges sitting on the dorsal metatarsal neck. The plantar fat pads remain anchored to the base of their respective proximal phalanx, and with the dorsal dislocation of the proximal phalanx, the plantar fat pad is pulled more distally. With the MTP joint capsule already weakened by the course of this disease, the metatarsal heads protrude through the capsule, leaving them to lie in a subcutaneous position. This can lead to increased plantar pressure and the formation of calluses.

In the hindfoot, synovitis, capsular and ligamentous laxity can lead to a progressive loss of the longitudinal arch resulting in the typical valgus deformity.[15] The foot then externally rotates to compensate for the lack of arch during gait.[16] This external rotation and valgus deformity, leads to contracture of the Achilles tendon. There is also a loss of the windlass mechanism in the plantar foot, leading to further inability to stabilize the arch during toe rise.[17] The gait pattern seen is a delayed heel rise, shortened step length, and decreased walking velocity.[16] In the past, it was felt that posterior tibial tendinopathy was responsibility for the valgus deformity, however electromyographic studies have demonstrated an increase in activity of the posterior tibial tendon in an attempt to stabilize the arch.[16]

DIAGNOSIS

Presentation and Clinical Features

Patients with RA often present with pain in the foot.[5,9] This pain is most frequently in the forefoot as a result of erosive damage to the cartilage and subsequent subluxation and dislocation deformities resulting in irritation with shoewear. Hallux valgus deformity results from the chronic synovitis and its effects on the joint complex. As the capsular structures attenuate, there is loss of stability of the first MTP. The progression of the disease and the eventual bony destruction within the joint also contributes to this instability resulting in a valgus deformity. There are claw-toe deformities of the lesser toes. The capsular weakening due to the disease process causes subluxation and eventual dislocation of the MTP joints of these toes. As the fat pads are translated more distally with the dislocated proximal phalanx, the metatarsal heads become more prominent leading to painful callus formation on the plantar surface of the foot. It is important to inspect the patients' shoes for signs of wear or excessive breakdown.

The patients with hindfoot arthropathy complain of "ankle pain," but on examination, it is localized to the sinus tarsi and subtalar joint. Destruction of the joint, increased capsular and ligamentous laxity, and tendonopathy all contribute to a valgus deformity of the hindfoot accompanied with increased pronation of the midfoot and forefoot. The deformity may be flexible or rigid. In excessive valgus deformity, patients may have pain generated from fibular stress fractures or fibular impingement on the calcaneus. The talus may be tilted into valgus, especially as the deformity progresses.

In terms of patients presenting with ankle symptoms, they may be related to an excessive hindfoot valgus deformity or isolated to the true tibiotalar joint. Often patients complain of a lack of motion and not pain.[18] This decreased range of motion leads to functional limitations in ambulation and stair climbing. Patients with RA have shorter stride lengths and slower walking velocities.[16]

Physical examination begins with an overall inspection of the patient's foot. This includes evaluating for bony malalignment, the presence of rheumatoid nodules, and any callosities or areas of increased wear. Splinter nail hemorrhages may be suggestive of rheumatoid vasculitis which may prompt a referral to a vascular surgeon. A careful assessment of the patient's sensory and vascular status is performed. Arteritis of the vasa vasorum of the cutaneous nerves can lead to peripheral neuropathy. The motor examination can identify weakness which may be indicative of spine involvement or specific tendon dysfunction. Palpation of the foot will identify painful joints. The midfoot joints are usually not symptomatic and rarely require surgical intervention despite degenerative changes seen on radiographs. Passively ranging the joints determines flexible versus fixed deformities. An overall examination of the patient weight-bearing may assess for the degree of malalignment. Evaluation of the hips and knees should also be conducted, as deformities at other joints, such as genu valgum, can lead to compensatory hindfoot valgus and forefoot varus. The patient's gait should be examined. The rheumatoid patient's gait tends to be shuffled with shortened stride length and decreased walking velocity.[16]

Initially, patients may present with a unilateral arthritis which progresses to a symmetric arthritis. It tends to affect the small peripheral joints and characteristically is associated with morning stiffness lasting at least 1 hour. The laboratory tests typically performed in the workup include rheumatoid factor which is typically positive in 85% of the patients with RA, an erythrocyte sedimentation rate (ESR) which is usually elevated, and the fluorescent antinuclear antibody test. This test is positive in less than half the patients with RA. Ninety percent of patients have an elevated C-reactive protein (CRP). This is not a specific diagnostic test, as CRP may be elevated in many acute disease processes. Complement levels are found to be elevated in the acute phase of RA but decreased in patients with RA and vasculitis. More recently, anti-cyclic citrullinated peptide antibody (anti-CCP) test has been used as a diagnostic test of RA. It has been found to be associated with more joint destruction and disease activity than rheumatoid factor;[52] however, a review of the quality of these studies investigating the use of anti-CCP as a diagnostic test of RA have found that the reporting quality of these studies may lead to bias and further studies are warranted.[53]

Radiographic evaluation includes weight-bearing anteroposterior, oblique, and lateral views of the foot as well as weight-bearing anteroposterior, mortise, and lateral views of the ankle. Initially, the only findings may be soft tissue swelling. With disease progression, there are marginal bony erosions and joint space narrowing. This is followed by subluxation and malalignment, ankylosis, and reactive sclerosis around those healing erosions. Nearly 80% of patients who had erosions on hand and foot films also had damage in their cervical spine.[19] It is important to correlate clinical findings of neck pain or neurologic abnormalities with the need to obtain dynamic cervical spine radiographs to evaluate for instability.

Magnetic resonance imaging (MRI) may be helpful in identifying specific joint involvement when physical examination finds diffuse synovitis and the examination is unclear. Additionally, computed tomography (CT) may assist in evaluating joint involvement.

Differential Diagnosis

The differential diagnosis when evaluating these patients includes other inflammatory arthropathies such as other autoimmune diseases and gout, tumor, or infection. As always, a thorough history and physical examination is performed. Radiologic tests are reviewed. The initial laboratory work-up includes a complete blood count with white blood cell differentiation, ESR, and CRP. A biopsy of the soft-tissue mass will aid in diagnosis. Histologically, there is synovial tissue angiogenesis and hyperplasia in the rheumatoid patient. Special staining techniques can identify rheumatoid factor from the tissue. Gout can be excluded by the lack of needle-shaped urate crystals located within polymorphonuclear neutrophils. Cultures will be negative helping to rule out an infection.

OPTIONS OF MANAGEMENT

Patients with symptomatic RA of their feet or ankles must initially be maximally medically

Table 1: Nonoperative interventions in the rheumatoid foot

Intervention	*Benefit*
Orthotic use	Pain relief Improved function
Shoewear modification	Accommodate deformity Distribute forces more evenly across foot Assists in correcting malalignment
Bracing	Accommodates deformity Useful in non-surgical candidates
Intra-articular steroid injections	Can be diagnostic Pain relief
Physical therapy	Helps to maintain joint motion
Medical synovectomy	Satisfactory results in a few studies

managed. Pharmacologic treatment involves three main categories of drugs: (1) Nonsteroidal anti-inflammatory drugs (NSAIDs); (2) Disease modifying anti-rheumatic drugs (DMARDs); and (3) Corticosteroids. NSAIDs are used mainly for pain control. They do not have an effect on disease progression. Corticosteroids may be used as an initial treatment to combat synovitis. They can provide improvement in a patient's symptoms while waiting for DMARD therapy to take effect. As their name implies, DMARDs are used to alter the course of the disease.

Conservative Options

The goals of nonoperative and operative treatment are the same: relieving pain, correcting or accommodating the deformity, and restoring or preserving function.

Nonoperative treatment is an important component of the overall management of the rheumatoid foot (Table 1). Altering a patient's footwear and the use of orthotics are the foundation of nonoperative treatment. In evaluating the type of orthotic to use, the patient's deformity guides the treatment. In patients who have flexible deformities, the orthotics need to be supportive in an attempt to re-establish a more normal foot alignment. In those patients with rigid deformities, the orthotics are accommodative and aim to decrease the plantar pressure and prevent soft tissue breakdown. Metatarsal pads placed proximally to the metatarsal heads relieve the plantar pressure from the heads. The decrease in forces through the MTP joints can allow for some resolution of the synovitis. Pain relief and improved function is seen in those patients who wear orthotics. Studies have demonstrated that there is no difference in function between custom-made orthotics when compared with standard orthotics[20,21] or improved pain relief and function with the use of orthotics when compared to wearing a shoe alone.[25]

Due to their deformity and possible sensory abnormalities, rheumatoid patients benefit from shoewear modification. Studies have shown that off-the-shelf specialist orthopedic footwear results in reduced pain and improved function as well as the gait pattern.[22-24] An extended steel shank can be added to the sole of a shoe to decrease the amount of force over the first MTP joint. Extra wide, extra depth shoes can accommodate hallux valgus or lesser toe deformities. These shoes may need to be stretched at the location of bony prominences. A rocker bottom shoe can improve forward propulsion with ambulation and relieve pressure in those patients with symptomatic midfoot arthritis. In the patients with hindfoot valgus deformity, a medial heel wedge can be built into the shoe or the orthotics. This decreases the impingement of the fibula along the calcaneus.

All shoewear and orthotic modifications are aiming to improve the overall alignment of the foot if the deformity is flexible or accommodate the fixed deformities. These modifications are used from the beginning of treatment and can help to decrease pain until the foot deteriorates to the point of requiring surgical intervention. In those patients who are not surgical candidates, more involved bracing may be needed.

For patients requiring more support around the hindfoot and ankle, a custom-made ankle foot orthosis with an anterior clamshell component helps to distribute the weight-bearing to the level of the calf. This brace may lead to skin breakdown over bony prominences with time. A double upright brace will similarly decrease the weight-bearing through the ankle but has less soft tissue irritation. These braces can be combined with accommodative orthotics and can be effective in treatment of patients who are not operative candidates.

Local corticosteroid injections decrease pain and swelling which allows improved function in the rheumatoid foot.[27] Ultrasound may be beneficial to help localize the symptomatic joint allowing greater pain relief with the injection.[26] Injections may be diagnostic as well as therapeutic, especially in surgical planning. This is not a long-term solution but can offer relief during an exacerbation.

Physical therapy to assist in range of motion exercises to maintain the motion of the forefoot, hindfoot, and ankle can be employed. There are no scientific studies looking at the effect these exercises have on pain or long-term function. Occupational therapy has been found to help to improve the function in the rheumatoid patient and teach joint protection.[32]

Medical synovectomy using a radioactive agent has been used in the foot and ankle. In small, retrospective studies, there have been satisfactory results; however, there were short durations of follow-up.[28,29] This is not a recommended method of treatment at this time.

Surgical Options

If after orthotic and shoewear modification patients continue to have severe pain or significant deformity with an inability to wear shoes, surgical intervention is indicated.

Surgical planning must be performed in the rheumatoid patient to allow for successful outcomes. Radiologic involvement of the cervical spine can be present in more than 80% of rheumatoid patients.[30,31] It is important that cervical instability is identified and treated prior to surgical intervention. Aspirin and anti-inflammatory medications should be stopped 1 week prior to surgery. Communication with the patient's rheumatologist should be considered regarding the stoppage of other disease modifying medications. Current literature shows that there is no statistically significant risk of wound breakdown in patients taking methotrexate, steroids, or both.[33]

In the forefoot, the aim is to restore the alignment of the first MTP joint to improve the weight-bearing function of the great toe and correction of deformities of the lesser toes to allow adequate padding of the metatarsal heads.

In treating the hallux valgus deformity of the great toe, the options are excisional arthroplasty, arthroplasty, or arthrodesis. Excisional arthroplasty can be performed by removing either the metatarsal head (Mayo's procedure) or excising the base of the proximal phalanx (Keller's procedure). These procedures may lead to a cock up deformity of the great toe, transmission of pressure to the lesser toes, forefoot instability, and decreased weight-bearing over the great toe. When compared with arthrodesis, resection arthroplasty patients have similar rates of satisfaction;[34] however, there are high rates of recurrence of deformity and return of pain over time.[35-38] This procedure is not favored over arthrodesis by the author (Figs 1A to C).

Joint replacement arthroplasty of the great toe has been performed using silicone, ceramic, and metal implants. The results of these implants are variable. While there have been a few small prospective studies that have reported satisfactory results,[40,41] these studies have had short durations of follow-up with recurrent deformity occurring. The high biomechanical demand on the first MTP joint can lead to osteophyte formation, osteolysis, and failure of the implant.[42,43] With the variable outcomes and short follow-up, joint replacement arthroplasty is not recommended.

Arthrodesis of the first MTP is the procedure of choice. Fusion allows for an increased amount of weight-bearing in the medial column. This improves the patients' balance and allows for a more stable platform for push-off during gait.[39] It also decreases the forces across the lesser MTP joints and protects the relocated plantar fat pad. The position of fusion and the stability of that fusion are key for obtaining good results.[44] The first MTP joint should be fused in a position of 20–30 degrees of dorsiflexion in relation to the first metatarsal or 5–10 degrees in relation to the floor, neutral rotation, and 10–15 degrees of valgus. A variety of fusion techniques may be used including threaded Steinman pins, lag screw compression, dorsal compression plating, or a combination of both (Figs 2A and B). With the newer locking plate fixation, arthrodesis is more reliable in osteoporotic bone. Depending on the type of fixation used, fusion rates can be as high as 100%.[44]

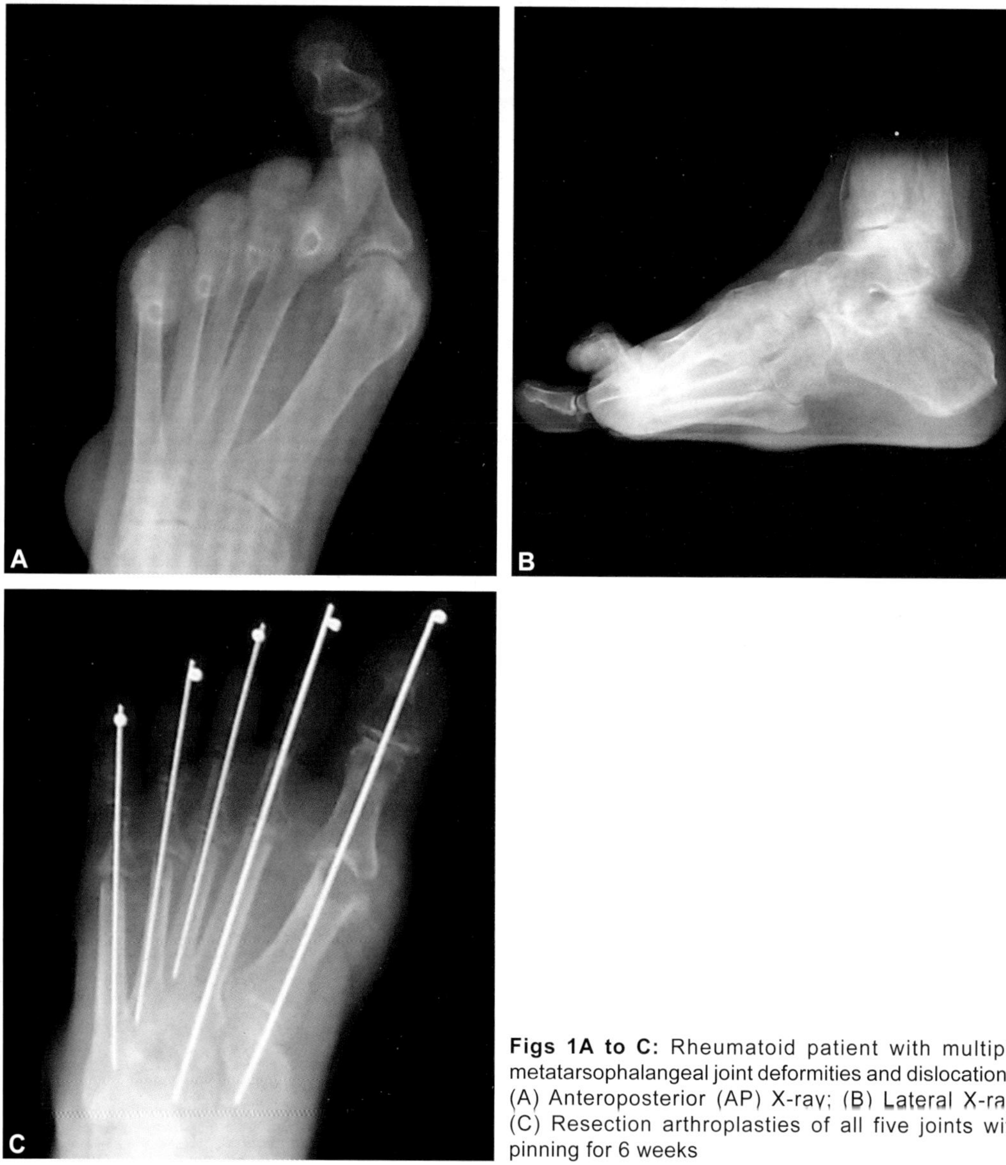

Figs 1A to C: Rheumatoid patient with multiple metatarsophalangeal joint deformities and dislocations. (A) Anteroposterior (AP) X-ray; (B) Lateral X-ray; (C) Resection arthroplasties of all five joints with pinning for 6 weeks

The goals of treatment of the lesser toe deformities are to realign the MTP and IP joints and provide padding of the plantar surface by relocating the plantar fat pad. This typically involves resection arthroplasty of the MTP joints, usually by resection of the metatarsal heads, either alone or in combination with the proximal phalanx. Recent literature has demonstrated arthrolysis of the lesser MTP joints in conjunction with first MTP fusion, when compared with lesser MTP resection, shows no significant difference between the groups in regard to use of orthopedic aides or shoewear, subjective rating, recurrent callosities, function, or walking capacity.[47] However, the literature on this technique is limited and resection arthroplasty remains the more common procedure. The procedure is usually performed through dorsal incisions; however, a transverse plantar incision has been utilized as well. Successful surgery requires adequate resection of the metatarsal head with cuts that are angled from dorsal distal to plantar proximal. This will decrease any plantar prominence and decrease the risk for callus formation or skin breakdown. The arc of the metatarsal length is gently decreased as you proceed

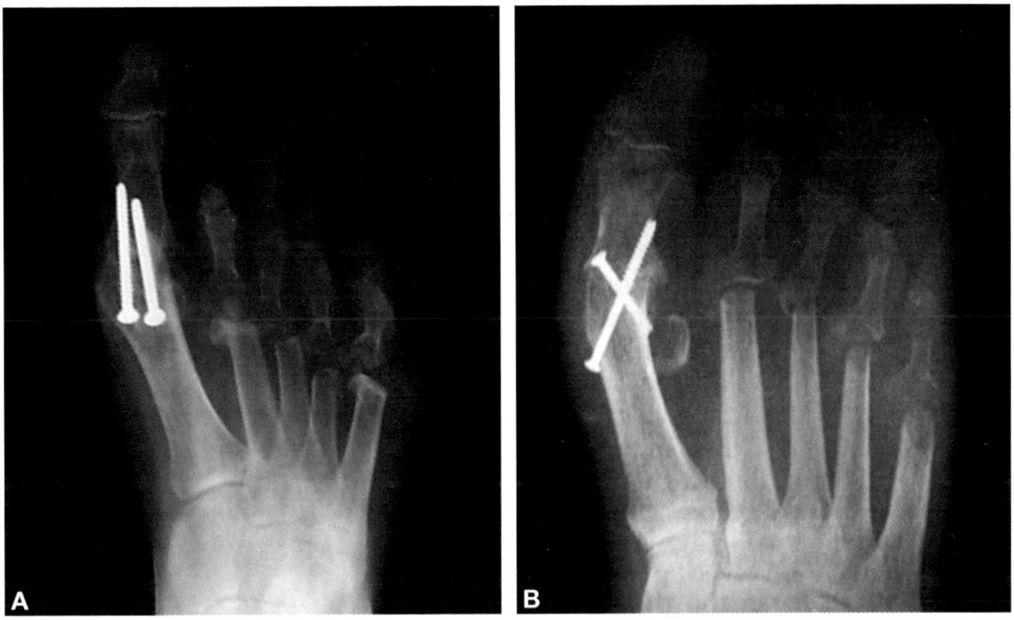

Figs 2A and B: Arthrodesis of the great toe metatarsophalangeal (MTP) joint associated with resection arthroplasties of the lesser joints. (A) 2 screw fusion technique. Note excessive length of great toe and recession of lesser toes; (B) Cross screw fusion of great toe MTP joint with more appropriate toe lengths

from the second to the fifth toes. Osteoclasis of the proximal interphalangeal (PIP) joints can be performed in fixed flexion contractures. The toes are then fixed with a 0.062 mm Kirschner's wires (K-wire) from the toe tip across the MTP joint to maintain the alignment. The wire is removed after 6 weeks.

This author's preference is to perform a fusion of the first MTP joint using a combination of a lag compression screw and a dorsal compression plate and resection arthroplasty of the lesser MTP joints. A popliteal block is placed in the preanesthesia area for the surgery and postoperative pain control. The patient is placed supine on the operating table. A bump is placed under the patient's buttocks to place the hip and lower extremity in a neutral position. An ankle Esmarch tourniquet is applied. If correction of the claw toe deformities of the lesser toes is planned, a calf tourniquet is used. A longitudinal incision on the dorsal aspect of the first MTP joint is made. Care is taken to identify the extensor hallucis longus tendon and retract it laterally. An incision is made over the dorsal capsule, and the capsule is freed up both laterally and medially off of the metatarsal head and base of the proximal phalanx. The plantar plate is also stripped off of the head of the metatarsal. A cone and cup reamer system is used. All osteophytes and reamed loose bone is removed.

The resection of the lesser metatarsal heads is performed at this point to avoid any unintended forces on the great toe fixation. Individual incisions are placed over the second and fourth webspaces avoiding the dorsal surface of the lesser MTP joints. Incisions over the joints themselves can lead to unintended contractures and recurrent malalignment over time. The incision is carried down to the capsule. The extensor digitorum longus and brevis tendons are tenotomized. The capsules (2–5) are opened sharply and the metatarsal heads are subperiosteally dissected free of attachments particularly the plantar plate. A small key elevator can release the plantar tissues. A microsagittal saw is used to perform a beveled resection of the head, beginning on the dorsal surface distally, and proceeding to the plantar surface proximally. The metatarsal head is removed. Often osteoclysis of the PIP or DIP joints can be performed to realign these joints; however, if necessary, a hammertoe correction is performed. The PIP joint capsule is opened longitudinally to protect the blood flow to the toe. The sagittal saw is used to resect the distal portion of the proximal phalanx and the proximal portion of the middle phalanx. The two ends of the bones are brought together. A 0.062 mm K-wire is used for fixation. The wire is driven from the tip of the toe across the corrected, realigned DIP, PIP and into the metatarsal shaft. Fluoroscopic confirmation of positioning is confirmed.

Returning to the great toe, the position of the fusion is established: 10 degrees of dorsiflexion in reference to the floor, slight valgus to sit next to a well-aligned second toe, and neutral rotation. A K-wire is passed from the medial proximal phalanx into the lateral distal metatarsal. The position of the joint is confirmed with fluoroscopy. A partially threaded, cannulated screw is then passed over the K-wire achieving compression across the joint. A pre-contoured dorsal compression plate is placed over the dorsal surface of the joint. It is held in position with K-wires. A locking screw is placed in the proximal phalanx. Then a non-locking screw is placed in the compression position in the metatarsal. The remaining screw holes are filled with locking screws. After irrigation of the wounds, the capsule of the first is closed with an absorbable 2.0 vicryl suture and all skin incisions are closed with nylon. A bulky dressing is applied with cast padding in between the toes for comfort. The patient is placed in a well-padded posterior splint and instructed to elevate the foot "toes above the nose" and no weight on the foot for one week. At 1 week, the patient is placed in a walking cast for five additional weeks with the sutures removed at 3rd week.

Excision of rheumatoid nodules is usually only undertaken when they occur in the incisional area for other more pressing surgical interventions. Recurrence of the nodules is common, hence the reluctance to do these procedures as an isolated surgical intervention. Nonetheless, they can be both disfiguring and dysfunctional and excision may then be undertaken. Such lesions occurring on the plantar surface and in the web spaces, over the medial eminence of the great toe, and over the fifth metatarsal head are examples of problematic sites potentially warranting surgical intervention (Figs 3A to C).

Rheumatoid involvement of the hindfoot results in a valgus deformity with compensatory forefoot supination. The prevalence of hindfoot involvement increases as the disease duration increases. CT evaluation of patients with RA revealed extra-articular involvement in 39%, subtalar involvement in 29%, and calcaneocuboid involvement in 25%. The motions of these joints are coupled, and it is rare to find isolated joint involvement. Surgical intervention is typically a triple arthrodesis although fusion of a single joint is considered if there is isolated arthropathy and adequate alignment. Isolated talonavicular arthrodesis has been found

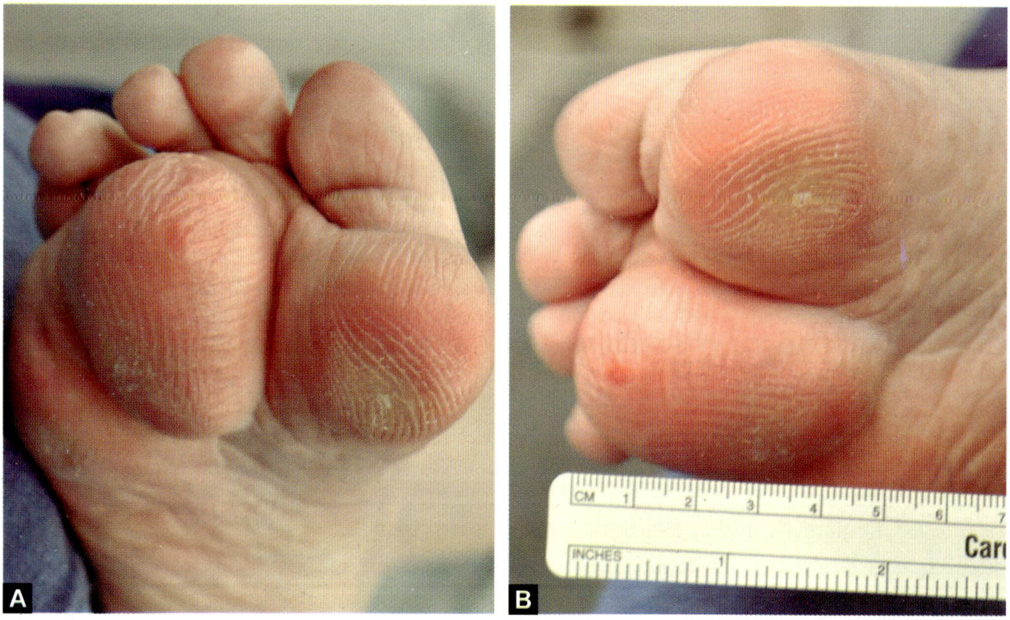

Figs 3A and B

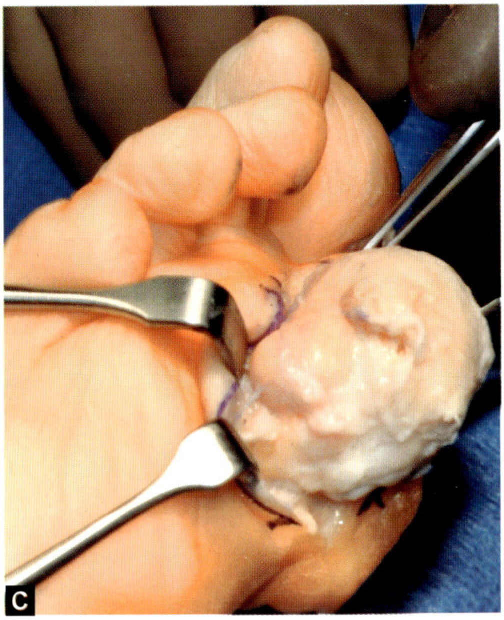

Figs 3A to C: Huge plantar nodule in rheumatoid patient; (A) Plantar view; (B) Oblique plantar view; (C) Operative excision

to have good results in 18 of 26 patients.[45] Fusion of a single joint decreases the symptoms at the surrounding joints in the hindfoot. Prior anatomic studies have found that fusion of the talonavicular joint limits subtalar motion significantly to less than 10% of its original motion.[46] The fusions are fixed with internal fixation and bone graft may be used if necessary. The patients are nonweight-bearing in a short leg cast for 6 weeks and are progressed to a walking boot or a weight-bearing cast until bony union occurs, usually about another 6 weeks.

The author will perform isolated single joint hindfoot arthrodesis if the clinical picture supports single joint involvement only. In those cases, the individual joint is fused (Figs 4A to C). In the vast majority of cases, these rheumatoid patients require triple arthrodesis to address their pain and correct their deformity (Figs 5A to D). The patient is placed supine on the operating table. A bump is placed under the patient's buttocks to place the hip and lower extremity in internal rotation to facilitate exposure of the subtalar joint. This can be removed during the talonavicular joint exposure. A thigh tourniquet is applied and inflated. Through an Ollier's incision over the sinus tarsi, the skin is sharply incised and then dissecting scissors are used to continue down to the extensor digitorum brevis (EDB) muscle and the extensor retinaculum. The EDB is incised to create a distally based U-flap to expose the subtalar, talonavicular, and calcaneocuboid joints. Care is taken to avoid injury to the sural and superficial peroneal nerves that course across that area. Careful skin retraction is also needed as the rheumatoid patient skin is thin and vulnerable to insult. A rongeur is used to remove the interosseous ligament. Currette and periosteal elevators are used to remove the articular cartilage off of the posterior, middle, and anterior facets of the subtalar joints, the calcaneocuboid joint, and the talonavicular joint. An ancillary anteromedial incision is made just medial to the tibialis anterior tendon over the talonavicular joint. The incision is carried sharply through the skin, and dissecting scissors are used down to the capsule of the talonavicular joint. A longitudinal capsulotomy is performed exposing the medial aspect of the talar head and navicular. This area is denuded of articular cartilage using a currette. The wounds are then irrigated with normal saline. Using a K-wire, each of the surfaces are drilled with holes to facilitate fusion of the subtalar, calcaneocuboid, and talonavicular joints. The foot is then positioned in plantar grade foot alignment with slight valgus, neutral rotation, and neutral internal and external rotation. The joints are stabilized with guidewires from the 7.3 cannulated screw system. The talonavicular guidewire is placed first, followed by the subtalar guidewires. The subtalar fixation is placed from the heel into the talar neck and a second into the talar body. The calcaneocuboid fixation is performed after the other two joints are stable with screw fixation. A staple has been adequate fixation for the calcaneocuboid fixation. Fluoroscopic imaging is used to confirm the alignment as well as visual inspection of the foot. Partially threaded, cannulated screws are then placed over the guidewires. Bone graft may be used as per the patient's needs. With the advent of locking compression plates for the talonavicular joint, this option is used in osteoporotic bone. This triple arthrodesis procedure is commonly combined with a tendo-Achilles lengthening. This is performed with no. 11-blade scalpel through the Hoke technique of percutaneous three hemi-section cuts in the Achilles. The joint capsules are then closed with 2.0 vicryl suture. The EDB muscle is re-approximated and sutured with 2.0 vicryl suture. The skin is then closed with nylon and the patient is placed in a short leg splint.

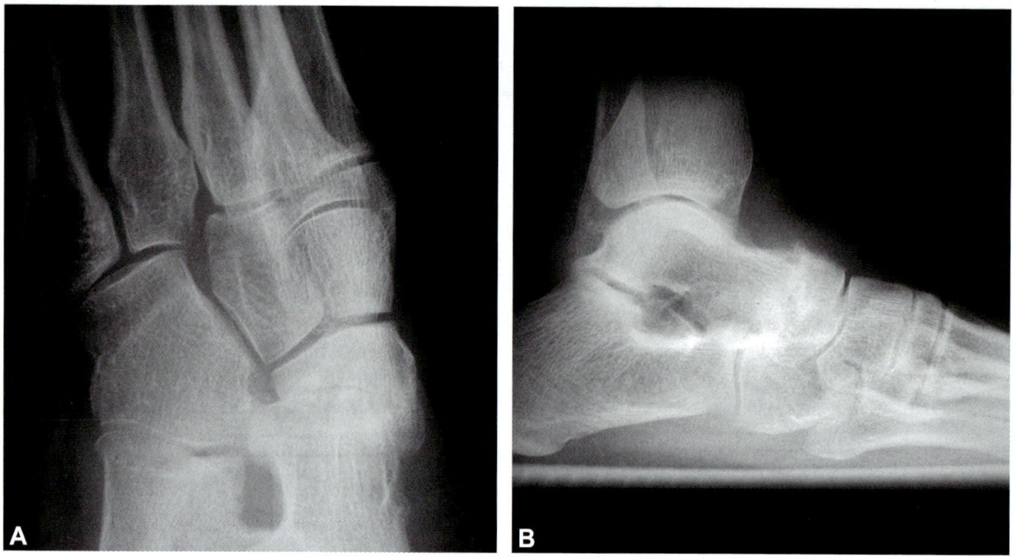

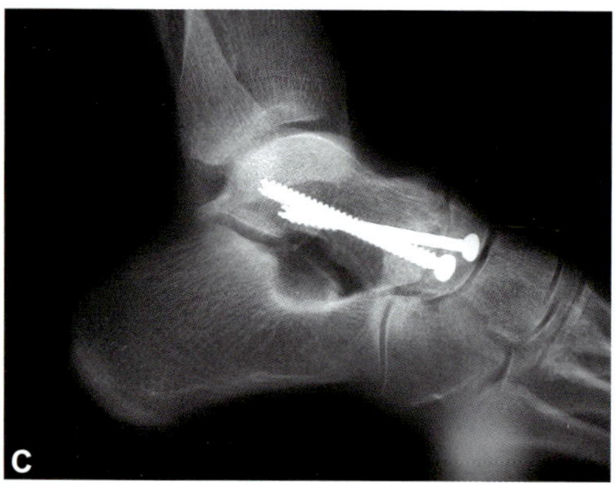

Figs 4A to C: Rheumatoid patient with isolated talonavicular disease. (A) Preoperative oblique; (B) Preoperative lateral; (C) Postoperative lateral of talonavicular arthrodesis

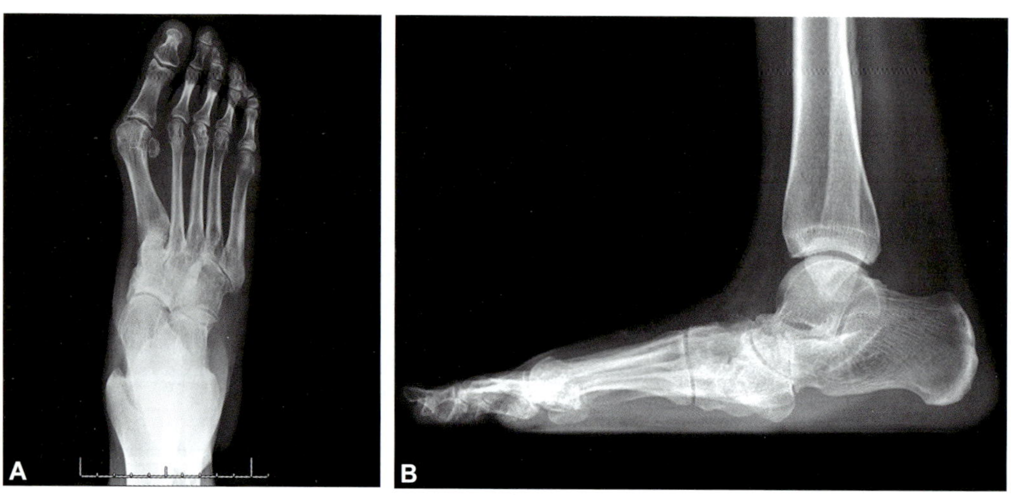

Figs 5A and B

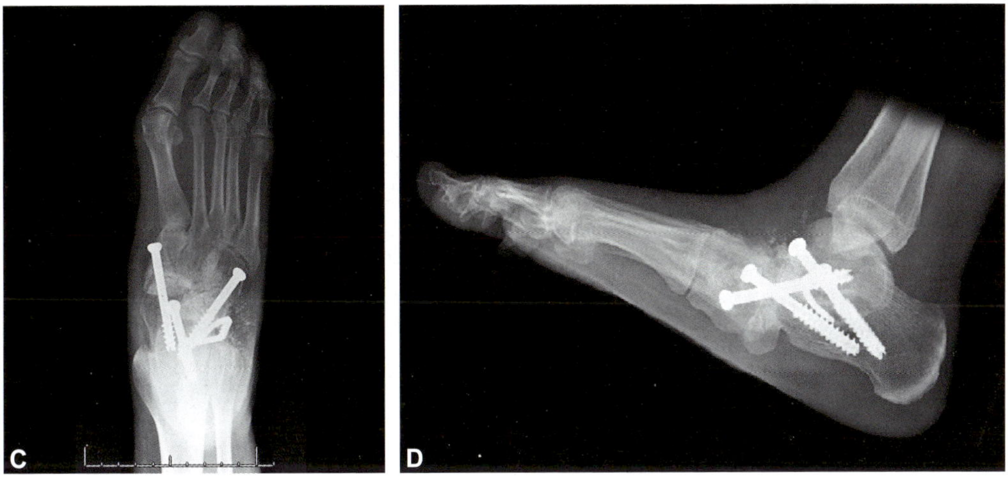

Figs 5A to D: Rheumatoid patient with subtalar and transverse tarsal disease. (A) Anteroposterior (AP) X-ray; (B) Lateral X-ray; (C) Postoperative triple arthrodesis, AP view; (D) Lateral view

Ankle involvement can be treated with synovectomy, arthrodesis, or total joint arthroplasty although the ankle is less commonly symptomatic. A triple arthrodesis should be considered prior to undertaking ankle surgery in the rheumatoid patient (Figs 6A to D). Synovectomy can be used for pain control in the symptomatic ankle joint. Akagi et al. found that after an average follow-up of 15 years, only 10% of ankles had a recurrence of their synovitis. While radiologic deterioration does continue after synovectomy, it is predominantly an osteoarthritic destruction.[48] Arthrodesis of the tibiotalar joint has been performed to relieve pain and correct the deformity of the ankle. The ideal position of fusion is neutral dorsiflexion, 0–5 degrees of valgus, and slight external rotation to match the contralateral side. Internal fixation is most commonly used with reports of good fusion rates and patient satisfaction. As the implants continue to improve, total ankle arthroplasty is being performed with better results and similar to the survivorship of ankle replacements for osteoarthritis (Figs 7 and 8).[49]

The author prefers to perform an ankle arthrodesis. The patient is placed supine on the operating table. A bump is placed under the ipsilateral hip to place the lower extremity into more internal rotation. A thigh tourniquet is used. A lateral incision is made over the distal fibula. The incision is carried out sharply through skin, down through the subcutaneous tissues and down to bone. Subperiosteal dissection of the distal fibula is performed, and then using a sagittal saw, the distal fibula is resected and morcellized later for bone graft. The anterior aspect of the distal tibia is subperiosteally dissected to expose the articular surfaces. The articular surfaces of the tibia and talus are denuded of cartilage with a combination of wooden handled elevators and curettes until subcortical bone is reached. An ancillary incision is made anteromedially just medial to the tibialis anterior tendon which is sharply dissected down to the joint. The joint capsule is opened and then any cartilage on the medial portion of the joint is denuded. The joint is thoroughly irrigated with normal saline and the joint surfaces are then drilled with a K-wire to facilitate fusion. The ankle is placed in a position of neutral to 5 degrees of dorsiflexion. The talar body is displaced as posteriorly as possible under the tibia and provisional fixation with guidewires from the 7.3 mm partially threaded cannulated screw set is obtained from the medial aspect of the distal tibia into the talar body. The position is confirmed fluoroscopically and a 7.3 mm screw is placed over the guidewire to obtain compression of the joint. A second guidewire is placed from the posterior aspect of the tibia into the talar neck. A partially threaded screw is placed over the wire. A third guidewire is placed from the lateral distal aspect of the tibia into the talus, and a partially threaded cannulated screw is placed over this wire. Fluoroscopic confirmation is confirmed. The wounds are irrigated with normal saline. The morcellized bone graft from the removed fibula is then placed in the anterior aspect of the distal tibia medially and laterally. The capsule is then closed

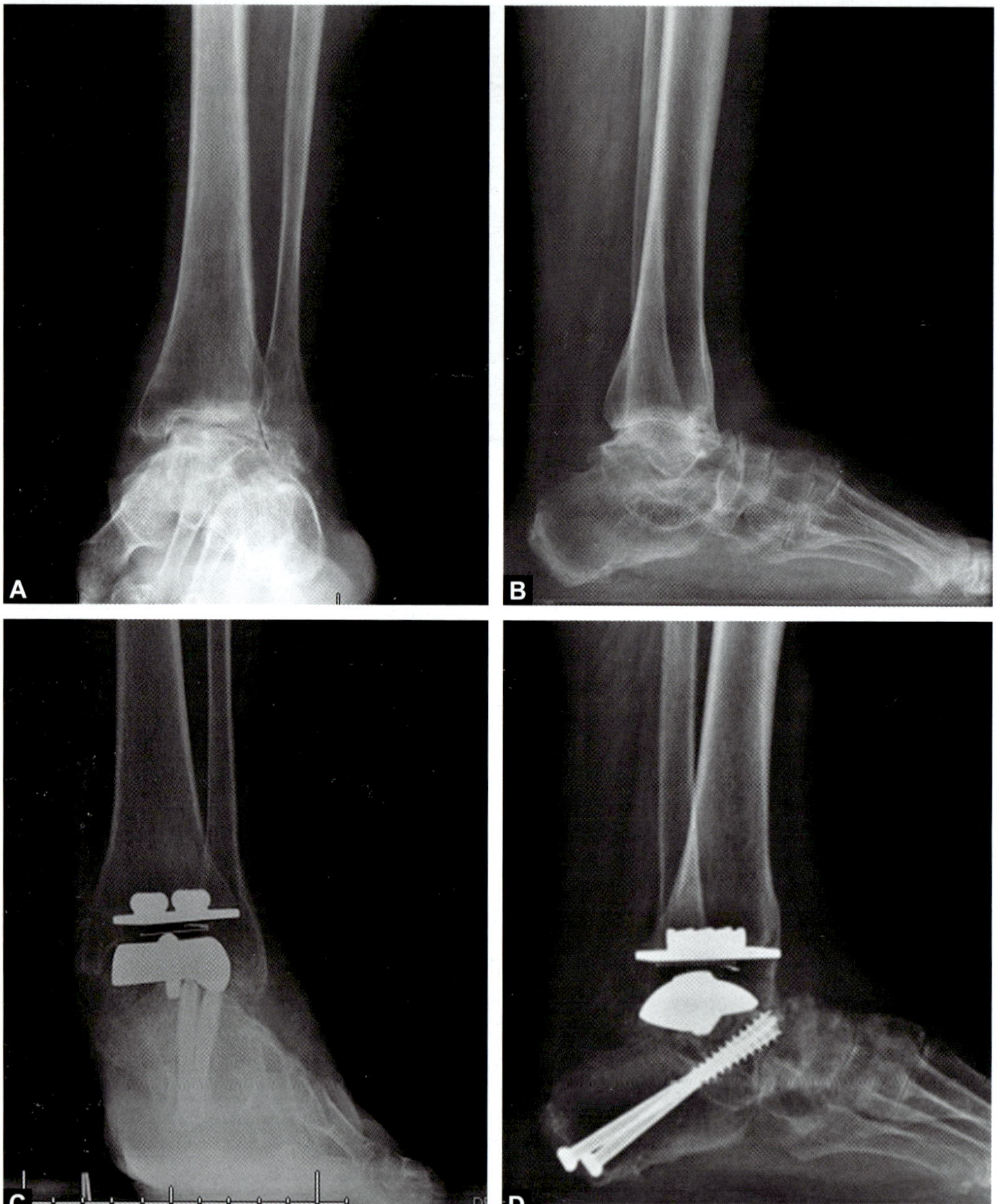

Figs 6A to D: Rheumatoid patient with extensive subtalar and tibiotalar disease (A) Anteroposterior (AP) X-ray view; (B) Lateral X-ray view; (C) AP view of arthrodesis of the subtalar joint with a STAR (Scandanavian total ankle replacement) total ankle replacement, AP view; (D) Lateral view

with 2.0 vicryl suture and the skin is closed with nylon. The patient is placed in a short leg splint in the operating room which is converted to a short leg cast in the office. The patient is kept non-weight bearing for the first 6 weeks followed by 6 weeks in a walking cast.

COMPLICATIONS

In regard to treatment of the first MTP joint, excisional arthroplasty is associated with recurrent malalignment of the great toe. This has been seen in as many 50% of patients.[37] These patients may go on

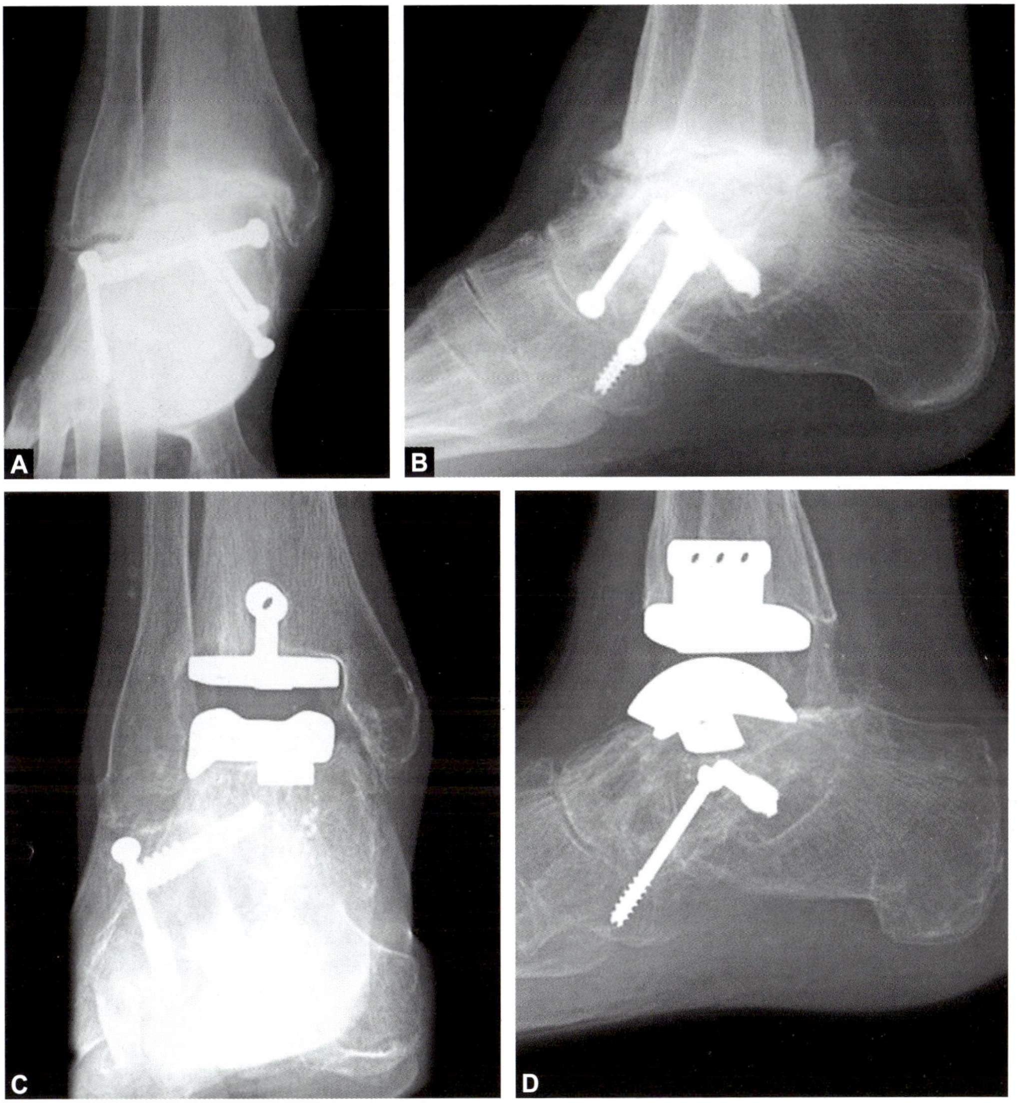

Figs 7A to D: Rheumatoid patient with severe ankle disease; S/P triple arthrodesis. (A) Anteroposterior (AP) view; (B) Lateral view; (C) AP view of Salto Talaris total ankle arthroplasty; (D) Lateral view of Salto Talaris total ankle arthroplasty

to spontaneously ankylose in a malaligned position. The salvage procedure would be converting to an arthrodesis. It is important to have good alignment of the toe for a successful fusion. The position of fusion and the stability of that fusion are key for obtaining good results.[44] Malalignment of the first MTP joint results in increased pressure on the lesser MTP joints leading to metatarsalgia of the lesser toes. This can also be seen if there is an inadequate resection of the metatarsal heads of the lesser toes. Additionally, metatarsalgia can be caused by plantar prominences from a poor arc of resection of the lesser toes resulting in the formation of a soft-tissue bursal swelling on the plantar surface of the foot. If this occurs, revision metatarsal head resection is indicated.

Fusion of the first MTP joint may lead to IP joint arthritis. If the fusion is in inadequate valgus or dorsiflexion, there are increased forces across the IP joint. The salvage procedure is revision of the MTP fusion to an appropriate position, fusion of the IP joint, or both.

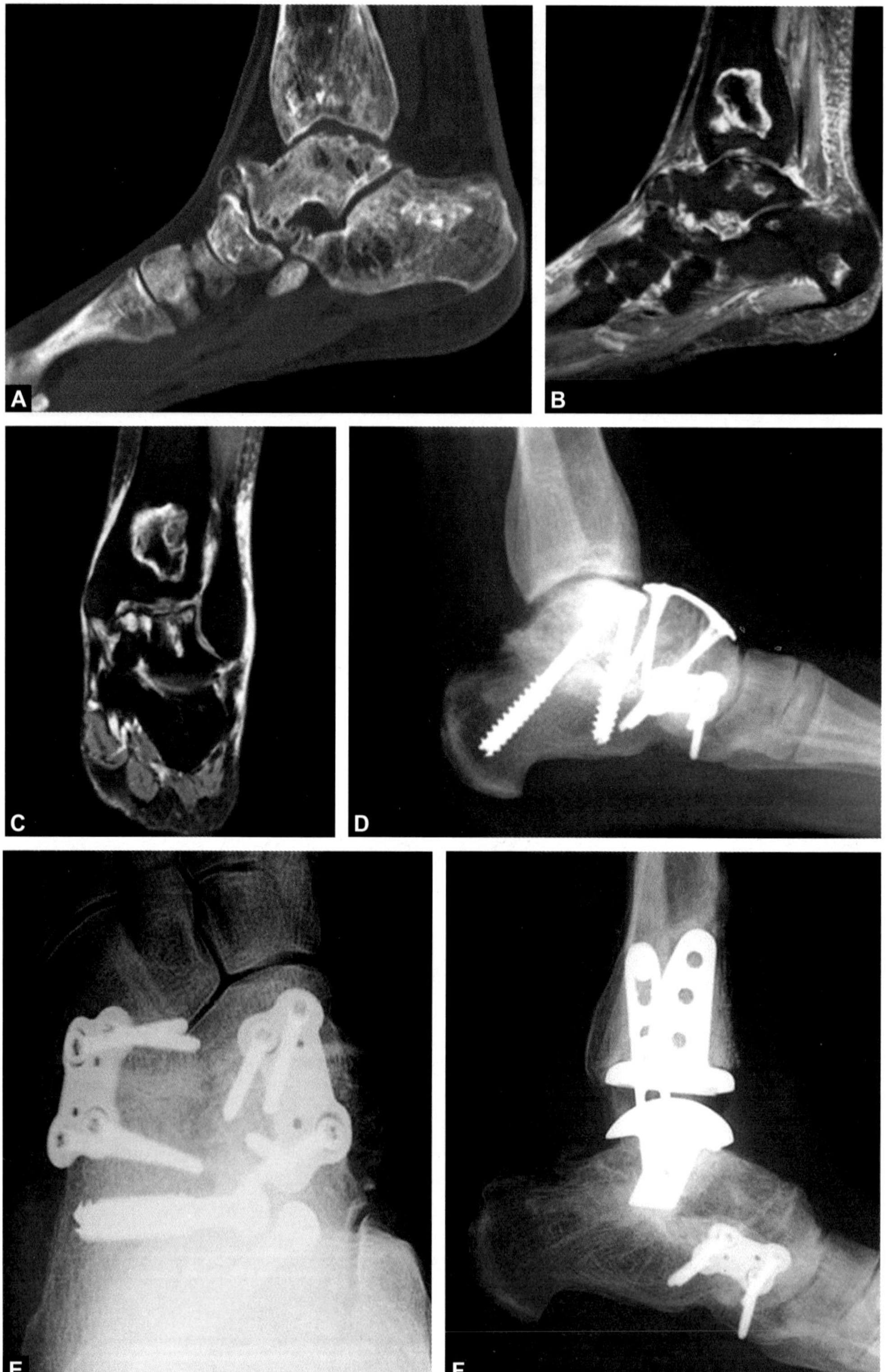

Figs 8A to F

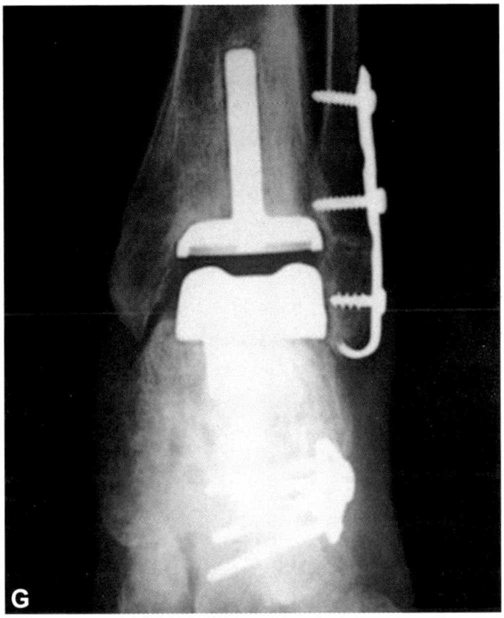

Figs 8A to G: Lupus patient on long-term steroids presents with bone infarcts in distal tibia and talus after a year on parathyroid hormone therapy. (A) Sagittal CT scan of patient with extensive arthritis involving ankle, subtalar and transverse tarsal joints; (B) T2 weighted MRI of sagittal (C) Coronal T2 weighted views of bone infarcts in tibia and talus; (D) Lateral view of triple arthrodesis using compression/locking plates for transverse tarsal joints; (E) AP view of foot; (F) Custom Salto Talaris® total ankle arthroplasty ("shark fin" tibial stem modification and 20 mm talar stem extension) for better purchase in bone, lateral view; (G) AP view of custom Salto Talaris® total ankle arthroplasty

There is a 5–10% incidence of nonunions of attempted arthrodesis of the first MTP joint. This may be a result of inadequate stabilization of the joint in a patient with poor bone quality. Revision arthrodesis with improved surgical fixation using a dorsal plate or crossed screws should be performed. Maintaining adequate postoperative immobilization is also important in achieving union.

As with all foot and ankle surgery, wound healing complications or infections can be present. Good surgical techniques and respecting the soft tissues is important. If a pin tract infection from exposed wires develops, local wound care with or without antibiotics may be used.

In a failed first MTP joint arthroplasty with implants, the implant should be removed. Bone grafting of any voids of bone should be conducted and a revision to first MTP arthrodesis is performed.

In the hindfoot, several complications can result with a triple arthrodesis. A sural nerve injury may result with a lateral approach to the hindfoot. Careful dissection during the lateral surgical approach will minimize this risk. Delayed wound healing may occur in 5–15% of patients. It is important to handle the soft tissues carefully and avoid extensive dissections. Superficial wound infections may occur in as many as 10% of patients. This may be associated with prednisone use, and again, careful handling of soft tissue is paramount. Nonunion of any of the joints in a triple arthrodesis can be seen. Talonavicular joint nonunion is the most common occurring in 3–5% of cases. Causes of malunion included inadequate preparation of the joint surfaces, surgical stabilization, and postoperative immobilization. The salvage procedure is a revision arthrodesis. Malunion or malalignment with residual deformity may be seen. This can be painful as the fibula continues to impinge against the calcaneus. It may result from unrecognized midfoot involvement, under correction of the deformities, or inadequate internal fixation. Revision arthrodesis is indicated. Another complication seen in the triple arthrodesis is progression of symptoms in the ankle. This may be seen if there is under correction of deformity. There may have been pre-existing ankle involvement that went unrecognized prior to surgery. The salvage surgery would be an ankle arthrodesis.

In the ankle, the complications are similar.[50] Sural nerve injury may result from lateral incisions. In a study of 130 ankle fusions, malalignment was the most common cause of failure.[52] Ninety percent of the fusions went on to solid, pain free union. Revision of the failed fusion was successful in 77% of their patients. Additionally, ankle replacements go on to failure at a rate of approximately 10% at 5 years.[51] An increased failure rate was seen in patients with malalignment greater than 10 degrees in the coronal plane. Component loosening may also lead to failure. The salvage procedure would be an ankle arthrodesis, which may be difficult due to the loss of bone stock.

REFERENCES

1. O'Brien TS, Hart TS, Gould JS. Extraosseous manifestations of rheumatoid arthritis in the foot and ankle. Clin Orthop Relat Res. 1997;340:26-33.
2. Smyth CJ, Janson RW. Rheumatologic view of the rheumatoid foot. Clin Orthop Relat Res. 1997;340: 7-17.
3. Koopman WJ. Prospects for autoimmune disease: Research advances in rheumatoid arthritis. JAMA. 2001;285:648-50.
4. Helmick CG, Felson DT, Lawrence RC, et al. Estimates of the prevalence of arthritis and other rheumatic conditions in the United States. Part 1. Arthritis Rheum. 2008;58(1):15-25.
5. Grondal L, Tengstrand B, Nordmark B, et al. The foot: still the most important reason for walking incapacity in rheumatoid arthritis: distribution of symptomatic joints in 1,000 RA patients. Acta Orthop. 2008;79(2):257-61.
6. Felts W, Yelin E. The economic impact of the rheumatic diseases in the United States. J Rheumatol. 1989;16:867-84.
7. Vainio K. The rheumatoid foot: a clinical study with pathologic and roentgenological comments. Ann Chir Gynaecol Fenn Suppl. 1956;45:1-107.
8. Müller-Lander U, Kriegsmann J, Franklin BN, et al. Synovial fibroblasts of patients with rheumatoid arthritis attach to and invade normal human cartilage when engrafted into SCID mice. Am J Pathol. 1996;149:1607-15.
9. Jaakkola JI, Mann RA. A review of rheumatoid arthritis affecting the foot and ankle. Foot Ankle Int. 2004;25(12):866-74.
10. Felson DT. Epidemiology of the rheumatic diseases. In: Koopman WJ (Ed). Arthritis and Allied Conditions: A Textbook of Rheumatology, 13th edition. Baltimore: Williams & Wilkins; 1997. p 6.
11. Kuper HH, van Leeuwen MA, van Riel PL, et al. Radiographic damage in large joints in early rheumatoid arthritis: relationship with radiographic damage in hands and feet, disease activity, and physical disability. Br J Rheumatol. 1997;36(8):855-60.
12. Firestein GS. The immunopathogenesis of rheumatoid arthritis. Curr Opin Rheumatol. 1991;3(3):398-406.
13. Van Zeben D, Hazes JM, Vandenbrouche JP, et al. Diminished incidence of severe rheumatoid arthritis associated with oral contraceptive use. Arthritis Rheum. 1990;33(10):1462-5.
14. Tandon VR, Sharma S, Mahajan A, et al. Pregnancy and rheumatoid arthritis. Indian J Med Sci. 2006; 60(8):334-44.
15. Spiegel TM, Spiegel JS. Rheumatoid arthritis in the foot and ankle-diagnosis, pathology, and treatment. The relationship between foot and ankle deformity and disease duration in 50 patients. Foot Ankle. 1982;2(6):318-24.
16. Keenan MA, Peabody TD, Gronley JK, et al. Valgus deformities of the feet and characteristics of gait in patients who have rheumatoid arthritis. J Bone Joint Surg Am. 1991;73(2):237-47.
17. Abdo R, Iorio L. Rheumatoid arthritis of the foot and ankle. J Am Acad Orthop Surg. 1994;2(6):326-32.
18. Michelson J, Easley M, Wigley FM, et al. Foot and ankle problems in rheumatoid arthritis. Foot Ankle Int. 1994;15(11):608-13.
19. Winfield J, Yang A, Williams P, et al. Prospective study of the radiological changes in hands, feet and cervical spine in adult rheumatoid diseases. Ann Rheum Dis. 1983;46(6):613-8.
20. Cho NS, Hwang JH, Chang HJ, et al. Randomized controlled trial for clinical effects of varying types of insoles combined with specialized shoes in patients with rheumatoid arthritis of the foot. Clin Rehabil. 2009;23(6):512-21.
21. Novak P, Burger H, Tomsic M, et al. Influence of foot orthoses on plantar pressures, foot pain and walking ability of rheumatoid arthritis patients—A randomized controlled study. Disabil Rehabil. 2009;31(8):638-45.
22. Fransen M, Edmonds J. Off-the-shelf orthopedic footwear for people with rheumatoid arthritis. Arthritis Care Res. 1997;10(4):250-6.
23. Hennessy K, Burns J, Penkala S. Reducing plantar pressure in rheumatoid arthritis: a comparison of running versus off-the-shelf orthopaedic footwear. Clin Biomech. 2007;22(8):917-23.
24. Williams AE, Rome K, Nester CJ. A clinical trial of specialist footwear for patients with rheumatoid arthritis. Rheumatology. 2007;46(2):302-7.
25. Hodge MC, Bach TM, Carter GM. Orthotic management of plantar pressure and pain in rheumatoid arthritis. Clin Biomech. 1999;14(8):567-75.
26. d'Agostino MA, Ayral X, Baron G, et al. Impact of ultrasound imaging on local corticosteroid injections of symptomatic ankle, hind-, and mid-foot in chronic inflammatory diseases. Arthritis Rheum. 2005;53(2):284-92.
27. Wallen M, Gillies D. Intra-articular steroids and splints/rest for children with juvenile idiopathic

arthritis and adults with rheumatoid arthritis. Cochrane Database Syst Rev. 2006;25(1):CD002824.
28. Barnes CL, Shortkroff S, Wilson M, et al. Intra-articular radiation treatment of rheumatoid synovitis of the ankle with dysprosium-165 ferric hydroxide macroaggregates. Foot Ankle Int. 1994;15(6): 306-10.
29. van der Zant FM, Jahangier ZN, Moolenburgh JD, et al. Radiation synovectomy of the ankle with 75 MBq colloidal 186rhenium-sulfide: effect, leakage, and radiation considerations. J Rheumatol. 2004;31(5):896-901.
30. Pellicci PM, Ranawat CS, Tsairis P, et al. A prospective study of the progression of rheumatoid arthritis of the cervical spine. J Bone Joint Surg Am. 1993;63(3):342-50.
31. Smith PH, Sharp J, Kellgren JH. Natural history of rheumatoid cervical subluxations. Ann Rheum Dis. 1972;31(3):222-3.
32. Steultjens EM, Dekker J, Bouter LM, et al. Occupational therapy for rheumatoid arthritis. Cochrane Database Syst Rev. 2004;1:CD003114.
33. Jain A, Witbreuk M, Ball C, et al. Influence of steroid and methotrexate on wound complications after elective rheumatoid hand and wrist surgery. J Hand Surg Am. 2002;27(3):449-55.
34. Torikai E, Kageyama Y, Suzuki M, et al. Comparison between resection arthroplasty alone and resection arthroplasty with arthrodesis of the first MTP joint for rheumatoid forefoot deformities. Mod Rheumatol. 2008;18(5):486-91.
35. Hamalainen M, Raunio P. Long-term follow-up of rheumatoid forefoot surgery. Clin Orthop Relat Res. 1997;340:34-8.
36. Fuhrmann RA, Anders JO. The long-term results of resection arthroplasties of the first metatarsophalangeal joint in rheumatoid arthritis. Int Orthop. 2001;25(5):312-6.
37. Vahvanen V, Piirainen H, Kettunen P. Resection arthroplasty of the metatarsophalangeal joints in rheumatoid arthritis. A follow-up study of 100 patients. Scand J Rheumatol. 1980;9(4):257-65.
38. Tillmann K. Surgery of the rheumatoid forefoot with special reference to the plantar approach. Clin Orthop Relat Res. 1997;340:39-47.
39. Beauchamp CG, Kirby T, Rudge SR, et al. Fusion of the first metatarsophalangeal joint in forefoot arthroplasty. Clin Orthop Relat Res. 1984;190: 249-53.
40. Pfeiffer WH, Cracchiolo A, Grace DL, et al. Double-stem silicone implant arthroplasty of all metatarsophalangeal joints in patients with rheumatoid arthritis. Semin Arthroplasty. 1992;3(1):16-24.
41. Shi K, Hayashida K, Owaki H, et al. Replacement of the first metatarsophalangeal joint with a Swanson implant accompanied by open-wedge osteotomy of the first metatarsal bone for hallux valgus in rheumatoid arthritis. Mod Rheumatol. 2007;17(2):110-4.
42. Cracchiolo A, Weltmer JB, Lian G, et al. Arthroplasty of the first metatarsophalangeal joint with a double-stem silicone implant. Results in patients who have degenerative joint disease, failure of operations, or rheumatoid arthritis. J Bone Joint Surg Am. 1992; 74(4):552-63.
43. Granberry WM, Noble PC, Bishop JO, et al. Use of a hinged silicone prosthesis for replacement arthroplasty of the first metatarsophalangeal joint. J Bone Joint Surg Am. 1991;73(10):1453-9.
44. Coughlin MJ. Rheumatoid forefoot reconstruction. A long-term follow-up study. J Bone Joint Surg Am. 2000;82(3):322-41.
45. Popelka S, Hromádka R, Vavrík P, et al. Isolated talonavicular arthrodesis in patients with rheumatoid arthritis of the foot and tibialis posterior tendon dysfunction. BMC Musculoskelet Disord. 2010; 11:38.
46. Astion DJ, Deland JT, Otis JC, et al. Motion of the hindfoot after simulated arthrodesis. J Bone Joint Surg Am. 1997;79(2):241-6.
47. Krause F, Fehlbaum O, Huebschle L, et al. Preservation of lesser metatarsophalangeal joints in rheumatoid forefoot reconstruction. Foot Ankle Int. 2011;32(2):131-40.
48. Akagi S, Sugano H, Ogawa R. The long-term results of ankle joint synovectomy for rheumatoid arthritis. Clin Rheumatol. 1997;16(3):284-90.
49. Kofoed H, Sørensen TS. Ankle arthroplasty for rheumatoid arthritis and osteoarthritis: prospective long-term study of cemented replacements. J Bone Joint Surg Br. 1998;80(2):328-32.
50. Mäenpää H, Lehto MU, Belt EA. Why do ankle arthrodeses fail in patients with rheumatic disease? Foot Ankle Int. 2001;22(5):403-8.
51. Loveday DT, Jackdon GE, Geary NP. The rheumatoid foot and ankle: current evidence. Foot Ankle Surg. 2012;18(2):94-102.
52. Elrefaei M, Boose K, McGee M, et al. Second generation automated anti-CCP tests beter predicts the clinical diagnosis of rheumatoid arthritis. J Clin Immunol. 2012;32(1):131-7.
53. Zintzaras E, Papathanasiou AA, Ziogas DC, et al. The reporting quality of studies investigating the diagnostic accuracy of anti-CCP antibody in rheumatoid arthritis and its impact on diagnostic estimates. BMC Musculoskel Disord. 2012;13(1): 113.

SECTION 9

The Diabetic Foot

Chapter Outline

49

The Neuropathic Foot

James J Sferra

ETIOLOGY

Diabetes afflicts multiple systems of the body, and diabetic foot disease represents a major concern in the overall well-being of those with the disease. Numbers are on the rise both globally and nationally as elderly and obese patients increase. In the US, the Center for Disease Control and Prevention (CDC) estimates that 25.8 million people (8.3% of the population) are affected with diabetes. Diabetes carries a 15–25% lifetime chance of developing involvement of the foot including ulcers, osteomyelitis, and Charcot neuroarthropathy.[1] Greater than 60% of nontraumatic amputations in the advanced medical world result from complications of diabetes. Identifying early signs of diabetic foot disease and appropriate treatment can prevent serious complications and eventual morbidity and mortality in this at risk population.

Due to the multisystem effects of diabetes, patients are best treated with a team approach. Often this requires input and coordination from an orthopedic surgeon, endocrinologist, vascular surgeon, physical therapist, orthotist, ophthalmologist, and infectious disease expert.[2]

PATHOPHYSIOLOGY AND NATURAL HISTORY

Ulceration occurs in the neuropathic foot due to repeated or prolonged biomechanical stress on soft tissues that have diminished protective sensation. Sensory neuropathy will affect about 75% of diabetics over their lifetime. The typical stocking-glove distribution begins distally and travels proximally in the extremities. Loss of large sensory nerves impairs light touch sensation and proprioception. Loss of small nerve fibers impairs perception of pain and light touch.[3]

A chronic, nonhealing ulcer permits an environment ripe for infection and eventual osteomyelitis. The evolution of disease is intimately tied to the vascular status of the individual. Many diabetic patients have peripheral vascular disease affecting both large and small vessels. This decreased blood flow combined with repetitive stress prevents the wound from healing. Over time, untreated ulcers progress to deeper wounds that may involve deep structures such as tendons, joints, and bone.[4]

Charcot neuroarthropathy is destruction of joints as a result of two kinds of neuropathy. Sensory neuropathy prevents the body from sensing trauma to the articulations of the foot with subsequent collapse and loss of the normal structure. Autonomic neuropathy results in loss of autoregulation of blood flow and the classic hyperemia seen in this form of the disease. The increased flow is thought to lead to high bone turnover with decreases in bone density. The result is elevated forces across weaker bones and eventual collapse (Table 1).

DIAGNOSIS

Use of Collated Data and Inductive Reasoning

The diabetic foot exam begins with a thorough history. Previous ulcerations, Charcot joints, and infections are critical when evaluating a new problem. History of other system involvement (such as hypertension, peripheral vascular disease, coronary artery disease, kidney disease, and retinal disease) is helpful in assessing the overall health of the patient and the degree to which the diabetes affects the body.

Table 1: Eichenholtz classification[6]

Stage	*Radiographic Features*	*Clinical Features*
I- Dissolution	Demineralization, periarticular fragmentation, dislocation	Acute inflammation: swelling, erythema, warmth
II- Coalescence	Absorption of osseous debris, organization and early healing of fragmentation, new bone formation	Decreased inflammation, swelling. Increased stability of fractures and joints
III- Resolution	Sclerosis, osseous or fibrous ankylosis. Radiographic smoothing of large fragments	Fixed deformity, stable and permanent enlargement of tissues, minimal daily changes in swelling and skin temperature

Testing for diabetic sensory neuropathy includes evaluation of light touch, proprioception, pinprick, and monofilament testing. The most common physical exam test is performed with a Semmes-Weinstein 5.07 monofilament. Ability to sense pressure with this size filament confers a reasonable amount of protective sensation (Fig. 1).

Visual examination of skin integrity should be thorough. All skin breaks and ulcers should be measured and probed for depth and extent. Color changes, hair distribution, and relative moisture also speak to the quality of the skin envelope. Ingrown nails and paronychia must also be evaluated as possible entry points for infection.

Observation of gait patterns is critically important. The clinician can see dynamic forces that are being exerted onto the foot and ankle. Evaluation of shoewear and orthotics for excessive wear will indicate areas that are being overloaded.

Vascular disease is common in diabetics with foot disease. Patients with dorsalis pedis and posterior tibial pulses that are diminished or absent should be screened further for vascular disease prior to any surgical procedure. Ankle-Brachial index (ABI) is an easily performed test that utilizes blood pressure cuffs and Doppler ultrasound probes. The pressure at which blood flow is permitted to the distal extremity is recorded, and the ratio across the ankle to that across the brachial artery is calculated. A measurement of 0.45 or greater is indicative of adequate blood flow to the foot to permit healing of a diabetic ulcer.

Absolute toe pressures greater than 40 mm Hg are another noninvasive test that is indicative of adequate flow distally. Transcutaneous oxygen measurements of greater than 30 mm Hg similarly suggest sufficient healing potential for diabetic ulcers. It is important to remember that no test is 100% accurate and reliable. Occasionally referrals to vascular surgery are required. When necessary, they may employ invasive testing and address occlusions.

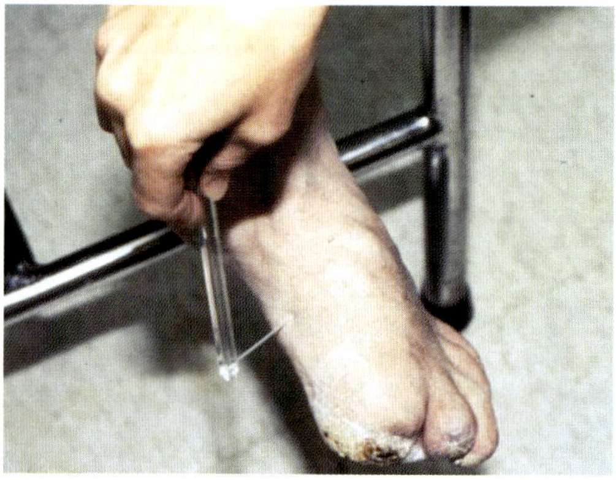

Fig. 1: Semmes-Weinstein pressure threshold monofilament testing

Foot deformities with prominent bony architecture often lay the foundation for soft tissue breakdown. When evaluating an ulcer, identification of joint contractures is of utmost importance. For example, a tight heel-cord and equinus contracture redistributes higher loads through the forefoot. Motor neuropathy manifests itself as claw toe deformities as a result of intrinsic muscle weakness. These toe deformities may predispose to ulcer formation on the plantar aspect of the metatarsophalangeal (MTP) joints or dorsally over the toe proximal interphalangeal (PIP) joints.

Autonomic neuropathy is another manifestation and can lead to abnormalities in skin temperature and sweating. Skin may become dry and scaly with progression to cracks. Loss of the normal neural control of blood vessels can lead to increased blood flow to the area and the hyperemia seen in Charcot neuroarthropathy. Patients with Charcot deformities may develop bony prominences as the foot collapses. Those with rocker-bottom feet are at high risk for development of chronic ulcers.

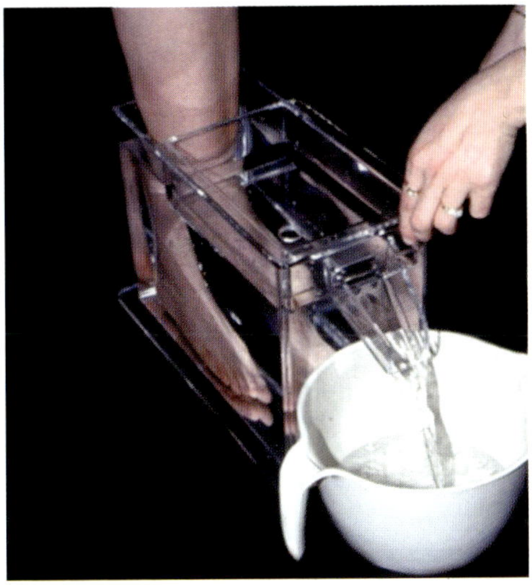

Fig. 2: Water displacement measurement device

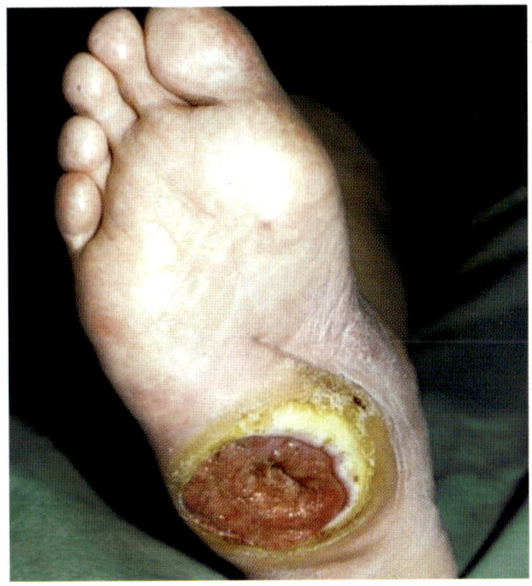

Fig. 3: Huge midfoot plantar ulcer which did respond to total contact casting

Table 2: Wagner classification and recommended management[7]

Stage	*Classification*	*Recommendations*
0	Pressure area with local skin changes, no opening	Footwear modifications
I	Open but superficial skin ulceration	Local wound care, footwear modifications
II	Full thickness ulceration of skin	Immobilization, local wound care, footwear modification
III	Full thickness ulceration with secondary infection	Add debridement and antibiotics
IV	Local gangrene	Local amputation, antibiotics
V	Extensive gangrene	Regional amputation, antibiotics

Following the progress of a patient with an evolving Charcot process requires some objective means to help determine when it is appropriate to move from casting to bracing, and perhaps, finally, to allow unprotected ambulation. Serial measurements of skin temperature have been recorded using skin thermistors and infrared readers. We have used water displacement testing to record the level of soft tissue edema. Although there are diurnal variations, a trend toward decreasing edema suggests resolution of the condition and a plateau indicates that a steady state exists. Increasing edema suggests that a regression to an earlier stage of management (i.e. returning to casting vs bracing) may be indicated. The technique for these measurements is simple. The patient steps into a container filled with water to the level of an outflow spout. The amount of runoff into a measureable beaker determines the reading of the moment. As the amount of edema varies, the outflow will vary (Fig. 2).

ULCERATION

Options of Management

Conservative

Nonsurgical treatment is the standard of care for patients with a new diagnosis of diabetic foot involvement. Most commonly a superficial ulcer is identified first. Appropriate treatment aims to halt progression and allow the soft tissue envelope to heal. A combination of shoe modifications and shoe inserts may redistribute forces on the foot and allow tissues to heal. Stage II and deeper ulcers may require greater immobilization to allow tissues to heal (Fig. 3). This is accomplished with a total contact cast or a Charcot restraint orthotic walker (CROW) (Table 2).

Total contact casting is the preferred technique for ulceration in the Charcot foot or ankle but

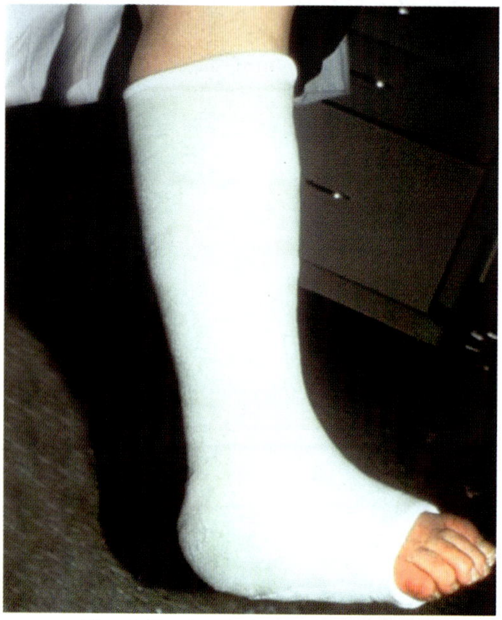

Fig. 4: Total contact cast (some are done with a closed toe)

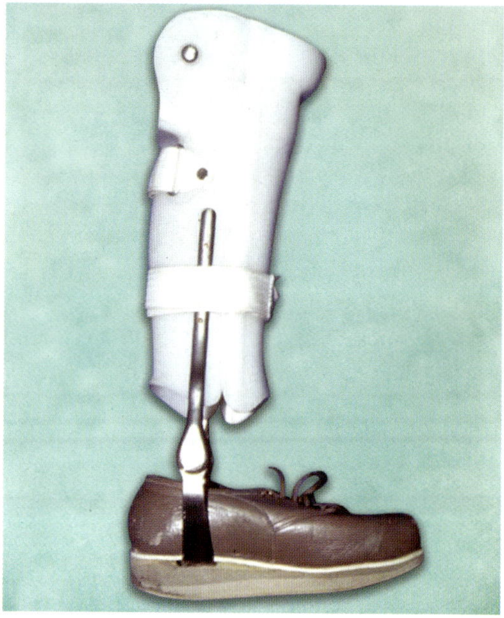

Fig. 5: Off-loading brace. PTB polypropylene upper component attached to shoe with double uprights

remains a labor-intensive endeavor (Fig. 4). Casts should be changed and wounds evaluated on a weekly basis for patients with Eichenholtz stage 1 disease (those at risk for deformity progression). Absence of protective sensation enables some patients to be less than fully compliant with removable braces. Casting ensures that patients are compliant with restricting weight-bearing activities. Once the disease process has reached the consolidation phase and the foot is felt to have reached its steady state, the patient may be transitioned to an offloading brace (Fig. 5) or a removable CROW boot (Fig. 6).

When ulcers become full-thickness (Fig. 3), the clinician must rule out underlying infection. Magnetic resonance imaging (MRI) scans are helpful in identifying osteomyelitis and fluid collections. Osteomyelitis by itself is not a surgical indication. In the absence of a soft tissue defect, the standard of care of uncomplicated osteomyelitis is medical with appropriate antibiotics. The vast majority of cases of osteomyelitis in the neuropathic patient population are associated with pressure ulcers. Treatment of these patients requires attention to the bone and soft tissues.

Surgeries

Surgical intervention on the neuropathic foot is considered for chronic recurrent ulceration, instability of articulations, deep infections, acute fractures, and progressive debilitating deformity. Surgery is individualized to the patient's anatomy and function. Goals of surgery are healing of existing and surgical wounds, creation of a stable segment capable of weight-bearing, achievement of a plantigrade foot, and/or improvement of alignment.

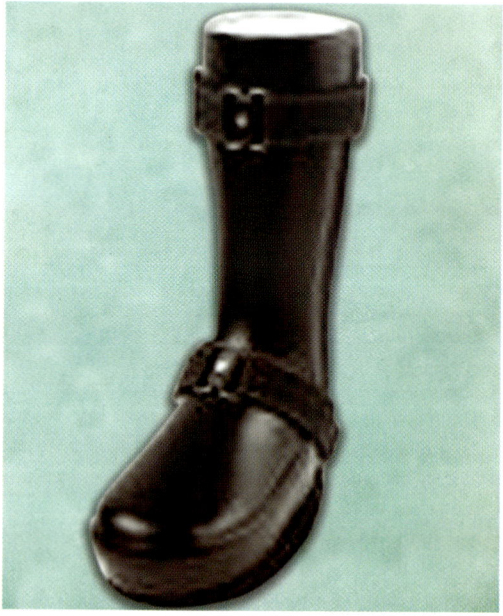

Fig. 6: The CRO walker or boot (Charcot Restraint Orthosis)

Neuropathic Unstable Ankle Fracture

Neuropathic patients who present with an unstable ankle must be treated differently from the ordinary patient.[8] Patients with diabetes have increased risk of malunion, hardware failure, and wound complications. Those with loss of protective sensation and compromised blood flow are especially at risk. Neuropathic patients often have decreased bone quality; therefore, typical fixation techniques must be augmented. The advent of locking technology has greatly increased the ability of the surgeon to create a stable construct in the absence of normal bone.

Preoperative planning is of the utmost importance. A computed tomography (CT) scan can be helpful in identifying comminution and posterior malleolus fractures. The surgeon should be prepared to add fixation as needed to achieve stability. Locking plates, Kirschner wires (K-wire), Steinman pins, external fixation, and syndesmotic screws should all be available, if needed.

The patient is positioned such that access to the medial and lateral ankle is possible. A large bump under the ipsilateral hip is often sufficient. Alternatively, a beanbag can be inflated with the patient in the semi-lateral decubitus position for access to the lateral ankle. It can then be deflated when addressing the medial ankle. This is especially helpful when approaching the posterolateral ankle for fixation of a posterior malleolus. A standard lateral approach to the fibula is used with care to protect the superficial peroneal nerve. If access to the posterior malleolus is needed, the incision is made just posterior to the posterior border of the fibula. A long incision is made to allow access to the posterior ankle. The interval utilized is between the peroneal tendons and the flexor hallucis longus (FHL). The FHL is retracted medially protecting the tibial nerve and posterior tibial artery. Fixation of the posterior malleolus should be addressed first. The fragment is reduced and clamped, and an antiglide plate is applied. Next the fibula is reduced and clamped. Care must be taken to avoid perforating the bone with sharp clamps. Iatrogenic fracture is common with neuropathic bone stock.

Locking plates are helpful in addressing poor bone quality, distal fibula fragments, and comminution. Syndesmotic fixation is routinely added for increased stability. Two or three screws are placed across four cortices and preferably placed through the fibula plate.

The medial malleolus is approached and the fracture is directly visualized. If the fragment is large, two compression screws are placed. Care is taken to avoid over-tightening the screws as this may split the fragment. An antiglide plate may be used for vertical fracture patterns. Tension band constructs are useful for small fragments. If fixation of the malleoli is suboptimal and there is fear of persistent instability, fixation may be augmented. Steinman pins may be introduced in retrograde fashion through the calcaneus and across the tibiotalar joint. These are routinely removed at 12–16 weeks. Alternatively, an external fixator may be placed to hold the tibiotalar joint in proper alignment. Neuropathic patients undergoing even a standard ankle fusion must be considered at risk for a potential Charcot reaction, and the means of fixation should be more substantial than in the usual patient (Figs 7A to D).

OSTECTOMY FOR CHARCOT ROCKER-BOTTOM DEFORMITY[9]

Ostectomy for Charcot rocker-bottom deformity is a relatively simple procedure compared to osteotomy and midfoot/hindfoot reconstruction. The goal is to remove the plantar prominence and heal the soft tissue envelope. This approach is ideally performed for stable deformities that have little chance to progress. It should not be used in patients for whom there is concern that the disease process has not fully run its course and consolidated. Care must also be taken to avoid destabilization of the foot by removal of structurally important bone, as this may lead to progression of collapse and deformity of the midfoot.

Rocker-bottom feet with bony prominences are frequently associated with either some history of ulceration or presence of an overlying ulcer. If surgical ostectomy is to be performed, the patient should undergo usual preoperative evaluation and be felt to have nutritional and vascular status to heal the surgical wound. An elliptical incision is typically used to remove chronically inflamed and fibrotic tissue. Care should be taken to ensure that primary closure is possible at the conclusion of the procedure. Incisions are ideally full-thickness to the bony surface in order to achieve a layered closure over the ostectomy site (Figs 8A to C).

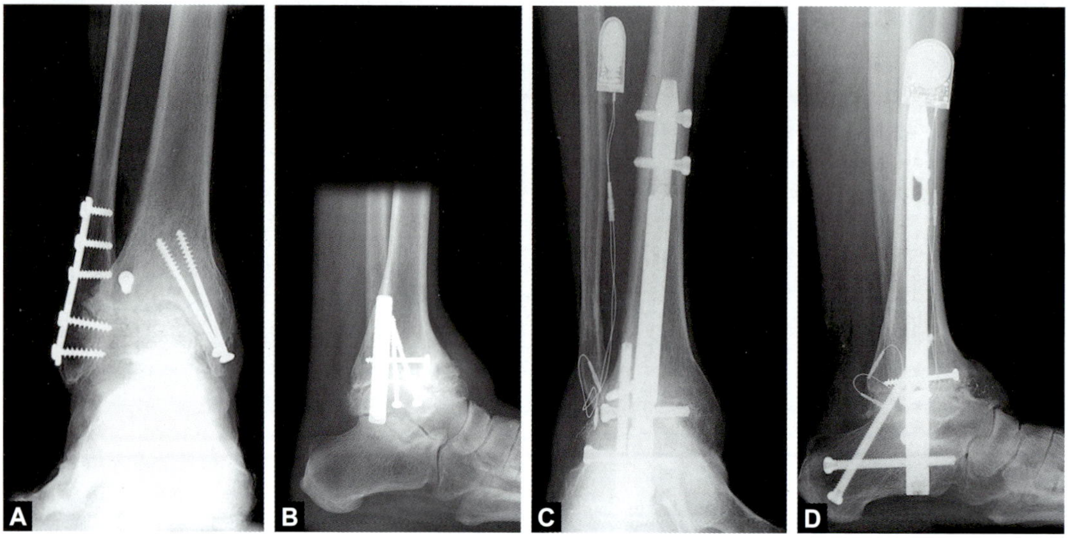

Figs 7A to D: (A) AP ankle in neuropathic patient with old repaired fractures and DJD of ankle and subtalar joint; (B) Lateral X-ray; (C) AP X-ray. Use of locking compression intramedullary rod with supplemental screw across joints and implanted bone stimulator for tibiotalocalcaneal fusion; (D) Lateral X-ray of tibiotalocalcaneal fusion

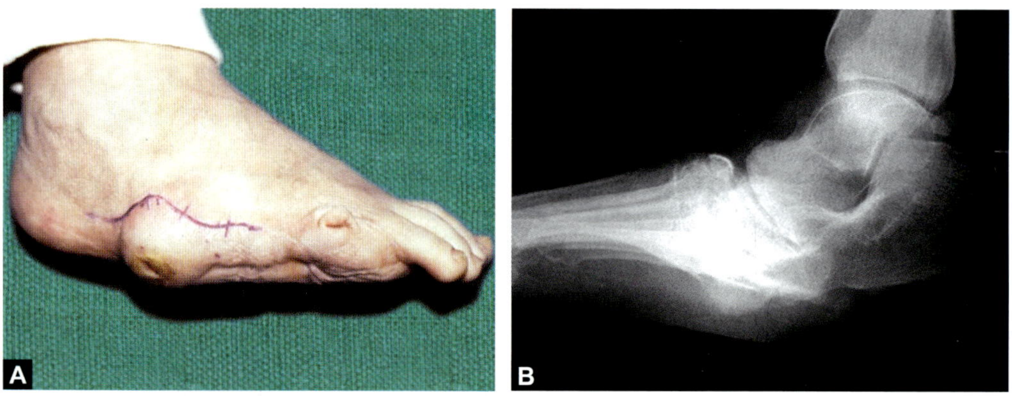

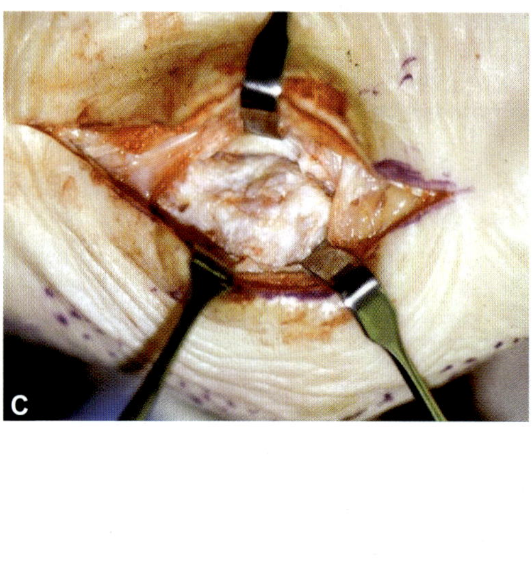

Figs 8A to C: Ostectomy for the Charcot midfoot. (A) Lesion with outlined incision; (B) Lateral X-ray with prominent plantar prominence; (C) Operative photo with plantar bone exposed

The bony prominence is exposed and removed with osteotomes, rongeurs, and rasps as appropriate. Care must be taken to avoid sharp edges that may lead to new ulcerations. Layered closure with absorbable suture is preferable. Skin is closed with nonabsorbable monofilament suture and is left in place until the wound is sufficiently healed.

Reconstruction of Rocker Bottom Charcot Deformity[10,11]

Surgical realignment and stabilization can transform severe Charcot deformities into braceable plantigrade feet. The complex deformities that develop in neuropathic patients are extremely challenging to reconstruct. Potentially devastating complications include nonunion, infection, recurrent deformity, and vascular compromise. If the patient encounters any of these, it almost certainly results in an amputation. Prior to undertaking reconstruction, patients must understand the inherent risks and be dedicated to complying with a lengthy postoperative treatment plan.

This procedure is best implemented as a limb-salvage procedure when bracing is no longer a durable option. Patients who have unbraceable and/or unstable feet often have a history of recurrent ulceration. Reconstruction and fusion in a plantigrade position aims to redistribute forces and reduce the risk of recurrent ulceration. Patients and surgeons should be aware that even after successful reconstruction has been achieved, lifelong bracing or custom shoe-wear with custom inserts is expected.

The typical pattern of collapse in these patients is through the midfoot with dorsal and lateral displacement (Figs 9A and B). The medial column is addressed first. Incision is made over the medial column in order to expose the talo-navicular, naviculo-cuneiform, and cuneiform-1st metatarsal joints. Care is taken to preserve tibialis anterior and its attachment. Cartilage and sclerotic bone are removed in preparation for fusion. Reduction of the joints are critical to achieve a plantigrade foot. A medially based wedge osteotomy of navicular or medial cuneiform is often required to address the abduction deformity. The medial column is stabilized with plates and screws. Assal and Stern[9] advocate using a medial column intramedullary screw in antegrade fashion from posterior talus into the 1st metatarsal shaft.

After realignment of the medial column, determination is made as to whether or not to prepare and fuse the remaining naviculo-cuneiform joints as well as the 2nd and 3rd tarsometatarsal joints. If they are reduced radiographically after the medial column is fixed, then they may be left alone. However, with deformity present, it is often necessary to access these joints in order to reduce the medial column. If this is the case, then the joints involved should be fused with plates and/or screws (Figs 10A to C).

Finally, the lateral column is evaluated. There is often collapse through the cuboid with dorsal displacement of the lateral column. These complex deformities frequently necessitate fusion of the lateral column to create a braceable plantigrade foot. A lateral extensile sinus-tarsi approach is utilized to prepare the subtalar, calcaneocuboid, and 4th/5th tarsometatarsal joints for fusion. Again plates and screws are placed in order to create optimal stability.

The advent of foot specific locking plates has been helpful in addressing these complex patients. Bone quality is often compromised, making locking

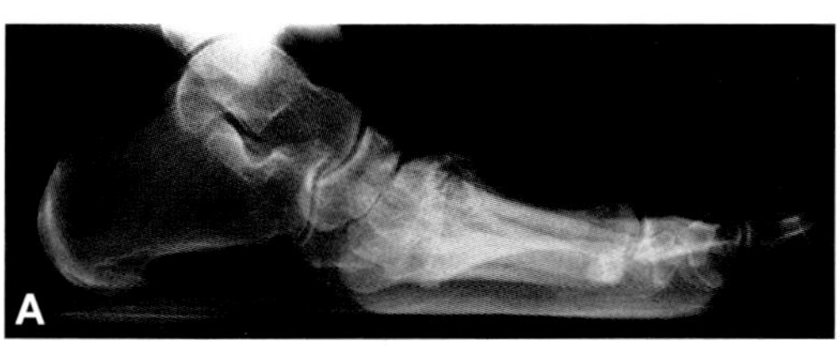

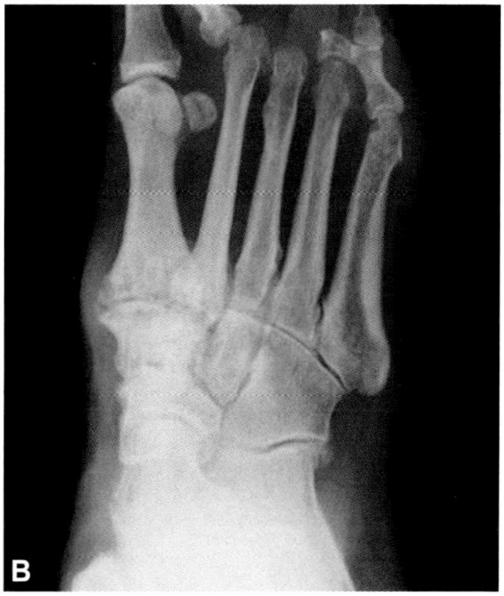

Figs 9A and B: (A) Midfoot Charcot lateral X-ray; (B) Note involvement of naviculocuneiform and tarsometatarsal joints on this AP X-ray

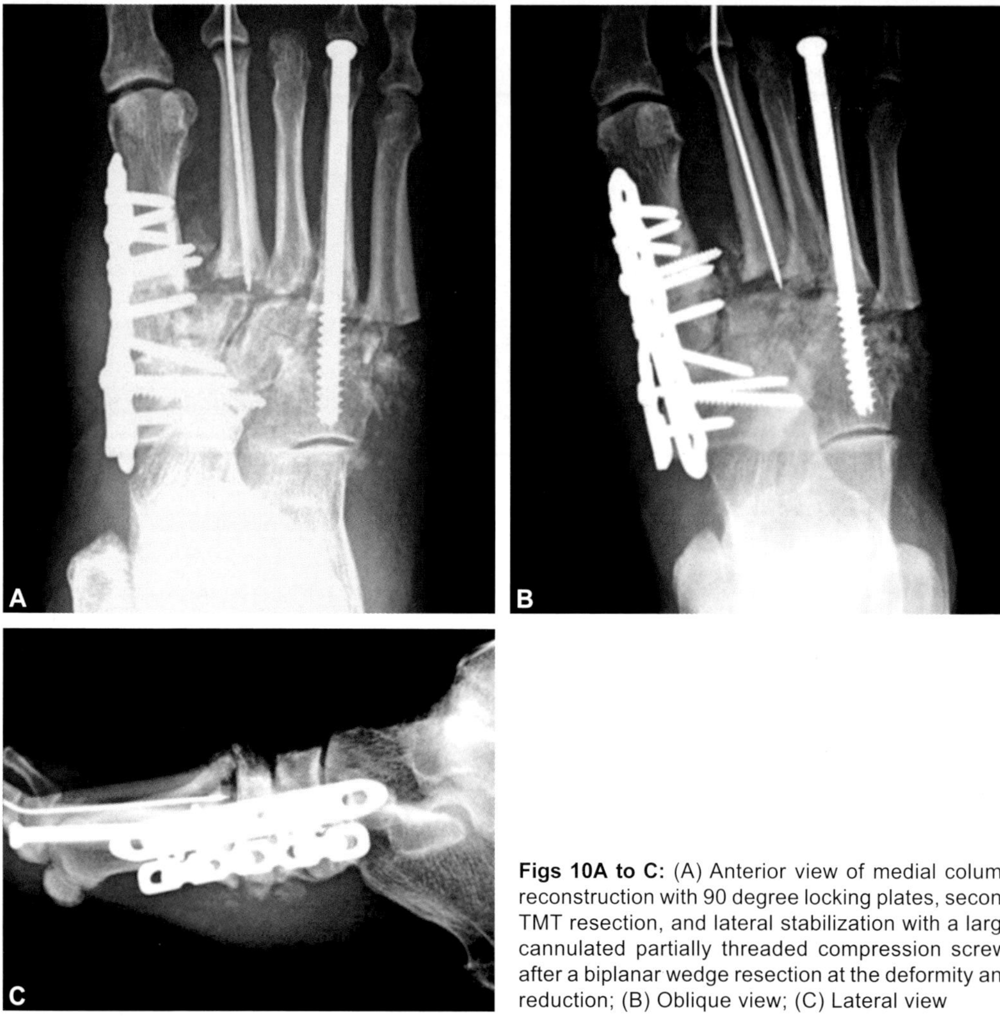

Figs 10A to C: (A) Anterior view of medial column reconstruction with 90 degree locking plates, second TMT resection, and lateral stabilization with a large cannulated partially threaded compression screw; after a biplanar wedge resection at the deformity and reduction; (B) Oblique view; (C) Lateral view

plates ideal. Cannulated screws and compression staples have also emerged giving the surgeon additional option for gaining fixation with the ultimate goal of fusion.

Bone graft is routinely used. Local autograft from joint preparation and osteotomies is utilized but usually insufficient. Cancellous allograft mixed with iliac crest aspiration is a technique used by the author to have enough bone graft for the many fusion sites while using the biological growth factors present in the patient's own iliac crest.

These patients are followed closely postoperatively with frequent weekly wound checks and cast changes for the first 3–4 weeks until the wounds are sufficiently healed and swelling decreased. They remain in a non-weight bearing cast for 4–6 months, and then transition into a walking cast or boot.

TIBIOTALOCALCANEAL FUSION (NAIL/PLATE)

Neuropathic deformities of the hindfoot may progress over time and result in arthritis and deformity of the ankle joint. In order to restore the anatomic axis and weight-bearing forces of the limb, it is sometimes necessary to fuse across the subtalar and tibiotalar joints. Retrograde intramedullary tibiotalocalcaneal (TTC) nails have been developed by multiple implant companies. They serve as load sharing devices and are positioned in the mechanically advantageous intramedullary canal. The fibula is routinely cut in oblique fashion proximal to the ankle joint and removed en bloc. It can be morselized and used for bone graft. Internal and external compression can be utilized to compress across both joints. Targeting devices can be used to minimize soft tissue stripping as the nail is locked in place. Achilles tendon lengthening is added as needed (Figs 11A to E).

Tibiotalocalcaneal fusion can also be accomplished with precontoured locking plates. These create fixed angle constructs and are a good option for poor bone quality or bone defects. Either fixation construct may be augmented with additional screws or staples.

Debridement

Deep infections of the diabetic foot and ankle are serious limb threatening conditions and may develop to be life threatening. Clinicians should be vigilant in evaluating and working up these patients with concern for infected wounds. Advanced imaging is helpful in determining the extent of the infection and during surgical planning. Deep infection in diabetics that involves tendons, joints, and bone is best addressed with thorough debridement.

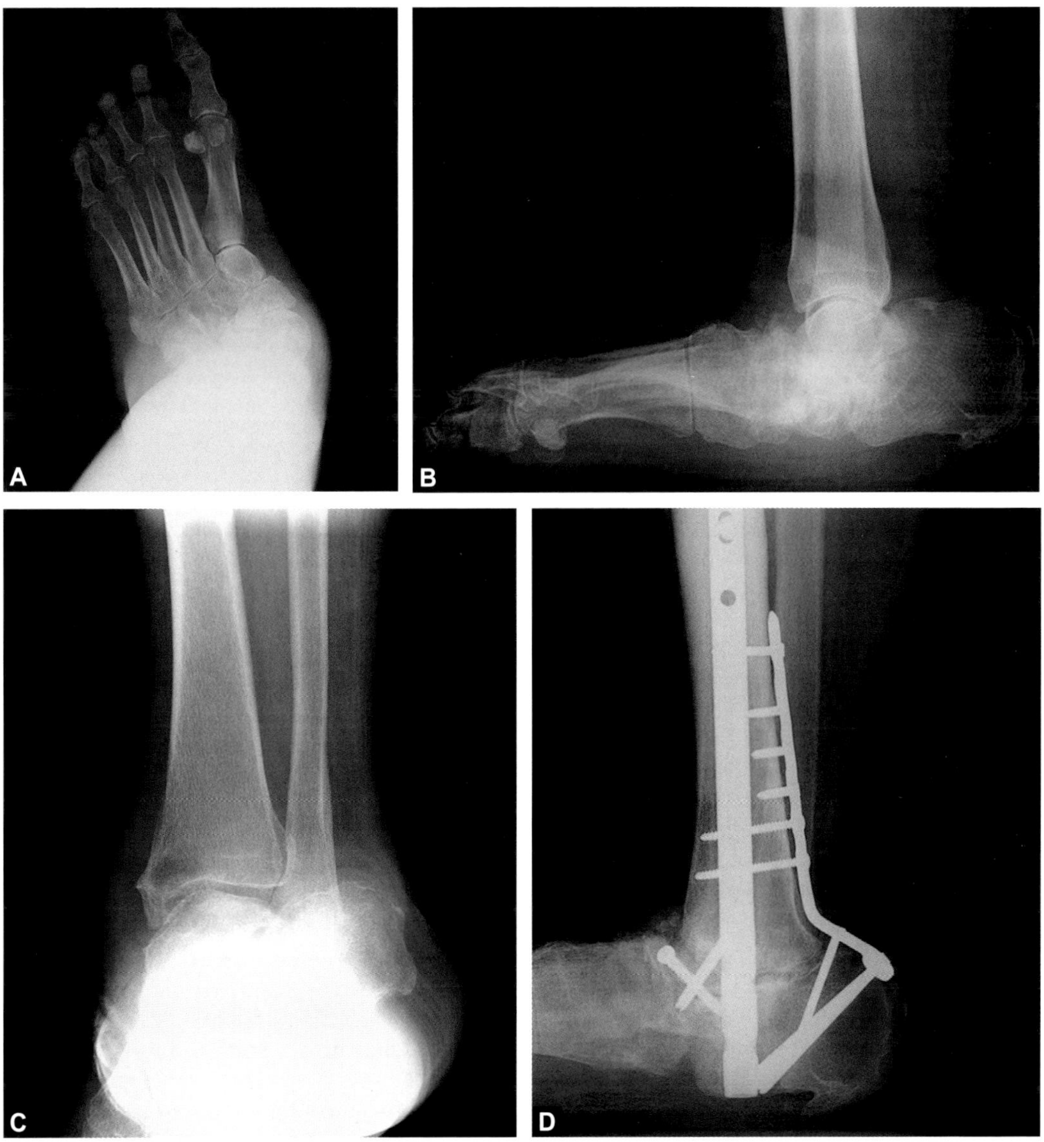

Figs 11A to D

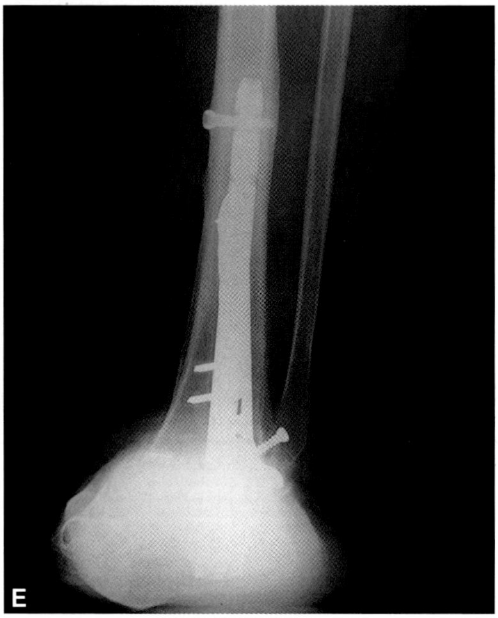

Figs 11A to E: (A) AP X-ray of Charcot foot with ankle and subtalar joint involvement; (B) Lateral X-ray; (C) Ankle view. Note intraarticular varus; (D) Lateral view with intramedullary locking compression rod and posterior locking plate with combination holes allowing locking or compression; (E) AP view of distal leg

Patients must be optimized prior to surgery with a thorough evaluation of their overall health by their primary care physician. Any cardiovascular or otherwise serious medical concerns need to be addressed prior to surgery with appropriate consultations.

Strict blood sugar control in the perioperative time period is critically important for wound healing. Noncompliant patients and unstable diabetics are often best controlled with an insulin drip immediately after surgery.

Surgical debridement is indicated for any deep abscess, necrotic bone or tendon, or recurrent ulceration that has failed maximal nonoperative treatment. Fluctuance with active purulent drainage requires open debridement to decompress the infection. Often loculations are present and can only be addressed in the operative suite.

Necrotic material in the wound base indicates limited healing potential. In order to achieve a healed skin envelope, the necrotic material must be removed. The entirety of the wound should exhibit healthy bleeding borders following the debridement. Primary wound closure is preferable when possible. This may require excision of underlying bony prominences.

Understanding the circumstances of how and why the ulcer initially formed is extremely important. Most ulcers will eventually heal after a thorough debridement with an appropriate period of non-weight bearing and immobilization. However, the rate of recurrence will remain exceedingly high if the causative factors are not also addressed. Close attention should be paid to shoe-wear, orthotic inserts, braces, bone alignment, and musculotendinous imbalances. For instance, plantar forefoot ulcers that exist in the presence of equinus contractures may benefit from heel-cord lengthening.

Procedure

The patient is positioned appropriately for direct access to wound. A tourniquet may be used, but gravity exsanguination is preferred to compression in order to avoid spreading infection proximally. Antibiotics are held at the start of the case until cultures are taken. Incisions are oriented such that extensile approaches can be made if more access is needed. Eliptical incisions are preferable to remove chronically infected and inflamed wound edges.

Sharp dissection will remove obvious unhealthy tissue. Healthy bleeding skin edges have the best opportunity to heal. Curettes and rongeurs are used to obtain a healthy bleeding base of bone and soft tissue. If needed, osteotomes and saw blades can be used to resect prominent bone. Cultures of soft tissue and bone are sent for aerobic, anaerobic, fungus, and acid-fast bacilli. Diabetics have compromised immune systems in the area of question and atypical organisms are more likely to be found than in the general population.

The soft tissues and bone are thoroughly probed and evaluated for loculations and pockets of infection. All deep fluid collections must be decompressed for eradication of the infection. Local joints should be accessed through a capsulotomy and evaluated for pyarthrosis.

The wound is thoroughly irrigated with several liters of normal saline through a bulb syringe, and bleeding is controlled. Deep layers are closed with absorbable suture and skin is closed with interrupted nylon. A splint is applied and the wound is evaluated within one week after surgery. An infectious disease consultation is obtained for deep abscesses and osteomyelitis. These patients frequently require intravenous antibiotics and close monitoring.

In the case of severe infections, even a thorough debridement may require a subsequent debridement in the next few days. Limb-threatening infections should be packed open to allow drainage with the expectation of repeat surgical debridement in the near future. Resection of additional bone can be beneficial in achieving a primarily closed wound. Strict elevation is critical to preventing excessive swelling that can compromise the wound. Healing the surgical wound is typically longer due to decreased local vascularity. Sutures should be left in place for 3 weeks or more depending on the amount of healing.

External Fixation

External fixation is a useful tool in reconstruction of Charcot deformities of the foot and ankle. Thin wire fixators stabilize bony segments in multiple planes and allow the surgeon the option to manipulate fusion and osteotomy sites in three planes over time. They can be applied in addition to standard internal fixation techniques described previously, or they can be implemented as the solitary mode of fixation.

External fixation is used as an adjunct to internal fixation in two cases: when traditional internal fixation fails to adequately stabilize the limb and when the patient is unable to comply with non-weight bearing status due to mental or physical limitations. Typically, these frames are removed when healing is visualized on X-ray and the added protection is no longer necessary. This can be anywhere from 3 months to 12 months or more.

External fixators are gaining popularity as the primary mode of fixation in some groups of high-risk patients: morbidly obese, immunocompromised, malnourished, osteomyelitic, and osteoporotic. The advantages of these devices are that they are sturdy, require less exposure and soft tissue stripping, and they leave no foreign material behind after their removal. These procedures are technically demanding and somewhat limited in stabilizing and compressing across multiple segments of bone. Pin tract infections can be troublesome but are easily treated with local wound care and antibiotics. Occasionally pins must be removed to prevent development of osteomyelitis. Because this technique is utilized in complex situations and patients with extensive comorbidities, unsuccessful outcomes frequently require revision to amputation.[5]

COMPLICATIONS/SALVAGE

Failure of major reconstructive efforts in the neuropathic patient often results in amputation. Unsuccessful outcomes must always be evaluated for infection. Nonunions may occur due to inadequate fixation, poor patient biology, or both. Revision of these complex reconstructions is exceedingly difficult and fraught with complications.

REFERENCES

1. Singh N, Armstrong DG, Lipsky BA. Preventing foot ulcers in patients with diabetes. JAMA. 2005;293: 217-28.
2. Aksoy DY, Gürlek A, Cetinkaya Y, et al. Change in the amputation profile in diabetic foot in a tertiary reference center: efficacy of team working. Exp Clin Endocrinol Diabetes. 2004;112:526-30.
3. Ross MA. Neuropathies associated with diabetes. Med Clin North Am. 1993;77:111-24.
4. Cameron NE, Eaton SE, Cotter MA, et al. Vascular factors and metabolic interactions in the pathogenesis of diabetic neuropathy. Diabetologia. 2001;44: 1973-88.
5. Pinzur MS. Neutral ring fixation for high-risk nonplantigrade Charcot midfoot deformity. Foot Ankle Int. 2007;28(9):961-6.
6. Johnson J. Surgical reconstruction of the diabetic Charcot foot and ankle. Foot Ankle Clin. 1997;2: 40-9.
7. Wagner FW. The diabetic foot. Orthopedics. 1987; 10(1):163-72.
8. Bibbo C, Patel DV. Diabetic neuropathy. Foot Ankle Clin. 2006;11:753-74.
9. Brodsky JW, Rouse AM. Exostectomy for symptomatic bony prominences in diabetic Charcot feet. Clin Orthop Relat Res. 1993;296:21-6.
10. Assal M, Stern R. Realignment and extended fusion with use of a medial column screw for midfoot deformities secondary to diabetic neuropathy. J Bone Joint Surg Am. 2009;91(4):812-20.
11. Johnson JE. Operative treatment of neuropathic arthropathy of the foot and ankle. Instr Course Lect. 1998;80:1700-9.

SECTION 10

Special Fracture Problems of the Foot and Ankle

Chapters Outline

50

Pilon Fractures

William Min, Jason Lowe

INTRODUCTION

Pilon fractures present a difficult treatment problem for the orthopedic surgeon. These fractures can occur from low-energy or high-energy mechanisms. Low-energy mechanisms are often the result of a rotational force that creates a spiral fracture pattern. High-energy mechanisms include axial loads that result in varying amounts of metaphyseal comminution and articular joint disruption. Pilon fractures are often complicated with soft-tissue injuries that help to dictate type and timing of fixation.[1] Careful preoperative planning is necessary for the operating surgeon to adequately treat these fractures. Rüedi and Allgöwer described important fixation points for operative management including reduction of associated fibular fractures to achieve adequate length, reduction of distal tibia fracture fragments through ligamentotaxis, correction of valgus deformity, reduction of the articular surface, bone grafting to metaphyseal defects, and medial buttressing to prevent varus deformity of the distal tibia.[2]

CLASSIFICATION

Pilon fractures are tibial plafond injuries that include varying amounts of comminution. Rüedi and Allgöwer described a classification system that included Types 1–3. Type 1 is a non-displaced T-type distal tibia fracture with intra-articular extension. Type 2 includes the T-type fracture pattern with displacement of the intra-articular fragments. Type 3 has multiple intra-articular fragments with varying levels of displacement.[2] AO classification of distal tibia/fibula fractures includes 43A for extra-articular fractures, 43B for partial articular fractures, and 43C for complete articular fractures with 1–3 for increasing levels of comminution.[3]

ANATOMY

Topliss et al. described six different major intra-articular fracture fragments of pilon fractures. These include (1) anterior, (2) posterior, (3) medial, (4) anterolateral, (5) posterolateral, and (6) die-punch.[4] The anterior fragment includes the majority of the anterior portion of the plafond. The posterior fragment includes a large portion of the posterior portion of the plafond. Combined anterior and posterior fragments constitute a lateral fracture fragment. The medial malleolus attachment is included in the medial fragment. The anterolateral fragment, otherwise known as the Chaput fragment, includes the insertion of the anterior inferior tibiofibular ligament. The posterior inferior tibiofibular ligament attachment is part of the posterolateral fragment. The posterolateral piece is also called the Volkmann fragment. Die-punch fragments are central, impacted lesions.[5]

PREOPERATIVE PLANNING

The soft tissues are evaluated at the initial presentation for any open injuries, abrasions, ecchymosis, and swelling. Open injuries are irrigated and debrided at the time of initial presentation. The soft tissues are again evaluated prior to definitive fixation in staged procedures for evidence of skin wrinkling. The soft tissue can take up to 3 weeks from the initial injury to improve enough for definitive fixation. Full-length radiographs of the tibia/fibula and radiographs of the ankle are part of the initial workup for a pilon fracture. Traction radiographs can be helpful in identifying the fracture pattern.[6] A computed tomography (CT) scan is necessary in most situations to elicit the different fracture fragments for operative planning.[5] Nonoperative therapy is only used if the fracture fragments are nondisplaced or the patient cannot undergo a surgical procedure.

SURGICAL APPROACHES

The anteromedial approach is used for medial plating of the distal tibia. The incision is made medial to the tibialis anterior tendon. There is no true internervous plane in this approach. The dissection is carried down to bone and through the extensor retinaculum distally. The saphenous nerve and long saphenous vein need to be protected during this approach.[7]

The anterolateral approach is needed for anterolateral plating of pilon fractures. The incision is made on the anterolateral portion of the distal tibia and the ankle. The internervous plane is between the extensor tendons of the anterior compartment and the peroneal tendons of the lateral compartment. The superficial peroneal nerve is protected in this approach.[8]

A posteromedial approach can be performed from a prone patient position. The incision is made medial to the posterior tibialis tendon and dissection is carried down medial to this tendon and posterior to the medial malleolus. A posterior arthrotomy is made to visualize the joint.[7]

A posterolateral approach is used to plate the posterior portion of the tibia. An incision is made lateral to the Achilles tendon. The internervous plane is between the flexor hallucis longus and the peroneus brevis.[7]

SURGICAL OPTIONS

Temporary Stabilization

Pilon fractures often have large amounts of soft tissue damage and swelling at presentation. A spanning external fixator with two pins in the tibial shaft and a transcalcaneal pin helps gain length, stability, and alignment of the fracture while the soft tissue envelope improves (Figs 1A to C).[8] The external fixator can also consist of a first metatarsal pin according to the surgeon's preference. The distal fibula can be plated at the time of the external fixator if the soft tissues allow and the surgeon prefers early fibula fixation to gain length of the distal tibia fracture. Alternatively, the fibula can be operatively fixed at the time of definitive tibia fixation.[9]

Definitive Fixation

The fibula is addressed first to determine length of the distal tibia and is fixed with a one-third tubular plate or a distal locking plate depending on the fracture pattern. The fibula incision is lateral or posterolateral depending on the approach planned for tibial fixation. The tibia and fibula can be fractured by a varus force causing a tension type break to the fibula with a simple or transverse pattern and a varus injury pattern to the tibia. An implant that is medially based is often necessary to counteract the varus force of the tibia. A compression type injury to the tibia and fibula creates more comminution in the fibula and a valgus injury pattern to the tibia. A lateral implant can counteract the valgus force. Primarily lateral or medial based implants may be supplemented with smaller implants on the other column according to the fracture patterns and level of comminution.[8]

The articular surface is addressed first and can be fixed through a medial or lateral approach depending on the fracture pattern. The articular surface can also be reduced through percutaneous methods. A reduction clamp or Kirschner wires (K-wires) (1.1 mm) can be used to hold the reduction while lag screw fixation is employed to secure the joint surface. Screw size can be 2.4 mm, 2.7 mm, or 3.5 mm cortical screws depending on the size of the articular fragments keeping in mind that a plate with distal fixation will be placed. Fluoroscopy is used to ensure adequate reduction of the joint.[10]

The articular block can then be attached to the metaphysis. A femoral distractor may be necessary to gain length of the tibia. In which case, the pins are placed in the tibia proximal to both the fracture and proposed plate and another pin is placed in the calcaneus. If an anterolateral plate is chosen as the implant necessary for the fracture pattern, the plate is slid proximally on the anterolateral portion of the tibia. The plate can be contoured as necessary to fit appropriately to the bone. A Cobb can be used to create a place for the plate. A well placed, proximal incision is made out of the zone of injury which is used to direct the plate into the correct position on the tibia. The plate is secured to the distal articular block first. Indirect reduction is then employed for the metaphyseal portion of the tibia. If adequate reduction is noted on fluoroscopic views, the plate is secured proximally with bicortical screws. This construct can be supplemented with a small medial construct (including a one-third tubular plate) if the fracture pattern necessitates it (Figs 2A and B).[10]

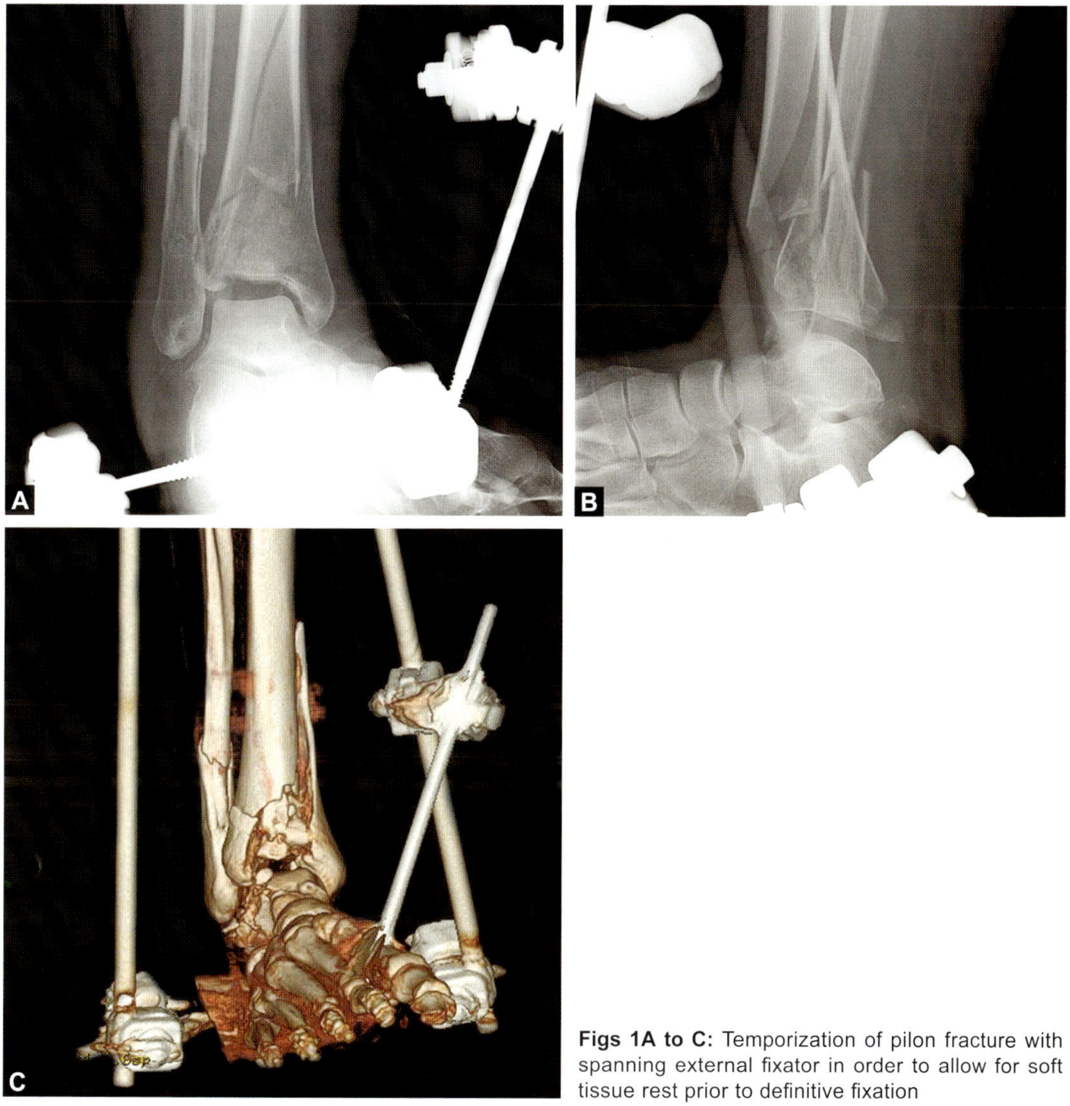

Figs 1A to C: Temporization of pilon fracture with spanning external fixator in order to allow for soft tissue rest prior to definitive fixation

Varus injury patterns are addressed through medial plating techniques. The medial plate is used as a buttress against varus forces on the tibia. Medial plates are often prominent and depending on the size of the bone being fixated, a 3.5 mm or 4.5 mm plate can be used and contoured to the bone from the medial malleolus proximally. The medial construct can be supplemented with a small lateral plate if the anterolateral fragment needs separate fixation (Figs 3A to D).[8]

Posterior pilon fractures are fixed through a posteromedial or posterolateral approach depending on the fracture orientation. The fractures are fixated by K-wires. They are then held in place by 2.7 mm or 3.5 mm screws used in lag technique in a posterior to anterior fashion.[11]

Locking plates can be helpful in patients with osteoporotic bone. They are also useful in situations where supplemental plates are precluded secondary to poor soft tissue quality. The locking plates can be applied with minimally invasive techniques.[12]

Tornetta et al. reported on the use of hybrid external fixation with limited internal fixation for treatment of complex pilon fractures. A limited incision was used over the joint to obtain a satisfactory articular reduction. Tension wires are used in the distal tibia fragments and 5.0 mm pins are used proximally along with a semicircular

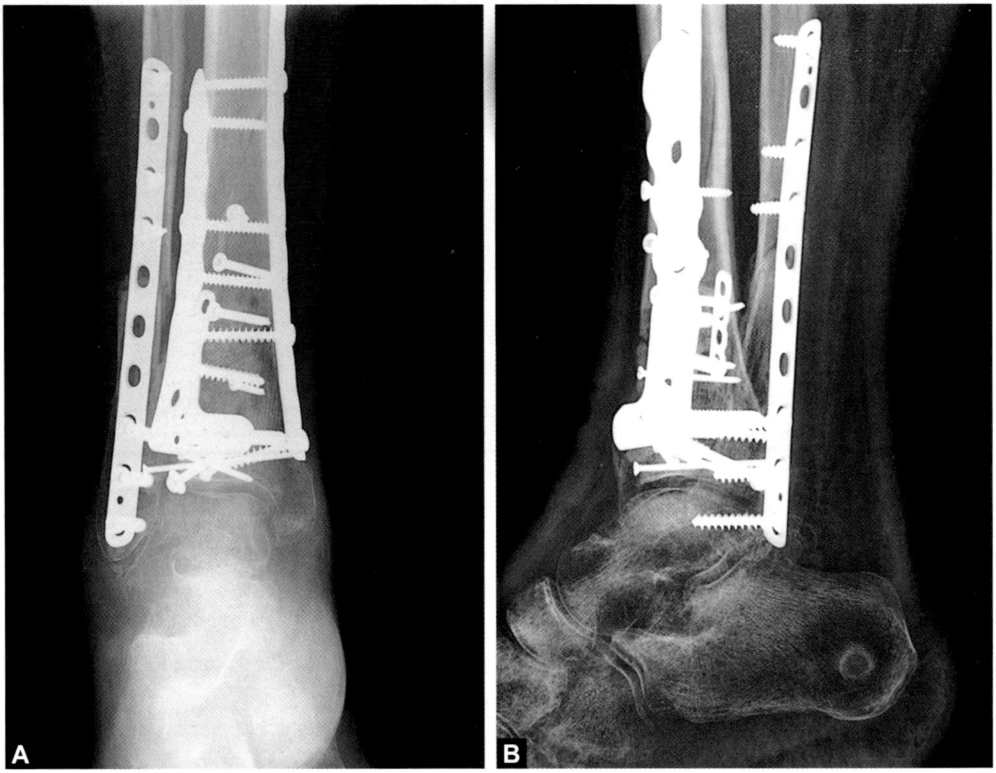

Figs 2A and B: Definitive fixation of pilon fracture with restoration of length through plating of fibula, independent screw placement for restoration of articular surface, and medial and anterolateral plating for distal tibia fixation

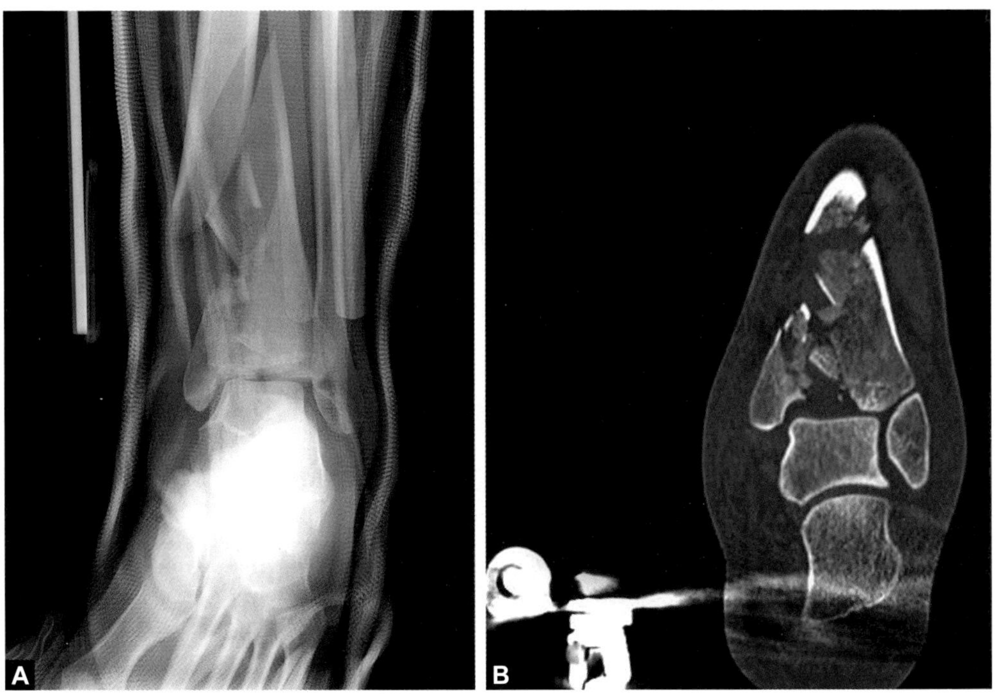

Figs 3A and B

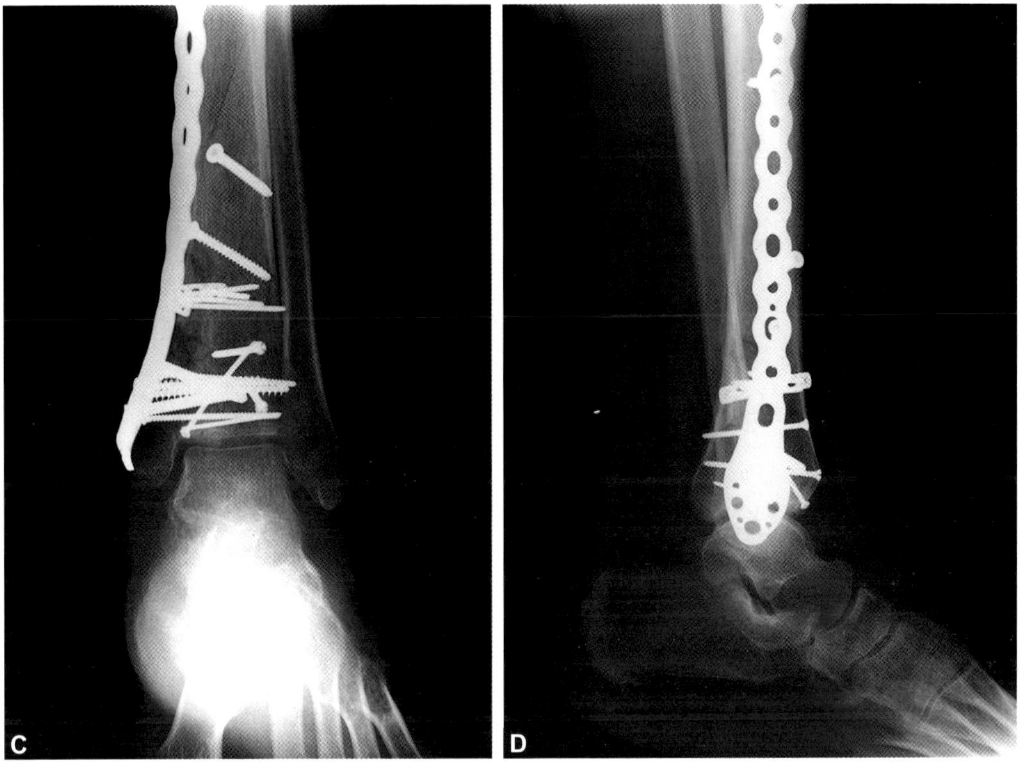

Figs 3A to D: Comminuted intra-articular pilon fracture with intact fibula underwent definitive fixation with independent screw fixation of articular surface as well as extra-articular metadiaphyseal fragment and minimally invasive placement of medial neutralization plate

frame. This construct is useful with pilon fractures with extensive soft tissue injuries that cannot withstand a large open procedure.[13]

Open injuries resulting in segmental bone loss provide a difficult treatment decision. Gardner et al. treated severe open injuries with an initial irrigation and debridement and external fixation. Antibiotic beads were applied with operative plate fixation. The beads were removed at a later date and the area was bone grafted which produced good results with healing.[14] Primary bone grafting with initial operative fixation is also an option if the soft tissues allow and there are no signs of infection.

COMPLICATIONS

Pilon injuries are often complicated by severe soft tissue injuries that may need plastic surgery intervention for coverage. Soft tissue compromise leads to higher rates of infection and wound break down. These complications are lessened with delay of definitive surgery until the soft tissue envelope has improved. Pin site infections occur with initial external fixation and hybrid external fixation constructs. Malunion and nonunion can be present with pilon fracture fixation. Ankle stiffness also complicates the postoperative course of pilon fractures and this can be decreased with earlier postoperative mobilization.[15] Postoperative arthrosis is also a complication of pilon fractures and may require later arthrodesis procedures.[15]

REFERENCES

1. Crist BD, Khazzam M, Murtha YM, et al. Pilon fractures: advances in surgical management. J Am Acad Orthop Surg. 2011;19(10):612-22.
2. Rüedi T, Allgöwer M. Fractures of the lower end of the tibia into the ankle joint. Injury. 1969;1:92-9.
3. Marsh JL, Slongo TF, Agel J, et al. Fracture and dislocation classification compendium - 2007: Orthopaedic Trauma Association classification, database and outcomes committee. J Orthop Trauma. 2007;21(10):S1-133.
4. Topliss CJ, Jackson M, Atkins RM. Pathoanatomy of the distal tibia fracture. J Bone Joint Surg Br. 2003;85B:246-9.

5. Topliss CJ, Jackson M, Atkins RM. Anatomy of pilon fractures of the distal tibia. J Bone Joint Surg Br. 2005;87B(5):692-7.
6. Griend RV, Michelson JD, Bone LB. Fractures of the ankle and the distal part of the tibia. J Bone Joint Surg. 1996;78A(11):1772-83.
7. Hoppenfeld S, deBoer P, Buckley R. Surgical Exposures in Orthopaedics: The Anatomic Approach. Philadelphia: Lippincott Williams & Wilkins; 2009.
8. Sirkin MS. Plating of tibial pilon fractures. Am J Orthop (Belle Mead NJ). 2007;36(12):13-7.
9. Sirkin M, Sanders R, DiPasquale T, et al. A staged protocol for soft tissue management in the treatment of complex pilon fractures. J Orthop Trauma. 1999; 13(2):78-84.
10. Colton C, Krikler S, Schatzker J, ed. et al. AO surgery reference. www2.aofoundation.org.
11. Amorosa LF, Brown GD, Greisberg, J. A surgical approach to posterior pilon fractures. J Orthop Trauma. 2010;24(3):188-93.
12. Bahari S, Lenehan B, Khan H, et al. Minimally invasive percutaneous plate fixation of distal tibia fractures. Acta Orthop Belg. 2007;73(5):635-40.
13. Tornetta P, Weiner L, Bergman M, et al. Pilon fractures: treatment with combined internal and external fixation. J Orthop Trauma. 1993;7(6): 489-96.
14. Gardner MJ, Mehta S, Barei DP, et al. Treatment protocol for open AO/OTA type C3 pilon fractures with segmental bone loss. J Orthop Trauma. 2008; 22(7):451-7.
15. Thordarson DB. Complications after treatment of tibial pilon fractures: prevention and management strategies. J Am Acad Orthop Surg. 2000;8(4): 253-65.

51

Unstable Ankle Fractures

William Min, Jason Lowe

INTRODUCTION

Ankle fractures are common injuries facing orthopedic surgeons. They result from a large variety of low- and high-energy mechanisms. Stable ankle fracture injury patterns do not displace with normal physiologic forces, while unstable fracture patterns displace with those same physiologic forces.[1] Some indications for surgery include multiple malleoli fractures and talar subluxation. Operative indications for other ankle fractures are subject to debate.

CLASSIFICATION

Lauge-Hansen created a classification for ankle fractures that is based on the deforming forces and the position of the foot at the time of injury. These include supination-external rotation, supination-adduction, pronation-abduction, and pronation-external rotation. Supination-external rotation first involves failure of the anterior-inferior talofibular ligament, then spiral fracture of the fibula at the level of the mortise, followed by rupture of the posterior-inferior talofibular ligament, and finally tearing of the deltoid ligament or a transverse fracture of the medial malleolus. Supination-adduction forces result in avulsion fractures of the lateral malleolus followed by vertical shear fractures of the medial malleolus. Pronation-abduction patterns often result in syndesmotic injuries. Avulsion medial malleolus fractures or deltoid ligament rupture occurs first. This is followed by failure of the anterior-inferior and posterior-inferior tibiofibular ligaments and finally a transverse fibula fracture at or above the mortise. This injury pattern also often results in lateral impaction injuries of talus. Pronation-external rotation injuries also often result in syndesmotic injuries. Transverse avulsion medial malleolus fractures or deep deltoid ligament ruptures occur first. These are followed by anterior-inferior talofibular ligament, a spiral fracture above the ankle mortise, and finally posterior-inferior talofibular ligament injury or a posterior malleolus fracture.[2] The Weber classification is used to describe lateral malleolus fractures. Weber A fractures are distal to the tibial plafond, Weber B fractures are at the level of the plafond, and Weber C fractures are proximal to the plafond.[3,4]

ANATOMY

The ankle joint consists of the tibiotalar articulation along with the distal fibula. Ankle fractures consist of distal fibula fractures, medial malleolus fractures, posterior malleolus fractures, syndesmotic injuries, and Maisonneuve injuries that can occur alone or in combination. The distal fibula fractures can have simple patterns including transverse, oblique, or spiral; however, they may also present as complicated fractures with comminution or butterfly fragments. The fibula is roughly four-sided. The correct length of the fibula can be determined by the incisura, the hollow portion of the distal tibia in which the fibula lies. The medial malleolus fracture can consist of transverse fractures or vertical shears. The syndesmosis consists of anterior-inferior tibiofibular ligament, interosseous ligament, posterior-inferior tibiofibular ligament, and inferior transverse tibiofibular ligament. Maisonneuve fractures involve fracture patterns that include syndesmotic injuries in association with proximal fibula fractures.[5]

PREOPERATIVE PLANNING

Lateral, anteroposterior (AP), and mortise X-rays of the ankle are necessary to evaluate the fracture pattern (Figs 1A and B). Full length tibia X-rays are also needed to look for a proximal fibula fracture.

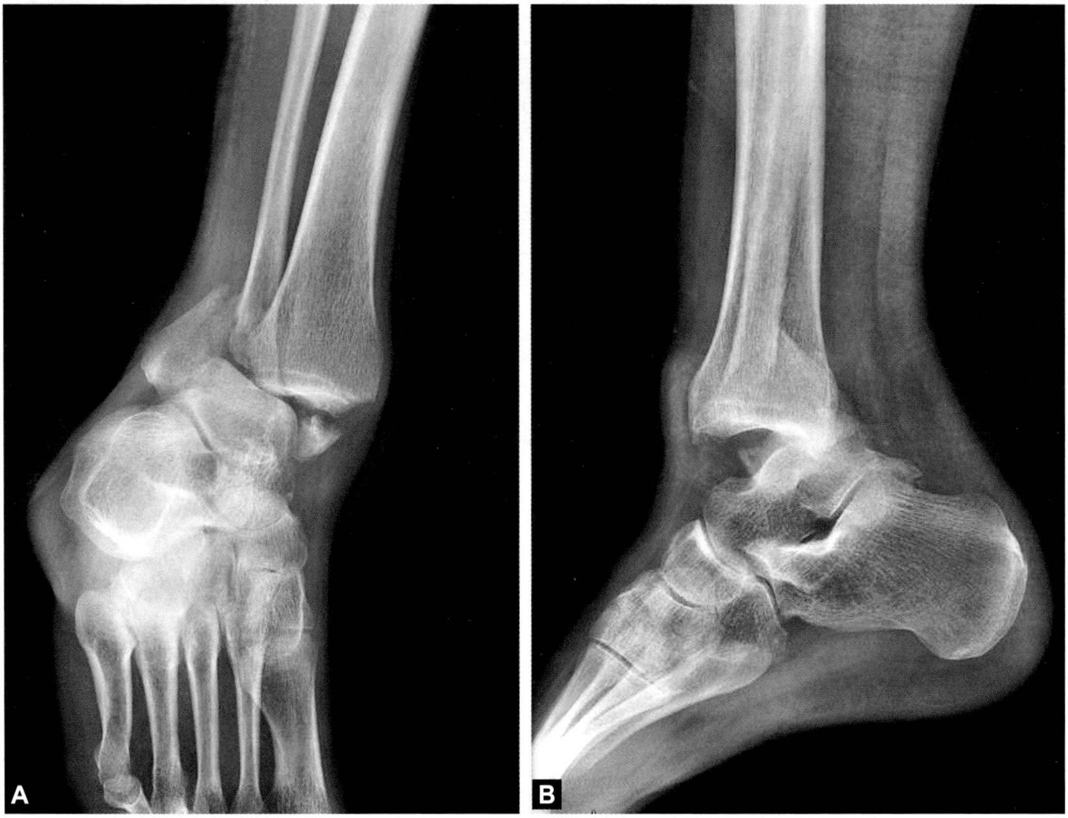

Figs 1A and B: Bimalleolar ankle fracture with tibiotalar dislocation

Closed reduction of subluxed or dislocated tibiotalar joints should be performed at the time of injury. Irrigation and debridement is performed initially for open wounds. The soft tissue envelope is evaluated prior to operative procedures on the ankle. The skin should wrinkle prior to operative management to help ensure that the skin will be able to be closed at the completion of the procedure.

Operative indications for ankle fractures include multiple malleoli fractures, open injuries, displaced fractures, syndesmotic injuries, and unstable fracture patterns resulting in tibiotalar subluxation or dislocation or medial clear space widening on X-ray. Nonoperative management is used for minimally displaced distal fibula fractures that do not demonstrate medial joint widening on external rotation stress views. Ecchymosis on the medial side of the ankle indicating deltoid ligament injury is not an operative indication. External rotation views are performed by holding the tibia and externally rotating the ankle while shooting a mortise X-ray. The medial clear space on this ankle is compared to a non-stress mortise X-ray. Positive stress X-rays with greater than 4–5 mm of medial clear space widening along with a distal fibula fracture are an indication for an operative procedure. Minimally displaced medial malleolus fractures in isolation also are treated nonoperatively if there is no displacement of the tibiotalar articulation or talar tilt. Posterior malleolus fractures can be treated nonoperatively if they are displaced less than 2 mm or constitute less than 25% of the articular surface.[6]

SURGICAL APPROACHES

The distal fibula is approached through an incision based over the lateral border of the fibula. Weber C ankle fractures may require incisions that extend to the level of the superficial peroneal nerve. The nerve is along the lateral border of the fibula, approximately 12 cm from the distal fibula tip. A posterolateral approach can be used to treat distal fibula fractures. The medial malleolus is fixed through an anteromedial incision that is made medial to the anterior tibialis tendon. The saphenous nerve and vein need to be protected with this approach. Posterior malleolus fractures can be approached from anterior to posterior or posterior to anterior. If approached from anterior to posterior, a percutaneous incision can be made on the anterior surface of the tibia. Blunt dissection should be used to dissect down to bone to avoid injury to the anterior neurovascular bundle.[7]

SURGICAL OPTIONS

Temporary Stabilization

External fixation can be used to stabilize unstable ankle fractures that cannot be closed reduced and whose soft tissues will not permit definitive fixation. An ankle-bridging construct can be used employing two tibial pins and a calcaneal pin with or without a first metatarsal or medial cuneiform pin. The goal is a reduced ankle mortise until the soft tissues allow definitive fixation with open reduction and internal fixation.[8]

Definitive Fixation

The patient is placed in a supine position. A bump is used under the operative hip to internally rotate the leg giving access to the lateral side and the fibula. When fixing the medial malleolus fracture, the leg is externally rotated. A small bump is placed under the distal lateral foot. This places a supination force on the ankle and helps reduce the medial malleolus fragment. The fracture can be fixed with or without a tourniquet.

Fibula Fixation

The fibula can be approached in several different ways. A pointed reduction clamp is useful in reducing simple fibula fractures. Lag screw fixation is used for an oblique fracture pattern. The lag screw is placed perpendicular to the fracture site and bicortical options include 2.0, 2.4, 2.7, or 3.5 mm screws. A one-third tubular plate can be used in a neutralization manner. The plate needs to be contoured to the lateral fibula to prevent malreduction of the fibula (Figs 2A and B).

Manual traction can be used to gain length of the fibula. This often is not enough if the fracture is shortened. In this case, a push pull technique can be used. Briefly, a one-third tubular plate is placed with a bicortical 3.5 mm screw placed in a hole distal to the fracture site. A 3.5 mm recon plate or a low contact-dynamic compression plate can be used instead of a one-third tubular plate. A 3.5 mm bicortical screw is placed proximal to the plate. A laminar spreader is then used to gain length by opening it between the screw and the proximal portion of the plate. After the length and rotation is restored, a bicortical screw is placed in a screw hole proximal to the fracture site. Three screws are placed proximal to the fracture and three screws are placed distal. Unicortical screws are placed distally at the level of the joint.[9]

Antiglide plating is useful for fixing oblique distal fibula fractures that are oriented in the proximal posterior to distal anterior direction. A one-third tubular plate is placed on the posterior fibula. It does not have to be contoured secondary to this surface being flat. A 3.5 mm bicortical screw is placed just proximal to the fracture site. The plate creates an axilla, which prevents proximal migration of the fracture. A 3.5 mm lag screw is then placed through the plate from posterior to anterior in the hole just distal to the fracture site. Two more bicortical screws are placed in the proximal portion of the plate. Cancellous screws of 4.0 mm can be placed in the remaining two distal holes.[10]

Bridge plating is used for comminuted distal fibula fractures. Plate choices include one-third tubular plates that are single stacked or double stacked if a stronger construct is necessary. Careful attention must be placed on the length and rotation of the fibula and may be achieved by push pull technique.

Distal fibula locking plates are useful for fibular fractures with a small amount of bone distal to the fracture site. They can also be used for osteoporotic bone. Locking screws can be used in each of the screw holes. The plates usually need to be contoured to accommodate the twist of the fibula.[11]

Medial Malleolus Fixation

Medial malleolus fractures need to be exposed and cleaned so that the anterior shoulder of the tibia can be visualized to assess the reduction. The joint can also be visualized and any debris should be removed. A K-wire hole is made just proximal to the fracture site. One tine of a pointed reduction clamp is placed in this hole and the other at the distal tip of the medial malleolus while a reduction maneuver of traction and supination is performed.

Transverse fractures are fixed with parallel screw fixation (Figs 2A and B). K-wires are placed through the tip of the medial malleolus, perpendicular to the fracture site, and into the proximal tibia. The

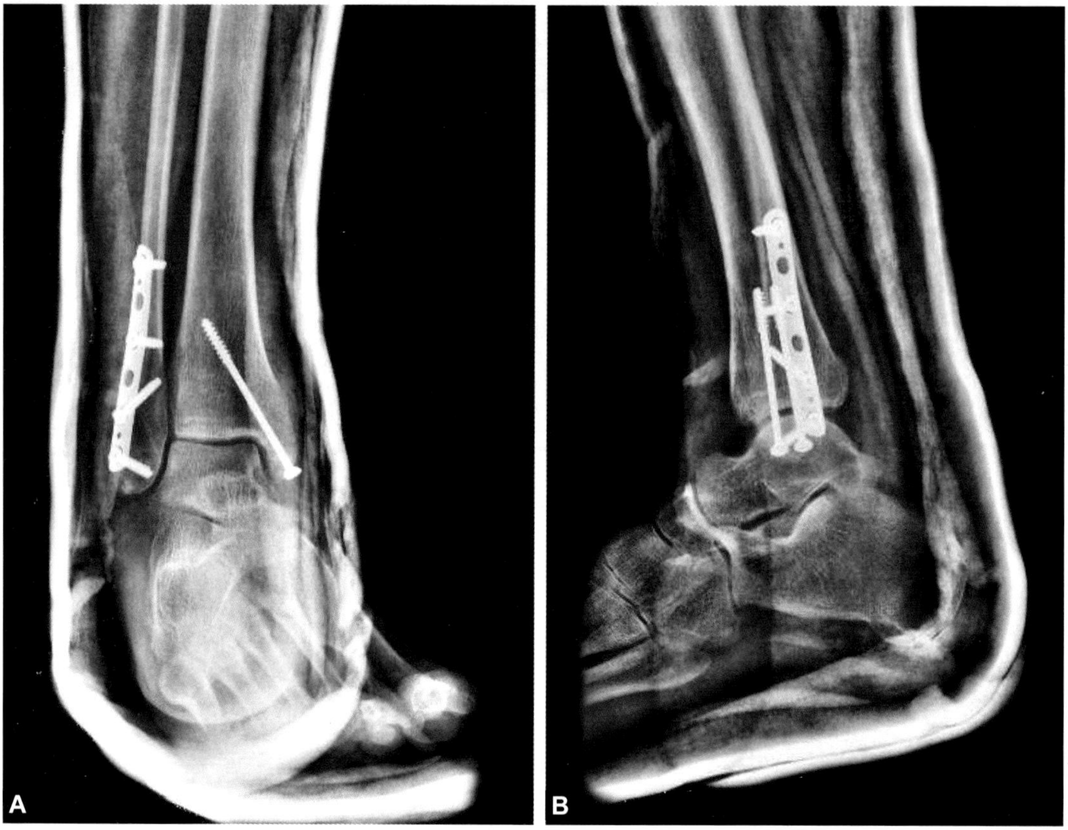

Figs 2A and B: Open reduction and internal fixation of bimalleolar ankle fracture with distal fibula plating and medial malleolar parallel screws

wires should be parallel on the anterior-posterior and lateral views and the wires must not enter into the ankle joint. A cannulated drill is used to drill through the near cortex. Cannulated screws of 4.0 mm are then placed over the wires. These can be used with or without a washer depending on the bone quality.[12]

Tension band technique is useful fixation for medial malleolus fractures. Two 0.45 mm K-wires are drilled perpendicular to the fracture site from the tip of the malleolus into the proximal tibia. A 3.5 mm bicortical screw is then placed from medial to lateral, proximal to the fracture site. A 20-guage wire is placed in a figure-of-eight fashion around the head of the screw head and around the bent K-wire tips.[13]

Vertical medial malleolus fracture patterns are treated with plate fixation. A one-third tubular plate can be contoured and placed in an antiglide fashion with two screws placed proximal to the fracture site. Plates can also be used on the medial malleolus in buttress mode.[12]

Posterior Malleolus Fixation

Posterior malleolus fractures require fixation if they are minimally displaced or greater than 25% of the articular surface. The fracture can be approached from a posterolateral approach and reduced by a Weber clamp or other large pointed reduction clamp. K-wires are then placed from posterior to anterior. Two cancellous 4.0 mm partially threaded cannulated screws are placed over the wires to compress the fracture. The screws can be placed percutaneously from anterior to posterior but only if the fracture can be reduced percutaneously. The screws can be placed with or without a washer depending on the bone quality.[14]

Syndesmotic Fixation

After fixation of the fibula, a Cotton test is performed to stress the syndesmosis. To perform a Cotton test, a towel clamp is placed on the distal fibula and externally rotated. If medial clear space widening or talar shift occurs on mortise X-rays when compared to unstressed mortise views, the syndesmosis requires fixation. Controversy exists on best fixation for the syndesmosis. The syndesmosis must be reduced prior to a screw being placed. A pelvic reduction clamp can be placed over the tip of the medial malleolus and on the distal fibula plate and compressed. Screw choice includes a 3.5 mm, 4.0 mm, or 4.5 mm cortical screw that is placed from the fibula into the tibia. The screw is aimed anteromedial secondary to the natural posterior position of the fibula in relation to the tibia. One or two screws can be placed through three or four cortices and can be placed through the plate. In the setting of a Maisonneuve injury, a two-hole one-third tubular plate may be placed on the fibula for placement of two syndesmotic screws. The distal syndesmotic screw should be placed parallel to the joint and 2 cm from the articular surface of the tibia.[15]

COMPLICATIONS

Hardware irritation on thin patients can be an issue postoperatively both from the fibular plate and the medial malleolus screws. A posterior fibula plate can irritate the peroneal tendons. Ankle fractures can lead to degenerative changes of the tibiotalar joint, some of which require a tibiotalar fusion at a later date. Wound healing problems are associated with ankle fractures more often in diabetics. Wound complications also occur after operating through edematous, tenuous skin.

REFERENCES

1. Tile M. Fractures of the ankle. In: Schatzker J, Tile M (Eds). The Rationale of Operative Fracture Management. New York, NY: Springer; 2005. pp. 551-90.
2. Lauge-Hansen N. Fractures of the ankle. III. Genetic roentgenologic diagnosis of fractures of the ankle. Am J Roentgenol Radium Ther Nucl Med. 1954;71(3):456-71.
3. Danis R (Ed). Les fractures malleolaires. Theorie et pratique de l'osteosynthese. Paris: Masson; 1949.
4. Weber BG. Die verletzungen des oberen sprunggelenkes, (2nd edn). Berne: Verlag Hans Huber; 1972.
5. Close JR. Some applications of the functional anatomy of the ankle joint. J Bone Joint Surg Am. 1956;38(4):761-81.
6. Griend R, Michelson J, Bone L. Instructional course lectures, the American Academy of Orthopaedic Surgeons – fractures of the ankle and the distal part of the tibia. J Bone Joint Surg Am. 1996;78(11): 1772-83.
7. Broudy A. Surgical approaches to the foot and ankle. J Bone Joint Surg Am. 1994;76(11):1757.
8. Antypas G, Konstas A, Kontogiannis G, et al. A two stages treatment of high energy fractures of distal tibia. J Bone Joint Surg Br. 2011;93B:364.
9. Minihane K, Lee C, Ahn C, et al. Comparison of lateral locking plate and antiglide plate for fixation of distal fibular fractures in osteoporotic bone: a biomechanical study. J Orthop Trauma. 2006;20(8):562-6.
10. Ostrum R. Posterior plating of displaced Weber B fibula fractures. J Ortho Trauma. 1996;10(3): 199-203.
11. Ricci W, Tornetta P, Borrelli J. Lag screw fixation of medial malleolar fractures: a biomechanical, radiographic, and clinical comparison of unicortical partially threaded lag screws and bicortical threaded lag screws. J Orthop Trauma. 2012;26(10):602-6.
12. Dumigan R, Bronson D, Early J. Analysis of fixation methods for vertical shear fractures of the medial malleolus. J Orthop Trauma. 2006;20(10):687-91.
13. Ostrum R, Litsky A. Tension band fixation of medial malleolus fractures. J Orthop Trauma. 1992;6(4): 464-8.
14. Gardner M, Brodsky A, Briggs S, et al. Fixation of posterior malleolar fractures provides greater syndesmotic stability. Clin Orthop Relat Res. 2006; 477:165-71.
15. McBryde A, Chiasson B, Wilhelm A, et al. Syndesmotic screw placement: a biomechanical analysis. Foot Ankle Int. 1997;18(5):262-6.

52

Talus Fractures

William Min, Jason Lowe

INTRODUCTION

Fractures of the talus rank second behind calcaneal fractures of all tarsal bones with an incidence of approximately 0.5%. The mechanism of talar fractures is a high-energy mechanism including a fall from height, motor vehicle accident, motorcycle accident, or other event causing forced dorsiflexion about the ankle. Talus fractures can be difficult fractures to treat for orthopedic surgeons secondary to their propensity to develop degenerative joint disease as well as avascular necrosis.[1]

CLASSIFICATION

Talar fractures are classified based on anatomic location and include head, neck, body, lateral process, and posterior process.

Talar Head

There is no formal classification system for talar head fractures. They comprise 5–10% of talus fractures and require a high index of suspicion. Pain over the talonavicular joint warrants further investigation and often times computed tomography (CT) imaging is necessary to make the diagnosis as plain films may be inconclusive. Two mechanisms have been suggested including axial loading on a plantarflexed foot leading to compression across the talar head and forced dorsiflexion with compression of the talar head against the anterior tibial plafond. Unrecognized fractures may lead to talonavicular joint instability and eventual post-traumatic arthrosis.[1]

Talar Neck

The Hawkins classification system (Type I–IV) is utilized to describe fractures of the talar neck. They account for 50% of all talus fractures. Type I fractures of the talar neck are nondisplaced. Displacement of even 1 mm should be classified as Type II. The ankle and subtalar joints remain congruent. The risk of talar body avascular necrosis is less than 14%. Type II fractures of the talar neck include subluxation or dislocation of the subtalar joint. This represents a spectrum from a minimally displaced talar neck fractures with subtalar subluxation to completely displaced fractures with subtalar dislocation. The risk of talar body avascular necrosis is 20–50%. Type III talar neck fractures are completely displaced with dislocation of both the subtalar and tibiotalar joints. The talar body is usually extruded in a posteromedial direction placing the tibial neurovascular bundle at risk. The talonavicular joint remains intact. Over 50% of Type III talar neck fractures present with open injuries usually over the anterolateral skin. The risk of talar body avascular necrosis is 75–100%. Type IV talar neck fractures are completely displaced with dislocation of the subtalar, tibiotalar, and talonavicular joints.[2,3]

Talar Body

The Müller AO/Orthopaedic Trauma Association (OTA) classification is used for talar body fractures. C1 fractures involve the tibiotalar joint. C2 fractures involve the subtalar joint and C3 fractures involve both joints.[4]

Lateral Process

Lateral process fractures occur from forced eversion. The fracture is often confused with an ankle sprain and is often called a "snowboarder's fracture". The fracture involves the subtalar joint and for larger fracture pieces can disrupt the lateral talar articulation with the lateral malleolus. The fractures are intra-articular and can be comminuted and also displaced.[5]

Posterior Process

Posterior process fractures of the talus are often confused with an os trigonum. An os trigonum is a developmental failure of the posterior tubercle fusing to the talar body.[6]

ANATOMY

The talar head articulates with the navicular. The talar body includes articulations for the medial and lateral malleoli and is located posterior to the lateral process. Behind the trochlea on the talar body is a posterior process in which the flexor hallucis longus runs behind. The talar neck lies between the head and the body. The lateral process is attached to the talar body and articulates with the subtalar joint.

The blood supply of the talus occurs from several different sources. Deltoid branches of the posterior tibial artery supply the majority of the body and the medial talar neck. Specifically the artery of the tarsal canal off the posterior tibial artery supplies a large portion of the talar body. The dorsalis pedis and peroneal arteries supply the talar neck and the lateral third of the talus.

Anterolateral blood supply to talar body is disrupted with Type I talar neck fractures. With Type II talar neck fractures the same anterolateral blood supply is disrupted along with the vessels from the sinus tarsi and tarsal canal. All three sources of blood supply are usually disrupted with Type III fractures.[7]

SURGICAL APPROACHES

Several approaches can be employed to reduce the talus. An anterolateral approach involves an incision made on a line parallel with the fourth metatarsal. After dissection through the extensor digitorum brevis, the lateral talus is visualized. The superficial peroneal nerve is at risk during this procedure.

The anteromedial approach incision extends from the medial malleolus to the base of the first metatarsal. The deltoid arterial branches must be avoided to protect the blood supply to the medial talar neck. These branches occur in the posterior portion of the dissection. This approach along with the anterolateral approach are used to access the talar neck.

A lateral approach can be employed for lateral process fractures. The incision is made in line with the peroneal tendons and anterior to the fibula. It is made over the midportion of the talus. This incision is marked with fluoroscopy prior to the incision. The subtalar capsule is then encountered and entered.

Posteromedial approach is used for posterior talar body fractures and posterior process fractures. An incision is made medial to the Achilles tendon and lateral to the posteromedial neurovascular bundle. The dissection is carried between the Achilles and the flexor hallucis longus.

A posterolateral approach is used for posterior talus fractures. The incision is made lateral to the Achilles tendon and posterior to the peroneal tendons. The sural nerve is at risk during this approach.

A transverse medial malleolus osteotomy allows visualization of the medial talus through an anteromedial approach. The medial malleolus can be secured at the end of the case with two 4.0 mm cancellous parallel screws perpendicular to the osteotomy site. The medial malleolus should be predrilled to allow for easier fixation at the completion of the case. The osteotomy level is made at the level of the ankle mortise. The deltoid ligament must be preserved to protect the talar blood supply. A lateral osteotomy can be made at the level of the ankle mortise to give visualization to the lateral talus.[8]

TREATMENT OPTIONS

Fractures of the talus are an orthopedic emergency if they are displaced or open. Open injuries are irrigated and debrided at presentation. Dislocations are reduced by closed means if possible. If talar fractures are irreducible, they are open reduced. An external fixator can be placed with 5.0 mm pins in the tibia and a transcalcaneal pin for talar fractures with severe open soft tissue injuries.

Fractures of the Talar Head

Nondisplaced and small articular fractures that do not result in talonavicular instability may be treated in a short leg cast for 6 weeks. Displaced fractures require open reduction and internal fixation. The talar head is best approached from an anteromedial incision with careful attention being paid as to not disrupt the vascular supply to the talar head. Partially threaded cancellous screws, headless compression screws, or bioabsorbable pins can be used to stabilize the fragment. The screws are placed from distal to the intact proximal talar body. Early motion should be initiated at 2 weeks after stable fixation; however, the patient is to remain nonweight-bearing for 6–8 weeks.[1]

Fractures of the Talar Neck

Nondisplaced fractures can be treated conservatively in a short leg cast for 6–8 weeks. Prior to initiating nonoperative treatment, a Canale view must be obtained to ensure the fracture is not displaced or malrotated. The Canale view gives a view of the talar neck and is taken with the foot in maximal plantarflexion and pronated 15°. Patients are not permitted to bear weight until follow-up radiographs demonstrate osseous remodeling.

Percutaneous fixation is also an appropriate option for minimally displaced fractures assuming no comminution in the talar neck is present. It is best performed via an anterior approach through two percutaneous incisions. Two, countersunk, parallel 3.5 mm or 4.0 mm cannulated screws should be placed perpendicular to the fracture medial and lateral in the talus.

Type II talar neck dislocations should be managed with immediate reduction, usually obtainable via closed maneuvers with the foot in plantarflexion, the knee flexed, a distraction force, and reversal of the force (Figs 1A to C). Type III and IV dislocations are often irreducible by closed means but an attempt should be made to reduce immediately closed at the time of presentation.

An anteromedial or anterolateral approach may be used for open reduction and internal fixation of the displaced talar neck. If manual distraction is inadequate, a femoral distractor may be placed in the lateral or medial calcaneus and tibia. The medial neck is most often comminuted versus the lateral side. Kirschner wires (K-wires) are placed for provisional stabilization. Careful attention should be paid to these K-wires because cannulated screws are placed over these wires for final fixation. A 3.5 mm cortical screw is placed anterior to posterior as a positional screw on the medial side when medial comminution exists. The lateral side does not usually have comminution and a 4.0 mm lag cannulated lag screw is placed for compression (Figs 2A and B).

Hawkin's sign is a radiographic indicator of talar revascularization which appears 8–10 weeks postoperatively. Biologically, it is a disuse osteopenia of the subchondral bone beneath the talar dome as seen on a mortise view radiograph. Presence of the Hawkin's sign is a favorable prognostic sign with regard to avascular necrosis. Partial weight bearing may be initiated once a Hawkin's sign is present. Full weight bearing is not permitted until radiographic healing is evident, usually by 12 weeks postoperatively.[2-4,9]

Fractures of the Talar Body

A combination of dorsiflexion and plantarflexion along with traction and a reversal of the forces will often reduce a dislocated talar body fracture. The approach is chosen based on the fracture pattern. Screw fixation can be employed with 3.5 mm or 4.0 mm screws. The majority of the talar body is covered with articular cartilage and thus screws must be countersunk. The screws can be placed from posterior to anterior or anterior to posterior. Posterior to anterior has been shown to be stronger in biomechanical studies. At least two screws are

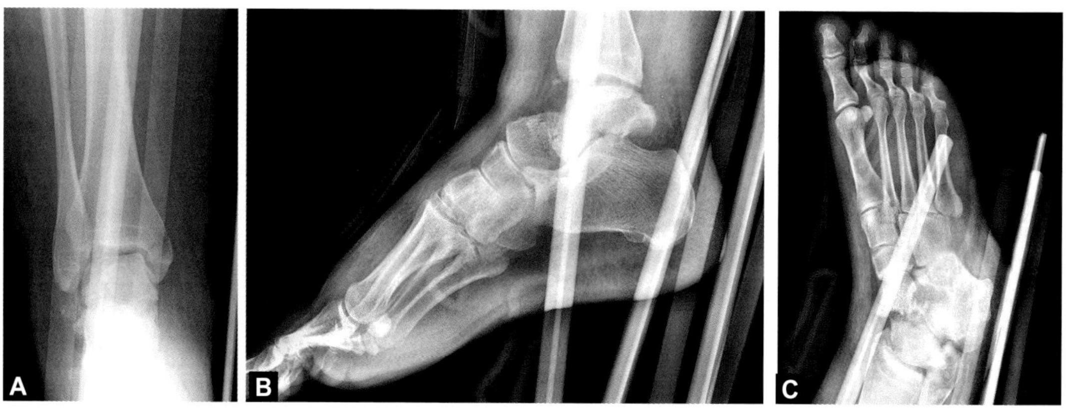

Figs 1A to C: Hawkin's Type II talar neck fracture

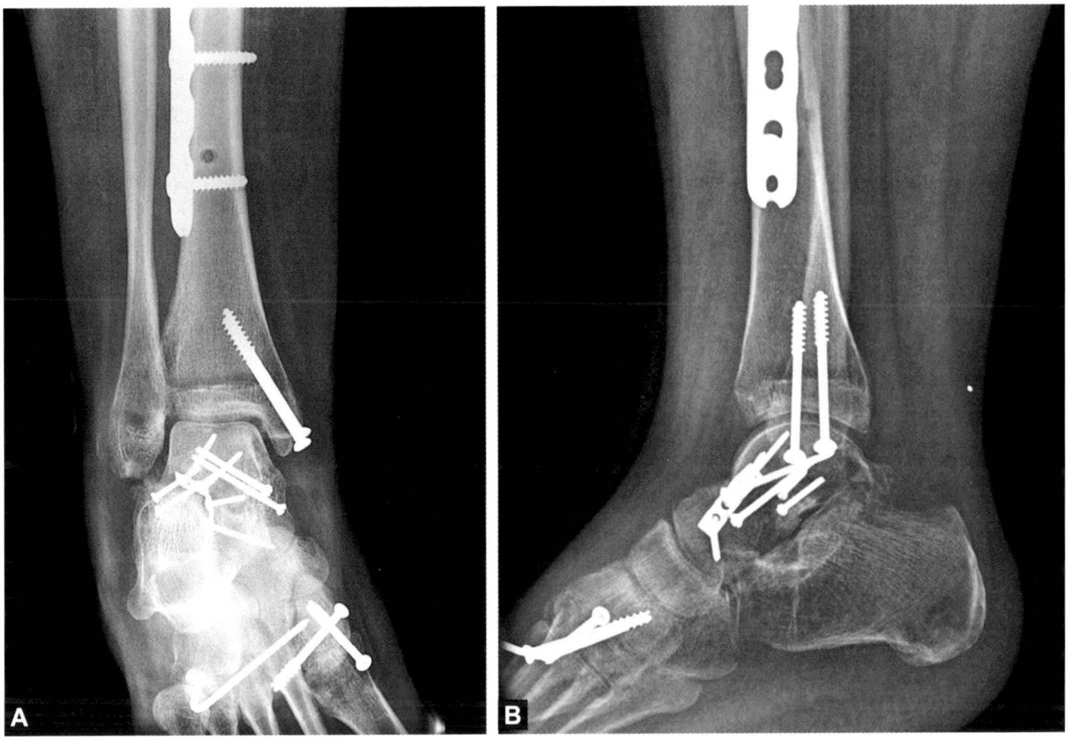

Figs 2A and B: Open reduction and fixation with independent lag screw and plate fixation of talar neck fracture

necessary for adequate fixation. A 2.0 mm plate can also be used for fixation. The plate may be placed on the medial or lateral side depending on the orientation of the fracture.[10]

Fractures of the Lateral Process of the Talus

Lateral process fractures are fixed through the direct lateral approach. These fractures are often small fragments and have associated comminution. A K-wire can be used for provisional fixation after a dental pick reduces the fracture. The K-wire is placed centrally due to the small nature of these fragments. If the fracture allows for two K-wires, they can be placed parallel to one another. A 2.4 mm or 3.5 mm cannulated screw is then placed over the K-wire for fixation. If the lateral process is too small to allow for two screws, a K-wire is placed as a second point of fixation to control for rotation. If the fracture is not operatively fixed and develops a non-union, the symptomatic fragment can be removed.[5]

Fractures of the Posterior Process of the Talus

A posterolateral or posteromedial approach is used to fix posterior process fractures. These fracture fragments are often small and control of the fragment is achieved by a K-wire used as a joystick. This K-wire is placed centrally in the fragment and drilled into the talar body. A 2.4 mm or 3.5 mm cannulated screw is placed over the K-wire for fixation. The posterior process fragment does not often allow for two screw fixation secondary to its size.[6]

COMPLICATIONS

Complications of talar fractures include osteonecrosis, post-traumatic arthrosis, and malunion. Osteonecrosis and arthrosis may lead to chronic pain and finally to an arthrodesis. Varus malunions are associated with displaced fractures of the talar neck that are not operatively fixed. Varus malunions lead to limited eversion.[1]

REFERENCES

1. Fortin PT, Balazsy JE. Talus fractures: evaluation and treatment. J Am Acad Orthop Surg. 2001;9(2): 114-27.
2. Hawkins LG. Fractures of the neck of the talus. J Bone Joint Surg Am. 1970;52(5):991-1002.
3. Canale S, Kelly F. Fractures of the neck of the talus. Long-term evaluation of seventy-one cases. J Bone Joint Surg Am. 1978;60(2):143-56.
4. Colton C, Krikler S, Schatzker J, ed. et al. AO surgery reference. https://www2.aofoundation.org.
5. Hawkins LG. Fracture of the lateral process of the talus. A review of thirteen cases. J Bone Joint Surg Am. 1965;47(6):1170-5.
6. Mehrpour SR, Aghamisirsalim MR, Sheshvan MK, et al. Entire posterior process talus fracture: a report of two cases. J Foot Ank Surg. 2012;51(3):326-9.
7. Mulfinger GL, Trueta J. The blood supply of the talus. J Bone Joint Surg Am. 1970;52(1):160-7.
8. Vallier H, Nork S, Benirschke S, et al. Surgical treatment of talar body fractures. J Bone Joint Surg Am. 2004;86-A:180-92.
9. Tyllianakis M, Karageorgos A, Papadopoulos A, et al. Surgical treatment of talar neck fractures. Evaluation of results. Eur J Trauma. 2004;30:98-103.
10. Vallier H, Nork S, Benirschke S, et al. Surgical treatment of talar body fractures. J Bone Joint Surg Am. 2003:85-A(9):1716-24.

53

Calcaneus Fractures

William Min, Jason Lowe

INTRODUCTION

Calcaneus fractures present difficult treatment issues for orthopedic surgeons due to their complications with both operative and nonoperative treatment. Calcaneus fractures include both intra-articular and extra-articular fractures. They occur from axial loads most often a fall from height and also from other high-energy mechanisms such as motor vehicle accidents and motorcycle accidents.[1]

CLASSIFICATION

Calcaneus fractures are classified in several different ways. Essex-Lopresti separated calcaneus fractures into extra-articular fractures and intra-articular fractures. Intra-articular fractures include joint depression and tongue type fractures. Joint depression fracture lines exit in or near the subtalar joint (Fig. 1). Tongue type fracture lines exit posteriorly and are often displaced by the attached Achilles tendon (Fig. 2). Extra-articular fractures include tuberosity fractures and anterior process fractures. Sanders created a classification based on the coronal computed tomography (CT) images of the calcaneus (Fig. 3). Type I fractures are minimally displaced. Type II fractures have two main articular fracture fragments with one fracture line. Type III fractures have three main articular fragments with two fracture lines and type IV fractures contain four or more articular pieces. The fracture lines include A, B, and C with A being the more lateral fracture line, B in the middle, and C a more medial fracture line.[2]

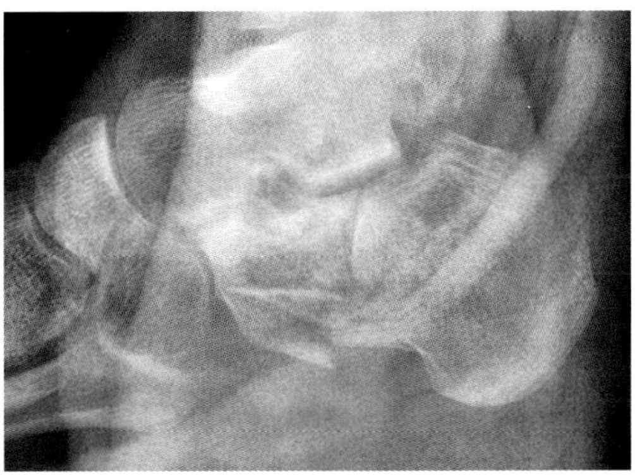

Fig. 1: Intra-articular fracture of calcaneus

ANATOMY

The calcaneus articulates with the talus as well as the cuboid. The anterior and middle facets form one articulation. The anteromedial sustentaculum tali is located inferior to the middle articular facet and remains a constant fragment after fracture. As a result of this fragment's inability to displace, it has been termed the "constant fragment". This fragment serves as the cornerstone to which later reconstructions are modeled. The posterior facet is larger and most often contains the major fracture lines. The lateral wall of the calcaneus is thin and the medial wall is thicker. The flexor hallucis longus and neurovascular bundle runs adjacent to this medial wall. The lateral calcaneal artery, lateral hindfoot artery, and lateral tarsal artery, which are branches of the peroneal artery, supply the lateral wall, skin, and soft tissue. The lateral calcaneal artery is important for the blood supply for the lateral corner of the incision.[3]

SURGICAL APPROACHES

A lateral extended incision is necessary for the majority of calcaneus fractures. The horizontal portion of the incision is made in line with the fifth metatarsal base. The vertical limb is made between the Achilles tendon and the distal fibula. These two limbs meet at a sharp corner. The

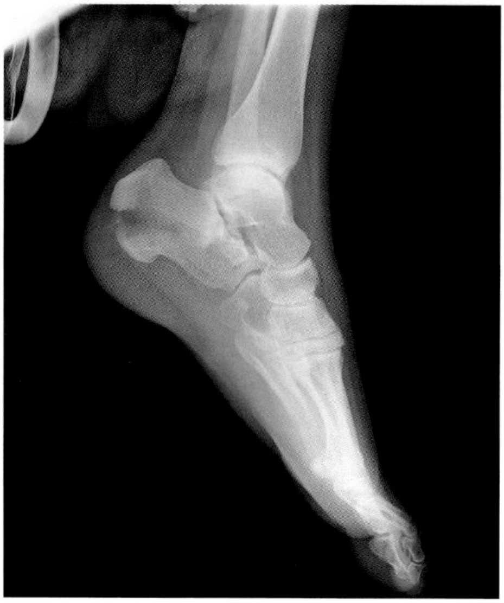

Fig. 2: Tongue type fracture of calcaneus necessitating emergent reduction and fixation to minimize soft tissue compromise

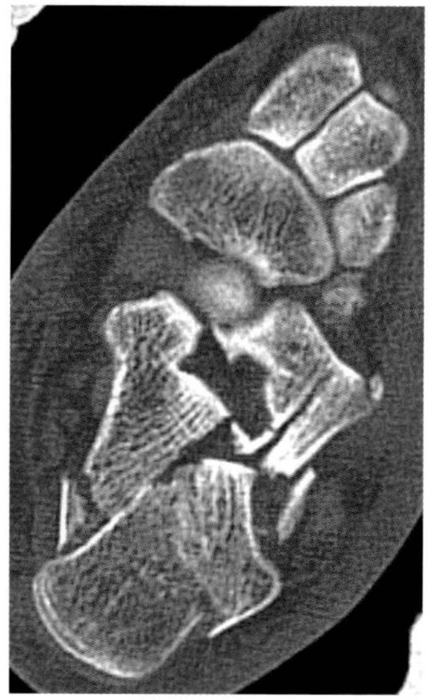

Fig. 3: Coronal CT scan demonstrating Sanders II intra-articular calcaneus fracture

corner of the incision is made sharp to bone. Full-thickness flaps are necessary in this approach to avoid wound-healing issues. The peroneal tendon retinaculum is released along with the talocalcaneal and calcaneofibular ligaments. The sural nerve and peroneal tendons are both contained within the flap. As the flap is raised, the sinus tarsi between the talus and calcaneus is exposed and the subtalar joint capsule is incised. Strict attention to flap handling is essential to avoid future wound complications. Instead of standard retractors, two to three 2.0–4.2 mm Kirschner wires (K-wires) are drilled into the talar body and used to retract the flap.[4] Closure of the wound after fixation is made over a Hemovac drain. Vicryl suture is used to approximate the subcutaneous tissue. Nylon suture is used for skin closure in an interrupted Donati suture fashion.

PREOPERATIVE PLANNING

Extra-articular fracture lines lead to varus or valgus malalignment, loss of heel height, and a widened heel. The intra-articular displacement can involve the calcaneocuboid joint, posterior articular surface, and anterior and middle facet surfaces. The primary fracture line starts posteromedial and extends anterolateral.[5]

A physical examination on a patient with a calcaneus fracture reveals large amounts of swelling and ecchymosis. X-rays of the foot should be taken including anteroposterior (AP), lateral, and a Harris heel view. The Harris view will demonstrate the varus or valgus malalignment of calcaneus fractures. A CT scan elicits the comminution of calcaneus fractures and helps plan best surgical management. A magnetic resonance imaging (MRI) is not useful in the acute setting but may be used to identify suspected calcaneus stress fractures.

Bohler's angle is often lost with calcaneus fractures. The angle is formed by a line extending from the posterior portion of the tuberosity to the most superior point on the posterior articular facet and a line from the superior portion of the posterior facet to the superior point on the anterior process of the calcaneus. A normal angle is from 20° to 40°. A decreased Bohler's angle indicates a loss of height of the calcaneus and disruption of the posterior facet. The critical angle of Gissane is measured from the anterior beak of the calcaneus and a line drawn along the border of the posterior facet. A normal angle measures from 120° to 145°.[6]

Patients over 60 years of age have worse outcomes with calcaneus fractures treated operatively than younger patients. Smokers and patients with other comorbidities also have poorer results. Factors including being male and involved in worker's compensation lead to worse results with operative treatment.[7] Definitive surgery cannot be undertaken until the swelling improves. The skin must wrinkle prior to the surgery.

TREATMENT METHODS

Nonoperative treatment in a splint or cast can be employed for calcaneus fractures with less than 2 mm of articular displacement and those fracture patterns that are not in varus or valgus malalignment. The patient will remain non-weight bearing in a splint, cast, or boot for 3 months. The initial splint or cast should be well padded to accommodate the significant edema encountered with acute calcaneus fractures. Nonoperative measures are also considered for patients that are over 60 years of age and patients that smoke cigarettes and have other comorbidities including diabetes or peripheral vascular disease.[7]

Open fractures are surgical emergencies that need to be debrided at the time of injury. Medial sided transverse tension wounds are most likely associated with calcaneus fractures. The displaced tongue-type fracture also presents a surgical emergency. The Achilles tendon displaces the calcaneal fragment superiorly and against the posterior skin of the foot and ankle. This leads to skin pressure, necrosis, and ultimately to open fractures.[8]

Tongue-type fractures are approached through the longitudinal posterior incision. A pelvic reduction clamp can be placed through this incision on the posterior tuberosity with the other limb of the clamp placed through a percutaneous incision on the heel pad onto the inferior calcaneus. The clamp is tightened and the superiorly displaced fracture is then reduced. Bicortical screw fixation is then used for fixation by way of two to three screws of 3.5 mm or 4.0 mm that are perpendicular to the fracture site (Figs 4A to C). The patient is then splinted in plantarflexion after the procedure to protect the repair.[8]

Open reduction and internal fixation builds off the constant sustentaculum tali fragment. This stays in position under the talus and thus the fractured parts can be pieced back to this fragment. The fracture is approached by first reducing the more medial fragments to this constant piece and then working posteriorly. The lateral wall can be removed and stored on the back table until the remaining fragments are reduced and provisionally stabilized with K-wires. The lateral wall is reattached prior to placement of a lateral plate (Figs 5A and B). The first important screw in the lateral plate is a bicortical screw from the lateral wall into the constant fragment.[9]

An external fixator may be applied to the calcaneus for definitive fixation. It can also be used to regain length and alignment prior to definitive fixation. Two tibial pins are placed from anterior to posterior. These are connected with pins placed in the posterior intact portion of the calcaneus. This can be a transcalcaneal pin if there is enough room. If space is an issue, 4.0 mm pins may be placed medially or laterally in the posterior portion of the calcaneus. Pins can then be placed in the first metatarsal base or medial cuneiform to give length on the medial side. A pin can be placed from the base of the fifth metatarsal into the fourth and third metatarsal, then attached by clamps and bars to the lateral calcaneus pin. This allows the surgeon to adjust length and pull the fragment out of varus alignment.[10]

Patients are to remain non-weight-bearing for 3 months after a calcaneus fracture with either operative or nonoperative therapy. Close attention is paid to the incision, especially the lateral corner, which is the most likely to break down or have healing problems. Strict elevation of calcaneus fractures is necessary, especially after operative treatment.

COMPLICATIONS

Wound complications are common after operative treatment of calcaneus fractures. Wound healing issues are most problematic at the corner of the lateral incision and can only be lessened by handling of the flap with care. Postoperative infections are also possible after operative therapy and are more likely after open injuries. Infections may require multiple debridements, long-term antibiotics, and skin coverage procedures. Patients often have difficulty with shoewear after calcaneus fractures secondary to the lateral wall blow out associated with the fracture and the resultant widened heel.[11]

Lateral impingement of the peroneal tendons can occur after both operative and nonoperative treatment of calcaneus fractures. Lateral wall blow out may also cause impingement after nonoperative treatment. The lateral plate may also cause impingement as well as scar tissue postoperatively. A lateral wall ostectomy can be performed after the fracture is healed to improve the impingement. The hardware cannot be removed for at least 1 year following the operation but can be removed if causing the impingement after 12–18 months.[12]

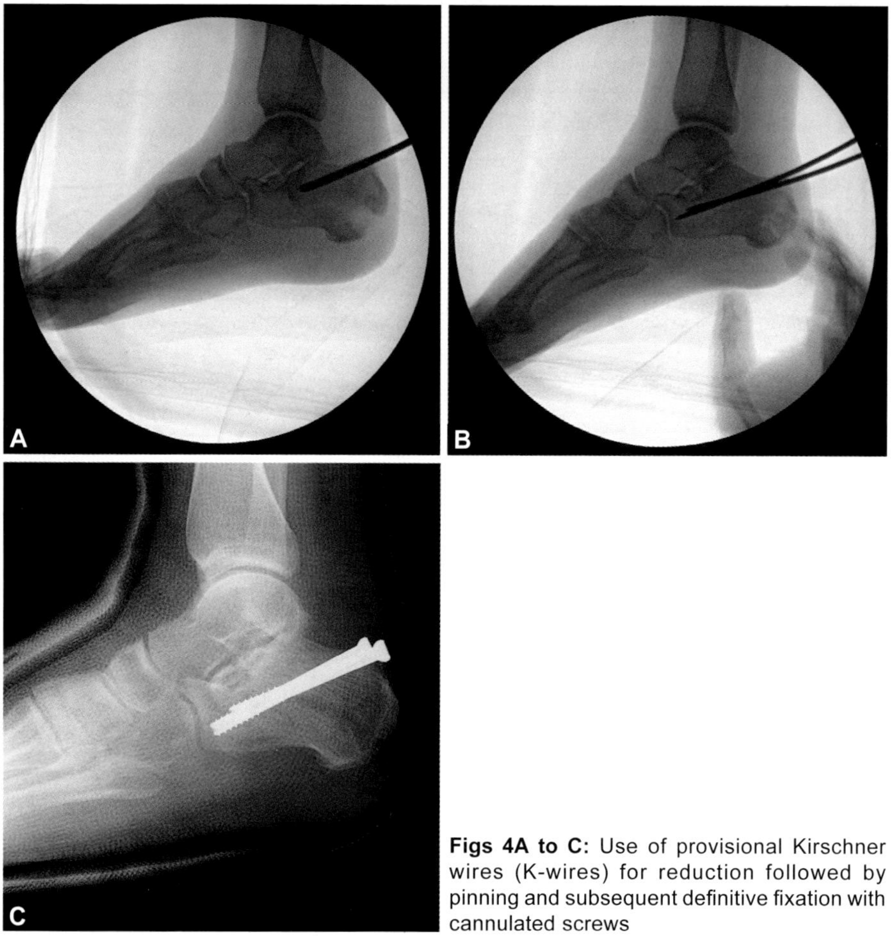

Figs 4A to C: Use of provisional Kirschner wires (K-wires) for reduction followed by pinning and subsequent definitive fixation with cannulated screws

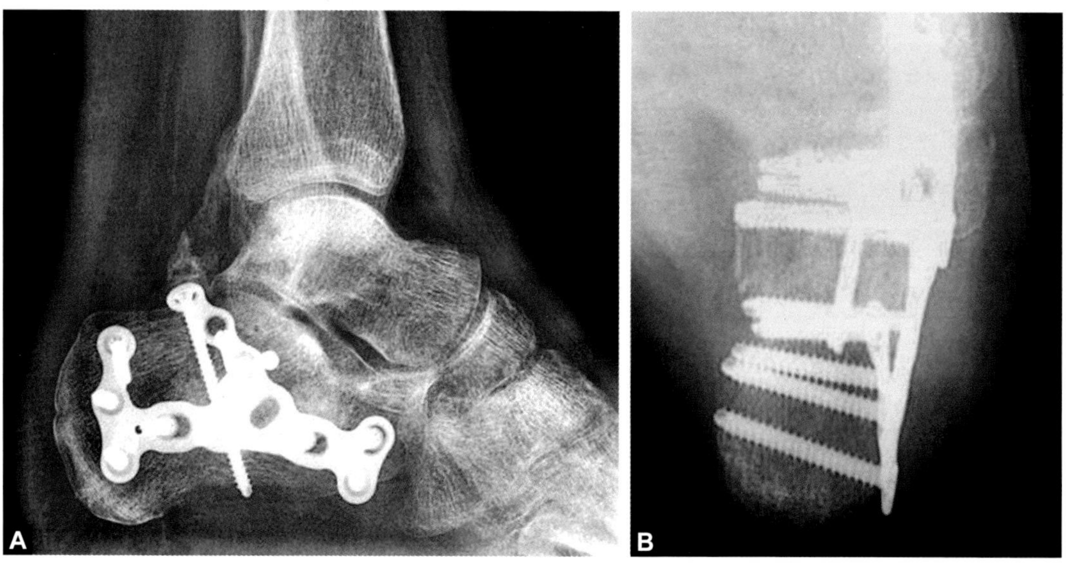

Figs 5A and B: Surgical fixation of intra-articular calcaneus fracture with lateral plating through an extensile approach

Patients often sustain malalignment of the heel after calcaneus fractures. Their hindfoot can be in varus or valgus. Valgus can also contribute to peroneal tendon impingement. After the fracture is healed, an opening wedge osteotomy on the lateral side of the calcaneus will correct the valgus deformity and improve peroneal tendon impingement. The posterior tuberosity can undergo an osteotomy to move it medially and thus help with the valgus deformity.[13]

Arthrosis is common after calcaneus fractures and most significantly affects dorsiflexion of the ankle. This is resultant of several factors. A calcaneus that does not undergo operative fixation loses height and can affect dorsiflexion. An osteotomy displacing the posterior tuberosity posterior and inferior can improve the height of the calcaneus and can aid in range of motion.

Subtalar arthritis is common after calcaneus fractures treated both operatively or nonoperatively secondary to the high energy associated with these fractures causing articular damage. If the degenerative joint disease of the subtalar joint becomes severe, a subtalar arthrodesis is performed. The previous calcaneus hardware is removed and a subtalar arthrodesis with screw fixation is performed. If the patient's calcaneus fracture was initially treated nonoperatively and lateral wall blow out with peroneal tendon impingement exists, an opening lateral wedge osteotomy or a medially displacing posterior tuberosity with a subtalar arthrodesis is performed.[14]

REFERENCES

1. Cave EF. Fractures of os calcis—the problem in general. Clin Orthop Relat Res. 1963;30:64-6.
2. Sanders R, Fortín P, DiPasquale T, et al. Operative treatment of 120 displaced intra-articular calcaneal fractures. Results using a prognostic computed tomography scan classification. Clin Orthop Relat Res. 1993;(290):87-95.
3. Bèzes H, Massart T, Devaux D, et al. The operative treatment of intra-articular calcaneal fractures. Indications, technique, results in 257 cases. Clin Orthop Relat Res. 1993;(290):55-9.
4. Lowery RB, Calhoun JH. Fractures of the calcaneus. Part I: Anatomy, injury mechanism, and classification. Foot Ank Int. 1996;17(4):230-5.
5. Sanders R. Intra-articular fractures of the calcaneus: present state of the art. J Orthop Trauma. 1992; 6(2):252-65.
6. Loucks C, Buckley R. Bohler's angle: correlation with outcome in displaced intra-articular calcaneal fractures. J Ortho Trauma. 1999;13(8):554-8.
7. Crosby LA, Fitzgibbons T. Intra-articular calcaneal fractures. Results of closed treatment. Clin Orthop Relat Res. 1993;(290):47-54.
8. Sanders R. Displaced intra-articular fractures of the calcaneus. J Bone Joint Surg Am. 2000;82(2): 225-50.
9. Letournel E. Open treatment of acute calcaneal fractures. Clin Orthop Relat Res. 1993;(290):60-7.
10. Talarico LM, Vito GR, Zyryanov SY. Management of displaced intraarticular fractures by using external fixation, minimally invasive open reduction, and early weight bearing. J Foot Ank Surg. 2004; 43(1):43-50.
11. Kerr PS, Prothero DL, Atkins RM. Assessing outcome following calcaneal fracture: a rational scoring system. Injury. 1996;27(1):35-8.
12. Chen W, Li X, Su Y, et al. Peroneal tenography to evaluate lateral hindfoot pain after calcaneal fracture. Foot Ankle J. 2011;32(8):789-95.
13. Didomenico LA, Haro AA, Cross DJ. Double calcaneal osteotomy using single, dual-function screw fixation technique. J Foot Ankle Surg. 2011; 50(6):773-5.
14. Radnay CS, Clare MP, Sanders RW. Subtalar fusion after displaced intra-articular calcaneal fractures: does initial operative treatment matter?: Surgical technique. J Bone Joint Surg Am. 2010:92:32-43.

54

Subtalar Dislocations

William Min, Jason Lowe

INTRODUCTION

Subtalar dislocations and peritalar dislocations are uncommon injuries. They compromise 1% of all dislocations in the body and result from high-energy mechanisms such as motor vehicle and motorcycle accidents.

CLASSIFICATION

Subtalar dislocations are classified according to the relationship of the foot position relative to the leg and ankle. There are four directions in which subtalar dislocations occur: (1) medial; (2) lateral; (3) anterior; and (4) posterior. Medial subtalar dislocations are the most common (65–80%). Lateral dislocations are most commonly associated with open injuries.[1,2]

ANATOMY

Medial subtalar dislocations occur as a result of an inversion force on a plantarflexed foot (Figs 1A and B). The resulting deformity places the calcaneus and remainder of the foot medially, while the talar head is prominent laterally. The skin may be tented on the lateral side and the foot resembles an acquired clubfoot. The sustentaculum tali acts as a fulcrum on the calcaneus to assist in the dislocation.[3] The calcaneonavicular (spring) ligament resists disruption and the force is translated through and ruptures the weaker talonavicular and talocalcaneal ligaments.[4] Most medial subtalar dislocations are reducible by a closed reduction. If the dislocation is irreducible, the peroneal tendons, extensor digitorum brevis, or talonavicular capsule can block the reduction.

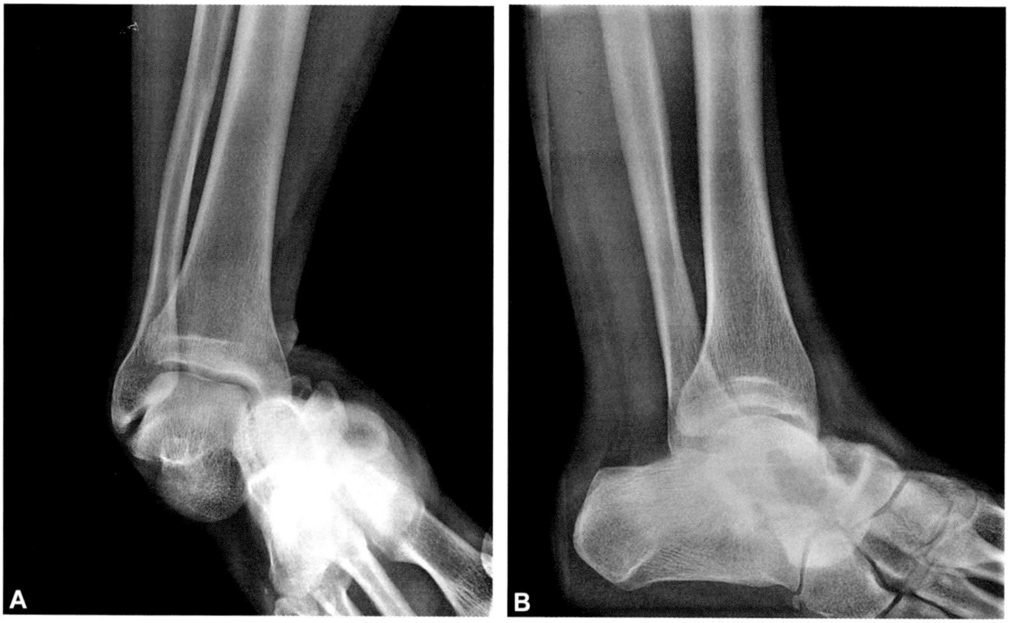

Figs 1A and B: Medial subtalar dislocation following high-energy trauma

Lateral subtalar dislocations occur as a result of an eversion force that causes the foot to pivot around the anterior process of the calcaneus. The calcaneus lies laterally and the talar head is prominent medially. The foot has a severe flatfoot appearance.[3] Lateral subtalar dislocations are associated with higher energy mechanisms and worse long-term prognosis. Over 50% present with open medial wounds. Frequently lateral subtalar dislocations are irreducible by closed manipulation as the posterior tibial tendon, flexor hallucis longus, or flexor digitorum longus blocks reduction.

SURGICAL APPROACHES

Medial subtalar dislocations are approached through an anteromedial incision over the talus. The interposed tissue is then removed and the dislocation is reduced. Lateral subtalar dislocations are approached through an incision over the sinus tarsi. The interposed tissue is removed and the lateral dislocation is then reduced.[5]

TREATMENT OPTIONS

In order to close reduce a medial or lateral subtalar dislocation, the knee must be flexed and the foot plantarflexed. For a medial subtalar dislocation, the foot is inverted. This deformity is exaggerated and the foot is everted to close reduce the subluxation (Figs 2A and B). Lateral subtalar dislocations are locked in eversion. This deformity is exaggerated and the foot is inverted to close reduce the dislocation. After the dislocation is closed reduced, the subtalar joint is usually stable. It can then be placed in a splint. If the medial or lateral subtalar dislocation is unstable, transarticular Kirschner wires (K-wires) can be placed from the calcaneus to the talus to stabilize the dislocation. A spanning external fixator can also be placed for open unstable subtalar dislocation.[6]

COMPLICATIONS

Complications after subtalar dislocations are directly related to the severity of the injury. Injuries with worse prognoses include open dislocations, high-energy injuries, delayed reductions, and intra-articular fractures. Conversely, uncomplicated dislocations with a stable reduction have an excellent prognosis. Pain when walking on uneven surfaces is a frequent finding when subtalar motion is limited after a dislocation.[7] Post-traumatic arthrosis is a common result, especially after lateral dislocations.[8] Tibial nerve injuries, posterior tibial tendon ruptures, articular fractures of the subtalar joint, and osteonecrosis of the talar body have all been reported.[8]

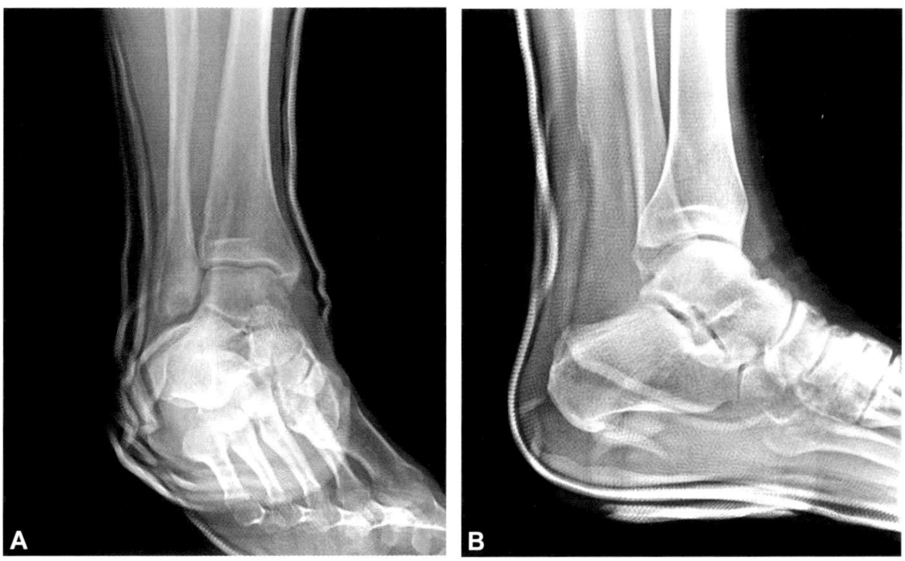

Figs 2A and B: Closed reduction and immobilization of subtalar dislocation

REFERENCES

1. Benirschke SK, Sangeorzan BJ. Extensive intra-articular fractures of the foot. Surgical management of calcaneal fractures. Clin Orthop Relat Res. 1993;292:128-34.
2. Letournel E. Open treatment of acute calcaneal fractures. Clin Orthop Relat Res. 1993;290:60-7.
3. Straus DC. Subtalar dislocation of the foot. Am J Surg. 1935;30:427-34.
4. Buckingham WW, LeFlore I. Subtalar dislocation of the foot. J Trauma. 1973;13:753-65.
5. Patnaik VV, Singla, RK, Gupta PN. Surgical incisions—their anatomical basis part III – lower limb. J Anat Soc India. 2001;50(1)48-58.
6. Milenkovic S, Mitkovic M, Bumbasirevic M. External fixation of open subtalar dislocation. Injury. 2006; 37:909-13.
7. Bibbo C, Anderson RB, Davis WH. Injury characteristics and the clinical outcome of subtalar dislocations: a clinical and radiographic analysis of 25 cases. Foot Ank Int. 2003;24:158-63.
8. Goldner JL, Poletti SC, Gates HS, et al. Severe open subtalar dislocations. Long term results. J Bone Joint Surg Am. 1995;77:1075-9.

55

Fifth Metatarsal Fractures

William Min, Jason Lowe

INTRODUCTION

The fifth metatarsal is the most common of the metatarsals to fracture. They comprise one quarter of all metatarsal fractures. While these fractures can occur from direct trauma, they most commonly are the result of sporting activities. Fifth metatarsal fractures can be complicated with delayed healing and nonunions.

CLASSIFICATION

Fifth metatarsal fractures are best classified according to the system proposed by DeLee.[1] The DeLee classification system divides the proximal fifth metatarsal into three anatomic regions or zones. Zone 1 involves the tuberosity and usually results in an avulsion fracture. Zone 2 involves the metaphyseal-diaphyseal junction and is caused by an adduction force to the forefoot. Zone 2 fractures are also known as Jones fractures. Zone 3 involves the proximal diaphysis often as a result of overuse. Each zone has a specific mechanism of injury, treatment, and prognosis thereby making it essential to correctly classify the fractures. A second classification system by Torg further subdivides proximal diaphyseal stress fractures (Zone 3) into three subtypes: (1) early union (Torg type I), (2) delayed union (Torg type II), and (3) nonunion (Torg type III). These subtypes are based on healing potential and radiographic appearance. Torg type II and III are less likely to heal nonoperatively.[2]

ANATOMY

The fifth metatarsal is made up of the head, neck, shaft, base, and tuberosity. The tuberosity projects laterally and proximally and lies in the subcutaneous tissue. The fifth tarsometatarsal joint is comprised of two articulations including the cuboid-fifth metatarsal articulation and the fourth-fifth intermetatarsal articulation. It is the most mobile of the tarsometatarsal joints allowing for the foot to accommodate to the ground in stance phase. The peroneus brevis attaches to the dorsal aspect of the fifth metatarsal tuberosity. The peroneus tertius attaches to the dorsal aspect of the proximal metaphyseal-diaphyseal junction. These muscle attachments make the fifth metatarsal unique in that it is the only lesser metatarsal with extrinsic tendon insertions.

The apophysis of the tuberosity should not be confused for a fracture in the adolescent patient. It appears as a smooth radiolucent line parallel to the metatarsal shaft in contrast to fractures, which are usually oriented in a perpendicular fashion.[3] In addition, two sesamoid bones need to be distinguished from an acute fracture. The os peroneum is found in the peroneus longus tendon on the lateral border of the cuboid and the os vesalianum is located in the peroneus brevis tendon just proximal to the fifth metatarsal base. The smooth contour of these ossicles make them easy to identify from acute injury.[4]

A single nutrient artery supplies the fifth metatarsal shaft and enters along the medial cortex at the junction of the proximal and middle third diaphysis. The base and tuberosity are supplied by epiphyseal and metaphyseal arteries. This creates a watershed area at the metaphyseal-diaphyseal junction leaving fractures in this region prone to delayed healing and nonunions.[5]

SURGICAL APPROACHES

The patient is positioned supine on a radiolucent table with a bolster under the operative hip. Under fluoroscopic guidance, a parallel line is drawn down the lateral border of the fifth metatarsal shaft using a Kirschner wire (K-wire). A 2 cm incision is made proximal to the tuberosity and inline with the shaft. The sural nerve lies directly under the skin incision and must be protected during screw insertion. The lateral band of the plantar fascia may be encountered; however, the peroneus brevis usually lies superior to the incision.

Diaphyseal fractures are approached through an incision at the junction of the plantar and dorsal skin. The short saphenous vein and sural nerve branches need to be protected during this approach.

TREATMENT OPTIONS

Indications for nonoperative treatment of fifth metatarsal fractures include nonathletes; avulsion fractures with less than 2 mm displacement (Zone 1); acute, nondisplaced Jones fracture (Zone 2); acute, nondisplaced metaphyseal or diaphyseal fractures, Torg type 1 (Zone 3). Nonoperative treatment consists of 6–8 weeks non-weight bearing in a short leg cast, followed by progressive weight bearing pending radiographic and clinical examinations. Callus formation should be evident in the medial to lateral direction by 6–8 weeks. However, radiographic signs of healing may lag behind resolution of symptoms. Pulsed-electromagnetic field therapy may be instituted if signs of delayed union are present.[2]

Operative treatment of proximal fifth metatarsal consists of intramedullary screw fixation with reaming of the canal and compression across the fracture site, corticocancellous inlay bone grafting, or a combination. Indications for surgical treatment include high-performance athletes, acute displaced fractures, and symptomatic nonunions. Surgery is contraindicated in patients with vascular compromise and local infection. However, diabetes is not a contraindication to surgery.

Using the surgical approach described above, a guidewire is inserted into the base of the fifth metatarsal adjacent to the cuboid articulation. The key to wire placement is "high and inside" position to ensure proper screw trajectory. The guidewire should not be advanced past the curvature of the fifth metatarsal. The canal is drilled from 3.2 mm to 5 mm depending on individual canal size. The canal is tapped, guidewire is removed, and a countersink is used at the tuberosity. A solid, partially threaded screw (5.5–7.0 mm) is advanced until all threads have crossed the fracture site. Screw diameter should be large enough to fill the canal.[6-8]

Diaphyseal fractures can be fixed with lag screw and plate fixation after reduction by a pointed reduction clamp. Lag screws of 1.5 mm are placed perpendicular to the fracture site. Multiple lag screws are used for fixation. A 2.0 mm plate is then used as neutralization construct. The plate is placed medially or laterally to avoid the extensor tendon.[9]

An alternative to intramedullary screw fixation is corticocancellous inlay bone grafting. Using the same surgical approach centered over the fracture site, a rectangular section of bone is removed from the fracture. The dimension of the section of bone to be removed is 0.7 cm × 2.0 cm. The medullary canal is reamed to remove sclerotic bone. An autologous corticocancellous bone graft measuring 0.7 cm × 2.0 cm is harvested from the anteromedial distal tibia. The graft is impacted into the defect created at the fracture site.[10]

FRACTURE PATTERNS

Avulsion Fractures (Zone 1)

Tuberosity avulsion fractures are the most common of the fifth metatarsal fractures. The mechanism involves an inversion injury with the foot in plantarflexion. The fractures are usually extra-articular and nondisplaced. Patients will complain of pain on the lateral border of the foot and tenderness over the styloid process of the fifth metatarsal.[11] Most tuberosity avulsion fractures heal with a course of nonoperative management. Patients may return to weight-bearing with resolution of pain. Prolonged periods of non-weight bearing have been associated with muscle atrophy, increased stiffness and lower outcome scores.[12]

In the rare case of symptomatic nonunions, small fragments are excised through a lateral incision. Larger fragments, displaced fractures (> 2 mm), and fractures that extend into the cuboid-fifth metatarsal joint should be bone grafted and internally fixed with tension band wiring, bicortical, or intramedullary screw placement.

Metadiaphyseal (Jones) Fractures (Zone 2)

The term "Jones fracture" has been incorrectly used in the medical literature to describe all fractures of the proximal fifth metatarsal. The definition of a Jones fracture is a transverse fracture at the junction of the diaphysis and the metaphysis without extension distally into the fourth-fifth intermetatarsal joint (Figs 1A and B).[10] The

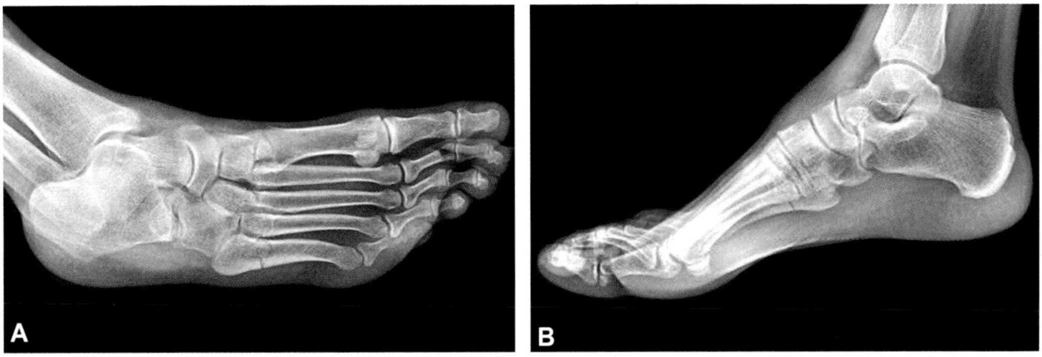

Figs 1A and B: Nondisplaced metadiaphyseal fracture of fifth metatarsal classically referred to as "Jones" fracture

mechanism involves an adduction force with the ankle plantarflexed. Nonoperative treatment may be considered in nondisplaced, Torg type I fractures (Figs 2A and B). Operative indications for Jones fractures include displaced fractures (> 2 mm), high-performance athletes, symptomatic nonunions, and the informed patient that prefers surgery to the risk of nonunion. The surgical treatment of choice is intramedullary screw fixation.

Diaphyseal Stress Fractures (Zone 3)

Stress fractures of the proximal fifth metatarsal have criteria the was outlined by DeLee which included (1) history of prodromal symptoms over lateral aspect of foot, (2) radiographic evidence of stress reaction, and (3) no previous treatment of fifth metatarsal fracture.[10] They are usually the result of increased duration/frequency of physical activity or training programs. Acute, nondisplaced fractures of the proximal diaphysis without widening, radiolucency, or periosteal reaction may undergo nonoperative treatment. Operative indications include fractures that display medullary sclerosis (Torg type II or III), periosteal reaction, displacement (> 2 mm), history of stress fracture (prodromal symptoms), and high-performance athletes. Fractures that display radiographic signs of hypertrophic nonunion can be considered for intramedullary screw fixation. Plate fixation with lag screws can also be used to stabilize this fracture pattern. Torg type III fractures benefit from corticocancellous inlay bone grafting.[2]

COMPLICATIONS

Complications from proximal fifth metatarsal fractures include delayed union or nonunion, sural nerve injury, refracture, and hardware prominence. Nonunions are more common with intramedullary screws of less than 4.5 mm, early return to sporting activities, inadequate grafting, and incomplete reaming of Torg type III fractures.[13] The dorsolateral branch of the sural nerve is within 2–3 mm of the screw head and needs to be protected during insertion.[14] Pain from sural nerve entrapment in nonunion fragments can also result. Refracture occurs after screw removal in the athletic patient. It is recommended that removal not be considered until the end of the athlete's career.[15] Hardware prominence is a direct result of the subcutaneous location of the tuberosity and is managed with shoe modifications.

SUMMARY

Fifth metatarsal fractures are common and warrant a course of nonoperative treatment in the nonathlete and nondisplaced fractures. Nonoperative treatment should consist of 6–8 weeks of non-weight bearing in a short leg cast. Radiographic and clinical examinations dictate progression to weight bearing. Signs of delayed healing or nonunion as outlined by the Torg classification should raise the discussion of surgical intervention. Surgical treatment of fifth metatarsal fractures is reserved for the high-performance athlete, displaced fractures (> 2 mm), and symptomatic nonunions. Surgical options include intramedullary screw fixation, open

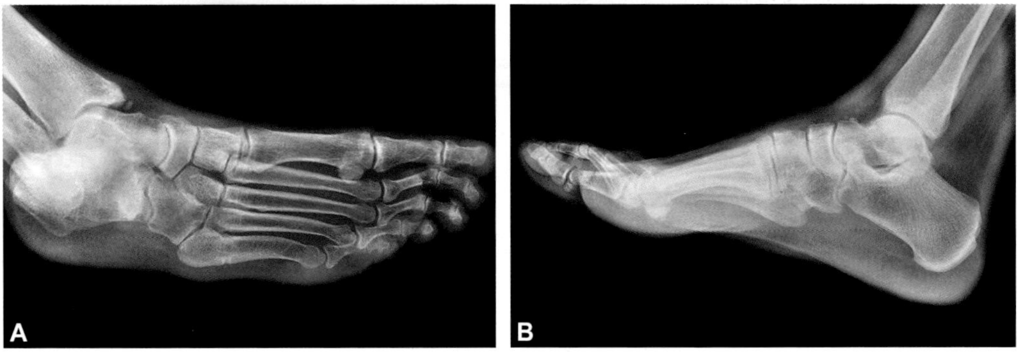

Figs 2A and B: Patient underwent closed treatment of fifth metatarsal fracture

reduction and internal fixation with plate and lag screw technique, and tricortical inlay bone grafting.

REFERENCES

1. DeLee JC, Evans JP, Julian J. Stress fracture of the fifth metatarsal. Am J Sports Med. 1983;11:349-53.
2. Torg JS, Balduini FC, Zelko RR, et al. Fractures of the base of the fifth metatarsal distal to the tuberosity. Classification and guidelines for nonsurgical and surgical management. J Bone Joint Surg Am. 1984; 66:209-14.
3. Quill G. Fractures of the proximal fifth metatarsal. Orthop Clin N Am. 1995;26:353-61.
4. Sarrafian S. Anatomy of the Foot and Ankle, 2nd edition. Philadelphia: JB Lippincott; 1993.
5. Smith JW, Arnoczky SP, Hersh A. The intraosseous blood supply of the fifth metatarsal: implications for proximal fracture healing. Foot Ankle. 1992;13: 143-52.
6. Hartog BD. Fracture of the proximal fifth metatarsal. J Am Acad Orthop Surg. 2009;17:458-64.
7. Ebraheim NA, Sabry FF, Haman S, et al. Anatomical and radiological considerations of the fifth metatarsal bone. Foot Ankle Int. 2000;21:212-5.
8. Kelly IP, Glisson RR, Fink C, et al. Intramedullary screw fixation of Jones fractures. Foot Ankle Int. 2001;22:585-9.
9. Vogler HW, Westlin N, Mlodzienski AJ, et al. Fifth metatarsal fractures. Biomechanics, classification, and treatment. Clin Podiatr Med Surg. 1995;12: 725-47.
10. Rosenberg GA, Sferra JJ. Treatment strategies for acute fractures and nonunions of the proximal fifth metatarsal. J Am Acad Orthop Surg. 2000;8:332-8.
11. Dameron TB. Fractures and anatomical variations of the proximal portion of the fifth metatarsal. J Bone Joint Surg Am. 1975;17:788-92.
12. Vorlat P, Achtergael W, Haentjens P. Predictors of outcome of non-displaced fractures of the base of the fifth metatarsal. Int Orthop. 2007;31:5-10.
13. Glasgow MT, Naranja RJ, Glasgow SG, et al. Analysis of failed surgical management of fractures of the base of the fifth metatarsal distal to the tuberosity: the Jones fracture. Foot Ankle Int. 1996;17:449-57.
14. Donley BG, McCollum MJ, Murphy GA, et al. Risk of sural nerve injury with intramedullary screw fixation of fifth metatarsal fractures: a cadaver study. Foot Ankle Int. 1999;20:182-4.
15. Wright RW, Fischer DA, Shively RA, et al. Refracture of proximal fifth metatarsal (Jones) fracture after intramedullary screw fixation in athletes. Am J Sports Med. 2000;28:732-6.

Index

Page numbers followed by *f* refer to figure and *t* refer to table